Ethics and Perinatology

EDITED BY

Amnon Goldworth

*Professor of Philosophy, San Jose State University,
Visiting Scholar, Stanford University School of Medicine, Department of
Pediatrics*

William Silverman

*Professor of Pediatrics (Retired) Columbia University
College of Physicians and Surgeons*

David K. Stevenson

*Harold K. Faber Professor of Pediatrics, Associate Chair,
Department of Pediatrics, Chief Division of Neonatal
and Developmental Medicine, Director of Nurseries,
Stanford University School of Medicine*

Ernlé W. D. Young

*Clinical Professor of Pediatrics and Medicine (Ethics),
Co-Director, Stanford University Center for Biomedical Ethics*

AND

Rodney Rivers

UK Advisory Editor

New York   Oxford   Tokyo
OXFORD UNIVERSITY PRESS
1995

Oxford University Press, Walton Street, Oxford OX2 6DP

Oxford   New York
Athens   Auckland   Bangkok   Bombay
Calcutta   Cape Town   Dar es Salaam   Delhi
Florence   Hong Kong   Istanbul   Karachi
Kuala Lumpur   Madras   Madrid   Melbourne
Mexico City   Nairobi   Paris   Singapore
Taipei   Tokyo   Toronto
and associated companies in
Berlin   Ibadan

Oxford is a trade mark of Oxford University Press

Published in the United States
by Oxford University Press Inc., New York

A catalogue record for this book is available from the British Library

Library of Congress Cataloging in Publication Data
Ethics and perinatology / edited by Amnon Goldworth . . . [et al.]
Includes bibliographical references and index.
1. Perinatology—Moral and ethical apsects. I. Goldworth, Amnon.
RG600.E845   1994   174'.2—dc20   94–13540
ISBN 0 19 262379 6

Typeset by the Electronic Book Factory Ltd, Fife
Printed in Great Britain on acid-free paper by
Bookcraft (Bath) Ltd, Midsomer Norton, Avon

Ethics and Perinatology

Foreword

John Lantos

Modern medicine is at a crossroads. A century of unprecedented technological achievement and scientific progress has led to abilities and achievements almost unimaginable a hundred years ago. Hospitals and health care have become a national obsession. The more health care we have and the healthier our population, the more health care we need and the more unacceptable any deviation from perfect health seems to be. Our tremendous progress doesn't seem to make us feel better, but instead only heightens awareness of our tremendous inadequacy. As Wildavsky put it, we are doing better and feeling worse.[1]

In spite of our success, our ignorance still knows no bounds. We still don't know why babies are born prematurely, why some children get necrotizing enterocolitis, how to prevent genetic diseases, or why we age. We will still ultimately develop poor health, degenerative diseases, and physical suffering, and we will still die. What, then, is the goal of medical progress? What achievements will we ultimately be able to point to as evidence that we have succeeded?

Neonatology exemplifies the paradoxical nature of medical progress as well as any other subspecialty area. Over the last twenty years, no other specialty has had such stunning success or such rapid progress. Improvements in birthweight-specific mortality rates can be measured in orders of magnitude. Basic science breakthroughs have been brought to the bedside. A medical specialty has been created where none existed before. Surely, neonatology should be judged one of the outstanding success stories of modern medicine.

And yet neonatology has always been one of the more ethically troublesome areas of medicine. As physicians have redefined the meaning of viability, they have also had to reconsider the meaning of parenthood, of family obligations, of personhood, and of the communities responsibility for those babies we choose to save or choose to let die. Physicians, parents, judges, insurance company executives, politicians, journalists, philosophers, and theologians have had to reexamine fundamental questions about the meaning of human community. In many contexts, and in many ways, they question whether neonatology is a dramatic success or a misguided effort.

One imagines the many voices in this societal dialogue as a Greek chorus, gathered around the bassinet of a tiny premature baby in a neonatal intensive-care unit, amid the beep and hum of monitors and intravenous pumps, the whoosh of ventilators, and the gurgling of suction machines, trying to conceptualize the symbolic meaning of the voiceless newborn.[2] What would she say if she could speak to us? What should we say on her behalf? Will she thank us someday? Are we torturing her? Is she worth it? Is she stealing money, time, and resources from other children? Can we let her die?

For some, more medical progress is the solution to these dilemmas. Each challenge can be seen as an isolated puzzle, the solution to which will put us closer to the ultimate success of the biomedical enterprise. Thus, if we can learn a better method to ventilate premature babies, or to treat genetic diseases, or discover a new, more effective, and less toxic cancer chemotherapy regimen or immunosuppressive drug, we will eventually be able to call the enterprise a success. For others, progress is becoming an illusory or chimerical goal, with each new medical endeavor creating more new problems than existed before, and requiring a larger societal commitment of time, money, and moral energy for a less and less defensible goal.[3]

The answers, of course, are neither simple nor one-dimensional. The voices in this book address these questions from many different perspectives and in many different modes of discourse. We hear clinical epidemiology, theology, philosophy, economics, law, and public policy. In some ways, the measure of our success may be our ability to talk to one another across disciplines, and to translate the messages from these different modes of discourse into something harmonious, rather than our ability to keep 400-gram premature babies alive. Technology is, ultimately, value-neutral. We must invest it with meaning. This book is an attempt to do that, and to determine what to call problems and what to call progress.

REFERENCES

1. Wildavsky, A. (1977). Doing better and feeling worse: the political pathology of health policy. In *Doing better and feeling worse*, (ed. J. H. Knowles, pp. 105–24. Norton, New York.
2. Lantos, J.D. (1989). The Hastings Center project on imperiled newborns: Supreme Court, jury or Greek chorus? *Pediatrics*, **83**, 615–16.
3. Illich, I. (1977). *Medical nemesis: the expropriation of health*. Pantheon Books, New York.

Preface

George Cattermole and John Goheen

Beginnings

Divine fire blazed
  with brilliant constellations
  and bright falling stars
While we sat in darkness and cold
  seemingly endless.

At last with pity good Prometheus
  carried a brand of fire
  stolen from the gods
To warm us.

We stirred up the fire in joy.

Apollo's son then commanded his
  serpents to encoil and caress
  our wounds
And when water boiled
  Asclepius knowingly
  mixed a potion of fresh herbs
  added some more for strength
Then turned and said
'Drink to relieve your suffering
  and cure your illness.'
Thence healing began.

The papers in this volume address ethical issues confronted by those caring for fetuses, newborns, and their families. The discussion is thus interdisciplinary, incorporating the views of professionals who bring a wide range of skills to the perinatal setting. Contributors include physicians, nurses, economists, legal theorists, ethicists, and philosophers. The editors have also included an international perspective, inviting authors from Canada, England, Scotland, Australia, and the United States to examine how perinatal medical, moral, and legal issues are dealt with in their societies.

The relatively recent and rapid development of new technologies and treatments for fetuses and newborns has dramatically lowered the birthweight/gestation survival threshold, and has resulted in a significant number of the sickest and smallest survivors suffering lifelong disabilities. Many perinatal tests and therapies have unproven risks and benefits, and, while there have been major advances, well-intentioned medical experimentation and guesswork have resulted in serious iatrogenic disorders.

At the same time, significant social and political developments have changed and challenged the traditional medical approach to pregnancy, birth, and infant-care. Maternal alcohol and drug abuse; concern for the rights of women, the unborn, and the handicapped; scarce resources; and the inability of many to pay for care all contribute to an extremely complex set of demands and choices. While many of these problems exist in other areas of medicine, the ethical quandaries they create can be intensified in perinatal care. The maternal–fetal and the parental–newborn relationships are unique, and can be medically and morally addressed in many different and conflicting ways.

Running through most of the chapters is an attention to the ethical role played by language and listening in treating newborns. Definitions become critical in this context; the choices of how to categorize patients and therapeutic procedures can involve normative and operative judgements which can determine whether or not a new life should continue. Whereas an organ transplant is by definition an act of mutilation, it can also be described as an act of charity on the part of the 'donor'. Religious and cultural convictions that can shape discourse are often tacit and difficult to formulate; terms and phrases such as 'futility', 'humane', 'person', and 'quality of life' are loaded with conflicting and problematic meanings which need to be clarified and understood if there is to be effective and honest communication between health professionals, patients, parents, lawyers, and lawmakers.

We find a solid consensus in these pages regarding the principle that the first and foremost responsibility of parents, proxies, and health-care providers is to serve the best interests of their patients. But we also find serious disagreement over how to answer the questions of what constitutes 'best interests' and how to reconcile conflicts between the perceived interests of newborns and the stated best interests of their parents and society. Because the fetus and newborn are unable to articulate their needs and values and have no history from which these can be surmised, others must speak for them and assume total responsibility for their health and lives. The dimensions of this responsibility are at once parental and personal, moral, medical, economic, and legal. The question of how they should be balanced in particular cases can be extremely difficult to answer.

None of the authors dissents from the principle that in matters concerning her fetus, the mother's autonomy and best interests should be unconditionally respected by fathers, health-care providers, the courts, and the law. The mother is not simply a 'fetal container', and because access to the fetus is possible only via 'interventions' into her body, her right to determine what may or may not be done to her must be respected. We learn, however, that this view is disputed by some, including health-care providers, for various reasons. To say that the mother's best interests should take precedence over those of her fetus does not imply, logically or morally, that the best interests of the fetus cannot or should not be considered. Although the 'sanctity of life' position is dealt with rather summarily in these pages, and is considered as an inadequate ethical basis for prescribing the relationship between a mother and her fetus, we do find examples of a 'paternalistic' approach to this relationship in medicine and law.

Ruth Macklin cites evidence showing that a significant number of physicians believe there are cases in which women who refuse medical advice (for example not to take harmful drugs while pregnant) should be detained against their will, and some doctors would in some cases support court orders for involuntary intrauterine transfusions for fetuses. We find also that in both the

United States and England there have been legal actions to force mothers to undergo caesareans, take medications, and receive insulin treatments in order to save their fetuses.

Two arguments are presented which are directly relevant to this 'paternalistic' approach to the maternal–fetal relationship. The first rests on pragmatic considerations regarding the consequences of judicial or legislative constraints aimed at forcing a woman to care for her fetus: for example, to criminalize non-compliance with treatment recommendations could drive women away from the medical establishment and prenatal care, and would in all probability discriminate against poorer women.

The second argument is far more controversial, and is at the center of a pitched philosophical battle in these pages. Does a viable fetus have a moral or legal status, and if so, does this status differ from that of a newborn or an adult? How, in fact and law, are we to determine when a fetus is viable? From differing viewpoints, Margaret Brazier and Alex Campbell question the paradoxical logic latent in the fact that English law allows for the destruction of a viable, probably abnormal, fetus, but confers full legal status on this same entity twenty-four hours later, after birth. Brazier claims that the law recognizes birth as the 'crucial watershed' not because a fetus lacks moral standing, but on the basis of the mother's autonomy.

Wayne Cohen touches on this point in acknowledging that underlying the belief that the mother's survival should be favored whenever possible is the value judgement that favors an 'actual' and 'independent' life over a 'potential' and 'dependent' one. Several reasons are noted for the failure to address clearly and consistently the moral status of fetuses and newborns, and Brazier pointedly and rhetorically asks whether or not neonaticide is distinguishable from homicide. While initially joining Alex Campbell and others in approving the absence of detailed formal regulations regarding the treatment of sick newborns, she concludes her paper by strongly advocating legal constraints on parents and health professionals to afford newborns the same rights as older persons.

In direct opposition to this position, Helga Kuhse argues for the need to distinguish between kinds of benefits and harms experienced by the perinatal patient and those experienced by the adults who care about and for them. A fetus or newborn experiences pain and pleasure, but in Kuhse's view these experiences are only momentary, and the newborn is incapable of desiring his or her own continued existence. We find a fundamental disagreement about whether or not fetuses or newborns can or should be considered as 'persons' and whether or not some very sick newborns can ever become persons. Kuhse believes that a newborn is closer to a fetus than a person, and, following a line of reasoning Brazier finds dangerous, she questions whether or not the best interests of a severely compromised infant with an 'admittedly short life-span' should 'count as much or more than the interest of those affected by its birth and care'. Rilke captures this insight in his poetry: to paraphrase, the flowers do not regret their wilting, it is for us to be their regret.

Kuhse concludes that we cannot assume that it is always in the best interest of newborns to continue a treatment involving prolonged and predominant pain. She is joined by Robert Weir in her view that death is sometimes in the best interest of a newborn, and that there are cases in which direct and intentional termination of life is medically and morally warranted. It could be argued that Kuhse proves too much. It is one thing to say that the best interests of newborns (those who are not, by definition, persons, and will not, according to diagnosis and prognosis, become persons) may dictate withholding or withdrawing life-sustaining treatments, or even euthanasia. It is quite another to say that healthy newborns are not persons, and therefore have no rights, or only those granted other animals. Her case studies supporting her claims deserve close scrutiny.

Weir stakes out what can be construed as a middle ground in this debate with the assertion that the 'principle of potentiality' is morally relevant and should entitle healthy fetuses and newborns to a *prima facie* claim to personhood and rights, including the right not to be killed, because they will subsequently acquire an actual person's moral and legal right to life. It may be true that a newborn is not a person; but it is truer to say that he or she is *not yet* a person.

Perhaps the most pressing and difficult problem dealt with in these essays is how to determine if and when life-continuing and even life-saving treatments are to be withheld or withdrawn from neonates. There are two basic questions here: who should make these decisions, and on what grounds should the decisions be based? An informed treatment decision consists of an 'objective' epidemiologically-based estimate of alternative probable health outcomes and of the 'subjective' evaluation of the harms and benefits attending these outcomes. David Thomasma poses the question of whether or not the 'objective' data may be 'themselves partially composed of subjective evaluative aspects': i.e., are not all data relevant data? He also explores the formidable difficulties involved in determining if and to what extent knowledge from previous studies 'fits' a particular patient's condition. John Sinclair and George Torrance address the need for improving ways in which both requirements can be met, outlining detailed methods and standards for the design and conduct of randomized trials, and providing models for the measurement, communication, and use of health-state preferences for both individual patients and health-care program evaluation.

The Federal legislation stemming from the Baby Doe regulations provokes and informs much of the discussion of how to decide if, when, and how to treat extremely compromised neonates, and several authors note that these regulations have had a beneficial effect in making us more aware of the rights of newborns and the handicapped. Ronald Ariagno critically clarifies the history, content, and scope of this legislation. This is important, given that several authors believe that neonatal care providers are sometimes overtreating because of fears of legal actions against them for withholding or withdrawing treatments from seriously sick newborns.

Alex Campbell is thankful that there are no regulations in the United Kingdom dealing with newborns; legislation is simply 'too blunt an instrument' to deal effectively and sensitively with perinatal treatment decisions. Although British courts have become involved in several controversial cases, they have relied upon the 'reasonable doctor' standard (what a reasonable doctor would do in similar circumstances) and the 'substituted judgement' standard (what reasonable people would want done to themselves to ensure an acceptable quality of life). Brazier and Kuhse call into question the legitimacy of the latter standard, on the grounds that it involves an imaginative impossibility. In contrast with the spirit of the Baby Doe regulations, the legal record in these matters in the United Kingdom reflects a more pervasive trust in the ability of health-care providers and parents to determine and act in the best interests of newborns, and an explicit reliance on 'quality of life' calculations.

Several authors argue persuasively that quality-of-life judgements are necessary components in decisions to withhold or withdraw life-sustaining treatments. With the notable exception of Brazier, there is general agreement that these decisions should be left to care-providers, parents, or proxies, with ethics committees acting in an advisory capacity, and court oversight requested in very difficult cases. There is, however, a wide range of opinion regarding the relevant considerations shaping these decisions and the weight given to the interests and desires of those making them. Brazier feels that the parent's claim to decide for their compromised child should carry less weight, the younger the child. A. G. M. Campbell is critical of those who would in all cases place the interest of the family as secondary, and believes that the family's desires and capacities regarding the future care of their infant are relevant. Mildred Stahlman and Albert Jonson emphasize the priority of the physician's moral and professional responsibilities as the infant's advocate, ranking family interests next, and finally those of society.

The relative and subjective meanings of 'benefits' and 'harms' are discussed by several authors. David Stevenson and Ernlé Young point out that, even though it is impossible to 'render absolute pronouncements about harm', there are cases where harms and goods are unambiguously understood, and that in these cases it is morally permissible to oppose parents if they advocate a course of action attended by more harm than good for the patient. They make an important distinction between harm and pain, pointing out that harm can occur without pain, and that the occurrence of pain is not 'sufficient for the conclusion that harm has occurred.' This distinction can shed light on the very complex area in which 'quality of life' judgements are made. A newborn suffering acute pain is obviously experiencing a poor quality of life; but it may well be morally justifiable to increase its suffering with measures that will make possible a future quality of life attended with significantly less pain. Joy Penticuff and Andrew Jameton discuss evidence that physicians can fail adequately to assess and manage infant pain, and identify several reasons for this. In evaluating these claims, readers should scrutinize carefully the case of Andrew Stinson cited by Penticuff and the Baby L case analysed by Ariagno.

Roberta Pagon and Nancy Jecker accept the terms 'futile' and 'inhumane'

as denoting meaningful criteria for treatment decisions, and attempt to
clarify their operational and ethical significance. Norman Fost complains
rather forcefully that this effort is misguided, claiming that the terms have
not been defined in a non-arbitrary way 'not subject to personal value
preferences', noting further that in the Baby Doe legislation the terms apply
to cases involving perpetual coma or immanent death despite full treatment.
The real possibility of misdiagnosis of such conditions as PVS (Permanent
Vegetative State) and whole brain death should also, he believes, caution
us in conclusions about futility, because labels can become self-fulfilling
prophecies. Fost's reexamination of Pagon and Jecker's analysis is guided
by his allegiance to the patient's best interest standard. The reader should
consider whether or not his application of this standard involves personal or
subjective judgements on his part, or yields significantly different practical
results. In this regard, it can be asked whether or not personal or subjective
judgements are always arbitrary; if they may not at times be unavoidable;
and, if so, how should they be dealt with?

    In a closely related discussion, both Joyce Peabody and Albert Jonson
consider and leave standing the ethical and practical problems confronting
those who would change the current medical/legal definition of death to
increase the number of transplantable organs. Were there to be a shift
from the definition of death as the irreversible loss of whole-brain function
to a definition of death as the irreversible loss of 'higher brain' function,
it could be possible to use the organs of anencephalic infants. Acknowledging that such a change may well be justifiable on 'speculative' ethical
grounds, Jonson nevertheless finds this unacceptable, basing his decision on
'pragmatic' considerations. What Jonson means here is unclear: a 'higher
brain' definition of death may exclude anencephalic infants from the rights
of autonomous rational persons, and thereby place them outside the scope
of Kant's dictum that we never treat persons as means only. However,
the dilemma may not be one of needing to choose between an ethics of
privacy and individual rights and an ethics of justice and utility. Johnson
cites convincing utilitarian considerations—the possibility of misdiagnosis; a
'slippery slope' leading to an overly inclusive donor pool; and the likelihood
of counterproductive confusion and distrust—which, taken together, may
well outweigh or block the benefits expected from the proposed change in
definition. Jonson's concluding remarks are powerfully suggestive. He notes
that the discovery that a 'vast part of the human genome is shared between
all human individuals' may help provide a basis for a more sharing and
just relationship between individuals. The influences of biology's expanding
understanding on the ethics of both caring and curing may be more profound
than we might expect. Had Aristotle had a better grasp of the 'facts of life' and
realized that mothers contribute more than menstrual matter to their fetuses,
he may have granted women a more 'rational' status in relation to men.

    There is wide agreement here regarding the crucial importance of providing
for and obtaining informed consent, in the contexts of both research and clinical settings. How a physician construes the meaning of 'informed consent' can

greatly influence how he or she communicates with a patient; the goal should be to guide, not to control, the proxy's decision. Amnon Goldworth identifies the shortcomings of the traditional 'professional practice' and 'reasonable person' standards, and argues for a 'subjective' standard of disclosure which requires that the values and interests of the particular patients and proxies help determine what information is material and relevant for shared treatment decisions.

William Silverman explains why the current requirements for 'study consent' are inadequate and potentially unethical on several counts, including their potential for discriminating against the poor by encouraging an inequitable distribution of the 'burdens of participation'. Both John Tyson and Goldworth join Silverman in calling for further research to determine what factors influence patients' preferences, what are the effects of providing information and obtaining consent in research and clinical contexts, and what the likely effects of merging study and customary consent would be. This should be done before Federal regulations governing research are extended to clinical practice, because they pose serious obstacles for clinicians desiring to carry out controlled studies of non-validated therapies.

The advantages of treatment 'teams' and what might be called 'informed agreement' between members of these teams are also discussed. Stevenson and Young point out that the process of reaching consensus among team members provides useful checks and balances which can guard against overly subjective interpretations. Relevant here is Cohen's emphasis on the importance of physicians' having a clear understanding of their own values and an ability to articulate them to patients, and, Young might add, to other members of a treatment team. Penticoff and Jameton explain the importance of recognizing nurses' capabilities in medical planning and decision-making. Judgements based on direct, 'hands-on', and personal experiences with newborns and their families can and should contribute to the medical and moral deliberations of treatment teams and ethics committees. In his extremely suggestive article, Jameton claims there exist 'basic power inequities' between nurses and physicians, and blames the failure to give nurses the decisional power they deserve on 'stale icons of gender'. Contrasting what he calls a 'process' approach to decision-making ('Let's talk and see what we come up with') with the conventional 'principled' approach ('How should we decide according to the principles of autonomy, justice, etc.?'), Jameton argues for the former, claiming that it is more conducive to humane decision-making in the perinatal context.

Tom Beauchamp and Thomasma elaborate on the problems inherent in the process of scientifically validating untested treatments, stressing the moral imperative that there be genuine 'equipoise' or 'balanced doubt' on the part of those designing and carrying out clinical trials. For informed consent to be authentic in these trials, it should include a shared understanding that there is such doubt about the efficacy of the proposed treatment. In the case of 'double-blind' studies where interventions are assigned by lot, genuine 'equipoise' and honest communication regarding it are ethically crucial. Richard Stevenson suggests that patients and their proxies should be informed of the comparative track records of available institutions in performing the considered treatments. Beauchamp further warns against clinician/researchers locating themselves in situations involving a possible conflict between their commercial self-interest and their professional responsibilities as scientists and physicians; the presence of a financial interest in the outcome of research can result in both bad science and bad care for patients. Gene Lewitt also cites evidence that some physicians' financial interests and fears are compromising their effectiveness as patient advocates.

The importance of prenatal care, both from a cost- and health-benefit perspective, is discussed in detail. From a nursing perspective, Penticuff identifies a wide range of proactive prenatal 'interventions', including pregnancy prevention and drug treatment programs—caring not only helps curing, it can prevent the need to be cured. Removing all financial barriers to prenatal care is justified on the ethical grounds of distributive justice and beneficence as well as on its cost-effectiveness. We find, however, that making prenatal care affordable may not by itself be sufficient for achieving improved health for mothers and newborns; obstacles such as lack of education and motivation and maternal substance abuse complicate the picture. In addition, Lewitt questions Harvey's economic justifications for expanded prenatal care, claiming that it is uncertain whether or not real cost savings would result. His reservations about the efficacy of prenatal care and his claims about the cost-effectiveness of such care warrant serious consideration. Peabody laments the lack of rational discussion of these issues, while at the same time observing that there is too much pressure 'to intellectualize such emotional issues as death and dying'. There is a similar ambivalence in her honest and provocative uncertainty about the moral wisdom of investing great amounts of time and money in 'hi tech' organ transplants in the midst of a widespread lack of medical resources for millions of impoverished youth.

Many authors regret the seemingly inevitable fact that economics can and does 'intrude' on the physician–patient relationship, and call for a more communitarian or 'society-wide' view which ensures rational balancing of equity and efficiency in perinatal care. Solutions to the pressing problems of increased costs and restricted access to health care involve the 'upstream' involvement of health-care professionals in the design, management, and allocation of health-care resources and systems. Responding to the concerns of Stahlman, Harvey, and others that rationing decisions do not belong in the hands of individual doctors, Lewitt argues that these decisions are made and must be made, and that health-care providers would be better off not to leave them solely in the hands of politicians, economists, and administrators. There is a growing awareness of the tension between efficiency and just distribution in the process of allocating and utilizing health resources, and several authors evaluate the Oregon 'experiment' from this perspective.

The discussion of a 'wider' view of professional medical ethics which obliges clinicians not simply to act as agents for patients and their families, but also to serve society at large should be of great interest to those in the United States who are following the Clinton Administration's health-care reform efforts. Relevant here is Stahlman's insistence that 'salvageable' infants must be treated without consideration of costs, and that this may only be possible if care-providers work for a change in national priorities. We are led to consider the potential danger of care-givers' resigning themselves to budgets and regulations set by those who are ignorant or insensitive to medical needs and preferences. There is a vital need for both medical professionals and patients to take an active role in shaping health policies.

The debates over the questions coalescing at the beginnings of life can only intensify as resources become scarcer and science and technology make possible increasing manipulation and control of living processes. Confronted by those new to life and yet close to death or severe harm, the authors of the following essays have grappled with the challenging questions of why and how and what we can do. Are there general principles and decision-making processes that can guide us in deciding who, how, and when to treat? How can treatments and research in the perinatal setting be carried out in both an effective and an ethical manner? What role should economic, legal, and religious considerations play in the design and delivery of perinatal health care? This volume offers a good beginning towards framing humane and just answers to these questions, and we encourage our readers to contribute their expertise, talents, and experience to continue the work.

Contents

Contributors

Ronald L. Ariagno Stanford University School of Medicine, Department of Pediatrics, 750 Welch Road, Suite 315, Palo Alto, CA 94304, USA

Tom L. Beauchamp Kennedy Institute of Ethics, Poulton Hall, Georgetown University, Washington, DC 20057, USA

Margaret Brazier Faculty of Law, Manchester University, Manchester M13 9PT, UK

Alex Campbell 34 Woodburn Crescent, Aberdeen AB1 8JX, UK

George Cattermole P.O. Box 71, San Gregorio, CA 94074, USA

Wayne R. Cohen Department of Obstetrics & Gynecology, Albert Einstein College of Medicine, Belfer Education Center, Room 510, 1300 Morris Park Avenue, Bronx, NY 10461, USA

Norman C. Fost Department of Pediatrics, University of Wisconsin Hospital, Madison, WI 53792, USA

Amnon Goldworth 4008 Laguna Way, Palo Alto, CA 94306, USA

Henry T. Greely Stanford Law School, Stanford, CA 94305, USA

Birt Harvey Lucile Packard Children's Hospital at Stanford, 725 Welch Road, Palo Alto, CA 94304, USA

David Harvey Royal Postgraduate Medical School, Queen Charlotte & Chelsea Hospital, London W6 0XG, UK

Andrew Jameton University of Nebraska, Department of Preventive and Societal Medicine, 600 S. 42nd Street, Omaha, NE 68198–4350, USA

Nancy Jecker University of Washington, Department of Medical History and Ethics, School of Medicine, SB-20, Seattle, WA 98195, USA

Albert R. Jonsen University of Washington, Department of Medical History and Ethics, School of Medicine, SB-20, Seattle, WA 98195, USA

Helga Kuhse Centre for Human Bioethics, Monash University, Clayton, 3168, Australia

John D. Lantos La Rabida Hospital, East 65th Street and Lake Michigan, Chicago, IL 60649–1396

Eugene Lewit The David and Lucile Packard Foundation Center for the Future of Children, 300 Second Street, Suite 102, Los Altos, CA 94022, USA

Ruth Macklin Albert Einstein College of Medicine, 1300 Morris Park Avenue, Belfer Building, Bronx, NY 10461, USA

Miranda Mugford National Perinatal Epidemiology Unit, Radcliffe Infirmary, Oxford OX2 6HE, UK

Roberta A. Pagon University of Washington, Division of Medical Genetics, Children's Hospital & Medical Center, P.O. Box C5371, Seattle, WA 98105, USA

Joyce Peabody Loma Linda University Medical Center, West Hall 123, Loma Linda, CA 92350, USA

Joy Penticuff School of Nursing, University of Texas, Austin, 1700 Red River, Austin TX 78701, USA

William A. Silverman 90 La Cuesta Drive, Greenbrae, CA 94904, USA

John Sinclair McMaster University, Chedoke McMaster Hospital, Department of Pediatrics, 1200 Main Street West, Hamilton, Ontario, L8N 3Z5 Canada

Mildred Stahlman Vanderbilt University Medical Center, Department of Pediatrics, Nashville, TN 37232–2370, USA

David K. Stevenson Stanford University, 750 Welch Road, Suite 315, Palo Alto, CA 94304, USA

Richard Stevenson Department of Economics and Accounting, University of Liverpool, Eleanor Rathbone Bldg., Myrtle Street, P.O. Box 147 Liverpool, L69 3BX, UK

David C. Thomasma Loyola University Medical Center, Medical Humanities, 2160 South First Avenue, Maywood, IL 60153, USA

George W. Torrance Centre for Health Economics and Policy Analysis, Department of Clinical Epidemiology and Biostatistics, McMaster University, 1200 Main Street West, Hamilton, Ontarion, L8N 325, Canada

Jon Tyson University of Texas, Department of Pediatrics, 5323 Harry Hines Blvd., F3 118, Dallas, TX 75235, USA

Robert Weir University of Iowa, College of Medicine, Biomedical Ethics, Room 110 MEB, Iowa City, IA 52242, USA

Ernlé W. D. Young Stanford University, Center for Biomedical Ethics, 701B Welch Road, Suite 222, Palo Alto, CA 94304, USA

1

Introduction: a thematic overview

David K. Stevenson, and Ernlé W. D. Young

I swear by Apollo, by Asclepius, by Health, by Panacea and by all the gods and goddesses, making them my witnesses, that I will carry out, according to my ability and judgment, this oath and this indenture. To hold my teacher in this art equal to my own parents; to make him partner in my livelihood; when he is in need of money to share mine with him; to consider his family as my own brothers, and to teach them this art, if they want to learn it, without fee or indenture; to impart precept, oral instruction, and all other instruction to my own sons, the sons of my teacher, and to indentured pupils who have taken the physician's oath, but to nobody else. I will use treatment to help the sick according to my ability and judgment, but never with a view to injury or wrong-doing. Neither will I administer a poison to anybody when asked to do so, nor will I suggest such a course. Similarly, I will not give a woman a pessary to cause an abortion. But I will keep pure and holy both my life and my art. I will not use the knife, not even, verily, on sufferers from stone, but I will give place to such as are craftsmen therein. Into whatsoever houses I enter, I will enter to help the sick, and I will abstain from all intentional wrong-doing and harm, especially from abusing the bodies of man or woman, bond or free. And whatsoever I shall see or hear in the course of my profession, as well as outside my profession in my intercourse with men, if it be what should not be published abroad, I will never divulge, holding such things to be holy secrets. Now if I carry out this oath, and break it not, may I gain for ever reputation among all men for my life and for my art; but if I transgress it and forswear myself, may the opposite befall me.[1]

Despite the distinctiveness of its invocations and the specificity of some of its admonitions, the origin of the Hippocratic Oath is shrouded in obscurity. Estimates of its actual date of origin vary from the sixth century B.C.E. to the first century C.E. Despite the authority which is often the concomitant of longevity, it is an Oath not taken easily by contemporary physicians without selective deletion from or modification of the variously translated text. The earliest extant references to the Oath, by Scribonius Largus (fl. 40 C.E.) and Erotian (fl. 60 C.E.), indicate that to them it represented an ideal, not an essential prerequisite. As such, however, it upholds themes that have stood the test of time. These themes are still of crucial importance to enlightened medical practice; some of them undergird the discussion of most of the discrete topics included in this present volume. In this introduction, we shall elaborate on three of these themes: the nature of the physician–patient relationship, especially in light of the emergence of respect for autonomy as a modern guiding biomedical ethical principle; the obligation to avoid causing harm to patients and the definitional difficulties this presents; and the distinctions between disease and illness, curing and healing.

THE PHYSICIAN–PATIENT RELATIONSHIP

The express concern with not doing things to alter the natural course of a disease that would occasion harm to a patient, the direction of attention toward the sick person and away from all exploitative or self-serving behaviour by the physician, and the insistence on confidentiality indicate that fundamental to the Oath is the conviction that patients are to be accorded respect by physicians treating them. As Duff and Campbell, drawing on the seminal work of Martin Buber, have pointed out, the ideal relationship between physician and patient is that of an 'I' to a 'thou', rather than that of an 'I' to an 'it':

In this view, each person is an individual, an 'I' who is embodied in a living organism. Also, each person is so related biologically and socially to significant others that there is a major other or 'thou' component within himself. Buber coined 'I-thou' to emphasize the close association between intrapersonal and intimate interpersonal conditions. He coined 'I-it' to refer more or less to person–object relationships. In general, I–thou relationships between persons imply nurture, intimacy, and full reciprocity between persons. Responsibility and power are shared, though not necessarily equally, because people differ in their capacities and interests.[2]

Although many of its textual details may be dated, the Hippocratic Oath affirms fundamentally that patients are to be respected as subjects, as 'thous', and never to be regarded as objectified 'its'. The form this respect has taken has changed with the passing of the centuries.

Ancient physicians who followed the teachings of Hippocrates would probably have distanced themselves from patients as a mark of respect. They would have refrained as much as possible from touching their patients, stressing instead observation and the use of all their senses to gather objective evidence about the disease process. Any symptoms would merely have been reported; talking with or touching a patient might have been confused with incantation or the ceremonious behaviors of other healers of the day. Thus, the ancient art of healing, as practiced by Hippocrates, was essentially a silent one, with the physician separated from the patient as a worshipper might be separated from a deity. However, the fact that this was done out of respect precluded the objectification of the patient; although treated at a distance, the patient remained a subject because of the physician's posture, which approached one of reverence.

The ancient separation between the Hippocratic physician and the patient also opened up a symbolic gap into which modern science inserted itself. With the introduction of laboratories and new technologies at the turn of this century, the distance between physician and patient first widened and then closed again, as physicians laid not their hands but their medicines and machines on patients. The giving and receiving of information and consent became prerequisites to practice; and the same ancient philosophy that had discouraged doing things to interfere with nature had strangely acquiesced across the centuries to more tampering with nature and invasion of the personal realm than was even imagined possible before. The irony of this is not fully appreciated without realizing that the Oath still imbues the physician–patient relationship with respect for nature and for the person who is in and of nature, and clearly admits through the admonition to do no harm a modern consideration that application of medicines and machines should be avoided if they do not serve the sick person.

Touching patients indirectly, not with hands that palpate various organs but with medications and machines, can erode the patient's subjectivity in the encounter with the physician. The patient can become objectified, an 'it' to be manipulated through the medical care system. 'I–it' medicine is not only impersonal, it is also paternalistic. The physician's (indirect) touching may not be informed by the patient's preferences, values, and over-arching life goals; instead, it signifies the extension of physician omniscience and omnipotence. This can lead, as David Rothman has argued, to physicians' becoming 'strangers' at the patient's bedside.[3]

But that is neither a necessity nor an inevitability. The emergence of the principle of respect for autonomy which, in the United States at least, occurred with increasing rapidity in the years following the Second World War, has served largely to restore subjectivity to the interactions between patients and their physicians. There is no doubt that it can also accelerate the process of objectification resulting from biotechnological advances; and ironically, respect for autonomy, when taken to an extreme, can objectify not the patient but the physician—treating her as an 'it' whose task is simply to do the bidding of the sovereign 'I'—the patient. However, respect for autonomy as understood within the context of 'I–thou' relationships generally preserves the 'thouness', the full subjectivity, of both parties. In such a form of the relationship, neither the physician nor the patient is sovereign, making unilateral decisions and imposing them on the other. Each respects the 'thouness' of the other (as well as of their respective selves); together, they negotiate treatment decisions—with the physician bringing to the decision-making process her specialized training and clinical experience, and the patient contributing his unique knowledge of personal preferences, values, and life goals.

Neonatal medicine, however, constitutes a clear exception to this general description. Although the infant might be respected as an independent 'thou', he is, and for the foreseeable future will be, incapable of dialogue. This could have the effect of his being regarded as an 'it'. Inevitably, he must be represented by an adult in the relationship with the physician. Usually, this representative will be the infant's parent or parents; on occasion, it will be a court-appointed guardian/conservator. The form of this relationship, between the physician and the infant's representative, will be crucial to the way in which the infant is touched and treated. The child's proxy may lack respect for the 'thouness' of the physician, treating her as an 'it' who is simply there to do his bidding, demanding either more or less in the way of treatment than medical judgment and expert opinion deem appropriate. Equally, the physician may objectify the infant, touching him only with medicines and machines because the physician–patient relationship can only be developed and expressed through an intermediary. Both errors can be detrimental to the patient. Both must be guarded against with unceasing vigilance. A clinical anecdote may be instructive in this regard.

The case involved an infant in a neonatal intensive care unit, whose care had become extraordinarily complicated because each day, the young parents of the infant (who were immigrants from Thailand) presented the treatment team with a different set of non-negotiable demands. On inquiry, it was discovered that within their Thai community the real locus of decisional authority was not parental, but lay with the head of the clan. The head of the clan spoke no English, and had not been to the hospital. As a displaced person, he was probably exerting more control within his community than would have been the case back in Thailand. In any event, cultural factors had objectified the relationship between the family and the treatment team. Any meeting of minds was problematic because, while there were encounters or transactions between the two parties, there was no true relationship. Only when steps were taken to bring the head of the clan into 'I–thou' contact with the treating physicians and nurses did it become possible to approach the ideal of respecting the personhood of the infant himself in the treatment decisions that were made.

The opposite case is that of the treatment team objectifying the patient because establishing a real relationship with the parent, parents, or proxy is too daunting a challenge. Parents can, at times, become the objects of the treating physicians' suspicion or even hostility: drug- or alcohol-abusing parents can be difficult people with whom to deal, especially when their behaviors in the prenatal period have resulted in fetal damage; grief-stricken parents can be aggressive and unreasonable; uneducated and immature parents can react to the medicalization of their infant in ways that may seem inappropriate to those more familiar with the hospital environment; and the personalities of the members of the treating team and those in the infant's family may simply be incompatible. Unless strenuous and conscious efforts are made by members of the treatment team to overcome difficulties of this sort, they can impede the attainment of the goal of respectful treatment as inspired by the Oath, with deleterious consequences for the infant concerned.

PRIMUM NON NOCERE

The abstention from 'all intentional wrong-doing and harm' is a Hippocratic legacy. A seemingly simple message, the admonition implies more than what is said. Although not explicit, one assumption is that harm is the consequence of an act, a doing; yet, in medicine, not doing something can also have detrimental consequences, indistinguishable, without the benefit of a historical perspective, from the harm resulting from an action. Both doing and not doing are categorically iatrogenic, once the physician–patient relationship is established. For example, death or injury can occur as the result of an error of either omission or commission. Thus, a simple charge to avoid doing things of any sort to patients is inadequate to ensure the avoidance of harm, even if the motto were strictly obeyed. Also, wrong-doing and harm cannot always be equated. There can be wrong-doing without harm and harm without wrong-doing. Moreover, the avoidance of wrong-doing does not guarantee that harm will be avoided and *vice versa*. The Oath assumes a physician–patient relationship and a set of complex interactions. These interactions are potentially or actually observable by the physician, the patient, or anyone else, from a variety of perspectives, and are describable in widely differing terms, ranging from physical to psychological ones. Harm must be understood from these observed interactions; and harm is thus an understanding or interpretation of observed events rather than simply a physical phenomenon.

Moreover, the understanding of harm implies a state, observed or imagined, from which there has been measurable change over a period of time. This notion of harm is complex because it admits a temporal dimension, a fundamental distancing which serves observation (one can also observe oneself) and interaction; harm cannot otherwise be understood to occur in any meaningful way. The occurrence of pain is not sufficient for the conclusion that harm has occurred. In fact, harm can occur without pain. Moreover, compliance with the charge to do no harm requires attendance over time, awareness or self-consciousness of at least one person (the distancing phenomenon), and a complex of interactions which is analyzable. Because harm is fundamentally contextual and perspective-dependent, its occurrence can only be confirmed by agreement or mutual understanding. Suicide is problematic in this regard; it is an open question as to whether or not death is a harmful event to the one ending his own life. However, a discussion of this issue would be beyond our scope.

The situation of the newborn patient is also challenging and anything but straightforward. Propositional communication and agreement with the infant are impossible; harm, therefore, cannot be confirmed through enquiry of the patient. None the less, since the physician, nurses, parents, or proxies are reflective beings, they can certainly agree as to whether their interactions with the newborn patient might be construed as nocent, and judgments about iatrogenic maneuvers can be made accordingly. Relative harms can also be assessed in this context and from various perspectives, if the avoidance of all harm is impractical or impossible. Finally, the occurrence of metabolic events, however they are measured, whether spontaneous or resulting from mechanical or chemical interactions caused by the physician, is not sufficient to postulate harm. That is, purely vegetative events cannot be called harmful in any meaningful sense, unless or until they are understood to be harmful by a non-vegetative, reflective consciousness. 'Good' or 'bad' do not exist at the level of pure action; they are only contrived by an observer of the action.

In summary, a concern to do no harm reflects a moral sense and is primarily a moral obligation to another person, actual or imagined, by a self-reflective sentient being engaged over time with that person, whether actual or imagined. The fetus or newborn is thus a legitimate beneficiary of the physician's Oath, but only by virtue of the physician's, parent's, or proxy's emotional engagement. *Primum non nocere* assumes such an informing and emotional engagement. It presupposes an 'I–thou' relationship between physician and patient, through sentient intermediaries.

Because interpretation is involved in the determination that harm is occurring, and because interpreting is an essentially subjective activity, it is inevitable that sometimes there will be differences of opinion about what constitutes harm to the neonate. Margery Shaw, for example, believes that

treatment is harmful if the quality of life after treatment is worse than it would have been without treatment and the child survives in either case. It is also harmful if it allows a child to live who would have otherwise died and the child is handicapped to such an extent that there is little or no opportunity to enjoy life.[4]

As we shall see in Chapter 15, 'Religious influences on decision-making', there are proponents of a sanctity-of-life point of view who would take issue vehemently with this assertion, admitting no quality-of-life considerations whatever into the decisional process. Beliefs about what constitutes harm, and when harm so construed is occurring, color different individuals' interpretations even of the same event. Whatever objective indicators there may be that an infant is being harmed (for example, irreversible damage to the lungs or intracranial hemorrhages), subjective factors will render absolute pronouncements about harm difficult to the point of being impossible. 'Judgment'—whether that of the physician, nurse, parent, or proxy—is value-laden, and often a synonym for subjective biases or beliefs.

Nevertheless, the fact that there is a treatment *team*, rather than a solitary treating physician, can be a useful check and balance against overly subjective interpretations—one way or the other. In this respect, many heads (and hearts) are often better than one. When a consensus begins to emerge among all who are participating in the care of an infant that the harms of continued treatment (or of non-treatment) are outweighing the benefits, then it becomes more difficult for any one member of the group to make claims to the contrary; increasingly persuasive arguments in support of such claims will be necessary. However, the dilution of responsibility through interactions of group members remains a potential risk when the decisions are made 'by committee'.

As Earl Shelp has pointed out, our choices often are between types or forms of harm rather than between harming and not harming.[5] No matter how we choose, there are times when some form of harm is inevitable. In such cases, harms must be balanced against harms—not only in degree, but also in kind.

These are the zones of ambiguity, where moral certainty is an unattainable goal and where reasonableness is the most for which we can strive. In such gray areas, where parents are going to have to live with the consequences of whatever they choose, it seems not only compassionate but wise to afford them maximal discretion in the decision-making process. Only where goods and harms are obvious and unambiguously understood does it make sense morally to oppose parents who choose what is harmful to the child or refuse the good. As Jonsen and Garland wrote more than a decade ago:

Diagnosis and prognosis are, by their very nature, probabilistic judgments. It is extremely difficult to forecast the ability of an endangered infant to participate in human experience; no single, clear criterion is available. Even as medical experience grows and skills improve, decisions will still be made without absolute certainty about outcome. While the moral certitude requisite for acting in good conscience does not exclude the possibility of error, it does require that judgments be based on reasonably strong evidence and that one act cautiously in the face of clear doubt.[6]

ILLNESS AND DISEASE, CURING AND HEALING

Eric Cassell has commented wisely on the distinction between 'illness' and 'disease', 'curing' and 'healing'.[7] In doing so, he draws heavily on insights derived from the Hippocratic tradition. His interpretation of that tradition may be summarized as follows.

'Illness' and 'disease' must be distinguished from one another on the basis of the Oath. Illness is that which is experienced by a person; it is a lived experience. Disease is the construction placed on a person's illness or malady as an explanation of it. Humorously, Cassell postulates that illness describes what the patient feels when he goes to the doctor, disease is what he has on the way home from the doctor's office. Organs become diseased; persons become ill.[8]

Our system of explanations for illnesses, our rational determinations that disease is present, owe much to the Greeks. 'Hippocrates is called the father of modern medicine primarily because he introduced the use of observation as a basis for the diagnosis and therapy of disease and rejected a system of medicine that depended entirely on magico-religious beliefs'. But, as Cassell goes on to show, the drive toward rationalism and objectivity prepared the way for the rejection of the spoken word in medicine and laid the groundwork for the deterioration of the physician–patient relationship from one that is profoundly personal into one that is increasingly impersonal. The more physicians concentrated on disease, the less attention they were able to devote to illness and to the person who felt ill.

If illness and disease are different, then curing and healing may also be quite distinct functions. Because devising a cure depends on understanding the etiology of a disease, that cure 'will be directed only against those objective manifestations of illness that our science has defined as a disease'.

Healing, in contrast, will occur when the person who has the disease is treated, not only with medicines and machines, but also with compassion and respect.

The state of being of the fetus or newborn is inextricably intertwined with that of the mother. Illness in the fetus or neonate cannot be elucidated through questioning; only through observing and probing can it be imagined. Disease, as it is understood by physicians, is a ready replacement for what ordinarily would be easily accessible to the asker. None the less, there is value in trying to fathom the illness of a fetus or newborn person, even if it cannot be ascertained through questioning, because there is both an objective and a personal aspect of the human circumstance in which dysfunction is experienced. The body always grounds the physician's inquiry and invites probing and tinkering with its machinery in order to return it to some understood order; but the body is more than something someone can observe and manipulate. It is lived in and experienced by the one whose body it is. Thus, whereas the what and the why of disease may drive scientific medicine, it may not be sufficient for knowing a person's illness (what ails a person). Scientific medicine casts the physician as curer, yet the physician who follows the Hippocratic ideal is to be a healer. Although injury or death may easily be construed in technical terms, these are actually personal matters:

'Medicine', Hippocrates said, 'is more necessary to philosophy than philosophy is to medicine.' Nature continually drives men to form theories that might give order to nature. But nature is not guided by the theories of men. For the physician, nature is portrayed in the sick. Our theories and constructs about sickness and disease have come and gone through the ages, but the sick have remained essentially the same. It is to them that the physician owes his allegiance and, ultimately, it is in them that the truth resides.[9]

The paradoxical vision of the physician is situated in practice. In an article by Schwartz and Wiggins, a phenomenological model of medicine yields a description of a practical discipline responding to the distress of human beings in the everyday-life world. Because it is a practical discipline, medicine is defined not as much by a body of knowledge as by the goals it seeks to achieve: promotion of health and the treatment of illness. These goals make medicine necessarily both a science and a humanism.

As Stevenson observed:

As scientists, we have been trained in the way of the scientific method and we have learned that it will provide solutions to many health problems, that science is necessary in modern medicine. As physicians, we must remember that we live in two worlds: the world of medical science, which provides us with our ideals (our models of understanding ourselves) and with real advances against disease, and the world of people, persons with instincts, with pain and suffering, hope and joy . . . we touch people and change their lives. Hippocrates was wrong about the laying on of hands.[10]

As editors, we hope this volume will inspire in practitioners of neonatal and perinatal medicine a renewed dedication to these twin goals: that of making their art at once more scientific and more humanistic. Each of the chapters represents the unique pairing of an experienced practitioner with another expert, both contributors having been chosen by the editors to comment on a particular topic of special interest to them. The author of the second article in each couple had the opportunity to read the article of his or her partner; they could thus comment directly in their own text on selected points already made, ensuring that certain issues would be re-emphasized, or make new points omitted by their colleagues, yet considered relevant to the discussion. We believe that the format of this text, with its integration of perspectives from physician and non-physician experts, makes this volume a unique and valuable resource to anyone interested in ethics related to the care of fetuses and newborns.

REFERENCES

1. L. Clendening, *Source book of medical history*. Dover Publications, Inc, New York (1960), pp. 14–15.
2. R. S. Duff and A. G. M. Campbell, 'Moral communities and tragic choices'. In R. C. McMillan, H. T. Englehardt, Jr., and S. F. Spicker (eds), *Euthanasia and the newborn: conflicts regarding saving lives*. D. Reidel Publishing Company, Dordrecht (1987), p. 277.
3. D. J. Rothman, *Strangers at the bedside: a history of how law and bioethics transformed medical decision making. Basic Books, New York (1991)*.
4. M. W. Shaw, 'When does treatment constitute a harm?' In *Euthanasia and the newborn*, p. 120.
5. E. E. Shelp, 'Choosing among evils'. In *Euthanasia and the newborn*, pp. 211–31.
6. A. R. Jonsen and M. J. Garland (eds), *Ethics of newborn intensive care*. Health Policy Program, School of Medicine, University of California, San Francisco (1976), p. 149.
7. E. J. Cassell, *The healer's art*. MIT Press, Cambridge, Mass. (1985).
8. Cassell, *The healer's art*, p. 230.
9. M. A. Schwartz and O. Wiggins, 'Science, humanism, and the nature of medical practice: a phenomenological view'. In C. E. Odegard, (ed.), *Dear Doctor. The Henry J. Kaiser Family Foundation*, Menlo Park, (1986), pp. 117–56.
10. J. K. Stevenson, 'The Surgeon, healer with work at hand'. *Archives in Surgery*, **124**, 1123–6 (1989).

2

Maternal–fetal conflicts: ethical and policy issues

2A   MATERNAL–FETAL CONFLICT I

Wayne R. Cohen

One of the great appeals of obstetrics for its practitioners and its aspirants is that medical decision-making affects simultaneously the well-being of mother and fetus. This duality confers a pattern of complexity on clinical problem-solving that is often intriguing and provocative. From this unique quality of obstetrics a number of abstruse challenges to modern bioethics have emerged.

Under most circumstances, the desire of the mother (the only member of the maternal–fetal dyad able to express opinions) and the goal of the obstetrician are coincident—to do what is possible to ensure a healthy outcome for mother and baby. Bad obstetric outcomes are mourned by both doctor and family, because the expectations of each have been frustrated, and the sense of loss is shared. It is not surprising, therefore, that few situations in obstetrics are more perplexing and cause more anguish for all concerned than those in which the best interests of the mother and fetus are in conflict; but few are more intellectually challenging and fewer still offer the opportunity for the practitioner to examine his or her own values and to address ethical issues of complexity and moment. Indeed, from these issues of maternal–fetal conflict have emerged a number of absorbing lessons relating to the ethical treatment of pregnant women.

SOURCES OF CONFLICT

For purposes of this chapter we shall define maternal–fetal conflict as any situation in which the intent or actions of the pregnant woman do not coincide with the needs, interests, or rights of her fetus as perceived by the obstetric caregivers. In order for a conflict to exist, the interests, rights, expectations, or desires of the mother and fetus must differ. They can do so only if the values of a third party (doctor, judge, father, social order, law, etc.) are conferred upon the fetus, which remains necessarily a passive participant in decisions that affect it profoundly. From one perspective, such situations can, therefore, be viewed as really conflicts between patient and health-care provider as much as between mother and fetus. As a consequence, these issues have forced obstetricians to confront a number of puzzling uncertainties concerning the role of paternalism in medical care and of the autonomy of the mother with regard to decisions that affect the health or life of the fetus she carries.

There are of course conflicts in which individuals other than the pregnant woman need not necessarily be involved. If a pregnant woman uses tobacco, ethanol, or cocaine she places her fetus at risk. In so doing, she makes a choice that puts her interpretation of her moral obligations to the fetus in conflict with the expectations of society at large. A mother might do the same by an act of omission, such as choosing not to seek prenatal care during the pregnancy. Such choices are bewildering to most observers, particularly because for the woman to choose otherwise, i.e. not to smoke or drink alcohol and to seek prenatal care, would place the mother at no excess risk. Maternal behaviors that might place the fetus in jeopardy are certainly discouraged in many ways; but our society has generally not placed itself in the position of forcing women to avoid activities that place their pregnancy at risk. The reasons for this may be manifold—economic, legal, political, personal—but underlying them is an implicit conviction that the pregnant woman has a moral right to autonomy in matters concerning her pregnancy. (In fact, this may extend to a legal right as well. A recent case [*in re* Valerie D., Conn. 1992] in which a pregnant woman was accused of child-neglect because she was using illicit drugs during pregnancy was overturned by the Connecticut Supreme Court. Similar cases in other venues have had the same result. There have been suggestions of forcing women to alter their lifestyles, including a recommendation of incarceration of drug-users for the duration of pregnancy to protect the fetus. Thus far the courts have been unwilling to intervene in this manner.) This societal mindset—tolerance of choices that do not harm other adults or already-born children—should be kept in mind as we ponder other kinds of situations in which choices concerning the fetus may place the mother at risk.

The concept of maternal–fetal conflict could be expressed more broadly to encompass any situation in which a decision or medical intervention designed to aid the mother or fetus places the other in potential jeopardy. Such situations are, in fact, commonplace. In fact, thus defined, the concept could encompass the majority of therapeutic or diagnostic decisions in obstetrics, because every decision made by doctor or patient requires weighing the risks and benefits to which mother and fetus will be exposed. In most such cases, the risks are low, and they and the benefits of the considered options can be reasonably quantified and balanced. Many potential conflicts thus have little practical importance in the sense that the doctor assists the patient in choosing among options, each of which may be perceived as reasonable. For example, the decision as to whether or not to use anesthetic medication during labor and delivery is rarely a source of significant conflict, even if doctor and patient differ in their views of the issue. Such medications have obvious advantages for some individuals, but do carry small and recognized risks of complications. The patient is generally given nearly complete autonomy in this decision, and in most cases the use of anesthesia or the avoidance of it is unlikely to have a significant effect on obstetric outcome.

Perhaps the most obvious situation of maternal–fetal conflict involves decisions about terminating pregnancy. These conflicts are nevertheless viewed by many as arising from quite different issues than those that occur later in pregnancy when the fetus is potentially viable. The decision to induce abortion is obviously one that values maternal health and interests over those of the fetus. In some respects, this is the least complex of the issues, because American society, by virtue of its current practice and its laws, allows the mother autonomy in resolving this conflict. The mother may choose to terminate her pregnancy before the third trimester in most states without a requirement to state or discuss the reasons for her decision. Such a choice presumes pregnancy and motherhood would be inappropriate incursions on her emotional, social, or physical well-being, and is made by the woman in the context of her personal moral value system. An obstetrician might advise induced abortion of a pregnancy in a mother with, for example, severe pulmonary hypertension or scleroderma nephropathy. (The former carries a high risk of maternal death and the latter of progression to chronic renal failure if the pregnancy continues.) In these situations, terminating the pregnancy kills the fetus to preserve the mother's life or health, a vivid example of a conflict between maternal and fetal interests; but to maintain the pregnancy may ultimately place both in jeopardy. Nevertheless, some mothers might choose to continue the pregnancy even under these adverse circumstances—a decision that may be baffling to some health-care providers, but which is accepted out of respect for the patient's expression of her own values.

More complex decisions, which have more subtle but still quantifiable risks, exist. For example, a woman with epilepsy who requires phenytoin to prevent *grand mal* seizures faces a dilemma. The drug is an acknowledged human teratogen. To take it during pregnancy eliminates the potential adverse consequences of seizures to fetus and mother, but exposes the fetus to the possibility of dysmorphism and even mental deficiency. The risks and the benefits of using and avoiding treatment can be assessed objectively and a decision reached. If the mother chooses not to take phenytoin against the advice of her physician, she has opted to assume risks that are primarily maternal (but to a smaller extent fetal as well) in order to avoid a recognized risk of malformation. Conversely, a woman might insist on continuing to take the drug during her pregnancy despite reassurances that the risk of recurrent seizures is low. Perhaps her own experience with complications of seizure activity might lead her to accept a fetal risk in exchange for eliminating one of her own. Numerous other examples of everyday choice-making that involve weighing risks and benefits to mother and fetus could be cited. For those in which risks are reasonably well understood and perceived to be relatively small, major conflicts between doctor and patient arise rarely. This is presumably because the doctor respects the patient's autonomy in these kinds of matters, and because the risks are small he or she is comfortable with either alternative.

ROLE OF THE HEALTH-CARE PROVIDER

Other kinds of choices that have the potential for affecting pregnancy are rooted in conflicts in which the outcome is less certain and in which there is almost always the involvement of a third party from the medical-care establishment involved in attempts at resolution. In most of these situations, the obligation of the obstetrician is to act or advise ethically, and this requirement is reasonably met by considering the ethical principles of beneficence and respect for persons (Beauchamp and McCullough 1984). The former dictates that the doctor be mindful of and act in what are perceived to be the best interests of mother and fetus; the latter allows the mother appropriate autonomy in the decision-making process.

We have been addressing primarily situations in which a pregnant woman makes a decision that places her or her fetus in potential jeopardy, and that runs counter to the physician's recommendations. There is another kind of maternal–fetal conflict that is less common, but can be even more disconcerting for the medical-care team. The doctor may be put in a position of deciding on a course of action that will preserve the life or health of the mother or fetus at the expense of the life or health of the other. Certainly the increasing use of living wills and health-care proxies may make these situations more rare, but they will occur, and can be bewildering for the health-care provider who has not rehearsed his or her response to such issues.

Consider the horrible dilemma of the physician confronted suddenly with an unconscious term pregnant victim of traumatic injury with hemorrhage and evidence of fetal asphyxia. To perform emergency cesarean delivery might spare the fetus but increase the risk of maternal death; to delay the cesarean condemns the fetus but might facilitate maternal survival. A decision might need to be made before the woman's next of kin or designated proxy could be consulted. Here the issues of autonomy are displaced to the physician, as neither mother nor fetus can participate in the decision.

In addition, the principle of beneficence is confounded; it must be violated for either mother or fetus. Indecision could result in injury to both. On what basis are decisions made in such situations? There exists a general presumption to favor the mother's survival whenever possible—a view to which I adhere. This requires placing a relative value judgment on the two lives, of favoring actual over potential, independence over dependence. It is not a choice made comfortably by most of us; moreover, some individuals, by virtue of their personal or religious beliefs would favor fetal over maternal survival. In any case, the outcome will rarely be certain at the time a decision is required, and many probabilities must be weighed.

The physician has first to consider the medical options. In this case there are two: intervene promptly to rescue the fetus from adversity and condemn the mother to probable death or disability from surgery she may be too unstable to endure; or reserve intervention to give the mother the greatest possibility of intact survival and hope (probably in vain) the fetus survives unaffected after exposure to the prolonged oxygen deprivation that may be the consequence of the maternal hemorrhage. It would be appropriate for the doctor to consider the patient's value system or previously expressed wishes in this regard. Often they will be unknown, but may be accessible in some circumstances. When a pregnant woman has a severe medical disease that could result in her sudden deterioration or death, these issues should be discussed sensitively but frankly with her when possible. If nothing is known of the patient's desires, the decision will probably be made on the basis of the doctor's own perspective. This will necessarily be colored by his or her own personal history, religious background, and moral values. All that can be asked of the physician is that he or she confront the issue squarely, weigh the conflicting obligations to mother and fetus, and choose the path that, accepting the ineffable uncertainty of the situation, seems like what ought to be done. Of those who judge the decision with hindsight, no less should be expected, because whatever the consequences of the decision it cannot be undone to test the outcome of the alternative.

COMMUNICATION AND IMPOSING VALUES

Effective communication between doctor and patient is obviously a requisite component of good medical care, and the importance of good communication in avoiding or resolving ethical conflicts is underestimated. Expert clinicians are able to modify the style and content of their discussions with patients so as to provide a clear explanation of the situation in a manner appropriate to the patient's ability to understand and to interpret the information. The content and nature of such discussions may differ depending upon the patient's level of education, what the physician perceives as the patient's style of emotional defense or adaptation, and her interest in participating in the process. These necessary variations in form and substance notwith-standing, one may reasonably ask what ethical imperatives should always be considered in the communication process, particularly as it relates to perinatal medicine and the conflicts we have been addressing.

Danziger (1978) identified a spectrum of interactional styles between doctors and patients that ranged from situations in which the physician acted simply as a provider of information with the patient a passive recipient to those in which both parties acted in a process of co-operative decision-making. It has been pointed out (Danziger 1978; McRae and Mervyn 1989) that when physician and patient bring different expectations to their communication there is the potential for conflicts to develop. When the physician is interested in merely providing information but the patient wishes to be an active partner in decision-making, or when the physician desires an interactive approach to the problem and the patient chooses to act merely as a recipient of information, there is the potential for problems and misunderstandings.

Many health-care workers argue that even the most well-educated layperson may not be able to understand complex medical issues in the way that a trained health professional can, and consequently patients should not always be allowed complete autonomy in decisions concerning their health. It is true that medical decisions have become increasingly complex. The moral burden of the physician to inform and educate every patient about her medical situation has increased in parallel. Some patients, whatever their ability to understand the issues, give the burden of the decision-making back to the physician by asking, 'What do you recommend?' or 'What would you do in my situation, doctor?' There are obviously a large number of issues at work here, not the least of which is the patient's need to displace or at least diffuse some of the guilt that may result from a decision that results in a bad outcome. Does the physician have a moral obligation to present his or her opinion to the patient?

A common example of this dilemma is the situation related to genetic amniocentesis. It is well known that the risks of fetal chromosome abnormalities begin to increase rapidly in women above the age of 35, and in the United States that age has generally been chosen as the one at which amniocentesis is offered or recommended. This has to do simply with the arithmetic of the situation. It is the maternal age at which the likelihood of finding an abnormality is approximately counterbalanced by the likelihood of injuring the pregnancy with the diagnostic procedure. Many physicians will recommend, even encourage, women to have this procedure (assuming, of course, that they would be willing to terminate a pregnancy found to be seriously affected), particularly in the older age-ranges. A woman at the age of 40 who delivers a baby has about a 2 per cent chance of the child having Down Syndrome.

Each of us brings a great number of individual social, cultural, religious, and personal biases to bear on the decision of whether to identify and abort a fetus with a congenital defect. For this reason, it would seem that the physician can best fulfill his or her ethical responsibilities by providing the patient with as much information as she requires with regard to the risks of the proposed procedure, the accuracy of its results, and the consequences of not having it performed, including an impression of what the life of an affected individual is like and what obstacles or benefits a family will meet by raising a seriously handicapped child. When some women are told of a 1 in 50 chance of having a baby with a serious genetic abnormality they leap at the opportunity to undergo a procedure to avoid such a possibility. Some physicians are surprised, however, to discover that a family may view a 2 per cent risk of a serious malformation as one that is small and worth taking. After all, there is a 98 per cent likelihood that the disorder will not exist (better odds than one gets in many of life's major decisions). Moreover, some families are better equipped emotionally, spiritually, and financially than others to cope with the stress of raising a child with a serious disability. Most doctors place intelligence and educability high on their personal and family value scale; some individuals and cultures have different expectations of their offspring.

The doctor will have opinions based on his or her own background and experience and perceptions of the patient's situation. Thus, the principle of beneficence requires that the patient be provided with the facts necessary for her to make a decision in the context of her own personal and family values; but the way in which information is transferred has a potential bearing on the decision. It requires presenting the facts of the situation in a neutral and dispassionate manner—a task that, considering the emotionally laden nature of the subject-matter, requires skillful communication. If, as happens frequently, she asks the physician, 'What do you think?' or says 'Do what you think is best', it is probably most appropriate to respond by saying that what might be best for me and my family is not necessarily best for you, and this is a decision that you must make. Thus the physician may be in the unusual and uncomfortable position of not giving advice. Considering the esteem in which many patients hold their doctors, the ability to usurp the patient's autonomy and impose one's own value system is difficult to resist. Sometimes it occurs not overtly but in subtle ways consciously designed to influence the patient's decision. Emphasis on words or phrases in a dialogue with the patient or even facial expressions or other body language can convey the doctor's opinion to the patient. Whether information can ever be given to the patient in a completely neutral manner is a matter of some disagreement among physicians. It seems to me there are great risks inherent in coloring the information in one way or another. The ethical thing to do is to resist these temptations.

These issues have to do with the degree to which the doctor should attempt to impose his or her own views upon the patient, and involve issues of control and paternalism. Armed with purely objective information, the patient should be able to reach a decision about whether to have the procedure. How should the physician respond when the patient asks, 'What do you think I should do?' Many physicians are tempted at that juncture to suggest what they think would be right for the patient or even to express what they themselves would do faced with the situation. I think that is wrong. Pregnant women should be capable of making these decisions based on their own value systems, and it is not fair for the physician to impose his or her own. It is, as has been stated previously, the pregnant woman who will live with the consequences of the decision. An acknowledged risk nevertheless exists in being too doctrinaire about this issue. Some women may need to share the burden of decision-making, and in some cases may not only choose to trust the physician to make a good decision, but may also feel he or she is in the best position to do so if the doctor is felt to have an ethical value system in accord with that of the patient. There is a difference between controlling and guiding. The former is to be avoided; the latter is to be commended as an important feature of doctor–patient communication. What is critical is that the patient be guided to explore her own values and reach a decision consistent with them. If the doctor is asked for a recommendation it should be made based on the context of the patient's values. However well-intentioned, persuading her towards the physician's values may not best serve her needs. This kind of counseling requires fine communication skills and often a lot of time. Mother, fetus and doctor will ultimately be well served by both.

What then should be the role of the doctor in assisting the patient with decision-making in the complex issues of maternal–fetal conflict in late pregnancy? Is it ethical for the physician to attempt to sway the patient's decision to coincide with his or her own? It would seem that the concept of preserving maternal autonomy and placing the fetus in the mother's ethical domain would militate against such persuasion except in so far as it may be necessary to insure that the patient has a clear understanding of the consequences of her decision.

ETHICAL OBLIGATIONS

Chervenak and McCullough (1985) pointed out that the fetus has interests that are addressed through beneficence-based obligations of the mother and physician; but that autonomy is not an issue for the fetus, since it is incapable of expressing or even having an opinion about what it might want. How is the scale weighing obligations of beneficence and of autonomy balanced? Should these issues perforce be considered of equal magnitude, and, if not, under what circumstances should one be considered to outweigh the other? When the conflict is between doctor and adult non-pregnant patient the issues are difficult, but can at least be defined with relative clarity.

Consider the Jehovah's Witness with hemorrhage who refuses transfusion of blood or blood products that the doctor feels might be life-saving. Some physicians would fully respect the patient's autonomy and, while doing everything short of transfusion to save her life, allow death to occur and not transfuse. Such an approach seemingly favors the patient's autonomy over the beneficence obligations of the physician to her; but viewed from a certain perspective, the harm that would occur from saving the life by blood transfusion (precluding eternal salvation) might be viewed by the patient to be as bad as or worse than death. To allow death does not thus necessarily represent a triumph of patient autonomy over the physician's responsibilities to cure. This view is difficult enough for most physicians to accept. Indeed for many it seems to betray all of their instincts, values, and noble intent. However dismaying that situation may seem, it becomes infinitely more complex if the bleeding patient is pregnant. Now the obligations of the physician to the fetus, who as yet has no religious values or beliefs, might counterbalance the wish to respect the autonomy of the mother, and some would opine that transfusion against the mother's wishes is justifiable as a moral obligation to preserve the best interests of the fetus. One's view of this conundrum depends on how one views the fetal–maternal relationship and the role of others in fostering it ethically. Decision-making would also be a function of how well one knows the patient. My own approach would be to acquiesce to the patient's desires if I knew something of them in advance of the situation and if I were certain there was no element of coercion (for example, by family members) in her decision. Were I ignorant or uncertain about either the depth of the woman's convictions or whether she arrived at the decision independently I would opt to transfuse and save the lives of mother and fetus if possible. In other words, I would adhere to Hippocratic doctrine and allow the principle of beneficence to prevail unless certain the patient desired otherwise.

The paradox inherent in that approach harks back to the issue of communication and prenatal care. An obstetrician may, after discussion of the patient's views, reasonably inform her that transfusion will not be administered under any circumstances; that transfusion would be given if the doctor felt it important; or that the doctor would avoid transfusion unless there were absolutely no other option to save the life of mother and fetus. The patient may reasonably (in fact, should) seek another physician if she is confronted with the latter two alternatives and finds them unsatisfactory.

THE MATERNAL–FETAL RELATIONSHIP

How can the maternal–fetal relationship be viewed from the perspective of applied ethics? There are three alternatives. The first is to assume that the mother and fetus are completely independent in the sense that the interests, rights, and goals of each are equivalent and sovereign. This view would require the physician or some other third party to act as the fetal advocate and for us to assume that such a person would always act in the best interests of the fetus. Second, one could assume that the fetus, being genetically derived from and for now inextricably a part of the mother, has not independent rights or interests, and that whatever occurs in the mother's interests carries the fetus along as a passive beneficiary or victim. This view would simplify much ethical decision-making because it restricts the physician's moral obligations of autonomy and beneficence to the mother. The third alternative is to assume that the mother and fetus are independent beings but that the mother has a special obligation to look after the best interests of the fetus in a way not different from the way in which one might expect her to exercise her moral obligations toward her children after birth.

The special difference between the two situations (mother–fetus or mother–child) resides in those dilemmas that require fetal interventions through the mother. Some of the perspective on this issue necessarily involves legal views of if and when the fetus becomes a person, and has thus conferred upon it the rights of personhood under the law. But as there is unlikely ever to be agreement on when and if personhood begins during intrauterine life, it seems that an ethical approach should not require a legal decision about whether a fetus is a person. It may, nevertheless, require a judgment by doctor and patient, which should be based on their own moral framework, and not upon any legal definition of viability, personhood, or independence. When doctor and patient hold legitimate but opposing views on this issue, preference should be accorded to the patient's will.

CONFIDENTIALITY AND PATERNAL CONFLICTS

Generally the physician's obligation to respect a patient's confidentiality is considered sacrosanct, even if she chooses therapy the doctor feels is not in her best interests or refuses that which is. Most physicians would agree not to involve third parties (for example, other family members) in a medical decision without the patient's acquiescence. Are there circumstances in which the patient's rights to privacy and to autonomy may be violated if the physician feels his or her obligations to promote the patient's well-being will be served best by involving third parties in the process? Such a party might be a health-care institution (with legitimate fiscal interests in the outcome), or members of the extended family, any of whom might in some cases claim a legitimate, even a compelling, interest in the outcome of the maternal–fetal conflict. Although it might be relatively easy to dismiss most such claims on the basis of the pregnant woman's autonomy and our moral obligation to support it, claims of one third party—the father of the fetus— are not so easily dispensed with. In fact, paternal–maternal or paternal–fetal conflicts do occur.

Situations in which a mother desires to abort or to keep a pregnancy are not infrequently disputed by the father. In such cases, the mother's moral autonomy is almost always respected, supported by the voice of law (*Roe vs Wade*, 410U.S.113 [1973]), which currently views the pre-viable fetus as essentially a part of the mother's body. This stance was recently upheld in *Planned Parenthood of Southeastern Pennsylvania vs. Casey* 1992, in which the United States Supreme Court held that paternal notification of intended abortion would impose an undue burden on women. The issue becomes more complex in the third trimester when mother and father disagree about whether to intervene in a pregnancy by, for example, cesarean delivery, *in utero* fetal therapy, or attempts to postpone pre-term delivery. Once delivered, a newborn is recognized legally and morally as an equally shared product of both parents. As the child is usually a genetically balanced composite of both, their interests in the child's well-being are usually given equal weight. However, before the moment of birth, with the fetus still enrobed in the mother's body, the father's wishes have often been ignored (except in so far as he may influence the mother's decision) or subjugated to those of the mother.

The issue is a curious one. From the perspective of a paternal advocate, the father may be viewed as having a legitimate stake and interest in the outcome of the pregnancy. After all, he participated in the decision to create the fetus (tacit in the sexual act or explicit as a conjoint decision with his partner), and may plan to participate in rearing the child, who is, from the genetic standpoint at least, as much his product as the mother's. Moreover, many fathers are actively involved in helping their partner cope with the experience of pregnancy (although mostly their support is welcomed but superfluous), and perceive themselves as having a major interest in optimal outcome, which, in this context, would mean a newborn with the ability to meet its inherited physical and cognitive potential. Yet despite these quite legitimate interests in outcome, cases of maternal–paternal conflict are virtually always decided on the basis of the pregnant spouse's desires. In other words, the doctor's moral obligations require that maternal autonomy should generally transcend paternal interest in the well-being of the fetus. Why should this be so?

The answer obviously resides in the uniqueness of the maternal–fetal relationship, a propinquity many consider inviolate from the standpoint of moral obligations to a pregnancy. What are the characteristics of the maternal–fetal relationship that make the mother's decisions about her autonomy and about the well–being of the conceptus take moral precedence over declared conflicting interests of third parties in the fetal outcome, even if the third party contributed genetic material to the fetus and can be demonstrated to have authentic and convincing interests in the welfare of the fetus?

For most of the pregnancy, although it is identifiably and genetically different from the mother, the fetus cannot survive without her, quite unlike the newborn, who could theoretically be reared successfully by anyone with the interest and will to do so. In late pregnancy, when the fetus would be perfectly capable of surviving if removed from the mother before the moment of spontaneous delivery, it cannot pursue this independent course without some intervention on the part of a third party (usually a physician); and any such intervention (cesarean section, induction of labor, forceps delivery, etc.) requires a physical intervention on the mother. Whether such a trespass on the body of another, be it major (for example anesthesia and cesarean section) or relatively minor (insertion of intravenous needle and production of uterine contractions to induce labor) should not be considered without the permission of the mother. To think or act otherwise would put medicine in the unconscionable position of forcing a patient to undergo a treatment for the benefit of another. Indeed, it seems reasonable to allow the individual who assumes all the physical and most of the emotional risks and burdens of a pregnancy the main role in deciding whether to permit interventions. Just as we give individuals choice over their own medical destiny, so should we give them control over that of their fetus. Sometimes this would mean subjugating the life and interests of one human to that of another—an uncomfortable choice at best, but one to which civilization is not altogether unaccustomed. The alternative would be to subjugate the rights and interests of the mother, and to make her right to control her own body less important than the interests of the fetus.

What does this stance mean in practical terms to the physician faced with a maternal–fetal conflict? Obviously, no rigid rules or protocols can (or should) be established for dealing with all the bioethical issues involving maternal–fetal conflict. To do so would invite simplistic, even thoughtless solutions to problems of bewildering complexity. Rather, each case must be analyzed individually; but a structure must exist within which all involved parties can frame their thinking about the situation so that decisions can be made with a clear awareness of the obligations each individual brings to the situation. The lack of such a framework invites chaos, impulsivity, and the false presumption that moral obligations have been identified and fulfilled.

The seemingly inexorable advance of technology has made medical judgments increasingly complex, and has added unexpected and challenging threads to the web of medical decision-making. For example, forms of artificial surfactant are now available for the treatment of respiratory distress syndrome of the newborn. If perfected, this drug will have remarkable life-saving potential for very premature babies; but it will also carry risks to be pondered by mother, obstetrician, and pediatrician as decisions about premature birth are considered. More daunting from the ethical standpoint is that techniques of intrauterine fetal surgery are being developed. Although largely experimental at present, it is likely that in the future physicians will have the ability to cure or improve fetal disease before birth by operating upon the fetus and, in so doing, on the mother as well. Such procedures will also need to be viewed in the context of the balance of potential welfare and infirmity to be sustained. However complicated and unprecedented are the medical decisions that may confront us in the future, our judgments will still be channeled by the same ethical principles, by the same blueprint for weighing opposing values and responsibilities that we have used for addressing today's and yesterday's moral dilemmas.

Ideally, the doctor has an obligation to understand the patient's value system and know whether it conflicts with his or her own. A bond of trust must be forged with the patient so that she understands the physician's own values and from what moral perspective he or she will make recommendations. This is a tall order, and cannot be accomplished in a short time. That is one of the important virtues of prenatal care. To develop a relationship of trust and clear communication and to anticipate conflicts and assess values through many encounters during gestation can avoid difficult contretemps during late pregnancy or labor.

The next issue of signal importance is that the physician understand that his or her moral obligations and medical priorities may at times seem discrepant with each other. Indeed it is the failure to appreciate, or at least to acknowledge this fact, that imports the anguish into issues of maternal–fetal conflict, and may also precipitate the dissolution of the doctor–patient relationship, rendering further communication and trust impossible. For example, a physician may view saving the life of a mother or fetus as an arresting medical priority; his moral obligation not to do so by blood transfusion if the patient has refused it results in a clash of values. At one level this conflict is between doctor and patient; at another it is between the doctor's moral and medical wills.

In a sense, a conflict of values is the provenance of most ethical dilemmas, and the most important step in resolving them is to acknowledge that many value systems exist, that most have legitimacy, and that what is considered moral behavior in one may be anathema to another. The obstetrician's responsibility may be said to be to foster the best possible outcome for mother and fetus in the context of the mother's value system. From that standpoint, the moral duty of the physician is not to optimize fetal outcome at all costs, because to do so might put the doctor's values in conflict with the patient's and might well require violation of the mother's physical or ethical boundaries against her will. To act in an ethical fashion in these conflict situations, the doctor really has a definable set of responsibilities. They are to assess the problem and identify alternatives accurately; to educate the patient in as unbiased a way possible as to the options and their consequences; to allow her, armed with the appropriate information, to decide the outcome of the situation; and to respect her choice as one made in good faith and grounded in her own moral context and world-view.

Critics of this approach to bioethical decision-making in obstetrics would argue that it ignores the fact, noted previously, that many patients return the decision-making to the physician and ask him or her to do what would be best. In so doing, the patient may be properly exercising her autonomy, presuming that she has considered all available options. In some respects, a voluntary choice of this sort implies that the patient shares the physician's value preferences. It has also been argued that not all value systems are equally moral, and that always to honour a person's wishes could lead to a slippery slope at some point on which morally repugnant decisions are tolerated. That is possible, but unlikely.

PROBABILITY AND DECISION-MAKING

It is important for the lay public to understand that virtually all medical judgments, decisions, and recommendations are based upon what the doctor feels is the probability of a particular outcome. Rarely is the outcome of a decision certain. The degree of certainty the physician can bring to a judgment varies, depending upon his or her own knowledge and experience (which under any circumstances have limits) and on what information is potentially available about the issue. Often the physician's concern and the patient's action are based upon what each, within his or her own value system, perceives as the ratio of benefits to harms inherent in the situation. It is especially vexing to conceptualize these factors in obstetrics, because the risks it seeks to reduce are in most instances relatively small. In addition to the fact that this makes answers to clinical problems difficult to determine and liable to error, the scale of the problem is one with which most patients are not familiar. For example, a cardiologist may advise a patient that a particular treatment will save one patient in four from death after myocardial infarction. Death is an end-point, and 25 per cent is a number most of us can grasp the significance of easily. In obstetrics, by contrast, many interventions are undertaken to reduce the risk of perinatal death by only a few per thousand, a scale most laypersons are not able to conceptualize as well, at least in terms of effects on their own health. The obstetrician must thus grapple with moral obligations to society as well as to the individual patient in ways that many practitioners do not. If electronic fetal monitoring were, for example, capable of saving the life of one baby per 1000 births, it would be unlikely to be advantageous to any individual patient; but applied to the more than 3 million births in the US annually it would have the potential to save 3000 lives—a number of some consequence. Decisions must be made on the basis of the degree of associated risk and benefit to the patient as well as to the population at large—a concept that it is difficult to communicate effectively to the individual patient.

As an example on a different scale, many obstetricians prescribe multi-vitamin and mineral supplements to pregnant women. Such medications have few and very minor risks (unless taken in great excess) and requirements for certain nutrients do increase during gestation, a balance of benefits and harms making their prescription reasonable. Whether supplements have a benefit to a woman eating a well-balanced nutrient-rich diet is not certain; but there is some evidence that supplementation in early pregnancy may reduce the risk of certain malformations. If a pregnant woman chooses not to take her supplements, she avoids a very small risk to herself and the fetus but precludes reaping some benefits for both. The general perception of medicine is that in this situation the potential benefits (though small) outweigh potential harms (even smaller), and vitamins and minerals are recommended. How should the physician respond to the patient who does not take her vitamins? In most cases, beyond some education and encouragement, nothing further is done. Certainly, no thought of coercion is entertained, because the benefits are small and uncertain and, in plain terms, not worth fighting over. How does this situation differ from that in which a pregnant diabetic woman chooses not to follow an appropriate diet and not to take insulin properly? Here the risks and benefits to both parties are better understood and much higher. There is convincing evidence that control of blood glucose within certain narrow limits during pregnancy is necessary to optimize fetal outcome. Indeed, failure to control glycemia can in some cases lead to severe fetal injury or death. The risks and benefits of not taking insulin or following a proper diet are much greater that those of not taking vitamins. Medical personnel would invest much more energy attempting to convince the diabetic patient of the virtues of proper treatment and the terrible risks of choosing to eschew it. Such an investment is ethically sound and does not override the patient's autonomy. To my knowledge the more extreme (and to me ethically questionable) approach of forcing a patient to accept treatment (by, for example, detention in a hospital or prison) has rarely, if ever, been taken. The exception would be patients clearly incompetent to make decisions. (The argument that any diabetic, pregnant or otherwise, who refuses treatment is mentally unbalanced is fatuous and, it seems to me, unfairly distorts the definable envelope of mental well-being.)

WEIGHING VALUES

The value system of most medically trained professionals makes them view attaining the best possible maternal and fetal outcome as a moral obligation—an outlook usually shared by the mother. Does the patient have the right to refuse treatment designed to benefit the fetus based on her own value system, and how far should or may the physician go to impose his or her values on the patient? This decision depends on several factors. First is the degree of perceived risks and benefits and the level of uncertainly associated with the situation. If the harms associated with refusal of treatment are relatively small or uncertain, patient autonomy is usually respected even if the doctor perceives the patient's decision to be irrational. If the probability of fetal harms to be accrued is more certain and the risks more serious (for example in the cases of a diabetic's not caring for herself or a patient's refusing treatment for syphilis) greater efforts are usually made to convert the patient's values so that she shares the moral stance of the physician with regard to obligations to her fetus. Although most doctors are indeed tolerant of patient autonomy (even when their choices conflict with those judged best by the doctor), the presence of a fetus alters thinking, and physicians often become fetal advocates.

Beyond weighing of risks and harms, another consideration has to do with the patient's ability to understand the risks. As has been noted previously, the complexity of medical information and technology and the related issues of informed consent and ethical problem-solving to be confronted have advanced in parallel. It is reasonable to assume that a degree of intellectual sophistication may be necessary to reach the most informed judgments about medical issues. All too often, doctors confuse knowledge with wisdom, and assume an uneducated person incapable of making a good decision about a complex issue. It is the physician's responsibility to explain the available facts, opinions, and potential risks and benefits of a situation to a patient in a manner she can understand. Uncommonly wise choices are frequently made by patients not endowed with much schooling, but possessing keen minds, common sense, and clear convictions about what is right for them and their families. Of course, sometimes patients with limited intelligence must confront quite complex problems. It is not easy to stand back and permit autonomy to such an individual; but our need to respect the patient's right to decide may compel us to do so, once we have fortified her with as much information as possible. Exceptions would include patients who cannot make an informed decision because of mental illness, subnormal cognitive abilities, or otherwise impaired mental function.

In such cases consultation with the patient's legal proxy would be desirable; but many such individuals do not have a legally appointed guardian, and the help of the courts may be required to be sure rights as well as interests are protected.

RESOLVING CONFLICTS

There are avenues to travel if the patient and doctor are at loggerheads over an issue of maternal–fetal conflict. If time permits, the patient's family, friends, or clergyman can (with her permission) be made aware of the situation and may help the patient to reach a decision. Other health professionals may also be asked to consult. An institutional ethics committee may discuss the issue and help with a resolution. In some instances, as a last resort, physicians or hospitals have asked the courts to intervene.

The prototypical situation that has provoked legal intervention has been when a mother refuses to submit to a cesarean section that the doctor feels is necessary to prevent fetal injury. Several situations have occurred in which the courts were requested to order a patient to undergo cesarean delivery (Fleischman and Rhoden 1989). In some cases, the patients had religious beliefs that precluded their consenting to surgery; in others, their personal value systems were at stake. In general, the courts have sided with the doctors, supporting the view that the state has a compelling interest in protecting the future of a viable fetus that overrides its duties to protect the mother from harm, inasmuch as the risks associated with cesarean section are small. The courts have thus felt that the state has a duty and right to value its moral obligations to the fetus over the mother's right of autonomy. This approach differs from that which the courts have taken in analogous matters concerning extrauterine lives. When a man whose life could be saved only by a bone-marrow transplant (*McFall v Shimp* Pa. D7C.3d90 [1978]) asked the courts to force his only genetically compatible but reluctant relative to donate bone marrow, they would not. The judge noted that, however unnecessarily cruel and morally vacant the relative's refusal might be, society could not force one member against his will to violate his own bodily integrity to save the life of another.

The difference between the two seemingly irreconcilable approaches to patient autonomy resides in the uniqueness of the maternal–fetal relationship to which we have alluded previously. The case involving the dying man also highlights the potential discordancy between moral and legal duties and codes. Although resorting to the courts is an understandable retreat for the embattled and frustrated physician, it risks substituting notions of legal rights for moral imperatives. It could be argued pragmatically that when a physician is reasonably sure what is best or right for the patient and she refuses to accede, any means of obtaining a good outcome is legitimate, as long as the risks of harm are small. Legal action can sometimes be justified in that way; but it is a cumbersome, time-consuming process, and does not absolve the physician from the need to perform a thoughtful, ethical analysis of the situation.

There is a practical issue inherent in these considerations that has not to our knowledge been confronted publicly. That is how one would go about performing, for example, cesarean section on a woman unwilling to have it but ordered to do so by the courts or a designated advocate. Would one drag her kicking and screaming to the operating room and physically restrain her in order to administer anaesthesia? It has been done, with the best of intentions and a good fetal outcome (Elkins *et al*. 1989); but it would seem nothing could be more repugnant to a physician sworn to protect the health and dignity of women than to force them to undergo major surgery against their will. To stand helplessly by without intervening might be equally difficult from the emotional standpoint, but perhaps preferable in terms of one's moral obligations.

One problematic aspect of recent court decisions that have allowed a recommended forced cesarean delivery is the concern of physicians who choose to respect a maternal decision to refuse therapy in a conflict situation. It is possible that as the law evolves, the physician may feel (or even be) obliged to bring these issues to the courts and seek an order to implement intervention. In other words, the physician may fear retribution in the form of a medical negligence lawsuit if a judicial resolution to a conflict is not sought, even if the doctor feels forced intervention would be ethically inappropriate. Thus, the involvement of the legal system represents a potential incursion on the rights of doctors and of patients to make independent judgements about difficult medical situations.

THE FETAL PROXY

It has been suggested that maternal–fetal conflicts might be avoided by having someone other than the parents or physician designated a fetal advocate (Clewell *et al*. 1982). Such an individual would be empowered to speak for the fetus in assenting to or refusing interventions. This proxy approach has some virtues, particularly for the specific situation of *in utero* fetal surgery, for which it was first recommended. The concept could, of course, be broadened to encompass many kinds of decisions affecting the fetus. It might minimize conflict, and remove the potential burden of anguish and guilt parents may feel when thrust unexpectedly into ethical dilemmas that demand difficult choices. It seems, however, that assigning an advocate acceptable to parents and physician might not be simple, and the approach merely reassigns responsibility. It does nothing to promote an ethical conclusion to the medical drama. It is, after all, the potential parents who will bear the lifelong burden of the decision long after the advocate has left the scene. As medical professionals, it would seem we would do better to invest our energies in educating, counselling, and coaching patients through this process. That effort, though it may sometimes be frustrating, even futile, should ultimately do more to preclude guilt and to promote ethical decision-making than would assigning a proxy. Furthermore, one can envision situations in which proxy decisions are invested with the same objections we have to the involvement of the courts. A fetal advocate might make a decision in conflict with the mother's desires, and physicians would be put in the position of forcing a patient to undergo a procedure against her will.

CODA

Dealing with cases of maternal–fetal conflict in obstetric practice can be a daunting task—far more difficult and challenging than discussing (or writing about) the germane theoretical issues. Some general guidelines for the perplexed can be formulated. As is the case for many ethical dilemmas, asking the right questions is more important than finding the answers; that is to say, the process of identifying, evaluating, and analyzing the problem should be the priority. Done well, it will lead to good decision-making.

Because ethical conflicts arise from clashes of value systems, the physician must have a clear understanding of his or her own moral values and be able to articulate them clearly to the patient. By doing so one can practice preventive ethics (Chervenak and McCullough 1990) when possible. Prenatal care affords the opportunity to explore the patient's value system, identify potential conflicts, and deal with them to avoid future crises. If solutions cannot be reached that are satisfactory to patient and doctor, consider referral to another physician whose beliefs are concordant with those of the patient. Always remember whose responsibility it is to make decisions, and adhere to the role of physician as counselor. Advising, educating, suggesting, and even advocating can all be legitimate roles for the physician. The boundary between these advisory functions and those of coercing, pressuring, and compelling is sometimes not obvious but it is always crossed with peril by the physician wishing to act ethically. It is the patient who will be most affected by the outcome of conflicts. That is not to imply that these choices do not affect the physician profoundly. They do; but it is the patient who will daily confront the enduring consequences of her choices.

Be sure all available facts, probabilities, and uncertainties are understood before decisions are made. Present this information to the patient in the most objective fashion possible, being especially certain she comprehends all available options and their consequences.

Finally, do not expect the resolution of ethical conflicts always to make all parties completely comfortable. Remember that despite their differences, patient and doctor remain partners in this process. No good is served by their becoming adversaries. The physician and patient should demand of each other that conflicts be addressed unhesitatingly, that the competing views of each be confronted, analyzed, and, finally, weighed so that a satisfactory resolution can be achieved. In so doing the moral autonomy and personal dignity of the pregnant woman will be best preserved and the physician's moral obligations to her best fulfilled. One can expect no more, and should tolerate no less.

REFERENCES

Beauchamp, T. L. and McCullough, L. B. (1984). *Medical ethics: the moral responsibilities of physicians*. Prentice Hall, Englewood Cliffs.

Chervenak, F. A. and McCullough, L. B. (1985). Perinatal ethics: a practical method of analysis of obligations to mother and fetus. *Obstet. Gynecol.*, **66**: 442–6.

Chervenak, F. A. and McCullough, L. B. (1990). Clinical guides to preventing ethical conflicts between pregnant women and their physicians. *Am. J. Obstet. Gynecol*, **162**: 303–7.

Clewell, W. H., Johnson, M. L. Meier, P. R. Newkirk, J. B., Zide, S. L., Handee, R. W., Bowes, W. A. Jr., Hecht, T., O'Keeffe, D., Henry, G. P., and Shikes, R. H. (1982). A surgical approach to the treatment of fetal hydrocephalus. *N. Eng. J. Med.*, **306**: 1320–5.

Danziger, S. (1978). The uses of expertise in doctor–patient encounters during pregnancy. *Soc. Sci. Med. (Med. Psychol./Med. Social)*, **12**: 356–67.

Elkins, T. E., Andersen, H. F., Barclay, M., Mason, T., Bowdler, N., and Anderson, G. (1989). Court-ordered cesarean section: an analysis of ethical concerns in compelling cases. *Am. J. Obstet. Gynecol.*, **161**: 150–4.

Fleischman A. R. and Rhoden, N. K. (1989) Ethical dilemmas in labor management. In *Management of labor*, 2nd edn (ed W. R. Cohen, D. B. Acker, and E. A. Freidman), pp. 551–71. Aspen Publishers, Rockville, Maryland.

McRae, M. C., and Mervyn, F. V. (1989). Contemporary issues in childbirth. In *Management of labor* 2nd edn (ed. W. R. Cohen, D. B. Acker, and E. A. Freidman), pp. 535–50. Aspen Publishers, Rockville, Maryland.

2B   MATERNAL–FETAL CONFLICT II*

Ruth Macklin

The phrase 'maternal–fetal conflict' has become familiar to perinatologists and scholars working at the intersection of medicine, ethics, and law. Yet the very notion is puzzling to many when they first encounter the phrase. In addition, it is rejected—perhaps surprisingly—by some feminists. The puzzled response is illustrated by an episode that occurred at a meeting of a medical school committee on appointments and promotion. A candidate for promotion to the rank of professor was presented to the committee as a leading contributor to the field of bioethics, specializing in perinatal law and ethics. One member of the committee asked what the candidate wrote about, and upon hearing the phrase 'maternal–fetal conflict', appeared both puzzled and amused. 'How can there be any such conflict?' he remarked, thinking of the fetus as a wholly dependent, passive form of developing life incapable of engaging in conflict. Others were similarly curious, and I outlined the array of circumstances, the sources of conflict described by Wayne Cohen in the preceding section of this chapter. Several of the listeners were fascinated, and at the conclusion of the meeting there ensued a heated debate on substantive issues among those who lingered to discuss these conflicts.

The response from some feminists of seeking to reject the idea of maternal–fetal conflict stems from the belief that pregnant women should not be characterized as doing battle with their fetuses. For one thing, women desire normal, healthy infants even when a pregnancy is unplanned. Therefore, they should not be stigmatized as being engaged in competition with the fetus during pregnancy. The language of 'maternal–fetal conflict' depicts an image of women hostile to pregnancy or to a healthy outcome, an image that is false and demeaning.[1]

Another reason for feminists' rejection of the phrase harks back to the unending controversy surrounding abortion and the right of women to self-determination regarding their own bodies. There is a legitimate concern among all advocates of choice that increasing deference to the fetus destined to become a child will lead to greater recognition of the 'rights' of fetuses in unwanted pregnancies, thus further eroding the right of women to choose abortion.

* Portions of this chapter are excerpted or adapted from two previously published works: 'The ethics of fetal therapy', in James M. Humber and Robert F. Almeder (eds), *Biomedical Ethics Reviews 1984* Humana Press (Clifton, NJ, 1984), pp. 205–23; and Chapters 3 and 4 of *Enemies of patients* (Oxford University press, New York, 1993).

A different yet related reason for seeking to reject the concept of maternal–fetal conflict is that it elevates the fetus to the rank of a *patient*. This
is worrisome to those who fear that treating the fetus as a patient co-equal
to the pregnant woman can result in a preference for the interests of the
fetus over those of the woman, thereby establishing grounds for overriding
her autonomy. Ruth Hubbard, a scientist and feminist writing about *in
utero* therapy, lamented the fact that the fetus is now being construed as
a patient:

It is clear that at this point pregnancy has become a disease with *two* potential
patients—the pregnant woman and her fetus—and of those, the fetus is
medically and technically by far the more interesting one. Already a recent
article in the *Journal of the American Medical Association* refers to the pregnant
woman as though she were merely the container in which the real patient—the
fetus—gets moved about.[2]

THE FETUS AS PATIENT

It may well be true that the reference to two 'patients'—the pregnant
woman and the fetus—creates an aura of tension. Although not necessarily
pernicious, the conceptualization of the fetus as a patient engenders controversy. One physician writes that these cases of conflict 'involve a struggle
between valid obligations to two patients, obligations that very rarely are
in opposition'.[3] Yet however rare such cases of conflict may be, when the
interests of one patient conflict with the rights or interests of a second, the
two become potential adversaries.

It is apparent from the medical literature that the fetus is thought of and
acted upon as a patient, a trend that became most pronounced with the
advent of fetal therapy. More than a decade ago, Canty and Wolf asserted
that 'the fetus has achieved recognition as a patient'.[4] Clewell *et al.* stated
that 'any proposed fetal treatment really involves two patients: the fetus and
the mother'.[5] Another leading team of fetal therapists, Harrison *et al.*, were
somewhat more tentative, concluding that 'the fetus with a treatable birth
defect is on the threshold of becoming a patient'.[6]

What follows from the fact that the fetus is being conceptualized and acted
upon as a patient? The answer depends, in part, on whether physicians
perceive their obligations to that patient as separate from and independent of
their obligation to the pregnant woman who is undeniably their patient. The
literature on this topic reveals a striking diversity of views. Ruth Hubbard
concludes that once construed as a patient, the fetus acquires 'rights' to
medical intervention, rights that may override those of the mother in the
eyes of the law. 'In this way the fetus's presumed "rights" as a patient can
be used to control pregnant women'.[7]

One bioethicist ties the concern about calling the fetus a patient directly
to the abortion controversy. John Fletcher points to a possible inconsistency

in encouraging fetal therapy on the one hand and respecting parental choice about abortion on the other: 'Is it not contradictory for physicians to speak of the fetus as a "patient", when one of the stipulations for that role is that physicians would not under any circumstances abandon such an individual?'[8] Fletcher bases his solution to this apparent inconsistency on a view of when it is proper to apply the term 'patient': 'The fetus with a treatable defect could not be fully considered a patient until separate from the mother, unless one took the position of being willing to coerce the mother to let the pregnancy go to term.'[9] This solution involves stipulating a definition of 'patient' that would be counterintuitive to many physicians. However, a more problematic feature of Fletcher's approach is that it raises the specter of abortion in the context of maternal–fetal conflict. Wayne Cohen takes the same approach when he identifies decisions about terminating pregnancy as 'perhaps the most obvious situation of maternal–fetal conflict'. Is this a valid maneuver?

I think the tendency to analyze ethical problems relating to maternal–fetal conflict in the context of abortion is a mistake, and should be resisted. To 'respect parental choice about abortion', as Fletcher puts it, is to grant ultimate authority to the parents to decide the fate of an organism dependent on the woman's body for its continued existence. The decision to abort is a decision to terminate that existence. The maternal decision to allow a pregnancy to go to term is an entirely different decision, made in different circumstances and for different considerations. It is no more inconsistent that some women choose to abort an unwanted fetus while others take as many steps as are necessary to ensure the birth of a normal, healthy infant than that some people choose not to have children at all while others choose to invest all their time, energy, and resources in their offspring.

The abortion controversy centers on the moral status of the conceptus, embryo, or fetus. To resolve the abortion controversy, opponents have to reach agreement on the point following fertilization at which the product of conception acquires rights, in particular, a right to life. No such agreement need be reached in the arena of maternal–fetal conflicts. There is widespread agreement, almost universal acknowledgement, that, once born, infants have a life that deserves protection from harm. The ethical question here focuses on what steps may be taken to seek to ensure that infants are 'well-born', that is, born as sound and healthy as possible.

A further point is worth noting in distinguishing maternal–fetal conflicts from the abortion controversy. In the context of abortion, as the pregnancy advances the ethical concerns grow correspondingly. In contrast, if the cause for concern is damage to the fetus likely to result in anomalies or developmental disabilities after birth, the early weeks and months are often the most critical time. Scientific evidence regarding the kinds of serious, irreversible damage that can be inflicted very early in pregnancy suggests that some of the worst consequences for infants can result from things that take place possibly even before a woman realizes that she is pregnant. The priorities that exist in the abortion context are almost reversed in maternal–fetal conflicts where the pregnant woman uses illegal drugs or alcohol, takes prescribed medications, or is exposed to environmental or occupational teratogens.

An intriguing analysis of the implications of treating the fetus as a patient is given by Ruddick and Wilcox,[10] who tie the issue to the type of contract (loosely understood) that can be negotiated between the woman and her physician. They propose three models of the therapeutic contract: 'gynecological', 'obstetrical', and 'pediatric'. According to the first contract, 'therapeutic decisions are to be guided solely by considerations of [the woman's] health, welfare, and desires'.[11] Presumably, this means that the fetus becomes a patient only if the mother so wishes. According to the second, or 'pediatric', contract that a woman might make with her obstetrician, the fetus is a patient by virtue of the woman's therapeutic contract. 'By extreme contrast with gynecological contracts, the woman's health is made secondary; therapy is to be guided by fetal considerations'.[12] The third contract, the 'obstetrical' one, is more qualified. On this model the commitment is to a successful outcome of pregnancy, namely, a healthy baby. 'Accordingly, under an obstetrical contract, the fetus is something between a full (pediatric) patient and a mere complication of a woman's (gynecological) condition. It is a provisional, or trial, patient with claims on the doctor's and mother's care . . .'[13]

Although this analysis is intriguing, the models are somewhat artificial, and probably nowhere exist in the pure forms in which they are depicted in the article. Perhaps more problematic from an ethical point of view is the worry that such 'contracts' could be treated as binding even if the woman decided to change her mind somewhere along the way. It is the nature of voluntary, informed consent to treatment that a patient may refuse the treatment or reverse an earlier implied consent. The Ruddick–Wilcox approach might presume too much in the way of a patient's advance consent to a course of medical management taking place over a prolonged period of time.

At bottom, the key question posed by construing the fetus as a patient is whether the interests of that patient can ever be permitted to override the rights and interests of the undisputed patient, the woman in whom the fetus is lodged. That is the crux of the ethical problem of maternal–fetal conflict.

PHYSICIANS' ROLE IN MATERNAL–FETAL CONFLICT

Although it is true that women hope for the best outcome of their pregnancy and most do behave in ways likely to achieve that outcome, that is not a sufficient reason to reject the concept of maternal–fetal conflict, as some feminists have urged. This is because the conflict is typically imposed from without: an attempt by a physician or health-care institution to coerce a woman into accepting what is deemed best for the fetus, or more correctly, for the child the fetus will become. A woman might not feel in conflict with her fetus, but some women are thrust into the role of adversary of their fetus by the attempts of others to control their behavior.

Physicians have recommended and sought to impose a number of different medical or surgical interventions on pregnant women, sometimes for the women's own benefit but usually for the sake of the fetus. Possibly the most common of these is cesarean section, which Wayne Cohen refers to as 'the prototypical situation that has provoked legal intervention'. Women refuse cesarean sections on religious grounds, because of fear of cutting, or for other reasons—some rational, others irrational. Questions are often raised about the competency—or to use a preferable term—'decisional capacity' of patients who refuse recommended treatments, within or outside the context of obstetrics. Although it is legitimate to raise the question of a patient's capacity for decision-making, it is a factual and moral mistake to construe as 'incompetent' patients who refuse doctors' recommendations, simply on the basis of those refusals.

A letter to the *New England Journal of Medicine* commented on an article by Kolder *et al.* which reported the incidence of court-ordered treatment of pregnant women.[14] The letter-writer accused the authors of 'skating over the issue of maternal competency'. The letter notes that 'maternal competency was established by a psychiatrist in only 3 of the 20 cases reported by Kolder *et al.* No evidence is given that the other 17 mothers were fully competent in deciding against medical intervention for their own welfare or that of their fetuses.[15] One presumption behind the doubts expressed by this physician seems to be that refusals of treatment should automatically trigger a psychiatric evaluation of the patient. A second presumption is that with more careful scrutiny, psychiatrists might well have found more of these women—perhaps all 17—less than 'fully competent' to decide.

The article to which the letter-writer referred reported on a national survey of the scope and circumstances of court-ordered obstetrical procedures. The survey found that court orders were obtained for C-sections in 11 States, for hospital detentions in 2 States, and for intrauterine transfusions in 1 State. Among 21 cases in which court orders were sought, the orders were obtained in 86 per cent. Of the women 81 per cent were black, Asian, or Hispanic, and 44 per cent were unmarried. Of the heads of fellowship programs in maternal–fetal medicine 46 per cent thought that women who refused medical advice should be detained, and 47 per cent supported court orders for procedures such as intrauterine transfusions.

The authors of this article argue that these procedures are based on dubious legal grounds, and that they may have far-reaching implications for obstetrical practice and maternal and infant health. Several objections can be raised about the legal procedures, as noted by George Annas, a leading authority on health law, who wrote an editorial in the same issue of the *New England Journal*. Commenting on the survey, Annas said:

In the vast majority of cases, judges were called on an emergency basis and ordered interventions within hours . . . The judge usually went to the hospital . . . When a judge arrives at the hospital in response to an emergency call, he or she is acting much more like a lay person than a jurist. Without time to analyze the issues, without representation for the pregnant woman, without briefing or thoughtful reflection on the situation, in almost total ignorance of the relevant law, and in an unfamiliar setting faced by a relatively calm physician and a woman who can easily be labelled 'hysterical', the judge will almost always order whatever the doctor advises.[16]

Along with other legal and ethical scholars who have studied this practice, Annas observed that 'Before birth, we can obtain access to the fetus only through its mother, and in the absence of her informed consent, can do so only by treating her as a fetal container, a nonperson without rights to bodily integrity ... Many women will quite reasonably avoid physicians altogether during pregnancy if failure to follow medical advice can result in forced treatment, involuntary confinement, or criminal charges.[17]

The results of the national survey stand in sharp contrast to a statement issued only five months later by the Committee on Ethics of the American College of Obstetricians and Gynecologists (ACOG). That statement said, in effect, that it is ethically unacceptable to coerce pregnant women and force them to undergo cesarean sections or other recommended procedures. The concluding paragraph of the committee statement reads as follows:

Obstetricians should refrain from performing procedures that are unwanted by a pregnant woman. The use of judicial authority to implement treatment regimens in order to protect the fetus violates the pregnant woman's autonomy. Furthermore, inappropriate reliance on judicial authority may lead to undesirable societal consequences, such as the criminalization of noncompliance with medical recommendations.[18]

Cesarean sections are not the only recommended medical procedure for which judicial intervention has been sought. A pregnant woman may be forced to take medication, such as penicillin, for the sake of fetal health. In a case that occurred in 1982, a court ordered a pregnant diabetic woman to receive insulin treatment despite her refusal on religious grounds.[19] Going back many years, Jehovah's Witnesses have been compelled to receive unwanted blood transfusions, including transfusions performed well before the onset of fetal viability. In a case that occurred in Jamaica Hospital in New York in 1985, a court ordered a Jehovah's Witness to be transfused when the fetus was only 18 weeks in gestation.[20]

It is inevitable that even when respect for pregnant women's autonomy is generally acknowledged, reasonable people will still disagree about particular cases. As Wayne Cohen observes in his discussion of pregnant Jehovah's Witnesses who refuse blood transfusions: 'One's view of this conundrum depends on how one views the fetal–maternal relationship and the role of others in fostering it ethically.' In an article I co-authored with a neonatologist colleague, we agreed on the resolution of maternal–fetal conflicts in a wide range of situations. But our article contained the following admission of our inability to arrive at complete agreement:

When it comes to established, efficacious treatments that pose low risk to the woman and great benefit to the fetus, such as blood transfusions given to the woman which are necessary to preserve the life or health of the fetus, we find ourselves in disagreement. One of us (A. R. F.) holds that it is acceptable for physicians to bring pressure to bear on the woman to accept the procedure, including the coercive step of seeking court adjudication. However, coercive measures should stop short of physically restraining or forcibly sedating a woman who continues to refuse treatment despite a court order that grants physicians permission to override her refusal. The other of us (R. M.) would allow persuasive efforts, emotional appeals, and other noncoercive means to convince a woman to accept a low-risk medical procedure for the sake of her fetus, but holds it unacceptable to invoke the force of law to override her refusal.[21]

Another unresolvable situation involving pregnant Jehovah's Witnesses began with an attempt by an ethics committee to devise a general policy for the hospital regarding treatment of Jehovah's Witnesses. The committee came to unanimous agreement about the treatment of adult nonpregnant patients with decisional capacity, adult patients lacking decisional capacity, and children of Jehovah's Witnesses. However, when it came to adult, pregnant Jehovah's Witnesses (at any stage of pregnancy) who refused blood transfusions, the committee was deadlocked and could formulate no usable policy statement.[22] This was the only time in its ten years' existence in which that committee was unable to reach a consensus on a matter of policy or on a recommendation in an individual case.

INSTITUTIONAL CREATION OF CONFLICT

Another category of maternal–fetal conflict must be noted, a category that falls outside the definition proposed by Wayne Cohen in his section of this chapter. That definition specified 'any situation in which the intent or actions of the pregnant woman do not coincide with the needs, interests, or rights of her fetus as perceived by the obstetric caregivers.' The category of exceptions to be noted here is that in which a health-care institution seeks legal coercion of a pregnant woman *even when* physicians are prepared to go along with the patient's request. Although information about the types or number of such situations is unavailable, one widely publicized case is worth reviewing by way of illustration.

The case occurred at George Washington University Hospital in Washington, DC in 1987. The patient was Angela Carder, a twenty-seven-year-old married woman who had recently been diagnosed as having a recurrence of cancer from which she had suffered intermittently since she was thirteen.[23] She had intentionally become pregnant in her desire to start a family, and had completed about 26 weeks. At the time these events occurred, Ms Carder's health was rapidly deteriorating. X-rays revealed an inoperable tumor in her lung. When she entered the hospital, she was asked if she really wanted to have the baby, and she replied that she did. She agreed to treatments intended to extend her life until at least her twenty-eighth week of pregnancy, at which time the potential outcome for the fetus would be greatly enhanced. As her condition worsened, her physicians estimated that she was unlikely to live for more than 24 hours. When asked again if she still wanted to have the baby, Ms Carder was somewhat equivocal in her reply. The fetus was then in 'a chronically asphyxiated state', which increased the chance that the fetus would die, or if it lived, would suffer permanent handicaps.

It was at this point that the hospital decided to go to court for a ruling on what was legally required. The trial court in the District of Columbia appointed a counsel for the fetus, and the District of Columbia was permitted to intervene on behalf of the fetus in the state's role as *parens patriae*—a role designed to protect vulnerable individuals unable to speak for themselves. On 16 June, 1987 a hearing was hastily convened in the hospital, with different attorneys representing the hospital, the fetus, and the District of Columbia; a lawyer for Angela Carder, the patient; several physicians from the hospital; Angela's mother, who testified; and her husband, who was too distraught to testify. No family member stepped forward to consent to a cesarean section. Her husband stood by her, her parents urged that a cesarean should not be done, and Angela's own physician was willing to abide by her apparent wishes, elicited while the hearing was still going on, not to have the surgery. During the course of the hearing, one of Angela Carder's physicians observed that the doctors did not want to perform a cesarean section on this patient.

The physicians caring for Angela Carder testified at the hearing that a cesarean section should not be performed because they did not believe that either Ms Carder or her family wanted it to be performed. However, the judge concluded that the patient had not clearly expressed her views in the matter, and that because she was now unconscious, she was unable to express her views. So the judge ordered the surgery to be performed.

In an affront to Angela's human dignity, the argument was offered that this patient was dying anyway, so it did not matter much if her life would be shortened in an attempt to salvage her fetus. The court-appointed attorney for the fetus began her argument by stating that 'we are confronted . . . with a need to balance the interest of a probably viable fetus, a presumptively viable fetus, age 26 weeks, with whatever life is left for the fetus's mother . . .' The attorney questioned 'what we will be depriving her [Angela] of realistically if we were to take measures to protect the life of the fetus at this point'.

The surgery was performed, and a baby girl was delivered. The infant died within two and one-half hours, and Angela Carder died two days later. In subsequent proceedings, the original court order was vacated, meaning that it would not stand as a judicial precedent, although of course the circumstances could not be reversed. The District of Columbia Court of Appeals stated:

If the patient is incompetent or otherwise unable to give an informed consent to a proposed course of medical treatment, then her decision must be ascertained through the procedure known as substituted judgement. Because the trial court did not follow that procedure, we vacate its order . . .[24]

This conclusion of procedural justice was buttressed by a further observation made by the court of Appeals. The court asserted 'that it would be far better if judges were not called to patients' bedsides and required to made quick decisions on issues of life and death'.[25]

The court of Appeals rejected the notion that the interests of the fetus must be balanced against the right of a pregnant woman to refuse an invasive procedure. The appeals court also dismissed the argument that under the substituted judgment procedure, Angela Carder would have consented to the cesarean section. The Court of Appeals declined, in addition, to accept the contrary arguments that Angela was competent and made an informed choice not to have the cesarean performed, or that, even if the substituted judgment procedure had been followed, the evidence would necessarily show that Angela would not have wanted the cesarean section. The appeals court opined: 'We do not accept any of these arguments because the evidence, realistically viewed, does not support them.'[26]

In addition to the challenge that led to the District of Columbia Court of Appeals vacating the court order that had required Angela to undergo a cesarean section, the American Civil Liberties Union filed a separate malpractice and civil rights case against the George Washington University Medical Center for its treatment of Angela Carder and for its decision to involve the court. As a result of the settlement, the GWU Medical Center developed a policy that now serves as a model for other hospitals to emulate.

The policy adopted by George Washington University Hospital places patient autonomy in the forefront. The policy states: 'We base our policies regarding decision making on this hospital's (and the medical profession's) strong commitment to respecting the autonomy of all patients with capacity.'[27] The policy adds that respect for autonomy does not end just because a patient refuses a course of action that physicians recommend. Moreover, the same ethical, legal, and medical standards that apply to non-pregnant patients also apply to the decision-making process with a pregnant patient.[28] The policy emphasizes the importance of counseling pregnant women and also urges that when a pregnant patient's decision 'appears unnecessarily to disserve her own or fetal welfare, great care should be taken to verify that her decision is both informed and authentic'.[29] When such circumstances arise, the physician should seek to explore reasons that lie behind the patient's decision.

Nevertheless, if all counseling and explorations with the patient fail, the ultimate decision is left to the woman. The policy states: 'When a fully informed and competent pregnant patient persists in a decision which may disserve her own or fetal welfare, this hospital's policy is to accede to the pregnant patient's preference whenever possible.'[30] The policy also addresses the issue of pregnant patients who are not capable of consenting to or refusing treatment in an informed fashion. In such cases, the document recognizes the authority of a surrogate for the patient, building in appropriate safeguards to protect the welfare of the patient and the fetus. The policy states that 'the hospital will accede to a well-founded surrogate's decision whenever possible'.[31]

Finally, and importantly, this model policy asserts that courts are an inappropriate forum for resolving ethical issues.[32] It endorses a strong commitment to keeping health-care decision-making within the patient–physician relationship. The policy concludes with the statement that 'it will rarely be appropriate to seek judicial intervention to assess or override a pregnant patient's decision'.[33]

The role of the lawyer appointed for the fetus in the Angela Carder case illustrates the perils of seeking to involve an advocate for the fetus. Wayne Cohen speculates that there may be some virtues in this approach, but also expresses the concern that a fetal advocate might make a decision in conflict with the mother's desires, with the result that physicians would end up forcing a patient to undergo a procedure against her will. If the Carder case is any indication, the overwhelming likelihood is that fetal advocates will in all cases argue vigorously for the right to life or health of the fetus.

PREGNANT WOMEN WHO USE DRUGS AND ALCOHOL

A strong movement has been joined by some physicians, prosecutors, legislators and others to coerce, detain, or incarcerate women who use drugs or abuse alcohol during pregnancy. Two different approaches attempting to use the force of law are 'pre-birth seizures' and 'post-birth sanctions'. The first seeks to control the behavior of drug-users during pregnancy, while the second seeks criminal penalties for women whose babies are born with damage alleged to have been caused by their drug-taking during pregnancy.

An advocate of the first approach is Dr Jan Bays, Director of Child Abuse Programs at Emanuel Hospital in Portland, Oregon. In an interview published in the *New York Times*,[34] Dr Bays was quoted as saying:

We must up the ante to criminalize or impose reproductive controls on people who are out of control. Addiction is the most powerful force I have ever encountered. You have to use all the guns you have ... The nice thing about jail is that moms get good prenatal care, good nutrition and they're clean ... But we can't force people into treatment, even if they're in jail. She can go out and have more children. So, people are talking about sterilization and that gets into reproductive rights.

A sobering reply was offered by another physician, Dr Ira J. Chasnoff, an expert on the effects of maternal drug-ingestion on the developing fetus and subsequently born infants, who is president of the National Association for Perinatal Addiction Research and Education. The *Times* quoted Dr Chasnoff as having said:

This is a short-term, knee-jerk solution. The temperance movement is creating such a level of frustration that people are beginning to lash out at the group with the least defenses—women, especially the minority poor ...

Criminalization of drug use by pregnant women won't accomplish anything in the long run. To develop punitive programs before we know the long-term effects of a mother's drug use on her children is ludicrous . . .

Furthermore, fear is not an effective deterrent because drug-using individuals are not reality-based and have strong denial mechanisms. They tell themselves they will never be caught.

These are the conflicting views of two medical experts on what approach to this problem is likely to be effective, as well as ethically acceptable. In addition, one might question Dr Bay's contention that in jail, 'moms get good prenatal care, good nutrition and [the jails] are clean'. In general, prisons provide little prenatal or gynecological care. In one episode in California, a woman in prison 'suffered severe abdominal cramping and bleeding for seventeen days without being allowed to receive treatment from an obstetrician; her son was born in an ambulance while she was being transported to an outside hospital, and lived only 2 hours.'[35] In another California women's prison, a woman who was six months pregnant 'suffered a miscarriage after she had been hemorrhaging and suffering abdominal pain for over three months. In spite of her critical condition she was only allowed to see an obstetrician/gynecologist on two occasions; as a result of the emergency nature of the miscarriage, she was also given a hysterectomy and is thus unable to have any more children.'[36] These are only two such episodes, but they suggest that imprisoning women for the duration of their pregnancy is contraindicated from a medical and health standpoint, as well as raising serious questions about the ethical permissibility of the practice.

Although law and ethics are not identical, they overlap. Laws are often made (or repealed) for ethical reasons. Sometimes moral obligations are transformed into legal obligations. An ethical analysis of this growing trend of attempting to impose legally mandated detention on drug-using pregnant women begins by looking at some of the negative consequences.

First, there are consequences that flow from the very act of incarcerating pregnant women. The negative consequences for the health of the woman and the future child could be serious, as is evidenced by the poor health care provided to pregnant women in corrections facilities. Among additional negative consequences rarely mentioned is the effect on the other young children of women forcibly hospitalized or jailed during their pregnancy.

Second is the consequence of eroding the relationship of trust between physicians and their women patients. When physicians are transformed from advocates and allies of their patients into agents of the State—reporting them to government officials—the prospect of a good physician–patient relationship is greatly diminished. This argument was made in the case of Angela Carder in an *amicus curiae* brief submitted by the American Public Health Association (APHA). The brief stated:

Rather than protecting the health of women and children, court-ordered caesareans erode the element of trust that permits a pregnant woman to communicate to her physician—without fear of reprisal—all information relevant to her proper diagnosis and treatment.[37]

A third likely result is driving poor and disadvantaged women (those statistically more likely to be identified and reported as drug-users) away from prenatal care, thus leading to even worse outcomes of pregnancy. This consequence was also mentioned in the *amicus* brief submitted by the APHA in the Carder case: 'An even more serious consequence of court-ordered intervention is that it drives women at high risk of complications during pregnancy and childbirth out of the health care system to avoid coerced treatment.'[38]

Yet this predicted consequence has been challenged by a public Solicitor in Charleston, South Carolina. Charles Condon, the Solicitor, used child-neglect charges against drug-using pregnant women in arrests beginning in 1989. By early February 1990, Mr Condon said that arrests had almost stopped because the hospital was seeing fewer cocaine babies once drug-using women perceived they faced the risk of jail. And, Mr Condon said, 'there is no sign that addicted women are avoiding prenatal care or having their babies out in the woods to avoid arrest'.[39] The prediction that drug-using women will be driven away from prenatal care is, like any other prediction, one that stands to be confirmed or denied by actual, empirical evidence. Although the evidence cited from South Carolina is based on very few cases, it cannot be altogether discounted. Neither can it be used as a sound indication of what is likely to happen elsewhere.

The arguments against legal coercion of drug-using pregnant women illustrate the divide between making moral judgments and imposing legal sanctions. To argue against incarceration or forced detention of pregnant women is not to condone their behaviour. Rather, it is to demarcate a line beyond which a moral obligation to the future child should not be transformed into a legal obligation.

There are at least two propositions to which all can assent. The first is that it is better for babies to be born healthy than unhealthy. Put another way, it is desirable for infants to be free from preventable diseases and developmental disabilities. This proposition is not meant to have any implications for those infants or children who are born with birth anomalies or diseases. It is perfectly consistent to hold that it is a better state of affairs for infants to be born healthy and sound than otherwise, and at the same time to maintain that infants born with disabilities deserve the same treatment and respect as healthy and able-bodied individuals.

The second proposition may appear somewhat less morally certain than the first, but I think it could also gain universal agreement. The second proposition is:

Once a decision is made to carry a pregnancy to term, pregnant women have a *moral* obligation to act in ways likely to result in the birth of a sound, healthy infant.

This second proposition is a corollary to the first. If it is better for infants to be born healthy than unhealthy, and if behaviour on the part of pregnant women can help to ensure that desirable outcome, then there is a moral obligation to act in ways most likely to bring about the desirable outcome. Nevertheless, the pregnant woman's moral obligation should *not* be transformed into a legal obligation, for the following reasons.

Firstly, like other moral obligations, the duty of pregnant women is contingent on a reasonable ability to comply. This stems from the philosophical precept *'ought* implies *can'*—before people can be assigned moral obligations to act or refrain from acting in certain ways, it must be physically and psychologically possible for them to act in those ways. What constitutes a 'reasonable ability to comply' with a moral obligation is often uncertain and open to dispute. In the case of addicted pregnant women, a number of different constraints might limit their ability to comply with the obligation to act in ways that promote the health of their future child.   If the woman is a heroin addict, she may not have access to a treatment program. If she is an alcoholic, she may have tried—and failed—to combat her alcoholism. If she is a crack addict, her addiction might overpower her wish to do what is best for her future infant. Furthermore, at present 'most alcohol and drug treatment programs exclude pregnant women. And poor women have an especially hard time finding help. One survey of treatment programs in New York City found that 87 per cent would not accept pregnant crack addicts on Medicaid.'[40]

In the more commonplace obstetrical situations, if a woman is a Jehovah's Witness, the strength of her religious belief may preclude her accepting a blood transfusion recommended for the well-being of the fetus. Another woman might refuse surgery out of religious convictions, an overwhelming fear of cutting, or having experienced a relative's death from an anesthesia accident. If she has been advised by her obstetrician late in pregnancy not to have sexual intercourse, a woman may be unable to resist her husband's insistence out of fear of violence on his part.

These or other circumstances can lead to legitimate questions about a pregnant woman's reasonable ability to carry out her obligation to promote the health of her future child. Applying the *'ought* implies *can'* maxim requires examining each individual circumstance to determine whether the obligation is one that the woman is capable of fulfilling.

In the absence of these sorts of extenuating circumstances, a pregnant woman's moral obligation is presumed to exist. A moral obligation to promote the health of the infant should *not*, however, be transformed into a legal obligation. Several different lines of arguments support this conclusion.

To begin with, not everything that is immoral should also be made illegal. Many actions are morally wrong, yet are not made subject to the force of law. To do so would convert our world into a completely legalistic one. Moreover, the intrusions into personal life that would be necessary for identifying and prosecuting people's failure to discharge their obligations would effectively eliminate the rights to privacy and confidentiality that we so cherish.

A different argument contends that legal coercion of pregnant women is too strong a response to their behaviour. In the case of therapeutic interventions, competent adults have a moral and legal right to refuse medical interventions that place them at risk. In the case of forced detention during pregnancy, the standards for taking away people's liberty by incarcerating them should be based on actual, serious harms already committed or a high probability of serious future harm to another existing person. Finally, legal coercion promotes social injustice because of the greater numbers of poor and minority women likely to be suspected, reported, or indicted for the alleged 'crime' of fetal abuse.

What about punishing women who used drugs during pregnancy after their babies are born? The arguments so far have primarily addressed the ethical issues pertaining to forced treatment of pregnant women and removal of their liberty during pregnancy. The alternative, more prevalent recent response is to seek to impose post-birth sanctions on women whose drug or alcohol abuse during pregnancy, or whose failure to comply with medical recommendations has been the probable cause of birth anomalies. Some writers have sharply distinguished the two situations, agreeing that forced interventions to protect offspring are a dubious public policy, yet arguing that post-birth criminal or civil sanctions for maternal behaviour that seriously injures offspring are justified.[41]

It is clear that a different set of arguments opposing legal coercion from those just outlined would have to be used in cases where pregnant women's behaviour has been the likely cause, or a contributory cause, of actual harm to a now-existing child. Still, I think an argument against post-birth sanctions can be made. Three ethical considerations, taken together with facts already mentioned, prompt a rejection of post-birth legal action.

The first consideration recalls the 'ought implies can' maxim. Drug- or alcohol-addicted women simply may not have it in their power to refrain from using these substances while pregnant, even if they are made aware of the likely imposition of legal penalties. Those who are informed and willing to enter a drug or alcohol treatment program are likely to find that treatment is not open to them. A determination that pregnant women should be held culpable and subjected to post-birth sanctions involves a decision to create a whole new category of criminals, and a crime whose perpetrators can only be women.

The second consideration points to the nature of the behaviour. Although it is arguable whether the behaviour of addicts and alcoholics is fully voluntary, it cannot be denied that when people use these substances they do so knowingly. But a large number of pregnant drug and alcohol abusers may still be ignorant of the consequences of their substance abuse on their future child. Women who use drugs and alcohol or engage in other medically non-compliant behaviour during pregnancy do not normally do so with the *intention* of harming their future child. Nor are they *deliberately* seeking to inflict harm either on the fetus or the child who will be born. While in the throes of addiction, addicts are not models of ethical behaviour. A craving for the drug takes precedence over everything. Given the fact that addicts have been known to kill their lovers, mothers, or children for a fix, it is not surprising to find little regard for a *fetus in utero*.

The third consideration is the harm to infants likely to result from punishing their mothers. Separating children from their mothers is likely to cause psychological harm, since alternatives such as foster-care are less than optimal. Mothers whose infants have been removed from their care are often reunited with them much later, further disrupting the continuity of parenting for a child. In addition, many women in this situation have older children at home, and they, too, will suffer from the separation if their mothers are imprisoned.

Taken together, these three ethical considerations lead to the conclusion that it is a bad idea to impose post-birth sanctions on women whose use of drugs or alcohol was a probable contribution to harming their infants. And although slippery-slope arguments must always be used with caution, there is a danger of expanding the conditions under which post-birth sanctions could be imposed on women for their behaviour during pregnancy: some alcohol ingestion as opposed to a lot; cigarette-smoking; continuing to work in an environment with known occupational hazards, such as a hospital operating room or delivery room; and so on. A professor of health law who defends legal penalties asserts that 'the desirability of post-birth sanctions should depend on the gains to children relative to the harms that might arise from such a policy'.[42] As individuals and as a society, we are notoriously poor at predicting the benefits and harms that are likely to arise from public policies. I surmise that holding women criminally responsible for their behaviour during pregnancy is likely to cause more harm than good. Proponents of legal sanctions suppose the reverse. Is there any empirical evidence that would lend weight to either prediction?

CONCLUSION

Recall the premiss that pregnant women have a *moral* obligation to refrain from behaving in ways that risk the health of their future child. None of the arguments against legal coercion serves to undermine that initial premiss. However, pregnant women are not the only ones who are under obligation. Duties fall to others, as well.

Recent research has demonstrated that fathers also contribute to their future children's health. The March of Dimes is sponsoring a number of studies to obtain further data on damages to sperm and the role damaged sperm plays in birth defects.[43] Evidence indicates that a man's exposure to toxins damages sperm, and also that cocaine can bind directly on to sperm and may be transmitted into an ovum. Animal studies showed that the offspring of males exposed to lead before mating had learning difficulties. Additional studies have correlated certain occupations of males with an increased risk of their wives' having miscarriages and stillbirths, as well as with an increased incidence in their children of brain cancer, leukemia, and spina bifida.[44] These data contribute to the mounting evidence of the role men play in the health of their future offspring, compelling the conclusion that they, too, have an obligation to minimize exposure to substances that could adversely affect their future children.

Physicians have an obligation to educate and counsel their women patients who engage in behavior that risks the health of their future children. As physicians and healers, their obligation to their patients embraces the duty to strive to maintain a good physician–patient relationship, free from threats or coercion. Rather than act as policing agents of the state in seeking to detect and report drug-use by pregnant women or positive screens in babies, doctors should be advocates of improved public policies in this area and help to work toward changing existing bad laws and introducing enlightened public-health measures. Moreover, as scientific evidence points to the contribution of damaged sperm to birth anomalies, physicians need to inform and counsel their male patients about these reproductive hazards.

Governments at every level have an obligation to ensure access for all women to adequate prenatal care, as well as to treatment programs to combat drug and alcohol abuse. Governmental actions that could result in driving drug and alcohol-using women away from prenatal care will very probably have the opposite effect from that intended: the more women who lack adequate prenatal care, the more premature and low-birthweight infants and infants with disabilities are likely to be born.

One price of upholding individual liberty in a free society is the occurrence of some tragic birth defects or impaired children, and the prospect of the death of a few viable fetuses. Although some tragedies are preventable, it is ethically unacceptable to seek to maximize prevention through legal coercion of the sort being proposed and already carried out with pregnant women. To seek to prevent some tragic illnesses and fetal deaths by erecting a system that pits physician against patient, makes criminals out of women who risk the health of their future children, and requires that women be sedated and strapped down to undergo cesarean sections or blood transfusions is desperate and extreme. An ethical analysis of maternal–fetal conflicts yields the conclusion that if legal coercion of pregnant women is ethically permitted and legally endorsed, a balance of *bad* consequences over good—both for women and for society generally—is likely to be the result.

REFERENCES

1. See, for example, Sherwin, S. *No longer patient*. Temple University Press, Philadelphia (1992).
2. Hubbard, R. The fetus as patient (MS, October 1982), p. 32.
3. Meeker, W. K. Letter to editor. *New England Journal of Medicine*, **317**(1987), 1224.
4. Canty T. G. and Wolf, D. A. Maternal ultrasound in neonatal surgery. *Pediatric Annals* **11** (1982), 888.
5. Clewell, W. H. *et al.* A surgical approach to the treatment of fetal hydrocephalus. *New England Journal of Medicine* **306** (1982), 1320.
6. Harrison, M. R. *et al.* Management of the fetus with a correctable congenital defect. *Journal of the American Medical Association* **246** (1981), 776–7.

7. Hubbard, p. 32.
8. Fletcher, J. C. The fetus as patient: ethical issues. *Journal of the American Medical Association* **246** (1981), 772.
9. Ibid.
10. Ruddick, W. and Wilcox, W. Operating on the fetus. *Hastings Center Report* **12** (1982).
11. Ibid., 11.
12. Ibid.
13. Ibid., 12.
14. Kolder, V. E. B., Gallagher, J., and Parsons, M. T. Court-ordered obstetrical interventions. *New England Journal of Medicine* **316** (1987), 1192–6.
15. Copeman, M. C. Letter to editor. *New England Journal of Medicine* **317** (1987), 1223–4.
16. Annas, G. J. Protecting the liberty of pregnant patients. *New England Journal of Medicine*, **316** (1987), 1213.
17. Ibid., 1214.
18. ACOG Committee Opinion. Number 55, Patient choice: maternal–fetal conflict (October 1987).
19. Cited in Rhoden, N. K. Informed consent in obstetrics: some special problems. *Western New England Law Review* **9** (1987), 82.
20. In the Matter of the Application of JAMAICA HOSPITAL for permission to transfuse blood into the person of Santiago X, Supreme Court, Special Term, Queens County, Part II, April 22, 1985.
21. Fleischman, A. R. and Macklin, R. Fetal therapy: ethical considerations, potential conflicts. In Weil, W. B. Jr. and Benjamin, M. (eds), *Ethical issues at the outset of life*, Blackwell Scientific Publications, Boston, 1987. pp. 144–5.
22. For a full report of this episode, see Macklin, R. The inner workings of an ethics committee: latest battle over Jehovah's Witnesses. *Hastings Center Report* **18** (1988), 15–20.
23. *In re: A. C.*, 533 A. 2d 611 (D. C. 1987). The account that follows is taken from the trial court transcript in the case; from an appeals brief filed by the court-appointed attorney for the fetus; an *amicus curiae* brief of the American Medical Association, the American College of Obstetricians and Gynecologists, and the Medical Society of the District of Columbia; and from the Opinion for the Court in the Hearing *En Banc* of the District of Columbia Court of Appeals (argued 22 September 1988 and decided 26 April 1990).
24. *In re: A. C.*, Appellant, No. 87-609, on Hearing *En Banc*, 1108.
25. Ibid., n. 2.
26. Ibid., 1109.
27. Appendix A to Settlement Agreement, Policy on Decision-making by Pregnant Patients at The George Washington University Hospital, 1.
28. Ibid., 3.
29. Ibid., 5.
30. Ibid., 6.
31. Ibid., 7–8.
32. Ibid., 9.
33. Ibid., 11.

34. Punishing pregnant addicts: debate, dismay, no solution. *New York Times* (10 September 1989), E 5.
35. NOW Legal Defense and Education Fund. *Facts on reproductive rights: a resource manual*, Fact Sheet #13, 'Punishing women for conduct during pregnancy'; cites Barry, Quality of prenatal care for incarcerated women challenged. 6 *Youth Law News* 1 (1985).
36. Ibid.
37. *In re: A. C.*, Court of Appeals, 1131-32.
38. Ibid., 1132.
39. Lewin, T. Drug use in pregnancy: new issue for the courts. *New York Times*, (5 February 1990), A14.
40. Ibid.
41. See, for example, Robertson, J. A. Letter to the editor, *New England Journal of Medicine*, **317** (1987), 1223; and Robertson, J. A. Fetal abuse: should we recognize it as a crime?' *ABA Journal* (1989), 38–9.
42. Robertson. Fetal abuse: should we recognize it as a crime?
43. 'Paternal–fetal conflict'. *Hastings Center Report* **22** (1992), 3.
44. Ibid.

3

Medical futility: decision-making in the context of probability and uncertainty

---

3A MEDICAL FUTILITY

Nancy S. Jecker and Roberta A. Pagon

INTRODUCTION

As soon as the baby was delivered, a large, whole-thickness piece of skin sloughed from one leg, leaving a large denuded area in which muscles and tendons could be viewed.[1] Now six days old, the tiny girl has been diagnosed with epidermolysis bullosa, a recessive genetic condition which causes blistering of the skin. She is unable to take fluids by mouth because of blistering of her mucous membranes. Third-degree burn-like erosions over her skin cause fluid and electrolyte imbalance problems and unremitting pain. Her condition is a lifelong disorder, for which there is no cure and no treatment to ameliorate the blistering and its effects.

Patients with epidermolysis bullosa have recurrent painful sloughing of skin that typically results in auto-amputation of fingers, contractures of limbs, and a constant need for total care. These blistering episodes are extremely painful, because they involve the full thickness of the skin. There has never been a case of spontaneous cure or prolonged remission. This particular baby has a severe form of the disease; she screams constantly when awake. A morphine drip provides sedation, and the baby sleeps intermittently for periods of up to five minutes. Physicians and Ethics Committee members debate the merits of providing fluid and nutrition through artificial means such as intravenous lines and gastrostomy. The parents ask that no efforts to prolong their daughter's life be undertaken.

How should physicians treat the family's request to withhold life-prolonging measures? The answer to this question will depend in part upon how physicians define medical futility, and how they weigh the inhumanity of prolonging suffering. The answer also will be influenced by physicians' attitudes toward the individual patient and family, and by a social milieu that attaches a special meaning to the plight of an imperiled child. Our society tends to view infants and small children as innocents, and so to regard any harms that visit them as gross injustices. For many health professionals, a sick child epitomizes the problem of evil: there can be no possible explanation for cruelties that befall children. This forces the conclusion that the universe is absurd or meaningless unless these harms can be removed.

In this chapter we wrestle with the problems of futility and inhumanity in medical decision-making. We propose that these terms have clear medical and moral meanings, and that they can serve as useful guides in the care of hopelessly ill newborns. We argue that certain psychological and ethical responses to cruelty or injustice in the neonatal intensive care unit (ICU) are warranted and useful. Others only heighten the anguish and compound the difficulties of medical decisions. Finally, we explore the problem of invoking futility and inhumanity under conditions of future uncertainty. We offer reasons for resisting a propensity to 'give the patient the benefit of the doubt', by using all modalities at one's disposal.

THE NEW MEDICINE

At the turn of the century most babies were born at home and sick infants were generally cared for, and either survived or died, at home.[2] Following the Second World War, new medical technologies became available to care for low-birthweight and premature infants, and medical developments, such as antibiotics, dramatically improved their care. Although mortality rates for sick newborns fell precipitously, morbidity remained a significant factor for many severely impaired infants. Thus some began to question whether newly developed techniques did, on balance, more harm than good. Others wondered whether life-saving medical care was being used merely to prolong dying.

By the late 1970s and early 1980s the issue of non-treatment of catastrophically ill newborns began to receive national media attention. The so-called 'Baby Doe regulations' promulgated in 1984 brought to a high point the ethical and legal dilemmas of appropriate treatment for infants with birth defects. The early version[3] of these regulations was eventually struck down.[4] The current 'Baby Doe regulations',[5] based on a 1984 amendment to the Child Abuse Prevention and Treatment Act,[6] allow withholding and withdrawal of life-sustaining treatment on the basis of both futility and inhumanity. Specifically, they identify three exceptions to required life-sustaining medical treatment:(1) an infant is chronically and irreversibly comatose; (2) provision of treatment merely prolongs dying and is not effective in ameliorating or correcting all the infant's life-threatening conditions; or (3) provision of treatment is virtually futile in terms of the survival of the infant, and the treatment itself under such circumstances is inhumane.

Despite these exceptions to maximal use of life-sustaining treatment neonatologists often feel compelled to treat handicapped newborns against their best judgment.[7] In a recent survey of 1007 members of the Perinatal

Pediatrics Section of the American Academy of Pediatrics,[8] neonatologists were asked to respond to three hypothetical cases of severely handicapped infants. Up to 32 per cent of respondents stated that maximal life-prolonging treatment was not in the best interests of the infants described, but thought that the Baby Doe regulations required such treatment. Some said that they felt pressure to over-treat such infants because of the regulations, new technology, and the legal climate, or through a combination of these factors.

DEFINING FUTILITY AND INHUMANITY

Despite misinterpretations of federal regulations and uncertainty regarding health professionals' ethical role, there are clearly cases where aggressive interventions are bad medicine. Neither legal nor ethical principles require provision of life-sustaining medical treatment to all imperiled infants. Nor does the law[9] or ethics[10] require individual providers to act contrary to conscience. Yet conscience is not self-certifying, and claims of conscientiousness should lead us to test conscience's leaning in the light of moral standards. We explore two standards of special relevance to imperiled newborns.

First is the standard of medical futility. It connotes that medical treatment is wasteful; even our best efforts will be useless and ineffective.[11] Futile situations elicit feelings of hopelessness and pointlessness; health providers who persist with futile efforts may feel a loss of professional purpose because their activities are leading nowhere. The second standard of inhumanity elicits quite different responses. It suggests that medical interventions provided without benefit rob patients of their very humanity. Inhumanity implies that medical care aimlessly prolongs a patient's pain or suffering, making the use of medical technologies a torture or punishment. Inhumanity suggests a failure to empathize with the sufferings of patients.

Yet to what, more specifically, do futility and inhumanity refer? We propose, first, that medical care can be futile in two distinct senses. Following Schneiderman et al.[12] we distinguish between quantitative and qualitative medical futility. Quantitative medical futility refers to situations in which the *likelihood* of a medical benefit's resulting from an intervention is extremely small. For example, treatment should be regarded as futile where there is less than one chance in one hundred of success. Qualitative medical futility indicates that the *quality* of outcome associated with an intervention is extremely poor. For instance, treatment that merely preserves permanent unconsciousness or total dependence on intensive medical care is qualitatively futile.

Inhumane medical treatment also refers to two quite different situations. First, medical treatment is inhumane where it aimlessly prolongs an already pain-wracked existence, or where it inflicts new pain or discomfort without benefitting the patient. For example, medical interventions are inhumane if they create intervals of nausea, retching, pain, or depression, or if they require invasion and injury of the body, without promising to help the patient.[13] A second sense of inhumanity denotes circumstances where life-prolonging medical interventions are applied to patients who lack the capacities that make continued existence *humanly* meaningful. Although such an existence is not painful, it can be undignified by virtue of falling sadly short of what human life ordinarily includes. Treatment that is inhumane in this second way may serve to continue the life of a patient who lacks 'indicators of humanhood'.[14,15] These include such qualities as consciousness, intelligent communication of thoughts and feelings, motor activity, and capacities of cognition and recognition. When such attributes are absent, and when an individual shows no evidence of enjoying life, treatment is inhumane. For instance, it is inhumane to prolong the life of a conscious stroke victim with the locked-in syndrome who has no control of motor activity and, hence, no means of controlling his or her environment or communicating voluntarily.[12]

Ordinarily, health providers anticipate that interventions will yield some benefit for the patient; hence determinations of medical inhumanity involve a carefully weighing of the burden of treatment against its estimated benefits. Where the chance of realizing a benefit for the patient is poor, the burden of treatment should be mild or abbreviated. An example is Trisomy 18, in which the odds of survival are very poor and humane medical care is confined to warmth, oral fluids, and sedation. As the chance of benefits to the patient increase, the burden of treatment can increase within limits, although it should not be prolonged indefinitely. For instance, in cases of severe trauma the chances of recovery are high, and full intervention is applied, despite the fact that it may be quite painful and dehumanizing initially.

Both kinds of inhumane treatment bear a resemblance to qualitative futility. Like inhumanity, qualitative futility refers to interventions where the quality of outcome associated with an intervention includes unrelenting pain or the absence of basic human capacities. However, qualitatively futile care differs from inhumane care because futility refers only to the extreme low end of a quality-of-life continuum. For example, unnecessary abdominal surgery may be inhumane, without being qualitatively futile. Similarly, ineffective chemotherapy that produces skin rashes, hair loss, and vomiting may be inhumane, but it does not indicate a quality of outcome that is below a minimally acceptable threshold. In other words, although a person experiences pain or discomfort, the existence associated with such interventions is well worth having.

Inhumane treatment also bears a likeness to quantitative futility. For an intervention to be inhumane, it must have little or no chance of benefiting the patient. By contrast, an invasive or burdensome medical treatment that promises to benefit the patient and improve the patient's condition is not inhumane. For this reason, it is not inhumane to invade and injure the body through surgery, or to prescribe medicines with untoward side-effects, when these hold out a reasonable promise of helping the patient. Nor is it inhumane to ventilate mechanically a comatose patient who has a reasonable prospect of recovery of consciousness. However, such actions would be inhumane if they are clearly not beneficial. A second noteworthy point is that treatment may be quantitatively futile without being inhumane. For example, it is futile in the quantitative sense to prescribe antibiotics for a cold, but it is not inhumane. Likewise, putting a cast around a bone that is injured but not broken is ineffective; however, it does not inflict suffering or indignity on the patient.

These definitions shed light on the case of the newborn diagnosed with epidermolysis bullosa who was described at the beginning of this chapter. First, there is every reason to think that a gastrostomy to provide food and nutrition will succeed in giving the tiny patient nutrients and hydration. However, gastrostomy may be futile in a different sense: the quality of outcome associated with it may fall well below a threshold considered minimal. Although the patient is neurologically intact, other features, such as the presence of severe unremitting pain and the impossibility of her ever leaving the hospital, support a judgment of qualitative futility. In addition, the prognosis for patients in her condition is early mortality, due to sepsis and inanition secondary to fluid and calorie loss across denuded surfaces. Thus, the gastrostomy procedure may only briefly prolong a tortuous existence.

How does the standard of inhumanity apply in this case? The fact that the infant is awake and neurologically intact creates the possibility that medical treatment is inhumane in the first sense described above: treatment merely prolongs a condition of conscious and irremediable pain. The extreme pain experienced from recurrent sloughing of the skin surely qualifies. Although a morphine drip sedates the patient briefly, she is not sleeping for any period of time and screams continuously when awake. What about the other sense of inhumanity? The infant in this case is not devoid of human qualities, such as consciousness or the ability to communicate with others. Nor will her condition prevent her from developing capacities such as self-awareness and the ability to use language. Therefore, medical care for this patient is not inhumane in the sense of continuing a life that lacks human qualities.

DECISION-MAKING UNDER UNCERTAINTY

Judgments of futility and inhumanity may be difficult to make in the perinatal setting, owing to diagnostic and prognostic uncertainty. In part, the problem of uncertainty admits of resolution through increased research on the outcomes of medical procedures for different populations of patients.[16] However, improved data will only reduce, not eliminate, the need to make medical decisions under uncertainty. There may be few reliable data about the efficacy of the newest forms of intensive care. Uncertainty is often compounded because very sick children suffer from multiple medical problems. In addition, there always exists uncertainty about the response of a particular patient to treatment because of individual biological variability, and because of variability in the expertise of care-providers. Thus, the actual outcome of a proposed treatment for a particular patient will always depend upon 'circumstances of persons, places, times and cultures'.[17]

Acknowledging medical uncertainty leads some to argue that physicians should 'give the patient the benefit of the doubt' and err on the side of treatment. Others, doubting the wisdom of this approach, worry that aggressive medical interventions may only perpetuate a meaningless or painful existence. What are the values implicit in these alternative strategies? What additional options exist?

To address these questions, it is useful to place the general problem of making medical decisions under conditions of uncertainty in broader perspective. One response to medical uncertainty calls for listing the various treatment alternatives and ranking each according to its worst possible outcome. According to this approach, the treatment one selects should be the one whose worst outcome is *superior* to the worst outcome of the other alternatives. The ethical basis for this approach is that physicians have a special ethical duty to avoid harming patients. Where some harms are unavoidable, this duty requires minimizing harm by choosing the outcome that is least bad.

Applying this general approach yields three more specific strategies.[18] Each reflects a different position about how 'worst possible outcome' should be defined. One strategy requires collecting statistical data that enables an across-the-board determination that certain categories of infants are unlikely to benefit from treatment; treatment is then not initiated on infants fitting that profile. This approach judges the worst possible outcome as saving an infant who will be severely impaired, and seeks to avoid this by identifying such infants in advance and excluding them from treatment. The trade-off this approach accepts is that some babies will die who could have thrived, although doctors and parents will never know which individual babies they were. One limitation of this approach is that statistical information about the outcomes of treatment for different patient-groups may be unavailable.

A second option involves beginning treatment for every infant that is potentially viable, and continuing active care until it becomes clearer that a particular infant will either die or lead a life of an unacceptable quality. In contrast to the first strategy, this second strategy assumes that the worse outcome consists of not making an effort to save an infant who would have survived and enjoyed a reasonable quality of life.

A final strategy also requires beginning treatment for every infant, but allows parents the option of terminating care before it becomes certain that a particular infant will either die or be devastatingly disabled. This approach takes an intermediate route and avoids identifying either saving a meaningless existence or failing to save a meaningful existence as the worst outcome. Instead, it solicits the input of family members in coming to terms with the 'gray area' of medical uncertainty. Parents are asked to provide information about which outcome *they* regard as the worst possible.

Is it worse to fail to rescue a viable infant whose life would be worth having, or is it worse to rescue a child who will go on to lead a painful and unwelcome existence? The advantage of the third option, which calls for individualized decision-making, is that it allows parents to participate in this determination. Although no one is entitled to insist on treatment that is clearly futile or inhumane, in situations of uncertainty about the outcome of medical interventions, parents should be intimately involved in the decision-making process.

FOUR CASE STUDIES

Having discussed the meanings of futility and inhumanity and reviewed the values implicit in rendering medical choices under uncertainty, we now discuss various ways in which these ideas emerge in actual cases presented to an Ethics Committee on which we both serve.

Case one

Michael was born at thirty-one weeks' gestation to his twenty-eight-year-old married mother. The pregnancy had been unplanned. At approximately twenty weeks' gestation an ultrasound examination revealed massive abdominal ascites, compression of the thorax, and polyhydramnios. It was felt at this time that the fetus was non-viable. Pregnancy termination was declined by the family, but stillbirth was anticipated. At thirty-one weeks' gestation, the mother went into spontaneous labor and an emergency cesarean section was performed. Michael was delivered in another city and remained there for nine days before being transferred to our institution. At birth he was severely compromised, requiring intubation, and cardiopulmonary resuscitation with intracardiac injections of epinephrine. Respiration was not established until 1000 cc of fluid had been removed from his abdomen. It was unclear how much asphyxia had occurred.

Michael was diagnosed to have the *prune belly syndrome*, a condition in which there is massive distention of the abdomen secondary to bladder-outlet obstruction. It appeared that Michael had posterior urethral valves which had blocked urine outflow from the bladder *in utero* until a time that they had 'ruptured', presumably secondary to increased bladder pressure. Because his bladder was dilated and flaccid, a suprapubic cystostomy tube was placed shortly after birth in order to drain his bladder. Renal function was abnormal initially, but subsequently improved. At six weeks of age he underwent fulguration of the posterior urethral valves following an episode of urinary retention. Because of abnormal-appearing ('echogenic') kidneys, the urologists were unable to give a clear long-term prognosis for renal function. One urologist anticipated that renal failure would occur at some point, perhaps late in adolescence, requiring either transplantation or dialysis; however, another urologist was more optimistic about the long-term outlook.

Michael had respiratory failure requiring intubation immediately after delivery. He remained on a ventilator throughout his entire hospitalization.

He appeared to have little primary lung disease, because he was ventilated with low-pressure settings and low levels of inspired oxygen; however, he had a small chest and no abdominal musculature, and it appeared that he lacked adequate diaphragmatic muscles to support independent respiration. At three months of age an attempt at extubation failed after several hours. Subsequently, a thoracic splint was placed in order to try to improve his chest-wall mechanics, and another brief trial of extubation was attempted two weeks later, which also failed within hours. The attending neonatologist and the attending pediatric pulmonologist felt that Michael had virtually no hope of being able to breathe independently and that he would require long-term mechanical ventilation via a tracheostomy. Because Michael was unable to gag or cough secondary to central nervous system dysfunction, the neonatologist and pulmonologist felt that the high risk for aspiration and recurrent pneumonia made him an unsuitable candidate for long-term ventilation.

Michael had evidence of prenatal neurologic compromise in that he had polyhydramnios, which is often an indication of inadequate sucking and swallowing *in utero* and, at the same time, had fixed joints (arthrogryposis), which can be caused by inadequate limb movement secondary to central nervous system dysfunction. In addition, he had a markedly abnormal neurologic examination, with no gag, no cough, severe hearing loss, and no visual tracking. He had no interaction with his environment, except to respond to pain. He had one seizure, and was treated with phenobarbital, which was in the therapeutic range and was not felt to contribute to his neurologic depression. Two cranial ultrasound examinations were normal. The attending neonatologist and a pediatric consultant from the Birth Defects and Neurodevelopmental Service were uncertain whether Michael's abnormal central nervous system examination was attributable to prenatal causes or perinatal asphyxia or both. Both doctors agreed, however, that he had severe neurologic impairment and that over time he had shown no neurologic recovery.

Michael's parents had difficulty adjusting to the various prognoses which had been offered. Because the family had been led to believe that Michael would be stillborn and that urologic surgery would be futile, they had wished no urologic intervention at the time of his admission. The hospital staff described the parents as angry and frustrated about the uncertainty of their son's prognosis. The parents had a strong extended social support network, including family and church members. They had little contact with the social work service, and had declined an offer of more extensive contact.

Because Michael was a poor tracheostomy candidate, the physicians and family decided unanimously to refrain from performing the tracheostomy and to discontinue ventilatory support when Michael was three and a half months old. Michael died shortly after life-support was withdrawn. Subsequently, an anonymous caller asked that the decision to withdraw life-support be reviewed by the Ethics Committee. The caller voiced two concerns about the decision to discontinue ventilatory support. First, Michael was medically stable at the time the ventilator was withdrawn. This suggested to the caller that the ventilator was not a futile intervention. Second, the caller expressed the related concern that it appeared inconsistent and arbitrary for the medical team to switch from aggressively treating Michael one day to withdrawing all treatment the following day. The underlying issue here appeared to be that some decline in the patient's medical situation should ordinarily occur prior to a judgment of futility. Otherwise, a futility judgment simply reflects a change in the physician's psychological attitude toward the patient, rather than a change in the patient's physical condition.

Case discussion

In this situation there was doubt that a tracheostomy would achieve the goal of facilitating mechanical ventilation and removing secretions. It does not follow, however, that treatment would be quantitatively futile. Quantitative futility requires that the odds of success are not only doubtful, but extremely poor. Certainly mechanical ventilation had been successful up to the time of the final decision. Let us suppose, for the purposes of discussion, that although there was a chance that the intervention would not succeed, there was also a reasonable chance that it would be effective. If we make these assumptions, can we conclude that tracheostomy and mechanical ventilation were not futile in the quantitative sense? Not before considering a further question: Would the physiological effects of treatment benefit Michael? Tracheostomy and artificial ventilation were quantitatively futile if they had an extremely slim chance of *benefiting* Michael in any way. Thus quantitative futility could not be ruled out even if it could be shown that these procedures would produce a favorable physiological *effect*.

The question of whether life-prolonging procedures would benefit Michael leads us to the related concerns of qualitative futility and medical inhumanity. In assessing these issues, two questions are central. First, was the quality of outcome associated with treatments, such as tracheostomy and ventilator support, inhumane in the sense of undignified? A second and related question is whether treatment is qualitatively futile i.e., whether the quality of outcome associated with treatment falls clearly below a minimally decent level. Let us consider these questions in turn. Did Michael possess qualities that enabled him to live a humanly meaningful existence? His severe neurologic impairment had so far shown no signs of improvement, and Michael had no interaction with his environment except to pain. Although there was disagreement about Michael's long-term prognosis, let us suppose that Michael's neurologic depression would neither improve nor worsen. In this case his permanent inability to communicate and to interact with the environment in any way suggests to us that medical care was inhumane. Mechanical ventilation and tracheostomy could achieve the effect of prolonging Michael's life, but would not enable Michael to lead a dignified and interactive life.

Turning next to qualitative futility, can we say that Michael's quality of existence is *so* poor that it is futile? Unlike the girl with epidermolysis bullosa that we described earlier, Michael was not in constant pain. However, he lacked capacities to recognize others or enjoy interacting with them or his environment. In light of these evaluations, we make the following assessments. First, the procedures in question were inhumane in another sense: they inflicted pain and discomfort without conferring a benefit on Michael. Second, even supposing that the tracheostomy and respirator could keep Michael's blood oxygenated, they had little or no chance of benefiting Michael. Thus, the procedure were futile in the sense of qualitative futility.

We conclude that the physicians' and parents' decision to withdraw ventilator support and for go a tracheostomy were ethically supported. The quality of outcome associated with these life-prolonging procedures did not benefit the patient.

Case resolution

The Ethics Committee's retrospective consideration of Michael's care re-affirmed the appropriateness of the medical team's prior treatment decisions. It also had a positive effect on addressing the anonymous caller's concerns about how medical decisions were made in this case. Although Michael was medically stable and his situation unchanged at the time the ventilator was withdrawn, what had changed was that the medical team had re-evaluated Michael's medical condition and the value of this treatment. They had arrived at a reasoned decision that continuing treatment was futile. Although treatment succeeded in physiologically stabilizing Michael, it did not benefit him in any broader sense.

Case two

Charlotte was an almost twelve-month-old girl with a chromosomal abnormality who had three major medical problems: a severe brain malformation involving absence of a significant portion of the brain, congenital heart disease with pulmonary hypertension, and Pierre Robin syndrome (a small jaw that impairs breathing). Charlotte developed progressive pulmonary disease that required almost constant hospitalization for the past two-and-a-half to three months. Intermittently she had required care in the pediatric ICU for ventilator support. The physicians caring for Charlotte concurred that further vigorous support of Charlotte was futile, because she had relentlessly progressive pulmonary disease and her growth was inadequate to allow her to 'outgrow' her lung disease. The parents, however, insisted that all efforts be made to support Charlotte, and were unwilling to accept options for limiting her care.

The attending physician provided the following history. Charlotte was admitted to the infant ICU shortly after birth for diagnosis and management of her birth defects. A chromosomal deletion was detected. The neonatologists caring for Charlotte discussed her poor prognosis with her parents and she was discharged home, presumably to die. When Charlotte had a respiratory arrest at home, her parents called 911; Charlotte was given emergency treatment and was admitted to the hospital. At that time, her parents denied any understanding of her grave prognosis and the decision to allow her to die.

An attending pediatrician from the Birth Defects Service became involved in Charlotte's care at that time. After much discussion, the parents made the decision to have a tracheostomy and gastrostomy performed to prolong her life and facilitate her management. Although the parents had been prepared for Charlotte's surgeries in the routine way, they appeared to be overwhelmed by the complexity of Charlotte's care. As a result, they did not return to the hospital for several weeks following Charlotte's surgeries.

Charlotte was eventually transferred to a nearby affiliated hospital, where the parents were trained for her home care after a contract between the parents and the hospital staff was agreed upon. The supervisor of the home-care program reported that Charlotte was discharged home with a full twenty-four hours of nursing care initially. When nursing care was reduced to twenty hours per day, there were gross deficiencies in Charlotte's care during the four hours that the parents provided care. Again, a contract between the parents and the home-care program was required in order to establish the parents' commitment to care, and it was reported that the mother eventually became quite good at Charlotte's care. Although Charlotte's father was fully trained, he never participated in his daughter's care.

Charlotte was stabilized at home with an average of sixteen hours per day of nursing care. Although she did not require ventilatory support, the supplemental oxygen that she received by tracheostomy was reaching the maximum level permissible in home care. At eight months of age recurrent respiratory infections prompted readmission to our hospital, where she remained almost exclusively over the next four months. While Charlotte was hospitalized, the attending physician, social worker, and home-health nurse supervisor met with the family to discuss the level of care appropriate for Charlotte. All physicians and nurses were in agreement that continued vigorous support in the pediatric ICU on a ventilator was futile in attempting to reverse her underlying problems and that it was appropriate to consider limiting her care. The possibility of weaning Charlotte from the ventilator, and not placing her back on it, even if her pulmonary function declined, was explored with the family. Previously, the family had found it difficult to participate in an entire care conference with the medical team, but on this occasion they remained for the whole meeting. At the end of the conference, they indicated that they were unable to make a decision, but would be back in touch with the social worker. They were offered the option of attending an Ethics Committee meeting, but indicated their discomfort at 'having another group of doctors make the decision for them'. When the family was contacted by the social worker five days later, the parents indicated that they still had been unable to arrive at a decision and reiterated that they would not attend an Ethics Committee meeting.

The attending physician requested that the Ethics Committee review the case in light of the medical staff's frustration in working with the family. At the time the review was requested, Charlotte was on a ventilator in the pediatric ICU. The attending physician summarized the problem. The family could not make a decision regarding Charlotte's care, and refused to allow others to help them in making a decision. A nurse felt that the parents were clinging to the supposed uncertainty of Charlotte's prognosis on the basis of the limited published experience with children with exactly the same chromosome abnormality. The attending physician pointed out that although Charlotte's chromosome abnormality was unique, her actual medical problems were commonplace. A social worker involved in the case stated that the family had felt 'vindicated' by the fact that Charlotte had not died when the doctors predicted she would. A second social worker pointed out that in the past the parents had been unwilling to assume responsibility ensuing from their decisions about Charlotte's care.

If the decision were made to continue with every effort to support Charlotte's life, she would no longer be a candidate for home care because of the high level of inspired oxygen required and because of the instability of her respiratory status, even on a ventilator. She was too medically fragile for foster-care placement. Respite care in a highly sophisticated medical setting might have been possible, although such resources for infants were extremely limited. Hence, the main option would be continuing her care in the hospital.

The Ethics Committee considered several options. The first option was to accede to the parents' prior request to continue full treatment. Under this 'hands off' option, the health-care team would not exert any pressure on the parents to reduce Charlotte's care. They would instead allow the parents to make up their own minds, in their own time and manner. A second option was confrontation with the parents. Confrontation would involve taking the family to court to establish their action as inhumane and abusive under the law. A third option was actively helping the parents to accept Charlotte's dying. This might involve discussing a 'no code' status with the family as a first step to allowing Charlotte to die. A second step might include discussing the possibility of not reinstituting ventilator support should Charlotte be weaned from the ventilator. Next, plans might be made to allow Charlotte to die in the hospital, rather than at home. Finally, the parents might be asked to abide by the terms of a contract of involvement with Charlotte during her hospitalization in order to aid in Charlotte's care and to have a meaningful basis for participation in treatment decisions. If the family refused to accept a contract or failed to follow through with its terms, this would provide a basis for future decision-making regarding Charlotte's case.

Case discussion

Continued aggressive support of Charlotte in the pediatric ICU was quantitatively and qualitatively futile because it did not provide a benefit to

Charlotte. However it might be thought that preserving Charlotte's life conferred a benefit on her parents. Although the medical team was in agreement that vigorous treatment of Charlotte was futile, should they be the ones to make a futility determination? Perhaps this decision should be left to Charlotte's parents. The first option considered by the Ethics Committee would be tantamount to letting the parents determine medical futility, because the parents would be granted sole authority to determine the course of care.

While it is sometimes ethically defensible to allow medical futility judgments to be made by a child's parents, there were several problems with this approach in Charlotte's case. First, Charlotte's parents were not capable of or willing to make a decision even when given the appropriate information in a clear, cogent, and understandable manner. Thus, continuing intensive medical treatment for Charlotte would not reflect the parents' wishes; it would reflect their non-decision. Non-decision is not unique. It may stem from the emotional nature of making a life-and-death decision for one's child, as well as the denial, shock, anxiety, depression, and fear such a decision provokes.[19]

A second reason why Charlotte's parents should not have been given responsibility for making treatment decisions is that their rights over Charlotte are not absolute. Although our moral[20,21] and legal[22] traditions give parents presumptive authority over the welfare of their children, this authority is qualified. Parental authority can be limited in order to protect a child's best interest.[23] This implies, on the one hand, that parents' wishes for aggressive treatment can be overridden if an infant's pain and discomfort would be frequent, long-lasting, and intense to the point of outweighing the positive experiences and pleasure.[24,25] On the other hand, any treatment that does not confer a benefit should not be continued. For example, treatment that merely sustains an unacceptably poor quality of life should be discontinued.[26] The notion of 'acceptable lives' is helpful here, and places the more abstract idea of 'best interest' in a biographical context.[27] Lives are defined by specific activities and relationships. For young children, these are primarily family activities and relationships. Charlotte would never reach adulthood, and her life as a child was confined to an intensive medical-care setting. It is doubtful that Charlotte's life would include the kinds of activities and relationships that make a child's life minimally worth living.

The third reason why the decision about Charlotte's care should not have been left exclusively to her parents is a consideration of the ethical limits of continued treatment of an individual for the benefit of others. It is sometimes morally permissible to continue treating fatally ill patients for the benefit of others if there is sufficient evidence that such treatment would be dignified by the nature of the relationship between the patient and the benefited third party.[28,29] However, it was far from clear that continuing Charlotte's medical treatment was compassionate toward her parents. Her parents had not stated that they wished present life-sustaining treatments to continue. Nor did their behavior give evidence that they were comforted by seeing Charlotte in the intensive care unit. Instead, they found relief in detachment and isolation from the hospital and from Charlotte.

The remaining options that the Ethics Committee considered were confrontation to establish that the parents' actions were 'inhumane and abusive' under the law, and helping the parents to accept Charlotte's death by reducing the level of her medical care gradually. While both options met the health-provider's responsibility to protect the patient's interests, only the latter showed compassion for the family's predicament. Although the pediatrician's *primary* responsibility is to the patient, the pediatrician also had responsibilities to the family unit.[30,31,32,33] However, meeting these responsibilities in Charlotte's case was rendered difficult because hostilities were present between the medical staff and the family. The medical team often felt they were held hostage by the family's apparently arbitrary demand that everything possible be done. In Charlotte's case, the goal became to facilitate, as much as possible, her family's transition to a new family structure in which she was absent.

Case resolution

The health-care team was intending to follow the third option and to bring about a positive outcome for the family. Soon after the Ethics Committee was convened, Charlotte's condition appeared to stabilize and she was sent home to be cared for by her parents. However, shortly after she went home she experienced an unexpected respiratory event and died. The suddenness of Charlotte's death made it more difficult for her parents to accept the loss of their daughter. The fact that Charlotte died at home, and under her parents' watch, also made it more emotionally trying for the family.

Charlotte's case illustrated to the Ethics Committee the need for a better policy for responding to situations in which parents are not able to make decisions about a child's medical care. In our experience, it is important for parents to involve themselves and take responsibility for medical decisions involving their offspring. When they are not able to do this, it often happens that full treatment is provided indefinitely. A better course, we believe, is to assign someone to act temporarily in place of the parents and on the patient's behalf. The difficulty with this approach, however, is that the law allows for appointing a guardian only if parents' medical choices constitute child-abuse or neglect. The legal system offers no remedy when parents are simply unable to decide. Thus there are few choices open to the medical team when parents are unable to reach decisions.

We recommend designing an institutional remedy for situations in which parents are unwilling to assume decisional authority. Ideally, an impartial review process should be available to identify parents who experience difficulty reaching decisions about a child's medical care. Individuals who participate in the review process should not be members of the medical team caring for the patient, but should instead facilitate communication between parents and medical staff and make hospital resources available to assist parents. Had a mechanism of this sort been in place for Charlotte's parents, they might have coped more effectively with the situation and have been able to exercise a decision about their daughter's medical treatment.

Case three

Samuel was born to a sixteen-year-old single mother who was a junior in high school at the time. The mother had insulin-dependent diabetes mellitus and had been hospitalized prenatally for management of the diabetes. Multiple congenital anomalies were noted at birth. The baby was transferred to our hospital for management. The mother and maternal grandparents lived in another State and could not accompany him. They were told by the transport team that he might have asphyxiating thoracic dystrophy, a lethal condition. The family requested that no extraordinary measures be taken in Samuel's care. His anomalies included tracheosoephageal (TE) fistula, multiple verte-bral and rib anomalies, absence of both thumbs, and absence of the left tibia with extra toes on the left foot. His heart, lungs, kidneys, brain, eyes, and ears were normal. The medical team felt at the time that he was a 'viable infant' and that his congenital anomalies were not life-threatening and should be managed in the usual way. The family was advised of this changed prognosis, and Samuel underwent repair of his TE fistula on day two with parental permission. Subsequently, Samuel became ventilator-dependent, but was unstable and required frequent resuscitations and ongoing intensive care. The family continued to be involved in Samuel's care from a distance. They visited the hospital when Samuel was three weeks old, at which time the mother expressed a desire for Samuel to be placed for adoption. Adoption proceedings were complicated by Samuel's racial background. Efforts were made to find a pre-adoptive foster-family in the vicinity of the hospital. It was anticipated that this family would have increasing involvement with Samuel should the medical plan include continued vigorous support. A physician with considerable experience with multiply disabled children assumed the role of continuity and parent-communication. The birth mother and her parents had kept in close contact with this physician by phone, and maintained their position that heroic measures should not be taken to support Samuel. The family frequently called the evening nursing staff and angrily criticized them for 'making Samuel suffer'.

The Ethics Committee met at the request of the social worker involved in Samuel's case with the agreement of his physicians. At the meeting, a social worker and some of the nurses caring for Samuel expressed the concern that Samuel was suffering. Samuel's recurrent need for sedation and/or paralysis was significantly interfering with his ability to interact. The question was raised as to whether it was appropriate to continue vigorous support. The specialists caring for Samuel felt that although many medical and surgical interventions to stabilize Samuel's upper airway had been tried, one viable option remained. At the time of the Ethics Committee meeting, a customized endotracheal tube was being fashioned in the hopes of stabilizing Samuel's airway to permit effective ventilation. Samuel had a large tracheal pouch at the site of his TE fistula repair that tended to be over-inflated so that the endotracheal tube compressed the trachea and prevented adequate air entry into the lungs. The hope was that the customized endotracheal tube would allow inspired gases to bypass the pouch, thus permitting adequate pulmonary ventilation. If this method was successful in stabilizing his airway, mechanical ventilation could be discontinued. He would require a tracheostomy indefinitely, and might require repeated hospitalizations. Substantial home-care services would also be needed. If Samuel's airway could not be stabilized, mechanical ventilation with frequent resuscitations would be the only way to keep him alive. The nursing staff expressed concern that Samuel was dying slowly, and that his physical and mental baseline dropped lower with each resuscitation. On these grounds, they questioned the appropriateness of repeated resuscitation. At the family's request, an outside consultant saw Samuel. The consultant concurred that active treatment was warranted.

The Ethics Committee agreed on the following recommendation: a care conference involving the nurses and physicians looking after Samuel should be convened seven to ten days after he was fitted with the customized tracheostomy tube in order to make decisions regarding his long-term care. It would be appropriate at that time to consider withdrawing or withholding care if it was felt that Samuel's suffering outbalanced the benefit or potential benefit of his care. Samuel's neurologic status as either brain-injured or not-injured would be irrelevant in this consideration.

Case discussion

Unlike the situation in Michael's or Charlotte's cases, the perception of the suffering of the patient was of paramount concern in this case. Also in distinction to the previous two cases, there was a debate about whether the treatment under consideration was futile. Since Samuel had an unusual deformity, it was virtually impossible to predict if he would benefit from the relatively novel approach of providing a customized endotracheal tube. Also, in contrast to the cases discussed previously, Samuel's case highlighted the difficulty of weighing the immediate cost of pain and suffering against an unpredictable long-term outcome. In attempting to find this balance, the perspectives of nurses and physicians were different. Nurses who provided Samuel's day-to-day care tended to focus on Samuel's present suffering and pain. The family was not present in the hospital and reflected a more detached perspective. Physicians tended to look ahead to the possible future benefit that an unconventional therapy might provide. The unconventional therapy reflected the lengths to which physicians will go in an effort to help a patient. While such efforts may reflect caring for the patient, they need to be weighed against the immediate ordeal to which the patient is subjected.[34] In this case, the burden of proof should not have automatically rested with those who favored reducing the level of care, but should have been shared by those who endorsed untried treatments. The purveyor of a heroic intervention should be expected to consider fully the significance of months of precarious care. Often, family members assume the role of challenging or questioning the medical team's tendency to continue treatment when the outcome is unclear. Unfortunately, in this case the family was unable to function as credible spokespersons for the child's best interest, and no substitute, such as a guardian *ad litem*, fulfilled this function either.

Case resolution

Three weeks after the Ethics Committee met, Samuel was fitted with a customized tracheostomy tube. Initially, he did well, but four weeks into therapy his airway was still tenuous, he had required several resuscitations, and it had become apparent that the team was no closer to resolving the issue of his long-term management. During that same four-week interval, Samuel's birth mother relinquished custody of Samuel to an adoptive family. Following this period of gradual decline, Samuel became septic and shocky over a four-day period. On the fourth day, a court order was obtained authorizing the hospital 'to decide to withdraw or withhold further medical support on behalf of Samuel'. Although the adoptive mother requested that more vigorous intervention be provided to Samuel (in the form of external chest compression), the attending physician determined that all support should be discontinued. The ventilator was removed and Samuel died in his adoptive mother's arms.

Case four

Neil was a seventeen-month-old boy with severe bronchopulmonary dysplasia (BPD), a chronic lung disease resulting from premature birth. He was hospitalized for all but one week of his life, initially in a neonatal ICU and subsequently in our hospital for twelve months. Neil was the 1100 gram product of a twenty-seven-week twin gestation. Because of his prematurity, he had respiratory distress, which had required ventilator support intermittently on five different occasions during his care in the neonatal ICU. His parents had strong negative feelings about the use of the ventilator, and every attempt had been made to manage him medically without ventilator support. He had not received ventilator support for ten months. Neil was discharged from the neonatal ICU, spent one week at home, and subsequently was admitted to our hospital for vigorous management of his respiratory status. His management had required essentially intensive care unit nursing while on a regular pediatric ward. He required oxygen therapy, nebulized medications every one to two hours, high-dose steroids, and continuous drip feeding via gastrostomy. In order to avoid ventilation, low-dose methotrexate, a previously untried therapy, was undertaken for eight weeks, between fourteen and sixteen months of age, in hopes of improving his respiratory status and minimizing the side-effects (poor growth) of steroids.

Neil's attending physicians on the pulmonary service regarded his respiratory status as deteriorating, since advancement of his medical therapy had been required to maintain the status quo. Since admission at twelve months of age, he had failure to thrive, with a total weight loss of 0.7 kilograms. Neil had never had a major central nervous system insult. On developmental testing at a corrected age of twelve months he was functioning at about the nine-month level. He was socially interactive.

Neil's parents had been appropriately involved in his care since birth. They had not been present during much of his admission to the hospital because they lived at a distance from the hospital and because they had other young children at home. They steadfastly maintained their wish that Neil should not be ventilated again. Options such as home ventilation were unacceptable to them.

The Ethics Committee was consulted by one of the pulmonologists because of the uncertainty of the medical care to be offered to Neil at this point. The pulmonologist indicated that Neil could not continue with the current mode of therapy, since he clearly was failing to thrive and was requiring high doses of toxic medications (steroids) with no improvement in lung function. The physician saw the two alternatives for Neil's care as including (1) mechanical ventilation, which might stabilize his lung condition and permit growth, which was considered the only long-term treatment for BPD, or (2) not ventilating Neil and allowing him to die. The dilemma posed by the first option, long-term ventilation, was that the long-term outlook for children with BPD who have been ventilator-independent and then become ventilator-dependent is unknown. Although studies suggest that about 50 per cent of such patients die, the long-term morbidity of the survivors is not yet known.

The social worker and pulmonologist involved in Neil's care indicated that the family's objections to ventilation were (1) that Neil's death was inevitable and they had lost hope for his survival; (2) that Neil was suffering; and (3) that while on the ventilator in the past Neil had required sedation to tolerate the mechanical ventilation, and they viewed this as 'no life'. The team of physicians caring for Neil did not reach a consensus about which course of therapy to pursue. The issues of futility and inhumanity were discussed at length during the Ethics Committee meeting.

Case discussion

The benefits of long-term ventilation for Neil were not known, and posed a difficult ethical dilemma. Such management is apparently regarded differently in different medical centres. Some centers reportedly are quite aggressive in pursuing long-term ventilator support for infants with BPD, whereas other centers do not provide that option. The inhumanity of Neil's treatment was also difficult to weigh. Initially, Neil was reported to be almost developmentally normal and socially interactive, with many 'good days'. Later, he had appeared to be suffering more and interacting less;

he had very few 'good days,', or even 'good moments'. Whether Neil would suffer more if placed on a ventilator was debatable. In the past he had become too agitated on the ventilator to make treatment effective without sedation. It was not clear if he would have the same response and require the same therapy should ventilator care be instituted long-term.

How should the medical staff have coped with the uncertainty surrounding Neil's case? Owing to the lack of empiric data about patients in Neil's situation, it was not possible to predict confidently the outcome of continuing his current treatment. Owing to a lack of consensus among the four pulmonary attending physicians caring for Neil, no specific recommendations had been made to the family regarding Neil's long-term management.

In hindsight, the Ethics Committee should have acknowledged and discussed openly the fact that people had conflicting views about what constituted the best medical advice. In the light of the gray area of medical uncertainty, a plan should have been developed to work with the family in reviewing the range of options open to them. One option that might have been presented to the parents was to place Neil on a ventilator until it became more certain whether he would survive with a quality of life that the parents regarded as acceptable. Under this approach, Neil's ventilatory status would be reconsidered when more data became available. A second option that might have been offered to Neil's parents was to withhold ventilatory support. If this option were offered, it would have had to be a genuine option that the medical team would respect. Such an option would have carried the risk that it might have been possible for Neil to have led a meaningful life, but he would have been allowed to die instead. In retrospect, the Ethics Committee might have decided that the considerable uncertainty surrounding treatment for BPD supported a presumption in favour of family decision-making.

Case resolution

Unfortunately, the goal of increasing the family's part in medical decision-making regarding long-term care was never realized. As the Committee was meeting, and unbeknownst to them, Neil's pulmonary condition deteriorated rapidly. In the course of receiving emergency care, Neil was intubated and transferred to the pediatric ICU. Shortly after the transfer, Neil died of influenza pneumonia.

Concluding remarks

In this chapter we have clarified the meanings of medical futility and inhumanity and discussed their ethical implications. We have argued that physicians are not required to offer, nor are patients entitled to receive, medical treatments that are futile or inhumane. Yet we have also indicated that in situations of significant medical uncertainty there should be a (rebuttable) presumption in favour of family decision-making.

Our case discussions bring to light several ways to enhance the process by which medical decisions are made. In Case One, we learned that the assessment of futility does not have to be crisis-driven. Cases One, Three, and Four illustrate the point that the evolving nature of the medical situation calls for constant reassessment of the family's role in medical decision-making. At the outset, families are often disenfranchised by the strong indications for aggressive medical care; but, as the medical indications become less certain, enfranchising the family becomes critical to good decision-making. Case Two teaches the need for staff to be alerted to the possibility that some families cannot make decisions, no matter how clear-cut those decisions appear to the medical team. We believe the legal system should provide more options for dealing with situations where parents are temporarily unable to make medical decisions. Case Three highlights the difficulties that arise when no family member or legal substitute is present to act as an advocate on behalf of the child.

All the cases we have discussed reveal a need to enhance communication between medical staff and parents of seriously ill children. One option is to activate an impartial review process as soon as staff express concern about parental decision-making. The outcome of such a process may be to make hospital resources, such as counseling services, available to parents. Such a review process would fill a unique function. In most institutions, social workers and chaplains are primarily invested in the needs of the family, and ethics committees tend to function largely to support medical staff, but no one is specifically assigned the task of bridging communication gaps between families and health professionals. Introducing a review process could encourage further discussion of the problems of futility, inhumanity, and uncertainty surrounding a given patient's care.

We recognize that even if one accepts these concepts and proposals, it will not be easy to implement them in the perinatal setting. The care of sick children is often intense and emotional. Medical optimism sometimes prevents health professionals and others from perceiving the problems of medical futility and medical inhumanity or actively managing these concerns. The ethics of the medical profession can encourage physicians to push technology to inappropriate levels. Among the values inherent in modern medical practice are faith in science, a commitment to conquering disease and forestalling death, and a desire to bend nature to one's will.[35] Thus, physicians may regard survival as evidence of professional skill, and view a patient's death as evidence of professional incompetence.[36] In the medical setting, prestige and praise are seldom lavished on those who do nothing, stand by, wait, or accept death.[37] Rather, health professionals are applauded for acting, intervening, and forestalling death. Once set in motion, these active, goal-directed virtues can easily acquire a momentum of their own. To balance and limit this tendency, virtues such as cautiousness, patience, non-recklessness, and humility must be honed; in the absence of these balancing virtues, more goal-directed values can assume excessive proportions.[38,39]

Only by continued reflection on cases that raise issues of futility, inhumanity, and medical uncertainty can health professionals grow more aware of the values inherent in modern medical practice and act to shape them. We hope this discussion may be a springboard for improved understanding and better care.

Acknowledgments

Drs. Craig Jackson and David Woodrum provided valuable assistance with this chapter.

REFERENCES

1. The cases described in this chapter are adapted from actual cases presented to the Ethics Committee of the Children's Hospital and Medical Centre in Seattle, Washington, during 1989 and 1990. The name of all patients have been changed to protect the privacy of patients, family members, and medical staff.
2. Cynthia Cohen. 'A history of neonatal intensive care and decision making.' *Hastings Center Report* **17**: 7–9.
3. Department of Health and Human Services. 'Nondiscrimination on the basis of handicap relating to health care for handicapped infants.' *Federal Register* **49**, 1984: 1622–54.
4. *Otis Bowen* v. *American Hospital Association et al.* U.S. Supreme Court. 106 S. Ct. 2101 No 84-15-9, June 9, 1986.
5. Department of Health and Human Services. Child abuse and neglect prevention and treatment program. *Federal Register* **50**, 1985: 14878–901.
6. U.S. Child Abuse Protection and Treatment Amendments of 1984, Public Law 98-457. Amendments to Child Abuse Prevention and Treatment Act and Child Abuse Prevention and Adoption Reform Act. Amendment no 3385. Congressional Record 1984; Senate S8951-S8956.
7. Ronald L. Ariagno and Ellen Wright Clayton.'Government regulations in the United States.' In Amnon Goldworth, William A. Silverman, David K. Stevenson and Ernle W.E. Young (eds), *Ethics and perinatology: issues and perspectives*. Oxford University Press, New York, 1993.
8. Loretta M. Kopelman, Thomas G. Irons, and Arthur E. Kopelman. 'Neonatologists judge the "Baby Doe" regulations.' *New England Journal of Medicine* **318**, 1988: 677–83.
9. *Brophy* v. *New England Sinai Hospital*. 398 Mass. 417;497 N.E. 2d 626 (1986).
10. Tom L. Beauchamp and James F. Childress. 'Virtues and conscientious actions.' In Albert Flores (ed), *Professional Ideals*. Wadsworth Publishing Company, Belmont, CA, 1988: 27–39.
11. Nancy S. Jecker and Lawrence J. Schneiderman. 'Futility and rationing.' *Amercian Journal of Medicine* **92**, 1992: 189–96.
12. Lawrence J. Schneiderman, Nancy S. Jecker, and Albert R. Jonsen. 'Medical

futility: its meaning and ethical implications.' *Annals of Internal Medicine* **112**, 1990: 949–54.

13. Susan Braithwaite and David C. Thomasma. 'New guidelines on foregoing life-sustaining treatment in incompetent patients: an anti-cruelty policy.' *Annals of Internal Medicine* **104**, 1986: 711–15.

14. J. Fletcher. 'Indicators of humanhood: a tentative profile of man.' *Hastings Center Report* **2**, 1972: 1–4.

15. Neil Buchanan. 'The very-low-birthweight infant: medical, ethical, legal and economic considerations.' *The Medical Journal of Australia* **147**, 1987: 184–6.

16. D. W. Overstreet, J. C. Jackson, G. van Belle, and W. E. Truog. 'Estimation of mortality risk in chronically ventilated infants with bronchopulmonary dysplasia.' *Pediatrics* **88**, 1991.

17. Raanan Gillon. 'Ordinary and extraordinary means.' *British Medical Journal* **292**, 1986: 259–61.

18. The three approaches discussed on pp. 7–8 are outlined in John D. Arras, David Coulter, Alan R. Fleischman, Ruth Macklin, Nancy K.Rhoden, and Bill Weil. 'The effect of new pediatric capabilities and the problem of uncertainty.' *Hastings Center Report* **17**, 1987: 10–13.

19. Lawrence J. Nelson and Robert W. Nelson. 'Ethics and the provision of futile, harmful, or burdensome treatment to children.' *Journal of Medicine and Philosophy*, in press.

20. Ferdinand Schoeman. 'Rights of children, rights of parents and the moral basis of the family.' *Ethics* **91**, 1980: 6–19.

21. Nancy S. Jecker. 'The role of intimate others in medical decision making.' *The Gerontologist* **30**, 1990: 65–71.

22. Nancy K. Rhoden. 'Litigating life and death.' *Harvard Law Review*, 1988: 375–446.

23. Earl E. Shelp. *Born to Die*. Free Press, New York, 1986, Chapter 3.

24. Carson Strong. 'The neonatologist's duty to patient and parents.' *Hastings Center Report* **14**, 1984: 10–16.

25. John J. Paris, Robert K. Crone, and Frank Reardon. 'Physicians' refusal of requested treatment.' *New England Journal of Medicine* **322**, 1990: 1012–13.

26. Nancy S. Jecker and Robert A. Pearlman. 'Medical futility: who decides?' *Archives of Internal Medicine* **152**: 1140–4.

27. William Ruddick. 'Questions parents should resist.' In Loretta M. Kopelman and John C. Moskop (eds), *Children and health care: moral and social issues*. Kluwer Academic Publishers, Dordrecht, 1989: 221–30.

28. Mark Yarborough. 'Continued treatment of the fatally ill for the benefit of others.' *Journal of the Americal Geriatrics Society* **36**, 1988: 63–7.

29. Nancy S. Jecker. 'Anencephalic infants and special relationships.' *Theoretical Medicine* **11**, 1990: 333–42.

30. Penny Williamson, Thomas McCormick, and Thomas Taylor. 'Who is the patient?: a family case study of a recurrent dilemma in family practice.' *Journal of Family Practice* **17**, 1983: 1039–43.

31. Howard Brody. 'Ethics in family medicine: patient autonomy and the family unit.' *Journal of Family Practice* **17**, 1983: 973–5.

32. Martin Livingston. 'How illness affects patients' families.' *British Journal of Hospital Medicine* **38**, 1987: 51–3.

33. Sanford Leikin. 'When parents demand treatment.' *Pediatric Annals* **18**, 1989: 266–8.

34. J. M. Duggan. 'Technological triumph—trivial pursuit.' *Australian and New Zealand Journal of Medicine* **19**, 1989: 506–8.

35. Nancy S. Jecker. 'Knowing when to stop: the limits of medicine.' *Hastings Center Report* **21**, 1991:5–8.

36. N. Pace, J. L. Plenderleith, and J. R. Dougall. 'Moral principles in withdrawing advanced life support.' *British Journal of Hospital Medicine* **45**, 1991: 169–70.

37. Nancy S. Jecker and Lawrence J. Schneiderman. 'Ceasing futile resuscitation in the field: ethical considerations.' *Archives of Internal Medicine* **152**: 2392–7.

38. Edmund L. Erde. 'The virtues of medicine: meaning and import.' In Earl E. Shelp (ed), *Virtue and medicine: explorations in the character of medicine*. D. Reidel, Dordrect, 1985: 201–21.

39. Stanley M. Hauerwas. 'On medicine and virtue.' In Earl E. Shelp (ed), *Virtue and medicine: explorations in the character of medicine*. D. Reidel, Dordrect, 1985: 347–56.

3B   MEDICAL FUTILITY: COMMENTARY
Norman C. Fost

INTRODUCTION

In their paper 'Medical futility: decision-making in the context of probability and uncertainty', Nancy Jecker and Roberta Pagon keep their promise to 'wrestle with the problems of futility and inhumanity in medical decision-making'. As in most professional wrestling-matches, the conclusion is apparent at the outset, and is clearly stated: '. . . that these terms have clear medical moral meanings, and that they can serve as useful guides in the care of hopelessly ill newborns'. I have never understood professional wrestling, so it is not surprising that I would not have predicted the conclusion of their match. That is, I do not find the concepts of futility and inhumanity to be clear or useful. On the contrary, I find them vague, arbitrary, and potentially hazardous, not just to clear thinking but to the welfare of patients, particularly critically ill newborns of the sort they describe in their detailed case discussions. I will try to make my disagreement clear, but not before commenting on a side-issue in this discussion, but one I consider even more important: the irrelevance of the federal 'Baby Doe regulations'.

THE IRRELEVANCE OF THE BABY DOE REGULATIONS

Jecker and Pagon state that the revised and current Baby Doe regulations 'allow withholding and withdrawal of life-sustaining treatment on the basis of both futility and inhumanity'. It is certainly correct that if the Baby Doe rules, and the statute on which they are based, regulated the practices of doctors and parents caring for seriously ill newborns, *then* futility and inhumanity would be the operative principles. But the fact is that the Baby Doe rules do not apply directly to doctors, parents, or hospitals. They are rules for State health departments seeking federal funds for child-abuse and neglect programs. The statute and the regulations require State health departments to provide assurances regarding how they will respond if they receive reports of the alleged medical neglect of infants. Absent such reports, States have no duty to seek out such events, to proscribe any particular decisions, or even to define medical neglect in any particular way.

Doctors, parents, and hospitals, absent a report of alleged medical neglect, are regulated only by whatever other laws apply to withholding and withdrawing of life-sustaining treatment. There are certainly laws that could be interpreted to apply to these decisions. My colleague John Robertson and I were the first to bring these legal hazards to public attention (Robertson and Fost 1976). But the law in theory is not the same as the law in practice. And the remarkable fact is that no doctor in the United States has ever been found liable, civilly or criminally, for withholding or withdrawing life-sustaining treatment from any patient for any reason.

On this point the authors and I seem to agree, but for different reasons. They apparently believe that the exceptions in the Baby Doe regulations—the stipulation that treatment may be withheld if it is futile or inhumane—offer a sufficient basis for letting a baby die, at least in some cases. They then present, in admirable detail, examples which would meet these permissible exceptions. While we agree that the law is tolerant of discountinuing care in the cases they discuss, the disagreement about the reasons is important in three regards.

First, I believe that a careful reading of the regulations shows that the terms 'futile' and 'inhumane' do not have the broad meaning ascribed to them by Jecker and Pagon. Rather, the terms are defined narrowly, applying only to situations of imminent death despite full treatment. If the regulations did apply to actual cases, they would not allow withholding of treatment for infants who had prospects for long life, no matter how brain-damaged, with the exception of cases of perpetual coma.

Second, by perpetuating the false belief that the Baby Doe regulations do apply directly to doctors, the authors may unwittingly aggravate the problem they appropriately denounce: namely, overtreatment of some infants. Much of this overtreatment is due to the false belief that there is a legal duty to provide it, as articulated in the Baby Doe regulations. The authors seem to be saying, 'Yes, you do have to pay attention to the Baby Doe regulations, but here's a way to interpret them as consistent with discontinuation of treatment.' I disagree with the premises that physicians should look to the regulations for guidance, and I believe that many, encouraged by hospital attorneys, will continue to interpret the regulations much more narrowly than the authors do.

Third, by acquiescing to the federal insistence that futility and inhumanity are the only justifications for withholding treatment, they give these words more power than they can bear, and distract attention from the more appropriate question: whether or not the patient's interests are being served, as best one can determine, by continuing treatment. It is this problem that is at the heart of their paper.

THE DEFINITION OF 'FUTILITY'

Since Jecker and Pagon intend that the concept of futility should not just be illuminating but practical, applicable to real cases and real laws, they offer definitions that presumably should allow the concepts to be applied in a consistent way. But the definition relies on other words, whose meaning is even less clear and less susceptible to consistent application.

Consider first their definition of *quantitative* medical futility. This, we are told, refers to a situation in which the 'likelihood of a medical benefit ... is *extremely small*' (italics added), for example<1:100. Why is 1:101 futile but 1:99 not? Why is 1:1000 futile? The numbers seem to be plucked from the air, with no rational basis. Since reasonable people will disagree about which numbers are the appropriate ones, the authors (or any other defenders of their favorite number) owe us an explanation of why treatment with a 1:100 chance of success should be considered futile. Since they do not offer us the completed syllogism, we can only surmise. One candidate explanation would be the following.

Perhaps the authors mean that even if the treatment were effective in 1 in 100 tries, it would not be worth it; the costs, broadly defined, of treating 99 patients without benefit would not be outweighed by the admitted benefit of success in 1 patient. But why is that not worth it? How does one determine how much cost is too much to achieve a defined benefit? The answer to that could be determined in a quasi-objective way; through careful cost–benefit analysis. But that creates more problems.

First, cost–benefit analysis would obviously be different for each condition, depending on the cost of the intervention, the value of the benefit, the severity of the condition, and other factors. PKU screening has a favourable cost–benefit ratio even though the 'chance of success' is less than 1:10 000 for each patient subjected to screening. In contrast, a very expensive intervention might have an unfavorable cost–benefit ratio even if success occurred 1:50 times. Finally, the definition of success or benefit is necessarily subjective. For some patients, survival for a year would be considered a benefit, even though the patient's productivity during that time might not be sufficient to conclude that the treatment costs were worth the benefits in objective terms. In summary, Jecker and Pagon's quantitative sense of medical futility necessarily involves qualitative judgments.

The concept of qualitative futility—meaning 'that the quality of outcome is extremely poor'—is more obviously dependent on subjective and personal notions of what benefits are worth certain costs. For some cases, such as the celebrated Wanglie family (Miles 1991), treatment which preserves the patient in a state of permanent unconsciousness is not futile. For their own personal reasons, they considered life itself to be a value, and their doctors could not deny that the treatment was medically effective in prolonging that life. Jecker and Pagon's other example of qualitative futility—total dependence on intensive medical care—is even more arbitrary. 'Intensive medical care' is not a self-defining term, and even treatments which everyone might consider intensive—such as home ventilator care—are hardly futile in all cases. Many patients totally dependent on such care find life worth living, with benefits that clearly outweigh the burdens in their own value system.

If there were any candidate condition for qualitatively futile medical care it would probably be the persistent vegetative state; i.e. there would probably be widespread support for the view that a patient or family asking for treatment in that situation was acting unreasonably. It is important to remember that many patients diagnosed as being in PVS are misdiagnosed. Even whole-brain death, a condition with much clearer criteria and much simpler methods of ascertainment, is commonly misunderstood and misdiagnosed (Youngner et al. 1989; Wikler and Weisbard 1989). If the chance of error were high, a request for continued treatment in the face of a *diagnosis* of PVS might not be so unreasonable. That is, continued treatment might not be futile. Jecker and Pagon may have intended to say that treatment for a patient *actually* in PVS might be considered futile; but the Wanglies and others obviously disagreed. It is unclear how one would determine the 'correct' definition of futility in such cases.

Because of considerations such as these some observers have concluded that futility can only be defined tautologically or that it should be abandoned as a useful concept in deciding whether or not continued treatment is indicated (Truog 1992; Wolf 1988). Wolf, for example, concluded that futility could only be defined narrowly, as 'failing to achieve a defined purpose' (Wolf). Lantos *et al.*, writing in 1988, found futility to be a useful concept in arguing that certain newborns should not be resuscitated (Lantos *et al.* 1988). By 1989, Lantos had concluded that futility was an ambiguous concept, with 'little consensus about how futility should be determined in practice' (Lantos *et al.* 1989).

THE DEFINITION OF 'INHUMANE'

If futility cannot be defined without reference to subjective and arbitrary values, then 'inhumane medical treatment' would seem even less viable as a moral construct in guiding decision-making. Jecker and Pagon's concept of inhumane treatment includes interventions which prolong the lives of patients who '. . . [fall] sadly short of what human life ordinarily includes'; i.e., patients who lack 'indicators of humanhood'. The futility of trying to define humanhood has been much discussed. Joseph Fletcher, who expended considerable thought on the subject, excluded children with Down Syndrome from the class of humans (Fletcher 1972), a judgment which was strongly repudiated by the President's Commission (President's Commission 1983), among others. The authors quote Fletcher's article, without criticism, as supportive of their own views.

Their example is illustrative: in the context of discussing treatment of patients who 'lack indicators of humanhood' they conclude, 'It is inhumane to prolong the life of a conscious stroke patient with the locked-in syndrome.' While it is unclear how one would know such a patient were conscious, I infer that even if such a patient were thinking the most brilliant and creative and human-like thoughts, he/she would be 'not human'.

Perhaps they only meant the patient lacked the indicators of humanhood;

that actually, he/she would be human. But if this is ambiguous to me, it may be ambiguous to others. It may be that some patients, perhaps most, would not want to be treated if permanently in such a state; but it is not clear that such a person is not human, or if not, why he/she would not qualify as a human. Defining such a person out of the class of humans would seem, at the least, arbitrary. Some would consider it inhumane.

LABELS AS SELF-FULFILLING PROPHECIES

Using such concepts as 'futile' and 'inhumane' involves dangers beyond the arbitrariness of the terms as applied in practice. They may also be self-fulfilling prophecies, as illustrated by the authors' discussion of trisomy 13. They consider treatment of such a child, other than comfort measures, to be inhumane because 'the chance of realizing a benefit for the patient is poor'. Withholding definitive treatment from such patients will usually guarantee early death, since they are commonly afflicted with life-threatening anomalies. But neonatologists have long been confronted with children who were considered non-viable (Fost et al. 1980).

In the 1960s, when I was an intern, a 1000-gram infant was considered non-viable, presumably because few if any in the hospital in which I worked had survived to discharge. Intensive treatment would presumably have been considered either futile or inhumane in Jecker's and Pagon's terms. As a result, in my hospital, medically necessary treatment was routinely withheld, and such infants commonly died. In other hospitals, other doctors were more aggressive—a policy eventually resulting in the present situation, in which most such infants are expected to survive. I do not mean to beg the questions of whether such treatment was morally warranted in 1960; whether appropriate safeguards existed for protection of infants from experimental treatment; or whether it is ever appropriate to 'volunteer' a non-consenting patient for experimental treatment that is unlikely to benefit him/her, but which may result in clear benefits for future patients. I only wish to make the point that labelling a situation futile or inhumane may predictably lead to decisions that will result in the patient's death, when a long and prosperous life may be more available than the decision-maker suspects.

There are many illustrations of this problem. New syndromes, such as Reye's syndrome and AIDS, are commonly diagnosed only in their most severe forms in the first cases. This selection bias may lead to the false conclusion that the outcome is worse than appears when a wider range of cases is included. The median life expectancy of a patient with HIV infection has mushroomed from 2 years to 10 years unrelated to advances in treatment, simply because diagnostic advances and better case-finding have resulted in earlier diagnosis, and diagnosis of patients with milder forms of the infection. What was once considered hopeless (?futile) has often become progressively hopeful. Labelling the patients as hopeless, and treatment as futile, can preclude discovery of the possibility of change.

THE LESSON OF THE ORDINARY/EXTRAORDINARY DEBATE

The authors acknowledge that there will always be uncertainty. What, then, is the value of labelling a treatment as futile or inhumane? If it will virtually always be the case that futile does not mean 'definitely unlikely to succeed', but only 'probably', then choices must be made.

Leon Kass taught us nearly twenty years ago that technology cannot do moral work. He was discussing the then-popular, now discredited, concept of 'extraordinary means'. Some writers of the day seemed to believe that, in the case of some treatments, we didn't have to decide whether we had a duty to use them; we only had to decide whether they met the definition of extraordinary means. If the intervention could be labelled as extraordinary, there was, by definition, no duty to use it. This concept arose from, and was most widely advocated by, Roman Catholic writers, following the teaching of Pope Pius XII in the course of discussing a Catholic physician's duty to use a respirator. History has shown us how elusive and evanescent those definitions were. Even if we conceded that a respirator constituted extraordinary means, whatever that meant at the time, few would consider it so today.

More important, even if it were extraordinary, in secular discussion an argument would be needed to explain why there was no duty to use it. Similarly, we now understand that some treatments that are quite ordinary, such as provision of food and water through a nasogastric tube, need not always be administered.

Just as the concept of extraordinary means failed to provide answers regarding when there is a duty to treat, the concepts of futility and inhumanity will fail for the same reasons. They cannot be defined, or have not to date, in any operational way that is not subject to personal value preferences. Because applying them will always involve uncertainty and choices, they will not help us avoid the untidy work of analyzing each case.

UNCERTAINTY IS NOT THE ONLY PROBLEM

After offering these terms, the authors acknowledge that uncertainty will make it difficult to apply them in the perinatal setting. Uncertainty is only one reason that defining treatment as 'futile' will not be dispositive. Consider, for example, the unusual case in which there is absolute certainty as to the diagnosis and prognosis. Certain patients who have been properly diagnosed as brain dead might qualify. When evaluated by competent clinicians, using widely agreed upon criteria, brain death should be one of the simplest diagnoses in all of medicine. When properly diagnosed, the prognosis is as certain as anything.[1] But even when there is complete

---

[1] I hasten to remind the reader that, as simple as it is, many highly skilled and experienced doctors just don't get it (Younger *et al.* 1989).

certainty as to the hopelessness of recovery, there are still choices to be made regarding continuation of 'life' support.

Several reasons could be proposed for maintaining the vegetative functions in such a patient. First, he may be a source of organs or tissues for transplantation. Second, as Gaylin suggested many years ago (Gaylin), maintenance of the living body might serve many other social purposes, including drug-testing; manufacture of useful biologic materials such as an antibodies; experiments on human physiology (Coller 1989; Fost 1980); or as a 'cadaver' for trainees to practice procedures. A family member or a physician might find some of these social purposes powerful reasons for maintaining mere biologic existence in a brain-dead patient. The certainty of the diagnosis of brain death would not therefore end the discussion of whether treatment should continue; rather, it would make such discussion possible.

CASE ONE: MICHAEL

The cases illustrate the imprecision and hazards of applying the concept of futility in the real world. In case one, a fetus, later to be known as Michael, was labelled as non-viable at 20 weeks' gestation. In other words, continuation of the pregnancy was considered futile from his perspective, presumably meaning he would not be able to survive outside the uterus.[2] But wait! Nine days after birth Michael is alive, if not well. Like many infants before him, he has traversed the boundary from non-viable to viable. The label non-viable apparently, in this case, meant something like 'seriously ill', or 'will need lots of high technology treatment'. Continuing the pregnancy was clearly not futile, in the sense of 'ineffective'. Was it inhumane? Did it rob Michael of his humanness? If it did, he seems to have recovered it. When we first meet Michael after transfer to the authors' institution he is an infant with prune belly syndrome, with the most pessimistic prognosis being renal failure 'at some point, perhaps in late adolescence'; a more optimistic expert thought he would do even better.

Despite these opinions, the parents were told that 'urologic surgery would be futile'. The meaning of futility is unclear in this setting. 'Ineffective' does not seem to apply, since the worst-case scenario assumed two decades of life, with treatment options for renal failure at that point. 'Inhuman' is not a word we usually apply to children who lose renal function in adolescence, or who require dialysis or transplantation thereafter. Presumably the futility label was meant to apply to his other disabilities—his respiratory failure or his severe retardation. Urologic surgery would be futile in correcting either of those. But that is either a tautology or a straw man. Urologic surgery is futile in all cases if we expect it to cure or benefit all bodily dysfunction.

[2] I assume this is what was meant by 'non-viable'. The authors do not tell us what definition they had in mind. Had they offered one, it would have presumably have been fraught with the same arbitrariness as the futility concept (Fost et al. 1980).

It is obvious to the point of triviality to call urologic surgery futile in this sense. I assume, therefore, that the futility applies to the other treatments, or to the idea of keeping him alive by any means. If that is what is meant, then that is what should be said: that Michael's life is not worth living, and no intervention, including feeding, will change that. Whether or not that conclusion is warranted is, of course, the central issue. My only point is that little light is shed on that central question by labelling the urologic surgery as futile.

In addition to distracting us (and perhaps the parents) from the central issue—is Michael's life worth living, regardless of the intervention—the futility label apparently alienated the parents because of its inaccuracy or ambiguity. They were told once—at 20 weeks' gestation—that he was a non-viable fetus. Then they were told that urologic treatment would be futile, although he might survive 20–40 years. At the least, they were entitled to be confused; at the worst, they had reason to lose trust in the doctors' predictive powers.

'Inhumane', according to the authors, means either painful without compensating benefit, or undignified because it's not a human life. It is not clear whether or how much pain Michael was experiencing. At one point we are told that Michael 'had no interaction with his environment except to pain', but later that 'Michael was not in constant pain'. How do we know how much pain he was experiencing, or whether it was treatable or manageable? As to dignity, it is yet another word requiring definition and instruction on how to apply it. Webster tells us it has to do with 'intrinsic worth' (Webster 1953). Can the authors provide some value-free non-arbitrarty guidance as to who or what has intrinsic worth? Is this a restatement of the concept of 'personhood', also not defined? Without operational definitions these words will be defined arbitrarily by those who use them as justifications for stopping treatment. Labelling treatment as inhumane or undignified does not constitute an argument for withholding it.

Finally, we are told that treatment was qualitatively futile because the quality of Michael's existence was so poor. Although 'not in constant pain he lacked capacities to recognize others or enjoy interacting with them or his environment'. Michael's ventilator was discontinued $3^{1}/2$ months after he was born, at 31 weeks' gestation. His adjusted age was 5–6 weeks. His inability to recognize others or enjoy his environment after 6 weeks of ventilator-dependent intensive care would not seem to warrant strong conclusions about his neurologic prognosis.

Perhaps the clinicians had other reasons to believe that Michael would not be able to interact with people and that therefore life had no benefit for him. If this were the case, it doesn't shed light to substitute 'undignified' as shorthand for this. It risks letting others use the word to mean anything they think it means, just as 'brain dead' is used by some to mean 'severely brain damaged', and 'vegetative' to mean something similar. We have enough time to say what we mean; to spell out the reasons why we think it is not in Michael's interests to be kept alive.

This, by the way, seems to be a 'best interests' argument. If it is, then the treatment would seem to be irrelevant. If he has no interest in living, what difference is it which treatment is keeping him alive? If he does have an interest in living, then the painfulness of treatment doesn't settle the matter.

CASE TWO: CHARLOTTE

In Charlotte's case, the claim of futility is apparently made because technology cannot do more than it is supposed to do. Charlotte's ventilator 'was futile in attempting to reverse her underlying problems and it was appropriate to consider limiting her care'.[4] Little light would be shed by the observation that the ventilator will not reverse her underlying problems, presumably referring to her missing brain substance or congenital heart disease. Ventilators are always futile in correcting those problems; no judgment is required in this case.

Presumably the authors mean to say that Charlotte's neurologic or cardiac problems are so severe that even if the ventilator succeeded in prolonging her life indefinitely it wouldn't be worth it because Charlotte was so impaired or handicapped from her other conditions. To put it another way, Charlotte had no interest in long life, presumably because she was so impaired neurologically that she could not appreciate any of the pleasures of life.

We can't tell if Charlotte's neurologic status was indeed so severe as to preclude experiencing pleasure. Nor can we tell if this is what is meant by the shorthand use of the word 'futile'. The effect of the label is to end the discussion, or at least to obscure the central issue: whether and why Charlotte had any interest in living. If she had no interest in living, questions should arise about all means of extending her life, including feeding. The ventilator is not the issue requiring definition; Charlotte's life, and her interest, are what require clarification.

Aggressive support, we are told, would be 'quantitatively futile because it did not provide a benefit to Charlotte'. Quantitatively futile, we were told, means that the likelihood of medical benefit is extremely small. But such treatment had already succeeded in keeping Charlotte alive for 12 months. The only medical benefit which the ventilator could hope to achieve is to maintain the ventilatory functions, primarily exchange of blood gases. Twelve months of life suggests that the ventilator had succeeded quite well in achieving its intended benefit. Why is 12 months of life not a benefit? How can futility be defined in a way that will tell us whether 12 months or 12 years of life is sufficient as to constitute a benefit? The answers to these questions are anything but clear; they seem inevitably subjective and personal.

Perhaps the authors mean that the treatment would be futile from that point on, that the prospect that she would live another day or week was extremely small. Just how soon death would have to occur to constitute confirmation of this notion of futility is not clear. Nor is it clear what the probability of death would have to be within this arbitrary period. The authors do not offer numbers, so we do not know what they mean by the term, nor we do know what conclusions to draw in light of subsequent events. We are told that Charlotte confounded the prognosticators by becoming so stable that discharge to home, a home that was previously considered inadequate, was not only considered but effected. We presume that this was not with the intent that she should die, but with the expectation that her parents were capable of keeping her alive. But again, the prognosticators apparently erred: shortly after she went home, she died.

I imply no criticism of the decision to send her home, or of the hazards of prognostication. I am no better at it. I only wish to make the point that calling her treatment futile short-circuits a complex series of judgments, some of which involve rough guesses regarding prognosis, and all of which involve subjective judgments about the interests of handicapped infants and the relative benefits and burdens of continuing treatment.

By 'qualitatively futile' we should understand that the quality of life was 'extremely poor'. As was previously stated, this is an opinion to which the physicians or authors are entitled. It is hardly a medical judgment, nor does the label 'qualitatively futile' shed any light as to why the authors' opinion on the quality of Charlotte's life should be preferred to the parents' opinion.

The authors do explain why they believe the parents should not have been given responsibility for deciding whether treatment should continue. It is the kind of argument which normally constitutes the essence of ethical reflection. It does not resort to shorthand, code-words, or shortcuts. I should say, lest I appear a curmudgeon or a vitalist, that I suspect my conclusions would be the same as the authors' if I knew all the facts. But I would not consider my intuitions to be a substitute for a argument, any more than calling treatment 'futile' can substitute for an argument.

CASE THREE: SAMUEL

It is always possible to find philosophers' cases that demonstrate the grayness of boundaries that surround all definitions. A critic of definitions may argue that dawn and dusk prove the uselessness of the concepts of night and day. But the difficulty of defining boundary cases does not reduce the utility of defining high noon as day and midnight as night. What is interesting about Jecker's and Pagon's cases is that they were not proffered by critics. They were selected, not as gray-zone cases, but as illustrations of the utility of the concept of futility. And yet they seem, to this reader, to highlight the ambiguity and hazards of the concept.

Samuel's condition, we are told, is 'lethal'. We are not told what is meant by this word, whether it means he will die from his condition in hours, days, weeks, months, years, or decades. We can assume, from the definition, that the probability of his dying, whatever the interval, is greater than approximately 1:100. The numbers are important, since the reason for assigning this label, I assume, is to anticipate the claim that life-sustaining treatment would be futile.

We are then told that this labelling of Samuel's condition as lethal is professionally disputed. Moreover, the authors, who previously described his condition, without equivocation, as 'lethal', later inform us that his deformity was sufficiently unusual that 'it was virtually impossible to predict if he would benefit from the relatively novel approach of providing a customized endotracheal tube'. This intervention is labelled 'heroic', apparently to support the conclusion that there was no obligation to provide the treatment. This recalls the now-abandoned practice of labelling treatments as 'extraordinary' as a bypass for the murky work of deciding whether they should be provided or withheld in a particular case.

CONCLUSION

'We have clarified the meanings of medical futility and inhumanity', the authors conclude. I wish it were so. Rather, I believe they have done something even more useful; they have clarified the ambiguity of these terms. They conclude that physicians are not required to offer treatments that are futile or inhumane; but the ambiguity of the terms seems to allow physicians to medicalize a subjective value judgment by labelling treatment as futile or inhumane. If treatment that can prolong life for 12 months (Case Two) is futile, why not 12 years? If physicians disagree (Case Two) how does it clarify the issue for one to label the treatment as 'futile' or 'inhumane' and the other to insist that it is effective and humane. This kind of debate reminds me of the less-than-persuasive response to 'Tastes great'; namely, 'Less filling'. As Truog et al. concluded, 'The rapid advance of the language of futility into the jargon of bioethics should be followed by an equally rapid retreat' (Truog et al. 1992).

With regard to Jecker and Pagon's observation on the need to include families more fully as early as possible, I can only agree. Similarly, their observations on the technophilic tendencies of modern medicine, the hazards of excessive medical optimism, and the often mistaken equation of survival with success are well founded and in need of reiteration. Their courage, candor, and clarity in publicizing their experiences in detail is essential to inform the public and policy-makers of the process, substance, and justifications of decision-making in hospitals. I have little doubt that discussions such as these will 'be a springboard for improved understanding and better care'.

REFERENCES

Coller, B. S. The newly dead as research subjects. *Clinical Research*, **37**:#3: 487–94, 1989.

Fletcher, J. Indicators of humanhood: a tentative profile of man. *Hastings Center Report* **2**: 1–4, 1972.

Fost, N. Research on the brain dead. J. Ped. **96** (#1): 54–6, 1980 (Jan.).

Fost, N. Treatment of seriously ill and handicapped newborns. *Critical Care Clinics* **2**: #1: 149–59, 1986 (Jan.).

Fost, N. Do the right thing: Samuel Linares and defensive law. *Law, Medicine and Health Care* **17** (4): 330–4, 1989 (Winter).

Fost, N. Chudwin, D., and Wikler, D. The limited moral significance of fetal viability. *Hastings Center Report*: 10–13, 1980 (December).

Gaylin, W. Harvesting the newly dead. Harpers, Sept 1974, 23–30.

Lantos, J. D., Miles, S. H. Silverstein, M. D., and Stocking, C. B. Survival after cardiopulmonary resuscitation in babies of very low birth weight. Is CPR futile therapy? *New Eng. J. Med.* 1988; **318**: 91–5.

Lantos, J. D., Singer, P. A., Walker, R. M. *et al.* The illusion of futility in clinical practice. *Am. J. Med.* 1989; **87** (July): 81–4.

Miles, S. H. Informed demand for 'non-beneficial' medical treatment. *New Eng. J. Med.* **325**: 512–15, 1991.

President's Commission on Ethical Problems in Medicine and Biomedical and Behavioral Research. *Deciding to forego life-sustaining treatment.* US Government Printing Office, Washington DC, 1983.

Robertson, J. A. and Fost, N. Passive euthanasia of defective newborns: legal considerations. *J. Pediatrics* **88**: #5: 883–9, 1976(May).

Truog, R. D., Brett, A. S., and Frader, J. The problem with futility. *New Eng. J. Med.* **326** (#23): 1560–4, 1992 (June 4)

Webster's New Collegiate Dictionary. G & C Merriam, Springfield, Mass., 1953.

Wikler, D. and Weisbard, A. J. Appropriate confusion over 'brain death'. *JAMA* **261**: 2246, 1989.

Wolf SM. Conflict between doctor and patient. *Law medicine and Health Care* **16** (#3-4): 197-203, 1988 (Winter).

Youngner SJ, Landefeld CS, Coulton CJ, *et al.* Brain death and organ retrieval. A cross-sectional survey of knowledge and concepts among health professionals. *JAMA* **261**: 2205, 1989.

4

Quality of life as a decision-making criterion

4A QUALITY OF LIFE AS A DECISION-MAKING CRITERION I

A. G. M. Campbell

INTRODUCTION

Perhaps the strangest of all the publications to follow the Baby Doe controversy in the United States is a report entitled 'Medical discrimination against children with disabilities' (US Commission on Civil Rights 1989). This bulky volume attacks the integrity and motives of those pediatricians and parents who together decide that life-sustaining treatments should be withheld or withdrawn from severely abnormal or damaged infants. What was accepted for generations as the exercise of 'reasonable medical discretion' in the face of a family tragedy is labelled as 'discrimination' against the handicapped and, in the Commission's view, as equivalent to the invidious discrimination practiced against individuals or groups on the basis of such morally irrelevant criteria as sex, race, colour, or religion.

The Commission is particularly opposed to 'quality of life' assessments in deciding about medical treatment, and many of the adverse comments about pediatricians seem to derive from the alleged inclusion of 'social judgements' in medical decision-making. The report emphasizes an interpretation of the law by the Department of Health and Human Services (the Federal agency charged with implementing the child Abuse Amendments of 1984), to the effect that '*the law does not permit life and death treatment decisions to be made on the basis of subjective opinions regarding the future quality of life of a retarded or disabled person*'.

It also records that nine major disability and medical associations have adopted 'Principles of Treatment' that also reject the use of quality-of-life criteria: '*Considerations such as anticipated or actual limited potential of an individual and present or future lack of available community resources are irrelevant and must not determine the decisions concerning medical care*' (Joint Policy Statement 1984).

The controversial nature of this report and some sense of its bias is apparent in the inclusion of a *Dissent* written by the committee chairman in which he criticizes the lack of any data about the dimensions of the problem 'during the very years when this report was being prepared at a cost of half a million dollars.' He also pointed out that failure to include the 'most sympathetic representation possible of the strongest counterarguments to the positions taken' would cause considerable damage to the report's credibility and concludes. 'the interests of handicapped newborns have been sacrificed to a political mission'.

In this chapter I shall argue that, in these difficult and poignant situations, quality-of-life predictions are not only inevitable but are necessary if pediatricians are to seek *on behalf of the infant*, the least detrimental of what may be several unsatisfactory options for treatment. Furthermore, if pediatricians are to help families to cope with the tragedy of abnormal birth, quality-of-life judgements are most important components of the detailed medical and ethical analysis that should precede any decision to withhold or withdraw life-sustaining treatment (see Chapter 6). To leave them out is to ignore the practical realities of caring for infants with catastrophic impairments, devalues the importance of compassion in medical decision-making, and reduces the doctor's role to that of a technician seduced by modern treatment imperatives and are blind to, or uncaring about, the possible adverse consequences for infant and family.

'Quality of life'

What is meant by 'quality of life' when used in this context? At the beginning it is perhaps worth emphasizing what it does *not* mean. To pediatricians it does not mean a utilitarian calculation of 'social worth' or value to the community, or even, as is often implied, consideration of the probable economic costs of long-term care to the family or State. Cost-effectiveness is relevant to technological innovation in any health service with finite resources; but the financial cost of treatment for an individual patient is not the primary concern of the doctor at the bedside. To a pediatrician, 'quality of life' means the infant's capacity for future health, development, and well-being, and the human costs that are likely to accrue with survival.

Thus when a pediatrician and parents consider the treatment options for an infant they are primarily concerned with the kind of future life that they want for the infant *in the infant's own interests*. Parents have high hopes for their infant. They wish, not for perfection or for some impossible ideal, but for a reasonable degree of physical and mental health. They hope that their child will be free of pain and suffering. Above all they desperately want reassurance that their infant will have sufficient brain function to allow sentience and cognition, and will be able to interact in human relationships. Like all parents they look forward to the time when their children can achieve at least some measure of independence and perhaps a family life of their own. Unless one believes rigidly in a 'sanctity of life' standard, it

seems self-evident that an 'infants best interests' standard must incorporate
quality-of-life considerations in any medical decision that seeks to maximize
benefit and minimize harm. Respect for the infant as a person and reverence
for life as most people wish to live it should require no less. Most persons with
experience of serious illness or disability recognize that there must be times
when early death is a preferable alternative to 'life' in the biological sense
of continuing vital processes, yet one where human functioning and capacity
are strictly limited or absent. *Granted that we can easily save the life, what
kind of life are we saving?* (McCormick 1974).

The 'data vacuum'

It has to be acknowledged that much of the debate about withholding
and withdrawing life-sustaining treatment takes place in something of a
medical and moral vacuum. With such individualized decisions it is difficult
to accumulate accurate data on 'undertreatment' or 'overtreatment'; and
almost impossible to find anything more reliable than anecdotal data on the
'rightness' or 'wrongness' of these decisions as viewed by the participants in
retrospect.

In 1973 it was reported that 14 per cent of the deaths in the Yale–New
Haven Hospital newborn unit had followed withdrawal of treatment (Duff
and Campbell 1973). Some years later a similar database was examined
in Aberdeen, Scotland, where the corresponding figure was 21 per cent
(Campbell 1982); and from 1981 to 1985 in the same area it was estimated
that out of a total of 185 deaths, intensive care had been withheld from 80
(43.2 per cent) and later withdrawn from 72 (38.9 per cent). Thus of the
105 infants who were treated intensively but who died within 4 weeks
of birth, 72, or almost 69 per cent, died following decisions to withdraw
intensive care, usually assisted ventilation (Campbell *et al.* 1988). Whether
this represents overtreatment or undertreatment it is difficult to say. It does
not necessarily mean that, in the United Kingdom, an increasing number of
babies were being denied the benefits of intensive care and allowed to die. In
neonatal units on each side of the Atlantic, the infant mortality in comparable
groups seems to be similar. Much larger numbers and more refined data
will be necessary to bring out any clear differences in policy. With new
knowledge and technology the diagnostic and prognostic implications of
many congenital abnormalities can be assessed with considerable accuracy
during pregnancy and after birth. Decisions to withdraw treatment can be
made on better facts and at an earlier stage than before, so that as the
absolute number of deaths falls there will be a proportionate increase in
the early deaths that follow withdrawal of treatment. Similarly, deaths
resulting from withholding life-saving resuscitation and assisted ventilation
will increase proportionately as more and more infants survive extremely
premature birth. Thus as perinatal mortality continues to fall, it seems
inevitable and proper for an increasing *proportion* of the deaths to result
from 'non-treatment' decisions when the futility and burdensome nature

of starting or continuing aggressive treatment become apparent to parents and staff. Attitudes to viability *can* affect the data on perinatal mortality (Fenton *et al.* 1990). American pediatricians are said to be more 'aggressive' than their European colleagues in their use of intensive care; but why has this made such little apparent difference to overall survival rates? We need to look in more detail at the deaths that occur during intensive care. Are the intensive care units and their populations really comparable? How does the *duration* of intensive care before death vary from unit to unit and from country to country? Is the *principal* effect of overtreatment the needless prolongation of dying rather than a significant increase in the number of handicapped children who survive? Could there really be little difference in actual practice between most American and most British units, just a reluctance in making this explicit in the legal 'climate' following Baby Doe?

The staff of acute facilities also need to be more aware of the long-term outcome of their treatment decisions. We need to know more about the quality of life of the survivors, particularly those who require various forms of continuing care. We also need to know more about the effects on parents and families, not only on those with handicapped survivors, but also on those who participated in decisions to allow their infants to die. Whatever the decision, it is these families who have to live with the consequences. Time is a great healer; but some lingering uncertainty about the wisdom of any such decision is inevitable. Understandably, there is great reluctance to re-open the emotional scars left by such traumatic experiences whatever the outcome. For the infant who dies, the loss and shared grief of family members is never forgotten, though most parents seem to adjust well and go on to have further healthy children. For parents whose child survived but is grievously handicapped the situation is much more poignant, particularly after a first pregnancy. It is difficult for parents to admit, even to themselves, that the child they have grown to love should have been allowed to die (Simms 1986). Unquestionably, some parents seem strengthened by the experience of bringing up a severely handicapped person; but others never adjust to the shock of abnormal birth or the effects of a devastating illness on their child, and remain for ever in a state of 'chronic sorrow' (Copley and Bodensteiner 1987). Some will express their bitterness at the 'broken promises of modern medicine'. A few will decide against having any further children, partly from the fear of recurrence and partly because they recognize that they would simply be unable to cope with the additional physical and emotional strain. They will always grieve for the 'normal' family they never had.

WHEN IS QUALITY OF LIFE AN ISSUE?

To anyone familiar with neonatal intensive care it is not surprising that concern about an infant's future quality of life should play such a prominent part in neonatal decision-making. The legacy of abnormal development or prolonged intensive care that parents fear most is 'brain damage', and what this might mean for their child. It follows therefore, that it is the condition of the infant's nervous system, especially the brain, that is the principal criterion used by pediatricians in determining whether to withhold or withdraw life-sustaining treatments.

When these dilemmas first came to public attention, the main focus of concern was the problem of faulty development, especially of the brain and spinal cord, with its potentially lethal and inevitably disabling consequences (Lorber 1971; Duff and Campbell 1973; Shaw 1973). In contemporary neonatal units, infants with congenital abnormalities, while still posing occasional dilemmas for pediatricians, have been overtaken in numerical significance by the problems of very immature infants, particularly those born at the limits of viability; and infants who have been damaged grievously by complications of pregnancy or birth, or even from the inherent hazards of neonatal intensive care. In addition, there are some degenerative disorders of the brain with just as devastating long-term consequences that do not become clinically apparent until later in childhood. Other particularly poignant quandaries are posed by those infants whose brains are intact but who have suffered irreparable damage to other organs.

For example, an infant may lose the major part of the intestine, but can survive through the use of continuous parenteral feeding. This technique when used long-term is fraught with complications, and can only be of temporary help. It therefore seems pointless to embark on such treatment if there is no hope of the infant's ever gaining adequate intestinal function for normal growth. The eventual recognition that treatment has failed and that it is necessary to make a heart-rending decision to stop treatment is particularly difficult and cruel after raised hopes that never had any prospect of fulfillment and after months or years of family bonding.

Infants of extremely low birthweight (ELBW:Φ<1000 gm)

Not all that long ago, 28 weeks' gestation age (birthweight~1000 gm) was considered to be the 'limit of viability' for infants born prematurely. Few infants under 1000 gm survived, and many of the survivors were abnormal at follow-up (Lubchenco et al. 1963). In the last three to four decades, developments in neonatal intensive care, particularly the increased availability of better and more appropriately miniaturized equipment for assisted ventilation, have made 28 weeks a meaningless standard. Tinier and tinier infants born earlier and earlier in gestation now have greatly increased chances of survival (Hack and Fanaroff 1989; Alberman and Botting 1991), and there have been equally encouraging improvements in morbidity, particularly among the relatively more mature. Pediatricians talk optimistically about the prospects for infants weighing under 1000 gm at birth, and there is some evidence that intensive care is justified, at least initially, for those infants who weigh more than 700 gm at birth. (Britton et al. 1981). For practical purposes 24 weeks' gestation (or >500 gm birthweight) is increasingly used as a more realistic 'marker' of viability, a trend reflected in the British Stillbirth Definition Act (1992), which reduced from 28 to 24 weeks the minimum gestation age by which a stillbirth (fetal death) is defined.

While it is true to say that most infants under 1000 gm will grow up to be healthy, for those under 700 gm birthweight at appropriate gestational ages (<26 weeks), the risks remain appreciable (Escobar *et al.* 1991). Below 700 gm, the prospects of future disabling handicap increase significantly with decreasing gestation age—a reflection of the immaturity of organ systems not yet ready for independent functioning and some indication that our treatments, however sophisticated, are still relatively crude.

Congenital abnormalities

Specific examples include the severe neural tube defects, such as open meningomyelocele, and primary brain defects, such as holoprosencephaly and hydranencephaly. Abnormalities affecting other organs, physically disabling though they are, do not usually pose such difficult problems, as, with appropriate treatment and support, they may be compatible with eventual good health and normal neurological development. Infants with congenital abnormalities involving several organs or systems are much more problematic. While each individual defect may be corrected, or at least ameliorated, by modern surgery, together they will seriously interfere with the infant's future health. For some infants who are born with a characteristic cluster of abnormalities, more complete diagnosis, by such techniques as chromosomal karyotyping, will confirm the presence of a syndrome such as trisomy 13 (Patau's syndrome) or trisomy 18 (Edwards' syndrome). In these infants a severe abnormality of the brain is always present, and early death is likely with or without treatment, so that a decision to withhold or withdraw life-sustaining treatment is less controversial (*Lancet* 1992). Indeed, once the diagnosis is confirmed, I believe that it is wrong to initiate or persist with aggressive treatment, as no real benefit to the patient will result. On the other hand, for infants with multiple abnormalities but with no evidence that the brain is abnormal or has suffered major damage, all necessary treatments should usually be provided. An important part of counselling and communication with parents is to familiarize them with what can be achieved by modern surgery, and how well children can adapt to the kinds of physical disability likely to afflict their child in future years.

Brain-damaging conditions

In addition to the damage suffered by premature infants discussed above, there will be a few infants whose developing brains are affected by a disseminated virus infection such as rubella or cytomegalovirus contracted early in pregnancy. There is also a numerically more important group of infants, born at term, and normally developed to that point, who, tragically, are damaged by hypoxic–ischaemic encephalopathy accompanying perinatal asphyxia, or infants who become subject to a brain-damaging metabolic disturbance such as hypoglycaemia during the neonatal period.

Diseases not apparent at birth

Some inherited metabolic disorders, for example Tay–Sachs disease or the Lesch–Nyhan syndrome, only become apparent during the early months or years of childhood, when the progressive degeneration of the brain becomes associated with extremely distressing clinical features and a deteriorating quality of life. In caring for these children, particularly troubling treatment decisions about the use of antibiotics, resuscitation, ventilation, etc. may occur at any time of their lives. A doctor has to be particularly cautious in advising on the best interests of someone who, while grievously afflicted, has become a loving and much loved member of the family.

'QUALITY OF LIFE' IN NEONATAL DECISION-MAKING

Is it ethical?

In the Hastings Center 'Guidelines on the termination of life-sustaining treatment and the care of the dying' consideration of quality of life is described as one of the most morally controversial issues in modern medicine (Hastings Center 1987a). The difficulties and dangers of adopting a 'quality of life' standard for those without decision-making capacity are acknowledged, '... but a failure to do so may condemn some patients to lives of indignity, pain, or burden that no person with decision-making capacity would choose.' ...'By allowing patients and their surrogates to make choices that consider "quality of life", we diminish the risk of forcing lives of pain, indignity, or overwhelming burden on those who are helpless.'

An infant's quality of life has always been an important consideration in society. In antiquity, infants did not achieve full rights, including the right to life, simply by virtue of being born, but had to show capacity for development in infancy and to demonstrate potential value to their community before being fully accepted. Drastic action was taken against any abnormal infants who did not have such potential. 'Both Plato and Aristotle, as well as the Stoics, Epicurus, and presumably Plotinus, accepted the morality of the exposure of infants, and presumably also abortion, on eugenic or sometimes on purely economic grounds' (Rist 1982).

In modern times the intentional termination of abnormal and even normal pregnancies has become widespread, and it has been pointed out that 'These biologic imperfections and what seem to be defects in parenting behaviour are not new. What is novel, over the few million-or-so years of human existence, is the idea that succor of all viable babies is a desirable social goal' (Silverman 1981).

To a remarkable extent the timing and manner of one's death is now dependent on technology, and using this technology responsibly is one of the biggest challenges of modern medical practice. Technological innovation simply has made it unwise and sometimes cruel to insist that an infant's right to life is absolute, or that, in all circumstances the interests of the family are secondary or should be ignored. The Hastings Center Newborns Project, *inter alia*, concluded: '*A moral framework acknowledging the centrality of quality of life considerations as reflected in a concern for protecting the best interests of children is appropriate for guiding decision making for children with severe disorders and diseases that prove unresponsive to medical interventions*' (Hastings Center 1987b).

Problems with quality-of-life criteria

A particular difficulty with assessing the quality of life for infants (and others who have never achieved decision-making capacity) is the necessity to have proxy decision-makers, usually the parents. One pediatrician/ethicist has pointed out the obvious conflict of interest that must exist when the child is seen as presenting a potential burden to the family, and how this should disqualify a parent as a suitable advocate (Fost 1981). Of course it is inappropriate for several reasons to leave the decision-making entirely to the parents; but my experience with parents and their thoughts and priorities at these sad and confused times does not support this rather cynical view, notwithstanding the recent history of child abuse in all its forms. There is the natural reluctance for surrogates, be they doctors, parents or other advocates, to make value judgements for another, particularly when, as with an infant or young child, that individual cannot indicate his or her own values and preferences in advance. There is considerable variation in what is viewed as 'quality', 'meaning', or 'happiness' in one's own life, which also must have some influence. But unless one favours making medical decisions on the basis of distrust, and unless there are compelling reasons to the contrary, it seems a better policy to *trust* that parents, and doctor(s) acting together will usually make decisions that are in the best interests of infants, with the courts available to deal with apparent abuses of trust or areas of irreconcilable conflict. Others seem to agree that the judgement of reasonable people may be used as an aid to morally acceptable decision-making. '*Reasonable people can be presumed to be drawing the line on the kind of life being preserved at the right place—in the best overall interests of the patient*' (McCormick 1978).

Another problem with quality of life is its very arbitrariness. In suggesting a formulaic approach, Shaw tried to improve the objectivity of the decision-making process by considering the 'quality' of one's life as expressed in a formula where **Quality of Life (QL)** = **NE** × (**H** + **S**) (Shaw 1977). This is meant to illustrate the relationship existing among the variables that influence one's life, where **NE** represents the patient's natural physical and intellectual endowment; **H**, the contribution of home and family; and **S**, the contribution from society. The formula was based on: '*how physicians and other medical professionals often tend to think about quality of life of* *patients in terms of their measurable or quantifiable physical or mental characteristics'.*

The formulaic approach, with its utilitarian overtones, has been criticized as a 'prescription for infanticide', and misinterpreted, sometimes deliberately, to imply a negative attitude to people with disabilities. It also appears to give undue weight to the social judgements that were condemned by the Commission on Civil Rights. Reducing a complex and, for each infant, a uniquely individual set of personal and family circumstances to a simple formula does not, and probably cannot, adequately convey the very different 'weightings' or values of each component; but this was never its purpose, as Shaw has emphasized. The formula was introduced merely to identify *'in broad terms'* those factors which affect quality of life, because Shaw believes, as I do, that they are *'not only relevant but central to humane medical decision-making'* and, that *'the QL equation, as a didactic instrument is intended to be an aid to decision analysis, not an algorithmic guide to clinical action, or a quantitative, event-related index such as the Apgar Score or the Glasgow Trauma Scale'* (Shaw 1988).

In advocating treatment or in considering its withholding or withdrawal in cases where considerable ambiguity is present the doctor may have to counter the swings of undue optimism and pessimism that will affect members of the intensive-care team and their judgements, and which, inevitably, will affect and influence the parents during their many interactions at the side of the incubator or cot. It is generally accepted that there is a presumption in favour of life unless there is no benefit to the patient. Any decision to withdraw intensive treatment, **not** basic care, must be made only after repeated review of all the facts of diagnosis and prognosis, and usually after much agonizing by the staff and parents. These infants are investigated intensively, often by many specialists; they are attended night and day by skilled nurses in the presence of anxious and emotionally exhausted parents who cling to every word of hope for survival. From their hours in the unit, and from their many discussions with the staff, they become trapped on a 'roller-coaster' of alternating unrealistic optimism and black despair. They become well aware of the implications of such problems as 'massive bowel infarction', 'chronic lung disease', and above all, 'brain damage'. They recognize what devastating effects these and other complications could have on their infant's future life, and they, like the staff, eventually come to recognize that there must be a time to 'draw a line' at the continued use of various 'heroic' resuscitative and other intensive measures to maintain life.

It remains my view that the key decision-makers must be the doctor who is identified as being primarily responsible for the infant's care and the parents (Duff and Campbell 1976; Campbell *et al.* 1989). The parents and the other family members from whom they may seek advice will have the most intimate knowledge of their family's particular circumstances, their strengths and weaknesses, their values and preferences, and, perhaps most importantly, of how the realities of family life will affect the upbringing of the infant, and perhaps the other children. The physician's duty is to present as much information as possible to the parents to help them to participate in the decision, not to put them in the position of having to take it by themselves. This information, often complex and difficult, even for professionals to understand, must be presented to the parents in a usable form, and certainly on more than one occasion, leaving ample time and opportunity for questions and wide-ranging discussion. Apart from the content of the information, it must be recognized that the attitudes of the doctor and other members of staff will have a powerful influence on the parent's views. Critics frequently say that the final decision is really the physician's, and that it is a sham to pretend otherwise. They argue that, if quality of life is being used as a criterion, the infant's future will be decided, not on what seems best for the infant, but on the values of the doctor. Examples of this kind of paternalism undoubtedly exist, but are likely to be obvious, and should be exposed by the kind of decision-making process described above. The 'paternalism' of a partnership in decision-making in which parents, having been provided with the facts and options, nevertheless want the doctor to express a view on the best course of action, is important to medical decision-making in most countries. Parents expect doctors to have done their 'home-work' on the facts of the case, and *trust* their doctor to put the infant's interests first. Everywhere it remains a fundamental tenet of ethical medical practice that the advice given by a doctor must be 'patient-centred' and free from the doctor's personal prejudices. However, providing information of this kind in a totally non-directive manner is probably impossible in practice, and may even be a disservice to those patients who expect advice *and* opinion at times of need.

Achieving the right balance of decision-making between the doctor and family can be a very taxing part of the work in a neonatal unit. These are, and must remain as primarily *medical* decisions. Leaning too much towards doctor dominance is seen as excessively paternalistic, whereas leaving all the decision-making to the parents places an enormous burden on them unfairly, and may merely reflect the discomfort of a doctor keen to 'pass the buck'. Such a 'cop-out' leaves parents isolated with a lingering sense of guilt that the decision may have been wrong. In discussing this dilemma, Strong offers the 'infant advocate argument' in support of decision-making by physicians, and indicates his belief that '*how physicians balance their conflicting duties to an infant and to its parents is the central issue in the controversy over decision making in the neonatal intensive care unit, not paternalism*' (Strong 1984). He defends the view that the infant-advocate argument justifies unilateral decision-making by physicians in certain cases, and argues that parents should have a voice in life-or death decisions. '*whenever there is evidence to justify a belief that saving the infant's life would place a heavy burden on the family.*'

Thus the question 'What is the anticipated quality of life for this infant?' can be reframed as 'Does this baby have the capacity for development to an extent that will allow him or her to "have a life" and not just merely "be alive"?' (Rachels 1986). Giving thoughtful consideration to this question is an important component of any 'due process' of decision-making, and seems a sensitive and compassionate part of seeking a resolution to an extremely poignant tragedy for an infant and family. It is a parent-centred approach that gives due weight to the role of parents in determining the nurture and upbringing of their children and recognizes the need for latitude and tolerance in making responsible choices within the context of individual families (Duff and Campbell 1973).

Is it legal?

The Baby Doe legislation did not fundamentally alter the law of the United States in relation to the treatment of abnormal infants, but the media publicity and political opportunism that followed this case and others left American pediatricians feeling vulnerable to legal harassment and possible penalty if reported under the Child Abuse Amendments of 1984. There seems little doubt that 'legalization' of this difficult area of medical practice created a feeling of compulsion towards more aggressive treatment for all infants whatever their condition, their future quality of life, or the views of their parents.

It is not surprising, therefore, that some pediatricians have over-interpreted the Baby Doe 'Rules' to protect their own interests (Levin 1985; Kopelman *et al.* 1988); and in a commentary included with the report of the US Commission on Civil Rights (see above), it was pointed out that *'there is no evidence of significant undertreating of severely handicapped neonates since 1985. If anything there is evidence of overtreatment'* (Engelhardt 1989).

Since these treatment dilemmas became matters of public controversy and debate in the early 1970s, lawyers have warned doctors that their failure to treat infants may expose them, not only to accusations of child abuse, but perhaps even of murder or manslaughter. The law prohibits anyone's taking active steps to cause death, but remains in a state of some uncertainty on the issue of withholding treatment and allowing a patient to die. It was suggested that the practices described by Duff and Campbell in 1973 would be in violation of the criminal law in almost every State in the USA (Robertson 1975). Others have pointed out that there would not be any legal liability for a failure to act unless there was a duty to act in the first place—in other words, unless there was a legal duty to provide the treatment that was withheld. In Scotland, for example, the equivalent provisions deal with 'neglect', and it is submitted that if a doctor has done all that was reasonable in the circumstances, it is not neglect, and hence not a breach of duty, to allow an infant to die (Campbell and Cusine 1981).

In the past few years there have been a number of opportunities for the courts to pronounce upon these issues on each side of the Atlantic. Academic lawyers have generally condemned decisions involving quality of life judgements, (Kennedy 1988); yet a number of court decisions seem to be based explicitly on just such considerations (see also Chapter 11). In some cases at least, the courts seem to have recognized that advances in life-saving technology have outstripped medicine's capacity to ensure that the benefits of this technology will always outweigh the burdens. Like the doctors, the judges try to conduct a careful balancing exercise in determining the course of action that best serves the interests of the patient.

In the landmark American case of Karen Quinlan in New Jersey, the court made a specific quality of life judgement: *'If the hospital ethics committee or other consultative body agrees that there is no reasonable possibility of Karen's ever emerging from her present comatose condition to a cognitive, sapient state, the present life-support system may be withdrawn'* (Rhoden 1985). And in overturning the original Baby Doe regulations, Judge Gesell specifically referred to the quality of the infant's life: *'None of these sensitive considerations touching on the quality of the infant's expected life were even tentatively noted. No attempt was made to address the issue of whether termination of painful, intrusive medical treatment might be appropriate where an infant's clear prognosis is death within days or months or to specify the level of appropriate care in such futile cases.'* In New York State, in the case of Baby Doe and two others that came to various courts, the eventual outcomes were also consistent with the application of quality of life standards (Steinbock 1984).

The quality of life issue was also seen from a different perspective recently where the parent's request for the continuation of aggressive life-prolonging treatment for a quadriplegic, blind, and deaf child was refused by the doctors and nurses because they believed it was futile, inhumane, and against the child's best interests. *'The court acknowledged that no physician or institution can be required to provide an intervention contrary to conscience. The subsequent willingness of another physician to care for the infant as the parent wished does not alter the moral or legal status of the medical team's refusal. The primary obligation of health care providers remains 'Do no harm'* (Paris *et al.* 1990).

Although legal interventions and the introduction of 'rules' for medical decision-making have been more prominent in the United States, it was in the *United Kingdom* in 1981 that a paediatrician was accused, tried, and eventually acquitted of attempted murder following the death of an infant with Down syndrome. In that case, it was clear that quality of life was considered to be important in the medical decisions taken. In an earlier case similar to Baby Doe, also heard by the Court of Appeal in 1981, the local authority was authorized to direct that an operation be carried out against the wishes of the parents because there was no evidence that the infant's life was going to be intolerable or 'so demonstrably awful' (Re B 1981). In several recent judgments the Court of Appeal has indicated that there can be circumstances where the quality of life would be so intolerable that treatment, without which death would ensure, could be withheld even though the child was not dying.

In one case heard, only because the child was already a ward of court, by the Court of Appeal in 1989 treatment 'to relieve suffering' was authorized, but it was made clear **that it was for the responsible doctors** to decide if they should do anything to prolong the infant's life. The Court considered that it would be in the child's best interests to ease her suffering, pain, and distress 'rather than to achieve a short prolongation of her life' (Brahams 1989). In another, that of a 16-month-old child who was *not dying*, the Court of Appeal authorized the doctors to withhold life-saving measures like ventilation should a life-threatening crisis occur in the future; and indicated that it would not order a doctor to treat a patient if, in his clinical judgment, to do so would not be in the patient's best interests (Brahams 1992).

In 1983, an examination of quality of life and treatment decisions was conducted in *Canada* by the Law Reform Commission (Curran 1984). The commissioners felt that medical treatment of the incompetent patient should be discontinued only for very serious reasons, as the legal prescription in favour of life should always be recognized. They went on to assert that under the federal law *'the value of human life should be considered not only from a "quantitative" perspective but also from a "qualitative" viewpoint and that it should be legally justified to consider quality of life when making 'substituted consent' for incompetent, seriously ill patients.'* They also considered three alternative mechanisms or models for ensuring consent and protection for patients in such situations—the *judicial model*, the *family or guardian model*, and the *medical* model. The commission, composed of leading Canadian lawyers, came down firmly in favour of placing the primary responsibility for decision-making on the physician treating the patient, and indicated that there should be no criminal liability on physicians for their decisions provided they were made *'on reasonable medical grounds under the circumstances, in the best interests of the incompetent patient and in conformity with other standards set by criminal law.'*

A review of the legal position on each side of the Atlantic includes a plea for better guidelines: *'towards establishing norms of parental and medical conduct which would be approved in litigation whether this be civil or criminal in nature'* (Mason and Meyers 1986). The authors suggest that guidelines must give primacy to fostering and preserving the lives of the newborn, but point out that this is not an absolute concept. *'Quality of life—not in the sense of social utility or worth but solely as judged by a physiological existence without intolerable pain or suffering—may properly enter such treatment decisions.'*

INTERNATIONAL VARIATIONS

The debate about forgoing life-sustaining treatment has largely been confined to 'developed' countries with health and social services of varying comprehensiveness and quality. Yet even under these circumstances, cultural and socio-economic considerations as well as the family and social resources must play some part in decision-making. In interviews with parents of children with Down syndrome, the parents argued that the degree of handicap of the child was the crucial factor in making the decision; but, in fact, the social class of the parents themselves was the only variable that was statistically significantly related to their opinions (Shepperdson 1983). It is unrealistic to pretend that differences in the prospects for severely brain-damaged infants in different countries and different communities can simply be ignored. For example, compare the likely future of a tiny infant with multiple problems born to a 15 year old single-parent teenager with a drug problem from an inner-city ghetto to that of a similar infant from a stable marriage who can be discharged to a relatively affluent suburban home with access to the full range of health and supporting services.

The United States

The original Baby Doe 'rules' required that, for hospitals to qualify for Federal funds, medical decision-makers must ignore an infant's actual or potential impairment when deciding treatment if the treatment is likely to prolong life and would have been prescribed for an infant without the impairment. It is easy to see the sense of this requirement where the disability is relatively minor, or where the treatment is straightforward and obviously beneficial. But such a non-discrimination principle is too simplistic and unworkable, and makes little sense for situations where there is catastrophic brain abnormality or damage. The idea that doctors and parents can disregard all impairments, no matter how devastating, is unrealistic and appallingly insensitive to the needs of some infants and families, particularly when it is unlikely that they will be provided with adequate help and facilities for long-term care.

Following medical and legal challenges to the original Baby Doe 'Rules' more flexible and conciliatory guidelines were issued. These include phrases more open to broader interpretation, like 'virtually futile' and 'reasonable medical judgment'. The revised 'rules', perhaps unintentionally, also seem to depart from a rigid sanctity-of-life position in that they allow exceptions to treatment for dying patients (life may be shortened by not prolonging dying). Most importantly, even this legislation acknowledges the importance of quality of life by permitting 'non-treatment' for infants who are 'clinically and irreversibly comatose'. Nevertheless, the basic intention remains intact: i.e. future impairments are irrelevant, and therefore abnormal, disabled, and potentially handicapped infants must be given all the 'medically beneficial' treatments that would be provided for normal infants.

The absurdity of an inflexible position in extreme cases is obvious. The legislation seems to permit the withholding of treatment from infants with, for example, anencephaly, but only because they are classified as 'dying'. On the other hand treatment seems to be required, and perhaps is mandatory, for an infant who will never be conscious, but cannot be said to be dying. Most people would probably agree that treating such an infant aggressively is wrong *because* of the nature of the impairment, i.e. permanent unconsciousness, and its effect on the quality of life. In the threatening legal climate in which they now practise, it is inevitable that some American pediatricians feel obliged, if only to protect their own interests, to provide all treatments possible for every infant. In so doing they must simply ignore the devastating impairments that will have major consequences for some infants and their families. Consider an infant with trisomy 13 who is neither unconscious nor 'dying' in the usual sense of that term. Should this infant's other defects, such as cleft palate and heart defect, be repaired by perfectly straightforward and 'medically beneficial' operations? Should the infant's life be artificially prolonged by assisted ventilation just to comply with the 'rules', when the parents, the doctors, and the nurses all believe that there would be no lasting benefit for the infant? Or is it right to say that, in the best interests of this infant and others similar, *'to adequately assess benefit, the nature of the life being preserved cannot be ignored'* (Rhoden 1985).

There was considerable opposition even to the revised Baby Doe legislation, though this was a compromise eventually agreed by lawmakers, some professional organizations like the American Academy of Pediatrics, and representatives of various advocacy groups. *'As such the law completely pleased none of these groups but was believed to be more acceptable than potentially more restrictive legislation threatened by its congressional authors'* (Stahlman 1986). Dr. Stahlman, a distinguished and vastly experienced neonatologist, also pointed out that *'The worst feature of the Baby Doe legislation is that it takes away the most necessary ingredient of the ethical practice of medicine, the conscience and sense of responsibility of the physician to his patient, and gives it to a committee.'* A number of organizations that promote children's health and welfare, but who were not consulted, also expressed concern and their conviction that these medical and ethical dilemmas could not be resolved in the patient's interests within a framework of legally mandated behaviour, but should be considered on a case-by-case basis.

The United Kingdom

As was indicated earlier, cases similar to Baby Doe have come to the attention of the British courts, but they have not stimulated any sustained demand for legislative action, nor have they led to any clarification of the law. In occasional polls of public opinion, it seems to remain the general view that family tragedies involving treatment dilemmas about abnormal infants should remain private matters for doctors and parents to decide together. As a result, British doctors, as indicated in the judgments discussed earlier, continue to have considerable discretion in taking decisions about life-sustaining treatment, and there is general agreement that quality of life considerations play an important part (Campbell 1982; Whitelaw 1986; Walker 1988). As one British neonatologist expressed it recently: *'I do believe that there are circumstances, albeit very rare, when it is ethically acceptable to withdraw life support from a baby whose life might be saved only by further prolonged discomfiture of neonatal intensive care, and in whom it is probable that substantial neurodevelopmental or physical handicap will radically limit the child's ability to participate in human experience and will render him or her forever dependent on a caregiver for everyday living'* (Chiswick 1991).

Canada

The Bioethics Committee of the Canadian Pediatric Society has issued its own advice on the treatment of critically ill newborns and older children (Canadian Pediatric Society 1986). The guidelines stress that all children have a justified claim to life and therefore to such treatment as is necessary either to improve or to prolong life, but go on to point out that the capacity to prolong life is now so advanced that *'there is a real danger that the prolongation of life will become the sole end, irrespective of the havoc it may wreak on other persons or desirable goals. The decision to use life-prolonging treatment must be guided by the best interests of the child.'*

Listed exceptions to the general duty of providing life-sustaining treatment include *'when the patient's life will be filled with intolerable and intractable pain and suffering'*. Strangely absent from this list, in spite of the preamble noted above, is any reference to conditions of permanent unconsciousness or the inability to interact with others.

Australia

A survey of the attitudes and practices of Victorian obstetricians and pediatricians demonstrated widespread agreement that doctors need not attempt to sustain the life of every severely handicapped infant, and that quality of life played a part in decision-making. Only two pediatricians (out of 111) and no obstetrician thought that life should always be sustained by all available means. The life prospects for the infant weighed heavily in decisions about treatment. In responding to the question, *'Under what circumstances do you consider that less than a maximum effort should be made to preserve the life of an infant?'* It was clear that most doctors do not do as much to sustain life if the infant's life will be of very poor quality (Singer *et al.* 1983).

New Zealand

A study in 18 hospitals showed that pediatricians gave consideration to the degree of disability, the disabled infant's future quality of life, and the family's quality of life in making decisions whether or not to provide treatment (Mitchell 1986). However most made it clear that the family's quality of life either was not important or was too unreliable a factor to merit much consideration. One commented: *'I do not find that the family's quality of life is a reliable factor because of the family's extraordinary coping strengths, out of all proportion to expectation.'*

The Netherlands

A recent report from the Dutch Society of Pediatrics entitled 'Medical action in neonatology' indicates that pediatricians in the Netherlands must take into account the expected quality of life when they consider whether to prolong the life of a seriously handicapped newborn baby (*British Medical Journal* 1992). Should the infant's life be judged 'non-livable', then the doctor, in close collaboration with the parents, with colleagues and with nursing staff may discontinue the treatment. Five criteria are used to test if the life of a baby is 'non-livable'. These are:

(1) the ability in later life to communicate verbally and non-verbally;
(2) the ability to look after oneself;
(3) the degree of dependence on medical support;
(4) the degree of suffering now and in the future; and
(5) the life expectancy.

The report states that a decision based on these criteria must be taken only with the greatest possible care. In the bigger Dutch hospitals these decisions are evaluated by the ethics committee, and the district public prosecutor may also be consulted. There is said to be a 'large degree of consensus' about these guidelines, but growing controversy about what to do with the babies who have very poor prospects but who are 'able to stay alive without medical action'. About 'active non-voluntary euthanasia in children there is no consensus in the Netherlands' (Visser *et al* 1992). Legally, if death is intended, it has to be categorized as unnatural, and will be investigated by the public prosecutor.

While acknowledging the pitfalls and dangers of subjective assessments made on behalf of a patient, most paediatricians in these developed countries, and probably in many others, recognize the importance of quality of life in this context, and believe it to be an appropriate part of responsible decision-making in the best interests of severely impaired infants and their families.

PROTECTIONS AGAINST BAD CHOICES

With such a complex interplay of attitudes in the emotional maelstrom that surrounds the tragedy of abnormal birth, it is inevitable that bad choices will occasionally result. The vast majority will be obvious, particularly as they are now usually made in large public institutions like teaching hospitals, and only rarely in the privacy of the home or a small hospital where there might be ignorance of modern advances in treatment and some lack of sensitivity to the current ethical 'climate'. Within major hospitals and especially within Intensive Care Units there is increasing consultation with a wide range of specialists who are up-to-date on new opportunities for successful medical and surgical management. In such a setting it is unusual to have to make these decisions in a hurry. In any setting, 'snap judgments' on quality of life criteria must be avoided.

The increasing complexity of decision-making itself provides some protection against bad choices, though, perhaps inevitably, moves to make the decision-making process more bureaucratic and more complex have created further problems and difficulties that have not necessarily been in the best interests of the patients that they were designed to protect. So many people may be involved that there can be serious delay in coming to a decision; and there are times when some decision is urgently needed. For example, referral of a difficult problem to the hospital infant Bioethics Committee, as currently practised in the United States, may compound delays unless the committee (or some key members) is organized to respond urgently to ethical emergencies at short notice. In a few hospitals these committees do not seem to be restricted to providing a broader forum for debate, or for setting policies and giving advice. They have taken on, or have been given, the responsibility for actually making critical decisions on difficult individual cases. Agreement, or even a consensus, may become impossible, so that, at best, the situation may be allowed to 'drift' in spite of the best efforts and good intentions of most members. At worst, particularly if there are legal or political implications, the interests of the infant may become secondary to the interests of committee members or the institution (Campbell 1992).

Perhaps the greatest protection for infants lies within the families themselves. The majority of parents have developed a strong attachment to their infant by the time of birth. Parents may think of the growing fetus as a member of the family long in advance of birth, although reluctant to 'tempt fate' by investing too many hopes early in pregnancy. To the mother in particular, the fetus is cherished as part of herself *and* as a 'person', however a philosopher or lawyer might define 'personhood'! The onset of fetal movements and other signs of the developing child create strong bonds that are reflected most poignantly in the acute grief experienced by mothers at the death of an unborn fetus and their resentment when they experience the callous and insensitive way in which hospital staff and others can sometimes react to the birth of a stillborn baby. In the neonatal period too, because their infant is very much a precious 'person' to them, they find it particularly difficult to countenance any decision to withhold or withdraw life-sustaining treatment. Yet it is precisely their concern for the kind of life that their infant will experience *as a person* that makes them willing to share in such an important but agonizing responsibility.

An infant's life has inherent value and dignity regardless of potential; but in the face of some of the worst injustices of faulty development, it seems wrong to most parents when so-called 'pro-life' groups call such decisions discriminatory, and insist that every infant has an absolute 'right to life', whatever the quality. It is particularly galling when families are subjected to intimidatory tactics and strident propaganda by lobbyists ignorant of the facts and the reasons behind particular decisions. These self-righteous moralists also do not have to live with the consequences. As it was cogently expressed by McCormick 'We *must avoid* **unjust** discrimination in the provision of health care and life-supports. But not all discrimination (inequality of treatment) is unjust. **Unjust** discrimination is avoided if decision making centers on the benefit to the patient, even if that benefit is described largely in terms of quality of life criteria' (McCormick 1978).

There are infants with abnormalities so severe that few, if any, with accurate knowledge would insist that life-sustaining treatment be continued. On the other hand there are infants with distressing but relatively minor problems where the vast majority, if not all, would agree that vigorous treatment is always indicated. Within this spectrum of abnormality or damage, there will always be some infants for whom no medical (or societal) consensus on the best course of action will emerge even after exhaustive debate. It is with these infants and children that the particularly difficult and controversial decisions arise, because so much depends on where 'a line is drawn' and who draws it. *'Lest patients in such "gray" areas be sustained coercively beyond a point at which many competent patients would say "halt", parents in consultation with physicians and possibly overseen by court review should be allowed some prudential leeway for interpreting a patient's best interest in context'* (Sparks 1988).

REFERENCES

Alberman, E. and Botting, B. (1991). Trends in prevalence and survival of very low birth weight infants, England & Wales: 1983–7. *Archives of Disease in Childhood*, **66**: 1304–8.

Brahams, D. (1989). Medicine and the law: Court of Appeal endorses medical decision to allow baby to die. *Lancet*, **1**, 969–70.

Brahams D. (1992). Life-sustaining treatment for brain-damaged child. *Lancet*, **339**: 1472–3.

British Medical Journal (1992). Dutch issue guidelines on handicapped babies. *British Medical Journal*, **305**: 1312–13.

Britton, S. B., Fitzhardinge, P. M., and Ashby, S. (1981). Is intensive care justified for infants weighing less than 801 gm at birth? *Journal of Pediatrics*, **99**: 937–43.

Campbell, A. G. M. (1982). Which infants should not receive intensive care? *Archives of Disease in Childhood*, **57**: 569–71.

Campbell, A. G. M. (1992). Baby Doe and forgoing life-sustaining tratment: compassion, discrimination or medical neglect? *In Compelled compassion (ed. Caplan A. L., Blank, R. H., and Merrick, J. C.), pp. 207–36 Humana Press*, Totowa, New Jersy.

Campbell, A. G. M. and Cusine D. J. (1981). On the death of a baby, Commentary 2. *Journal of Medical Ethics*, **7**: 13–18.

Campbell, A. G. M. Lloyd, D. G. and Duffty, P. (1988). Treatment dilemmas in neonatal care: Who should survive and who should decide? *Annals of the New York Academy of Sciences*, **530**: 92–103.

Canadian Paediatric Society (1986). Treatment decisions for infants and children. *Canadian Medical Association Journal*, **135**: 447–8.

Chiswick, M. L. (1991). Ethical considerations of starting and stopping life support in newborn babies. *Pediatrics in Europe*, **1**: 17–19.

Copley, M. F. and Bodensteiner, J. B. (1987). Chronic sorrow in families of disabled children. *Journal of Child Neurology*, *2: 67–70*.

Curran, W. J. (1984). Quality of life and treatment decisions: the Canadian Law Reform Report. *New England Journal of Medicine*, **310**: 297–8.

Duff, R. S. and Campbell, A. G. M. (1973). Moral and Ethical Dilemmas in the Special Care Nursery. *New England Journal of Medicine*, **289**: 890–4.

Duff R. S.and Campbell, A. G. M.(1976). On Deciding the care of severely handicapped or dying persons: with particular reference to infants. *Pediatrics*, **57**: 487–93.

Engelhardt, H. T. Jr. (1989). Comments on the recommendations regarding Section 504 of the Rehabilitation Act of 1973 and the Child Abuse Amendments of 1984. In *US Commission on Civil Rights: medical discrimination against children with disabiliteis, pp. 158–65. Government Printing Office.* Washington, DC.

Escobar, G. J., Littenberg, B., and Petiti, D. B. (1991). Outcome among surviving very low birth weight infants: a meta–analysis. *Archives of Disease in Childhood*, **66**: 204–11.

Fenton, A. C. Field, D. J. Mason, E., and Clarke, M. (1990). Attitudes to viability of preterm infants and their effect on figures for perinatal mortality. *British Medical Journal*, **300**: 434–6.

Fost, N. (1981). Counseling families who have a child with a severe congenital anomaly. *Pediatrics*, **67**: 321–4.

Hack, M. and Fanaroff, A. A. (1989). Outcomes of extremely low birth weight infants between 1982 and 1988. *New England Journal of Medicine*, **321**: 1642–7.

Hastings Center (1987*a*). Guidelines on the termination of life-sustaining treatment and the care of the dying. *Hastings Center, Briarcliff Manor, New York*.

Hastings Center (1987*b*). Report of the Hastings Center Project on Imperiled Newborns. *Hastings Center Report*, **17**(6): 5–32.

Joint Policy Statement (issued by the American Academy of Pediatrics) (1984) Principles of treatment of disabled infants. *Pediatrics* **73**: 559–60.

Kennedy, I. (1988). Treat me right: essays in medical law and ethics. *Clarendon Press, Oxford pp. 144–5*

Kopelman, L. M. Irons, T. G. and Kopelman, A. E. (1988). Neonatologists judge the "Baby Doe" regulations. *New England Journal of Medicine*, **318**: 677–83.

Lancet (1992). Editorial: Clinical management of Trisomy 18. *Lancet*, **339**: 904.

Levin, B. W. (1985). Consensus and controversy in the treatment of catastrophically ill newborns. In, *Which babies shall live? (ed. T. H. Murray and A. L Caplan) pp.169–205. Humana Press, Clifton New Jersy*.

Lorber J. (1971). Results of treatment of myelomeningocele. *Developmental Medicine and Child Neurology*, **279**: 299–301.

Lubchenco, L. O. Horner, F. A. Reed, L. H., Hix, I. E., Metcalf, D. ,Cohig, R. Elliott, H. C. and Bourg, M. (1963). Sequelae of premature birth. *American Journal of Diseases of Children*, **106**: 101–15.

McCormick, R. A. (1974). To save or let die: the dilemma of modern medicine. *Journal of the American Medical Association*, **229**: 172–176.

McCormick, R. A. (1978). The quality of life, the sanctity of life. *Hastings Center Report*, **8**: 1 (February) 30–6.

Mason, J. K. and Meyers, D. W. (1986). Parental choice and selective non-treatment of deformed newborns: a view from mid-Atlantic. *Journal of Medical Ethics*, **12**: 67–71.

Mitchell, D. R. (1986). Medical treatment of severely impaired infants in New Zealand hospitals. *New Zealand Medical Journal* **99**: 364–8.

Paris, J. J. Crone, R. K. and Reardon, F. (1990). Physician's refusal of requested treatment. The case of Baby L. *New England Journal of Medicine*, **322**: 1012–14.

Rachels, J. (1986). *The end of life: euthanasia and morality. Oxford University Press.*

Re B (a minor) (1981). *Weekly Law Reports* 1421 CA.

Rhoden, N. K. (1985). Treatment dilemmas for imperiled newborns: why quality of life counts. *Southern California Law Review*, **58**, 6: 1283–1347.

Rist, J. M. (1982). *Human value: a study in ancient philosophical ethics.* Brill, Leiden, The Netherlands.

Robertson, J. A. (1975). Involuntary euthanasia of defective newborns: a legal analysis. *Stanford Law Review*, **27**: 213–69.

Shaw A. (1973). Dilemmas of "informed consent" in children. *New England Journal of Medicine*, **289**: 885–90.

Shaw. A. (1977). Defining the quality of life: a formula without numbers. *Hastings Center Report*, **7**, 5(October): 11.

Shaw. A. (1988). QL revisited. *Hastings Center Report*, **18**, 2 (May): 10–12.

Shepperdson, B. (1983). Abortion and euthanasia of Down's syndrome children—the parents' views. *Journal of Medical Ethics*, **9**: 152–7.

Silverman, W. A. (1981). Mismatched attitudes about neonatal death. *Hastings Center Report*, **11** (6): 12–16.

Simms, M. (1986). Informed dissent: the views of some young mothers of severely mentally handicapped young adults. *Journal of Medical Ethics*, **12**: 72–4.

Singer, P. Kuhse, H. and Singer, C. (1983). The treatment of newborn infants with major handicaps. *The Medical Journal of Australia*, **2**: 274–8.

Sparks, R. C. (1988). To treat or not to treat: Bioethics and the handicapped newborn. *Paulist Press, New York.*

Stahlman, M. T. (1986). Medical ethics and the law. *Pediatric Research*, **20**: 913–14

Steinbock, B. (1984). Baby Jane Doe in the courts. *Hastings Center Report*, **14**, 1(February): 13–19

Strong, C. (1984). The neonatologist's duty to patient and parents. *Hastings Center Report*, **14**, 4 (August): 10–16.

US Commission on Civil Rights (1989). *Medical discrimination against children with disabilities. Government Printing Office, Washington DC.*

Visser, H. K. A. Aartsen, H. G. M. DeBeaufort, I. D. (1992).Medical decisions concerning the end of life in children in the Netherlands. *American Journal of Diseases of Children,* **146**: 1429–31.

Walker, C. H. M. (1988). Current topic—"officiously to keep alive". *Archives of Disease in Childhood,* **63**: 560–4.

Whitelaw, A. (1986). Death as an option in newborn intensive care. *Lancet,* **2**: 328–331.

4B QUALITY OF LIFE AS A DECISION-MAKING CRITERION II

Helga Kuhse

Introduction

Professor A. G. M. Campbell puts it well when he suggests that quality-of-life judgments, far from being viciously discriminatory, are a necessary ingredient of a patient-centered approach to medical decision-making at the beginning of life. To ignore quality-of-life considerations, he says,

is to ignore the practical realities of caring for infants with catastrophic impairments, devalues the importance of compassion in medical decision-making and reduces the doctor's role to that of a technician seduced by modern treatment imperatives and blind to, or uncaring about, the possible adverse consequences for infant and family. (p. 83)

In this companion piece, I shall agree with much that Professor Campbell has to say. Whilst there will be some substantive disagreement between us on what a patient-centered quality-of-life approach entails, the main aim of my paper is not to highlight areas of agreement or disagreement, but to sharpen the focus on the central issue raised by Professor Campbell: the connection between quality-of-life judgments and a patient-centered treatment perspective.

In passing, I shall also comment on the claim by the US Commission on Civil Rights, referred to by Professor Campbell with a sense of outrage (pp. 82–3), that the practice of allowing some severely impaired infants to die constitutes invidious discrimination against the handicapped, akin to racism or sexism.[1]

Quality of life vs. Sanctity of life

There is a school of thought—I want to call it the 'sanctity-of-life view'—which rejects quality-of-life considerations as a criterion for medical decision-making. According to the sanctity-of-life view, all human lives, regardless of their quality or kind, are equally valuable and inviolable. Consistently applied, the sanctity-of-life view would entail that life and death decisions, in the practice of medicine, must not be based on the quality or kind of life in question.

The sanctity-of-life view locates the value of life in human life *qua* human life, that is, in the continued existence of a human organism. The other approach—the 'quality-of-life' view—locates the value of human life in some valuable characteristic or characteristics, such as self-consciousness, rationality, the capacity to relate to others, the ability to experience pleasurable states of consciousness, and so on.[2]

I share with Professor Campbell the view that the 'sanctity-of-life' view is an implausible ethical doctrine. It has a philosophically unsound basis and, consistently applied, would require health-care professionals to prolong the lives of all patients with equal vigour—even if their doing so would not be in, or would be contrary to, the patient's best interests.

Whilst the sanctity-of-life view has long shaped traditional western religious and moral thinking and has had a profound influence on the law,[3] practising doctors have largely rejected the view that they have a duty to prolong life as such. Rather, doctors have generally taken the view that they have a primary duty to act in their patients' best interests.

Professor Campbell's approach to the treatment of severely impaired newborn infants is no exception. His overall account and repeated reference to the 'infant's (best) interests' suggests that he understands a 'quality of life' approach as one which focuses first and foremost on the best interests of the infant, although he also acknowledges that the family's interests must not be ignored in such cases.

As things stand, there is an unresolved tension between Professor Campbell's patient-centered 'best interest' approach and his apparent desire not to ignore the interests of the family unit. After all, there might well be a conflict between the interests of a family to structure their lives unencumbered by the heavy burden that caring for a severely impaired infant may impose, and the infant's putative 'right to life', or interest in survival. A consistently applied 'best interests' standard would be oblivious of the interests of the family, that is, of the negative effects the infant's survival might have on the parents, or on any of the other members of the family.

I shall set this problem aside for the moment, but will return to it later. First, I want to examine the rather slippery notion of decision-making 'in the infant's best interests'.

'In the infant's best interests'

For the purposes of our subsequent discussion, we should explicitly note a somewhat obvious point: when we are discussing quality-of-life criteria to justify decisions to provide or to forgo life-sustaining treatment, we are in fact speaking about criteria that will determine which infants will live and which infants will die. Put in terms of an approach that attempts to locate the right-or wrong-making features of such treatment decisions in the infant's best interests, this entails that a non-treatment decision is right when it is in the infant's best interests, and wrong when it is not. In other words, in all those cases where a decision is made to allow an infant to die, it must be the case that death, and not continued life, is in the infant's best interests.

Now, one might want to debate the question of whether we can ever rationally choose death, or whether death can ever be in a patient's best interest. I shall, however, not enter this debate here. For the purposes of our discussion, I shall take it as given that there are *some* lives so impoverished or filled with pain and suffering that it would be rational, and in a patient's best interests, to choose death.[4]

In suggesting that non-treatment is sometimes in an infant's best interests, Professor Campbell seems to agree. So does the prestigious American President's Commission. After advocating, in its much-discussed report *Deciding to forego life-sustaining treatment*[5] the 'best interests standard' for the treatment of severely disabled infants, the Commission accepts that there are some disabilities and impairments so severe 'that continued existence would not be a net benefit to the infant'.[6]

Now, if there are some conditions when it is in a severely impaired infant's interest to die, then it seems clearly wrong to label such practices viciously discriminatory. Whilst doctors and parents, in allowing these infants to die, use 'discrimination' to distinguish between infants that should be treated and those that should not, they are doing so on the basis of the morally relevant criterion of whether or not continued life is in the infant's best interests. This type of discrimination is required by morality, not condemned by it. It is clearly different from, for example, racism or sexism, which is based on the morally irrelevant consideration of the colour of a person's skin, or her sex.

But even if there is, *pace* the Commission on Civil Rights, agreement that it is *sometimes* morally proper to use quality-of-life considerations as the basis for allowing a severely impaired infant to die, there is no agreement as to when this is the case. This disagreement is not merely a matter of prognostic uncertainty about the severity of particular medical conditions or the probability of successful medical interventions, but also, and more fundamentally, a matter of peoples' differing interpretations of how the term 'the infant's best interests' should be understood.

There are two main approaches that I want to discuss. One approach, that advocated by the previously mentioned US President's Commission, understands 'best interests' in terms of the infant's 'well-being'. On this account, continued existence is thought to be in an infant's best interests if the infant's future life is likely to contain a positive balance of benefits over burdens. The second account, that apparently advocated by Professor Campbell, places primary importance on the infant's potential for mental development. On this cognitivist account, mere 'well-being' does not appear to be enough. Rather, there must also be a reasonably intact brain, which will allow the infant to 'have a life', rather than merely 'be alive' (p. 84)[7]. In other words, and if I understand Professor Campbell correctly, the infant must ordinarily have the potential to develop (some of) the characteristically human cognitive capacities possessed by normal adults—

rationality, self-consciousness, the capacity to relate to others, a sense of the past and the future, and so on.[8]

There are important differences between the approaches advocated by the President's Commission and by Professor Campbell. As we shall see, they will give rise to sometimes incompatible life-and-death decisions for certain categories of impaired infants. Moreover, both approaches have their own difficulties. In addition to that, they do, however, also share a common problem: neither approach can account for, or anticipate, how a surviving and mentally competent patient will judge the quality of his or her life. This problem, I shall suggest below, points to a more fundamental difficulty in both 'best interests' approaches to medical decision-making at the beginning of life. There is no connection between the 'best interests' of the infant and the 'best interests' of the older competent person into whom the infant may grow.

Interests and consciousness

The US President's Commission and to some extent also Professor Campbell (see below) rely on a close link between interests and affective states of consciousness. Patients have interests because they are capable of experiencing certain pleasant and unpleasant mental states. This applies to infants as well. Like all conscious beings, infants have an interest in well-being, that is, in experiencing positive mental states, such as pleasure and well-being, rather than states characterized by pain and discomfort.

A life in which there is a net balance of well-being over pain and suffering is, according to the President's Commission, in the infant's best interests. A life in which pain and suffering predominate is contrary to the infant's best interests.

Professor Campbell's 'best interests' account is more difficult to capture. Whilst he suggests that there is a link between an infant's 'best interests' and 'the infant's capacity for future health, development, and well-being' (p. 84), he seems to place primary emphasis not on 'well-being' as an affective mental state, but rather on the infant's capacity for cognitive development. He repeatedly suggests that 'brain damage' is a reason for non-treatment (pp. 86, 87–8) , whilst 'multiple abnormalities', without evidence 'that the brain is abnormal or has suffered major damage', do not ordinarily constitute an adequate reason for non-treatment (p. 86).

The approach advocated by the President's Commission thus locates the infant's best interests in 'well-being', whilst Professor Campbell's approach places primary emphasis on the infant's 'cognitive potential'.

Which approach is the correct one? The answer is important because it will give rise to different treatment decisions for certain groups of infants.

Whose point of view?

When seeking to define criteria for a patient-centered quality-of-life approach to medical decision-making at the beginning of life, it will not be long before the question of the appropriate point of view will be raised. Should we judge matters from our point of view, that is, the point of view of the rational adult, or should we judge matters from the perspective of the impaired infant?

A respectable philosophical tradition has it that we should, in such circumstances, put ourselves into the other's shoes. Only then will we be able to properly evaluate and consider the interests at stake.[9] The President's Commission agrees. To adopt the perspective of the rational adult, the Commission notes, may well be prejudicial to a proper evaluation of the interests of the infant.[10] After all, what may look like a misfortune from our present perspective, may not be a misfortune when judged from another. One of Thomas Nagel's examples illustrates the point:

Suppose an intelligent person receives a brain injury that reduces him to the mental condition of a contented infant, and that such desires as remain to him can be satisfied by a custodian, so that he is free from care. Such a development would be widely regarded as a severe misfortune, not only for his friends and relations, or for society, but also, and primarily, for the person himself. The intelligent adult who has been *reduced* to this condition is the subject of the misfortune. He is the one we pity, though of course he does not mind his condition.[11]

In other words, whilst you, the reader, and I might well regard it as a great misfortune if illness or accident were to reduce our mental capacity irreversibly to that of an infant, and whilst *we* might under the circumstances prefer death over such an impoverished existence, it does not follow that such an existence is a misfortune for, or contrary to the best interests of, an infant.[12]

This raises a problem for cognitive best-interests accounts, including that advocated by Professor Campbell. For whilst it may be true that parents and doctors regard severe 'brain damage' as a particularly serious defect in an infant, which, in their view, warrants non-treatment (pp. 86, 87–8) it does not follow that brain-damaged existence is contrary to the best interests of the infant.

Professor Campbell acknowledges that 'quality-of-life'-based criteria of decision-making have been criticized on the grounds 'that the infant's future will be decided, not on what seems best for the infant, but on the values of the doctor'. (p. 90) He also acknowledges that it will be difficult for doctors to offer advice which is entirely free from personal prejudices, but then goes on to say that it 'remains a fundamental tenet of ethical medical practice that the advice given by a doctor must be "patient-centered"' (p. 91).

In focusing on cognitive potential, rather than on an infant's well-being, Professor Campbell does, however, not seem to adopt a patient-centered approach. After all, an infant who is able to experience affective conscious states, such as pleasure or pain, might be said to have an interest in experiencing pleasure and in not experiencing pain. It might also be said to have an interest in continued existence if its future life is likely to contain more pleasure than pain, irrespective of its potential for cognitive development. This lends an initial credence to the view that 'well-being', as advocated by the President's Commission, rather than 'cognitive potential', as advocated by Professor Campbell, is the appropriate best-interests standard to adopt.

If this conclusion were correct, it would also seem to follow that the charge of 'discrimination', levelled by the US Commission on Civil Rights against the practice of allowing some severely impaired infants to die, might well be justified—at least in all those cases where this decision is based solely on the infant's mental impairment and lack of cognitive potential, rather than on the 'best interests' approach advocated by the President's Commission. But we should not too readily embrace this conclusion.

It is true that in focusing on the infant's well-being as the basis for its 'best interests' approach, the President's Commission has clearly identified a criterion that is morally significant. It matters, morally speaking, whether an infant's life (or, indeed, the life of any other conscious being) is likely to be characterized by states of well-being, or by pain and discomfort. Whether that being also has the potential for cognitive development is a separate question. As Jeremy Bentham so aptly put it some two centuries ago when considering the interests of non-human animals who lacked distinctly human cognitive capacities, 'The question is not, Can they *reason*? nor, Can they *talk*? but, can they *suffer*?[13]

Jeremy Bentham was, however, not concerned with arguing that non-human animals, on account of their capacity to experience painful and pleasant states of consciousness, have a 'right to life', or an interest in their own continued existence. Rather, Bentham was focusing on the question of 'moral standing'.[14] A being's capacity to experience pleasurable and painful states of consciousness, he was arguing, is a morally relevant capacity which affords those beings entry into the moral sphere, making them 'morally considerable' in their own right.[15] But, to be morally considerable or to have moral standing is not, as we shall see, the same as having an interest in one's own continued existence, or a 'right to life'.

I shall return to this fundamental point in a later section of this paper. First, I want to show where a consistently applied 'best interests' standard, as advocated by the President's Commission, would lead in practice.

Well-Being

Take the following 'worst-case' scenario, described by John Robertson: A profoundly retarded, non-ambulatory, blind, and deaf infant spends the few years of his life in the back-ward cribs of a state institution. Whilst many people would probably want to say that continued existence is not in such an infant's best interests, this point is denied by Robertson. Such a child, Robertson contends, is so different from us—and has such different desires and wants—that we can't be sure that life might not, after all, be in the infant's best interests.[16]

Robertson is correct. Provided such a severely retarded infant is not experiencing physical pain, it is difficult to reach the conclusion that non-treatment is justified on the grounds that the infant would be 'better off dead'. As John Arras notes, if we imagine that the child were able to take part in a dialogue, he might admit that his back-ward existence isn't much, but then go on to say that [1]It's better than nothing. They feed me, change me, occasionally cuddle me. And I'm not in any pain to speak of. So why not just play out the meager hand that I've been dealt?'[17]

Whilst an infant or older retarded child is not, of course, capable of such thought-processes, this imagined dialogue shows that even a very marginal existence need not be contrary to an infant's best interests. Similar reasoning can be applied to many other apparently hopeless medical conditions as well—for example trisomy 13 or 18. Whilst Professor Campbell rejects aggressive treatment in these cases on the grounds that 'no real benefit for the patient will result' (p. 87), the account advocated by the President's Commission might well lead to a different conclusion. Provided the infant does experience a net balance of benefits over burdens over the admittedly short span of its life, continued existence would, on this criterion, still be in the 'infant's best interests', and it would be wrong to withhold life-sustaining treatment, until and unless the point were reached where future burdens would predictably outweigh future benefits.

Something seems to have gone terribly wrong in the Commission's exclusive focus on the impaired infant's 'well-being'. What this account suggests is that the infant's simple interest in experiencing the occasional cuddle, the satisfaction of being fed and changed perhaps, counts for as much or more than the generally more complex interests of all those affected by its birth and care. This conclusion is not only counterintuitive, but also, as I shall later suggest, ethically unsound.

Professor Campbell would certainly want to agree that the family's interests ought to play a role in medical decision-making (pp. 99–100). He might, however, also want to argue that the exclusive focus on 'well-being' was flawed right from the start. After all, a supporter of the cognitive-potential approach might say, the presence or absence of such characteristics as the capacity to think, to communicate, to act autonomously and morally, to relate to others, and so on, is also highly relevant from the moral point of view, and must be regarded as a necessary and perhaps sufficient condition for the provision of life-sustaining treatment.[18]

But there is, as we shall see, a serious problem that must be confronted by anyone who believes that the 'best interests' approach can be grounded in an infant's cognitive potential.

Cognitive potential

If an infant is severely mentally impaired and will never become a competent adult person, there is a continuity of interests across the infant's, the child's, and the adult's lifespan. The infant's and adult's interests are exhausted by the President's Commission's criterion of well-being. The infant and adult has an interest in experiencing pleasurable states of consciousness and an interest in not experiencing unpleasant ones.

When it comes to infants who have the capacity for cognitive development, however, things become much more difficult. There is a morally significant break between the simple interests of the infant, and the more complex interests of the competent older child and adult, which include an interest in self-determination and the autonomous structuring of one's life. Whether a competent but severely physically impaired person will or will not find her quality of life acceptable will not only (and sometimes not at all) depend on whether she experiences a considerable degree of pain and discomfort, but also on her own perception of what the 'good life' for human beings entails, and on whether such a life is open to her.

This means that 'quality of life', understood as 'well-being' and/or 'cognitive potential', is a poor predictor of whether continued life is or is not in a future adult person's best interests.

Some severely physically impaired survivors regard their lives as very much worthwhile. Writing in the *Journal of Medical Ethics*, Mrs Alison Davies thus notes that according to a recently proposed bill, advocating law reform for the selective non-treatment of severely impaired infants, she should have been allowed to die when an infant, on account of the potential quality of her life:

I am 28 years old, and suffer from severe physical disability which is irreversible. I was born with myelomeningocele spina bifida.

I have suffered considerable and prolonged pain from time to time and have undergone over 20 operations thus far, some of them essential to save my life. Even now my health is at best uncertain. I am doubly incontinent and confined to a wheelchair and thus, according to the bill, I should have 'no worthwhile quality of life'.

... My parents were encouraged to leave me in the hospital and 'go home and have another', I owe my life to the fact that they refused to accept the advice of the experts.

Despite my disability, I went to an ordinary school and then to university, where I gained an honours degree in sociology. I now work full-time defending the right to life of handicapped people. Who could say that I have 'no worthwhile quality of life'? I am sure that no doctor could have predicted that despite my physical problems, I would lead such a full and happy life.[19]

Alison Davies is correct when she suggests that it is very difficult, if not impossible, for doctors to pre-judge the quality of life of a severely physically disabled but mentally competent adult. Not everyone who once was a severely impaired infant agrees that his or her life should have been prolonged at the time. Some survivors believe that the physical pain and suffering they were made to endure whilst an infant or child was so severe that their future life cannot make up for it.[20] Others believe that certain non-medical criteria, such as parental love and support, are essential for a satisfactory quality of life. As Anne McDonald, suffering from a severe form of cerebral palsy, has put it: 'I could have had a happy life despite my disabilities if I had been loved ...I love the life I now lead, even though I am severely disabled. However, I still believe I should have been killed rather than being locked away [in a state institution] for fourteen years.'[21]

Accounts such as these suggest that it may not always be unjust or viciously discriminatory to allow a severely impaired infant to die—at least not if one takes seriously the views of those who believe that they should have been allowed to die when they were still infants. On the contrary, to keep such an infant alive would fail to take seriously the best interests of the future adult.

But what about those severely physically impaired survivors who are now grateful that their lives were sustained whilst they were still infants? Would it, for example, have been discriminatory and unjust to allow Alison Davies to die, given that she is now glad to be alive? One might initially think that the answer must be 'yes'. I do, however, want to reject the conclusion that one can speak of 'discrimination' in such cases.

The reason is not merely that cognitive potential and physical well-being are less-than-perfect predictors of a person's future quality of life (which entails that we cannot always predict how a survivor will judge our efforts to keep her alive whilst still a severely impaired infant), it is also— and much more fundamentally—that the infant does not as yet have the perspective, and interests, of the future adult. This means that we are making quality-of-life judgments for someone who, in one sense of the term, does not as yet exist.

This brings me to the fundamental philosophical reason for my rejection of both Professor Campbell's and the President's Commission's understanding of the 'best interests' standard in terms of either well-being and/or cognitive potential.

AN ALTERNATIVE ACCOUNT[22]

Interests and the direct wrongness of actions

I believe that the question of how we ought, morally, to treat severely impaired infants cannot ultimately be answered satisfactorily in isolation from such fundamental philosophical questions as: What makes human life valuable? and Why is it wrong to take human life, but not wrong (or not as wrong) to take the lives of other living things, such as chickens, pigs, trees, or cabbages? Before we have given an answer to questions such as these, we are lacking an adequate foundation for discussing such issues as abortion, euthanasia, and the forgoing of life-sustaining treatment on the one hand, and the killing of non-human animals and other living things on the other[23].

Let us approach the issue in the following way. Many people hold the following intuitions: It is wrong to kill an adult person who wants to go on living, but it is not wrong, or not as wrong, to kill a wide range of non-human animals for a variety of human purposes. People also believe that it is very wrong wantonly to torture, say, a kitten; but not wrong, or not as wrong, painlessly to kill a kitten. Why should this be so? An ethics focusing on the interests of different human and non-human beings can make sense of these widely held intuitions.

The philosopher Michael Tooley has provided an appropriate ethical framework.[24] He believes that the wrongness of an action is related to the extent to which the action prevents some interests, desires, or preferences from being fulfilled. This basic principle explains both why it is *directly* wrong (i.e., a wrong done to the being) to inflict pain, and why it is *directly* wrong to kill a being who has a desire to go on living. Any being capable of feeling pain can have a desire that the pain cease; but only a being capable of understanding that it is a 'continuing self' can have a desire to go on living. Tooley suggests that we reserve the term 'person' for those beings who are continuing selves, and I shall from now on follow this example.

If neither, say, kittens or fetuses are persons, this can explain why it is not directly wrong to kill them painlessly. Kittens and fetuses are not the kinds of beings who can desire their continued existence. It also explains why it is directly wrong to kill a person, or torture a kitten(or a fetus capable of experiencing pain): the killing thwarts the person's desire to go on living; and the torturing thwarts the desire of the kitten (or fetus) that the pain cease.

This has direct implications for the practice of medicine, not only as far as the morality of directly ending a patient's life is concerned (a point to which I shall return later), but also when it comes to the *prolongation* of life. If we ask why it is normally a good thing to extend the life of a person, the answer is clear: because the person values her own life and desires her own continued existence. (It also explains why it is *not* directly wrong to allow a person to die, if—perhaps because she is terminally ill—she no longer desires her own continued existence.)

Newborn infants are not capable of desiring their own continued existence. In many morally relevant ways, they are more like fetuses than like persons. They have no desire to continue to live because they have no concept of their future life. There are no links, either of memory or of anticipation, between the separate moments of their existence. This means that one major reason for preserving the lives of persons—the fact that continued life is what they desire or want—will not apply to newborn infants. It also means that, strictly speaking, we cannot even say that continued life is in a newborn infant's interests. It is true, of course, that an infant may, if all goes well, grow into a happy child and adult and judge her life worthwhile; but, as we have already seen, this is not always the case. Moreover, and that is the crucial point, the person's life is not linked at the mental level with the life of the infant. The infant and the child are physically the same organism, but the child is a *person*, in the full sense of the term, and the newborn infant is not.

This means that infants (like kittens and fetuses) do not have an interest in their own continued existence, that they do not have a 'right to life', and that it is not *directly* wrong to refrain from preserving their lives. (Although it may, of course, be wrong for other reasons—for example, because the parents very much want their infant to survive, or because a worthwhile life will now not be lived.)

Infants, like kittens and sentient fetuses, do, however, have other interests. They are, at least soon after full-time birth but quite possibly earlier on,[25] able to experience pain and discomfort, and they can feel hungry and cold. They can therefore be said to have an interest in not experiencing pain and discomfort, and in being warm and well-fed. Doctors sometimes pay insufficient attention to these basic interests,[26] either because their focus is on survival,[27] or because they think that infants are not able to anticipate or remember pain.[28] That newborn infants are not able to anticipate or remember pain does, of course, follow directly from the view I have defended: that infants are not continuing selves. None the less, this gives us no good reason for ignoring an infant's moment-by-moment experience of pain, or for treating it less seriously than the momentary painful experiences of a person.

Those who argue that medical decision-making for seriously ill or impaired infants should be based on 'the best interests of the infant' do not necessarily dispute that an infant's pain and suffering should count—at least, not if the notion of 'best interests' is understood in terms of the infant's well-being. But this pain and suffering, supporters of this view might say, can be outweighed by future benefits. In other words, while it may be necessary to inflict some temporary suffering on an infant or child in our efforts to keep it alive, this is justified by the future well-being likely to be experienced by the child.

But this type of argument must face a serious objection. It is not only, as we noted above, that the future person may think that the pain and suffering she endured as a child cannot be outweighed by her now worthwhile life; it is also that infants are not persons with an interest in their own continued existence. If this is correct, then it is not plausible to hold that the infant's painful experiences will be balanced out, for the infant, by future states of well-being, or the worthwhile life to be lived by a person. There are no connections, at the mental level, no overlapping strands of memory and of anticipation between the life of the infant and the life of the child or adult. This is not simply a matter of the limit of the length of recall, or of the range of anticipation of the infant. Rather, the life of an infant (and of all those who will not achieve cognitive functioning beyond the level possessed by an infant) is a matter of moment-to-moment experiences. This means that the lives of those of us who are persons are not linked, at the mental level, to those our infant selves. It also means that the interests of our infant selves are not our interests, and our interests now were not those of ourselves as infants.[29]

This does not, of course, entail that it is never justified to inflict some degree of pain and discomfort on an infant in our efforts to keep it alive. The decision may be justified if it ensures the future well-being of an incompetent child or adult, or makes possible the existence of a future person, glad to be alive. It may also be justified because the parents very much want their infant to survive. But in all these cases the justification is not that the infliction of pain and suffering was in the *infant's* best interests; rather, it lies in the satisfaction of the interests of others. Hence, if a treatment required to keep an infant alive causes prolonged pain and discomfort, then it would be better to say that it is administered, not in accordance with, but *despite* the best interests of the infant.

Let us return to the case of the severely physically and mentally impaired child described above, who spends his time in the back ward of a state institution. As we noted, if such a child is adequately cared for, and suffers no pain, life would (whilst not strictly in his interest) at least not be *contrary* to his interests. He may experience states of well-being during and after feeding, and would quite possibly enjoy the occasional cuddle and back-rub. The picture changes dramatically, however, once considerable pain and suffering would need to be inflicted on such a child in our efforts to keep him alive. Such efforts would be contrary to his best interests because they would not, and could not, be outweighed, for *him*, by future states of well-being. Hence, whilst it would not have been directly wrong, on the view I am defending, to allow the child to die (provided the infant's suffering during the dying process is adequately relived), it might well have been directly wrong to sustain such an infant's life by way of procedures which impose a severe burden on the child.

If the view I have outlined is correct and infants do not have an interest in continued life, then this would provide grounds for the widely held belief (also shared by Professor Campbell) that it is sometimes morally proper for parents and doctors to allow a handicapped infant to die, not only when life, with or after treatment, is dominated by pain and therefore contrary to the infant's best interests, but also when life, while not strictly in the infant's interests, would not be contrary to them.

This is not to deny, of course, that it would, other things being equal, be a good thing to keep every infant alive who is likely to experience states of well-being, or who is likely to grow into an autonomous child and person.[30] But in medical practice, as elsewhere, other things are seldom equal. The birth of a severely handicapped child can dramatically affect the life of the parents and the siblings.[31] It can also be costly in terms of medical and other social resources. This means that many important interests are at stake, and not merely the short-term interests of the infant. It would be wrong to disregard these other interests altogether. To do so would be incompatible with any principle of the equal consideration of interests of all those affected by the decision—and such a principle is fundamental to ethics.[32]

Conclusion

In conclusion, let me return to the charge of discrimination, levelled by the US Commission of Civil Rights against the practice of using quality of life as a basis for decision-making for seriously impaired infants. It seems that this charge would be justified in almost all cases—if, that is, it were the case that infants have an interest in their continued survival. Whilst the charge of discrimination would not apply to severely impaired infants whose life is dominated by pain and discomfort, it could none the less justifiably be applied in most cases.

As we have seen, however, the concept of 'the infant's best interests' is more complex than is sometimes appreciated by those who appeal to it to justify treatment or non-treatment decisions for severely impaired newborn infants. Whilst there are many reasons why an infant's level of impairment is morally significant, and may justifiably result in the decision to allow the infant to die, the justification can only very rarely be based on the claim that our doing so is in the infant's best interests.

The charge of discrimination can be met, however, by showing that impaired infants (or indeed any infants) do not have a 'right to life', or an interest in their own continued existence. This means that it is not discriminatory or wrong to allow a severely impaired infant to die, even if the infant would experience states of well-being, or grow into a person who would one day be glad to be alive. In almost all cases, the justification for allowing severely impaired infants to die is thus not found in the 'quality' of the impaired infant's life, as the term is ordinarily understood, but rather in the different *kinds* of life possessed by infants and persons.

One final point needs to be made. It is often thought that there is a morally relevant distinction between different kinds of treatment, where 'extraordinary' or 'disproportionate' treatments may justifiably be withheld from a patient, whereas 'ordinary' or 'proportionate' means must always be employed.[33] Professor Campbell, too, seems to appeal to a distinction of this kind. He holds that 'aggressive treatment' (p. 85, 95) and 'intensive treatment' but 'not basic care' (emphasis in original) may sometimes be withheld or withdrawn. If we understand 'aggressive treatment' and 'intensive treatment' as treatment which is painful or burdensome to the infant, whereas 'basic care' is not, this distinction would be morally relevant, from a patient-centered best-interests perspective.

This is, however, not how the distinction is ordinarily understood. Rather, those who appeal to the distinction typically assume that there is an *intrinsic* moral difference between, for example, 'ordinary' and 'extraordinary means' of treatment—irrespective of how these treatments affect particular patients. Whilst I do not believe that this is a plausible view, I shall not attempt to argue for this conclusion here.[34] For our purposes, we should merely note that a patient-centered 'best-interests' approach would always focus on the interests of the patient, not on means of treatment. In other words, if it were decided that an infant's life is such that an early death is in the infant's best interests, then *all* life-sustaining treatments should be withdrawn—irrespective of how one might want to classify them on a scale or ordinariness or extraordinariness.

More than that. If it is in an infant's best interests to die, then it would be best, from the infant's point of view, if its unpleasant mental states were to cease as soon as possible. This could be achieved through the adequate and continuous administration of painkilling drugs or narcotics, or through the direct and intentional termination of the infant's life.

As in the case of the distinction between 'ordinary' and 'extraordinary means', it is widely believed that there is an intrinsic and morally relevant difference between intentionally ending a patient's life (killing the patient) and allowing the patient to die. If a patient's interests are, however, best served by being killed rather than by merely being allowed to die, then killing the patient would be required by the 'patient's best interests' approach.[35] One might, of course, want to reject this conclusion on the basis that it fails to equally consider the interests of all others affected by this decision,[36] but this presupposes that it can be shown that intentionally ending the patient's life *would* in fact adversely affect the interests of others—and that assumption is not universally shared.

NOTES AND REFERENCES

1. US Commission on Civil Rights: *Medical discrimination against children with disabilities*, Government Printing Office, Washington DC, 1989.
2. See Helga Kuhse: *The sanctity-of-life doctrine in medicine—a critique*, Oxford University Press, 1987. See also: Richard A. McCormick: The quality of life, the sanctity of life, *Hastings Center Report*, Vol. 8, February 1978, pp.30–6.
3. See, for example, S. H. Kadish: respect for life and regard for rights in the criminal law, in S. F. Barker (ed.): *Respect for life in medicine, philosophy, and the law*, Johns Hopkins University Press, Baltimore, 1977, pp.63–101; and E. W. Keyserlingk: *Sanctity of life or quality of life—in the context of ethics, medicine, and law. Study written for the Law Reform Commission of Canada*, Law Reform Commission, Ottawa, 1979.
4. See, for example Bernard Williams: The Makropoulos case, in James Rachels (ed.): *Moral* Problems, 2nd edn, Harper & Row, New York, 1975, pp.410–428.
5. President's Commission for the Study of Ethical Problems in Medicine and Biomedical and Behavioral Research: *Deciding to forego life-sustaining treatment—ethical, medical, and legal issues in treatment decisions*, Government Printing Office, Washington DC, March 1983.
6. Ibid., p. 218.
7. Professor Campbell is here drawing on James Rachels: *The end of life-euthanasia and morality*, Oxford University Press, 1986.
8. Professor Campbell does not refer to these characteristics. The importance he attaches to 'brain damage', however, suggests that it is capacities such as these which determine treatment/non-treatment decisions.
9. See for example R. M. Hare: Moral thinking—*its levels, method, and point*, Oxford University Press, 1981, Chapter 5.
10. President's Commission for the Study of Ethical Problems in Medicine and Biomedical and Behavioral Research: *Deciding to forego life-sustaining treatment*, op.cit., p. 219, fn.79.
11. Thomas Nagel: 'Death' in James Rachels(ed.): *Moral problems*, op.cit., p. 405.
12. See also John Robertson on this point in Involuntary euthanasia of defective

newborns, *Stanford Law Review*, Vol. 27, 1975, p. 254. I owe this refernce to
John D. Arras: Toward an ethic of ambiguity, *Hastings Center Report*, Vol.
14, April 1984, p. 30.

13. Jeremy Bentham: *The principles of morals and legislation*, Chapter 17,
Section 1, 1789. The quotation is reprinted in Tom Regan and Peter Singer:
Animal rights and human obligations, 2nd edn, Prentice Hall, Englewood
Cliffs, NJ, 1989, p. 26.

14. For a good recent discussion of 'moral standing' see Tom L. Beauchamp: The
moral standing of animals in medical research, *Law, Medicine & Health Care*,
Vol. 20, 1992, pp. 7–16.

15. The term is Kenneth E. Goodpaster's. See On being morally considerable,
The Journal of Philosophy, June 1972, pp. 308–25.

16. See Note 12.

17. See John D. Arras: Toward an ethic of ambiguity, p. 31.

18. John D. Arras: ibid.

19. In Helga Kuhse and Peter Singer: *Should the baby live—the problem of
handicapped infants*, Oxford University Press, pp. 144–145.

20. For some examples, see p. 145 of Helga Kuhse and Peter Singer: *Should the
baby live?*

21. See Anne McDonald: If we keep babies alive, we must give them a life
worth living, in *Proceedings of the Conference—The Tiniest Newborns*:
Survival-What Price?, Centre for Human Bioethics, Melbourne, 1984, p. 61.

22. In this section I draw heavily on a previously published article: Helga Kuhse:
Severely disabled infants: sanctity of life or quality of life?", in W. A. W.
Walters (Guest Editor): *Baill iere's clinical obstetrics and gynaecology—
international practice and research, human reproduction: current and future
ethical issues*, Vol. 5, September 1991, pp. 752–755.

23. See Helga Kuhse: *The sanctity-of-life doctrine in medicine*, Chapter 5.

24. Michael Tooley: *Abortion and infanticide*, Oxford University Press, 1983.

25. See Susan Tawia: When is the capacity for sentience acquired during human
fetal development?, *The Journal of Maternal–Fetal Medicine*, Vol. 1, 1992,
pp. 153–65.

26. See J. W. Scanlon: Barbarism, *Perinatal Press*, Vol. 9, 1985, pp. 103–4.

27. S. Rovner: Surgery without anaesthesia: can premies feel pain?, *Washington
Post*, 13 August, 1986.

28. P. McIntosh: Doctors seek pain relief for patients who can't say how much it
hurts, *The Age* (Melbourne), 22/9/1986.

29. Peter Singer: Life's uncertain voyage in P. Pettit, R. Sylvan, and J. Norman
(eds): *Metaphysics and morality*—Essays in honour of J. J. C. Smart, Basil
Blackwell, Oxford, 1987, pp. 154–72.

30. Here we must, however, also note the following point. If the reason for
preserving an infant's life is that the infant has the potential to grow into
a happy child or autonomous adult, then this very same reason could also be
extended to any action or omission which has a high probability of resulting
in the existence of a happy child or autonomous person—sexual intercourse
under circumstances when conception is likely to occur, and refraining from
having an abortion. This means that in so far as one wanted to object to a
decision not to preserve the life of the infant, because of the potential of

that infant, one would also have to object, just as strongly if other factors are equal, to a decision to avoid having a child at all—either by using a contraceptive, by having an abortion or by mere voluntary abstention at times when conception would be likely to occur.

31. See for example M. Simms: Severely handicapped infants, *New Humanist*, Vol. 98, 1983, pp. 1–8; and S. Kew: *Handicap and family crisis*, Pitman, London, 1975.

32 Peter Singer: *Practical ethics*, Cambridge University Press, 1979, Chapter 2.

33. Sacred Congregation for the Doctrine of the Faith: *Declaration on euthanasia*, Vatican City, 1980.

34. See Helga Kuhse: *The sanctity-of-life doctrine in medicine*, Chapter 4.

35. See Helga Kuhse: Death by non-feeding: not in the baby's best interests, *The Journal of Medical Humanities and Bioethics*, Vol. 7, 1986, pp. 79–90.

36. See note 32.

5

The use of epidemiological data for prognostication and decision-making

5A   FROM PROBABILITY TO PREFERENCE

John C. Sinclair and George W. Torrance

INTRODUCTION

The first part of this chapter will review the physician's role in using epidemiologic data in predicting the future course of disease (prognostication) and in deciding whether medical intervention is likely to do more good than harm. By epidemiologic data we mean data obtained from *groups* of patients with the same disorder who have been observed over the time-course of their disease, or who have been subjected to treatment. By reference to such data, the physician infers the *probable* course of events if he/she should simply observe his/her patient, or intervene with treatment. Although the viewpoint adopted in this chapter is primarily that of the individual physician caring for the individual patient, we will also consider, when relevant, the factors which enter when comparable decisions are to be made from a societal viewpoint—for example in the planning and financing of treatment programs based on the health-care needs of populations.

The key word in the preceding paragraph is the word 'probable'. The idea that observation of or experiments involving previous similar cases can provide a basis for predicting future events is fundamental to the science of epidemiology. The idea is based on the concept of a series: that is, if a sufficiently long succession (or series) of similar objects (or patients) is observed, a kind of order gradually emerges, 'not fixed or accurate at first, but which tends in the long run to become so'.[1]

The *probability* of an event's happening presupposes such a series. For example, let the probability that a newborn baby will survive to one year of age be 99 out of 100. The larger series comprises all newborns, the smaller all newborns who live to one year. Then the chance or probability that any given newborn will live to one year is 99/100. Note that, even in the face of this very high probability, we cannot say with certainty that the next newborn in the larger series will live to one year; in fact, the next one may die.

Given an infinitely large series, we may be sure that the probability is exactly 99 in 100. However, given only a few thousand, or only a few hundred in the series, we become progressively less sure of the exact probability, because random error is playing a larger role. In medicine, probabilities can never be based on anything close to a series of infinite size. Consequently, all estimates of probabilities in medical science are subject to imprecision. The degree of imprecision is quantitated by calculating the confidence interval (see below) around the point estimate for probability.

The applicability of a probability estimate to a specific patient depends on how closely that patient resembles those in whom the probability was determined. Temporal, geographic, socioeconomic, biomedical, and other differences may reduce the generalizability of probability estimates. For example, returning to the chance of the newborn's surviving to one year, it will be found that in some countries the probability of surviving to one year is much lower, and in others, somewhat higher than 99 in 100. These different probabilities are calculated by substituting a series of the right kind—in this case, for example, previous births within those specific countries. It is a central problem in medical care to judge whether probabilities, even highly precise ones, generated from previous or concurrent observation or experiments in other patients are based on a 'series' relevant to decision-making in one's own patient.

Epidemiologic data can provide, at best, a set of probabilities that are valid, reasonably precise, and applicable to one's patient. However, even in this utopian situation, the physician may not have a sufficient basis for decision-making. Specified health outcomes may be valued differently by different patients, and if these values could be measured, they could have a critical impact on decisions concerning the preferred choice of medical action.

Silverman anticipates this latter dimension in his Foreword to *Effective care of the newborn infant*:[2] 'Given the growing number of interventions available in neonatal medicine and the complexity of mixed medical and social consequences of these actions, decision-making is becoming increasingly difficult. The first requirements for rational decisions in the face of uncertainty are the probabilities that specified events will occur after proposed courses of action. There is, therefore, a desperate need for "best available" forecasts of expected outcomes of alternative interventions to provide neonatologists with the quantitative information they can use for replies to parents' questions; and to begin a discussion with them that will lead to a decisive value judgement: the choice between alternative courses of action.'

Therefore, we conclude Part A of this chapter with a consideration of health-state preference measurement and its application to epidemiologically-based estimates of probabilities for health outcomes.

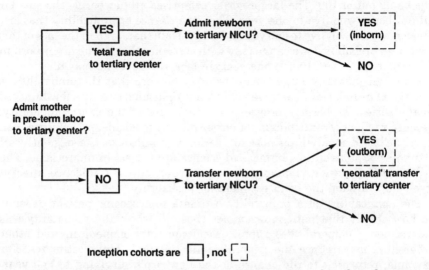

Fig. 5.1 Are low-birthweight babies better off being transferred, as fetuses, to be born in the teriary center rather than being transferred after birth? Note that the common 'inception' point in maing this comparison is at the point of decision whether or not to transfer the mother in pre-term labor.

MAKING A PROGNOSIS

The events which occur beginning with the biologic onset of a disease or condition and ending with the 'outcome'—for example intact survival, survival with permanent disability, or death—constitute the natural history of disease. Within this frame, there is the point at which the physician or other health professional interacts with the patient, makes a diagnosis and, on the basis of what he/she knows about the likely clinical course of the disease, makes a *prognosis*. The prognosis is a probabilistic judgement—specifically, an estimation of the relative probabilities that the patient will develop each of the alternative outcomes of the natural history of the disease.

Because a prognosis consists of probabilities, it should not be made simply by informal recall of one's previous clinical experience of similar cases. Rather, a prognosis should reflect a 'best estimate' derived from review of all valid prognostic studies which are applicable to the patient. Critical appraisal criteria have been advanced for judging the validity of reports in the literature concerning clinical course and prognosis:[3]

1. Was an 'inception cohort' assembled?

A valid study of clinical course and prognosis requires that patients be identified at an early and uniform point in their disease or condition. Thus, an inception cohort could comprise, for example, consecutive births

Table 5.1 Survival of extremely-low-birthweight livebirths
($\leqslant$ 1000 g)

McMaster Health Region, 1977–1980[5]		
Hospital of birth	No.	Per cent
Delivered at tertiary center	92/171	54
Delivered at community hospitals	25/84	30
Transfer neonate to tertiary center	25/42	60
No transfer	0/42	0
Total survivors	117/255	46

in a defined population, or consecutive babies discharged home alive from a neonatal intensive care unit. It is not difficult to find examples of a failure to define the inception point in prognostic studies in the clinical literature. For example, a number of studies have compared the survival of low birthweight (LBW) infants born within a tertiary care center ('inborn') with low birthweight infants transported to the tertiary care center after birth at an outlying hospital ('outborn').[4] The common inception point in such a contrast is the point at which the decision is made to transfer, or not transfer, the mother to the tertiary care center. As is apparent from Fig. 5.1, the comparison of the outcomes of LBW infants who are 'inborn' vs. 'outborn' gives an incomplete and biased view of the outcomes of the cohorts which are generated from the common inception point.

2. Was the referral pattern described?

In order to judge whether the patients described in reports of natural history and prognosis resemble one's own patient, any selection filters should be described. Since the advent of 'regionalization' in neonatology/perinatology, it can readily be appreciated that the referral process can generate hospital-based patient samples (for example, those found in tertiary care centers) that can be very different from those found in the general population. An example of the impact of such referral patterns in our own region is shown in Table 5.1[5]. During the years 1977–80, there were 255 livebirths weighing less than 1000 g in the McMaster Health region, of whom 117 survived (46 per cent). However, among those delivered at community hospitals, survival ranged from 0/42 (0 per cent) in those not transferred to 25/42 (60 per cent) in those transferred to the tertiary care center; overall, survival rate was 30 per cent among those born at community hospitals in the region, versus 54 per cent among those delivered at the tertiary care center.

3. Was complete follow-up achieved?

Ideally, the clinical outcome of all patients in the inception cohort should be known. This goal is seldom achieved, and a loss-to-follow-up rate of 5 per cent or even 10 per cent is commonly encountered, even among the most carefully conducted studies of natural history and prognosis. In a review of published reports of follow-up studies of surviving very-low-birthweight babies, Escobar and co-workers[6] found that among reports of 85 cohorts in which the incidence of cerebral palsy was calculated, the per centage of infants lost to follow-up ranged from 0 to 53 per cent, with a median of 10.9 per cent; thus, at least one-half of studies in this series had a loss-to-follow-up rate which exceeded 10 per cent.

The problem presented by loss to follow-up is that those who are lost cannot be assumed to be random deletions from the inception cohort, and therefore those that are retained may no longer be representative of the original cohort. Patients may be lost to follow-up for a number of reasons which are non-random: death, institutionalization, adoption, mobility, and exceptionally good or exceptionally poor health are just a few. The operation of selection bias due to loss to follow-up has been demonstrated empirically in the field of neonatal follow-up: for example, in a German follow-up study of at-risk infants, the incidence of cerebral damage was twice as high (10/49: 20.4 per cent) in infants who did not return for a 6-month follow-up examination as in infants who did present at the follow-up clinic (35/347: 10.1 per cent).[7] As a rule of thumb, studies in which the loss-to-follow-up rate exceeds 10 per cent should be viewed with suspicion, particularly if the risk of adverse outcome is low; the lower the risk, the greater the potential for distortion of results stemming from loss to follow-up.

4. Were objective outcome criteria developed and used?

The outcomes, and how they were ascertained, need to be described explicitly and objectively. This applies to biomedical terms such as cerebral palsy and chronic lung disease, and also to functional concepts such as disability, impairment, and handicap. It is necessary not only that such outcomes be explicitly defined, but also that the operational criteria for their ascertainment be consistently applied.

5. Was the outcome assessment 'blind'?

Outcomes should be assessed by examiners who are unaware of the risk factors for the outcome. Blinding of the examiner to prognostic factors in the patient controls a form of bias in assessing outcome termed the diagnostic suspicion bias, whereby a more detailed or intensive search for an adverse outcome is undertaken in patients with, as compared to without, the prognostic risk factor. The operation of this bias has been demonstrated empirically in the scoring of a videotaped neuromotor examination in infancy.[8]

6. Was adjustment for extraneous prognostic factors carried out?

A factor which is a determinant of the outcome, which is associated with the exposure or risk factor, but which is not the risk factor under study is, in this sense, an extraneous prognostic factor, also known as a 'confounder'. For example, differences in racial distribution, socioeconomic class, or geography can confound the relationship between birthweight class and outcome. Multivariate analysis with appropriate adjustment for such extraneous prognostic factors may be necessary in order more accurately to determine the prognosis associated with a risk factor, and also to avoid incriminating other factors which, in themselves, are not causally related to outcome.

Typically, the application of the foregoing critical appraisal criteria considerably reduces the number of reports on the basis of which a prognosis is to be made. The effect of the application of these criteria has been to maximize the *validity* of the information on which the prognosis is based. However, two important issues remain—*precision* and *applicability*.

By *precision*, we mean the range of random error of the prognostic statement. When the sample size of a prognostic study is small, any prognostic conclusion must be imprecise. For example, the incidence of retinopathy of prematurity $\geq$ Grade III among survivors of extreme prematurity (gestational age 24–27 weeks) has been reported to be 15/70 (21.4 per cent).[9] One way of expressing the precision of this estimate is to calculate its 95 per cent confidence interval. The 95 per cent confidence interval of a proportion is that proportion $\pm$ twice its standard error. The standard error of a proportion p based on a sample of n patients is $\sqrt{p\,(1-p)/n}$. Thus, the standard error of 15/70 is $\sqrt{0.214(0.786)/70} = 0.049$ or 4.9 per cent, and the 95 per cent confidence interval around our prognostic estimate of 21.4 per cent is 11.6 per cent, 31.2 per cent. This interval indicates that if the observation just reported were to be repeated 100 times, the true value would be expected to be included within the calculated confidence interval on 95 occasions. Because the interval (11.6 per cent, 31.2 per cent) is rather wide, we cannot make a very precise prognostic statement based on this single report. We might be able to improve the precision, however, if we could derive a 'typical estimate' of prognosis from all comparable valid reports. Quantitative methods for combining the results of several studies, called 'meta-analyses', have been developed and applied particularly for summarizing the effect of treatment (see below), but are also needed in the field of prognosis. We may expect to see such reports increasingly in future.

The *applicability* to our patient of prognostic studies in the literature has already been considered in part. For example, we have discussed in this context the relevance of the inception point, the referral pattern, and the operational definitions for the outcome criteria in applying the results of reports of prognosis. However, there is an additional important issue to consider—that of secular trend. Particularly in a rapidly developing field such as neonatology, patient outcomes can change substantially over time. For example, birthweight-specific survival rates among low-birthweight

infants increased greatly during the 1970s and 1980s.[10] The likely effect
of this trend is that a prognosis for survival of low-birthweight babies
derived from reports of previous experience would underestimate the current
expectation for survival. As another example, rates of cerebral palsy among
survivors of very low birthweight also increased during this time-period,[11]
so that the current risk for cerebral palsy among survivors could have been
somewhat underestimated on the basis of reports of prior experience. There
is a need, not well met at present, for developing methods which incorporate
data concerning current trends in important outcomes in making 'on-line'
prognostic forecasts.

DECIDING WHETHER TO INTERVENE

Medical treatment constitutes an intervention in the natural history of
disease. The questions to be asked about any treatment are:

1. What is the magnitude of the baseline risk (i.e. without treatment,
   what proportion of patients like this one will experience an adverse
   outcome?)?
2. Is there an effect of treatment (i.e. is there an effect that is real, and not
   due to chance?)?
3. What are the direction and size of the treatment effect?
4. Are there unwanted side-effects attributable to the treatment?
5. What is the relevant viewpoint(s) for valuing clinical outcomes: patient
   only, patient and family, patient and all others even remotely affected?
6. From the relevant viewpoint(s) what is the value of each clinical outcome,
   good and bad, and what is the overall net value of all the outcomes taken
   together? That is, on balance, does treatment for this patient do more good
   than harm?
7. What is the relevant viewpoint(s) for valuing economic outcomes: patient
   and family, hospital, third-party payer, health-care system, society?
8. From the relevant viewpoint(s) what are the economic costs and the
   economic benefits of treatment? Is the net economic cost positive or
   negative, and how large?
9. If the treatment does more good than harm but has a positive net cost, is
   the excess good sufficient to outweigh the excess cost?

To obtain answers to these questions is not a simple matter. Research may
sometimes result in a wrong answer because of systematic error (bias) or
random error (imprecision). Even valid conclusions from research can be of
limited generalizability to clinical practice. Thus, the physician needs to be
concerned not just with the published results of clinical research concerning
treatment, but also with the methodological issues of bias, precision, and
applicability.

Table 5.2 Structure of a study to evaluate the effect of a treatment

		Event	No event	Total
			Outcome	
Exposure	Treated	a	b	n_1
	Control	c	d	n_0
		m_1	m_0	T

Event rate in treated group = a/n_1

Event rate in control group = c/n_0

Event rate ratio (ERR) = $\dfrac{a/n_1}{c/n_0}$

Event rate difference (ERD) = $a/n_1 - c/n_0$

Proportionate event rate difference = $1 - \text{ERR}$

Number needed to treat = $\dfrac{1}{\text{ERD}}$

Expressing the effect of treatment

Table 5.2 displays the structure of a typical study which seeks to evaluate treatment. There are two exposure groups (labelled 'treated' and 'control') and two possible outcomes (labelled 'event' and 'no event'). The physician places particular emphasis on studies in which patients are assigned to the treated or control groups by a random (or quasi-random) procedure. An event may be any outcome, such as occurrence of disease, complication of disease, or death.

Such a study design permits answers to the clinically relevant questions, cited above, concerning the effect of treatment:

(1) the magnitude of risk in the absence of treatment is given by the event rate in the control group, c/n_0; and

(2) the effect of treatment is given by comparing the event rate in the treated group with that in the control group. This comparison is expressed as either the *event rate ratio* (ERR), $a/n_1 \div c/n_0$, or the *event rate difference* (ERD), $a/n_1 - c/n_0$. In studies of the etiology of disease, the event rate ratio is known as the relative risk (or risk ratio) and the event rate difference is known as the risk difference.

These measures of treatment effect convey different (and to some extent complementary) information. The event rate ratio indicates the *relative*, but not absolute, magnitude of reduction in the event rate. The ERR's complement $(1 - \text{ERR})$ gives the proportionate event rate difference. Thus, an ERR of 0.60 represents a 40 per cent reduction in the rate of events in the treated group relative to the rate of events in the controls.

The event rate difference, on the other hand, indicates the *absolute* magnitude of reduction of events. For example, an ERD of -0.20 represents an absolute 20 per centage-point reduction of events in the treated group. The reciprocal of ERD (1/ERD) indicates the number of patients one needs to treat in order to prevent one patient with an event. This latter measure is particularly relevant when considering whether to use a treatment which is effective but whose effect is bought at considerable cost (in the form of clinical side-effects and/or economic cost). In the example here, 1/0.2, five patients need to be treated to prevent one with an event.

Bias

The fundamental goal of clinical research concerning the efficacy and safety of treatment is that it should obtain an unbiased answer to the question posed. By 'bias' we mean a force which leads to an answer which is systematically different from the truth.

Most studies on treatment or prevention use designs which can be classified into one of five categories. These designs are listed below in order of ascending methodologic rigour:

- single case reports;
- case series without controls;
- non-randomized studies using historical controls (i.e. observational studies comparing current patients who receive the innovative treatment with previous patients, typically from the same institution or from the literature, who did not);
- non-randomized studies using concurrent controls (i.e. observational studies comparing contemporaneous patients who did or did not receive the experimental treatment); and
- randomized controlled trials (experimental studies).

The case report or case series (without controls) are the designs most prone to bias. The absence of a control group opens the door to fallacious interpretation: any change in the clinical course of patients in a case series is attributed to treatment, even when the change would have occurred in the absence of treatment.

Studies which utilize controls provide a much more valid basis for reaching conclusions about the effect of treatment. However, the performance of a controlled study is not in itself a sufficient guarantee of a valid result. Biases can seriously impair studies using either historical or non-randomized concurrent controls.[12]

The randomized trial is the strongest design for evaluating the effect of treatment. It offers maximum protection against selection biases which can invalidate comparisons between groups of patients because of 'confounding'. A confounder is an extraneous characteristic which is a determinant of the outcome and is unequally distributed between the treatment groups being compared. In non-randomized studies, one attempts to control confounding

by strategies such as exclusion of patients with certain characteristics, stratification according to risk at the time of sampling, matching, or stratification
or adjustment in the analysis. However, these techniques require that the
source of confounding be known. In clinical medicine, the confounders
are often unknown; a presently unknown confounder may be discovered
tomorrow. It is the unique property and strength of randomization that it
has the capacity to allocate not only known but also unknown confounders
in an unbiased manner.

Several features of the design of a randomized trial deserve emphasis: (1)
There must be an *a priori* hypothesis, stated in quantitative terms, and
susceptible of disproof. This requires a predetermined sample size based on
estimates of (a) the hypothesized clinical effect of the new treatment and (b)
the investigators' predetermined probabilites of (i) missing a real treatment
effect and (ii) incorrectly identifying the treatment as being effective. (2) The
allocation process should be truly random and impervious to code-breaking
or tampering. (Quasi- random allocation procedures such as alternate, day of
week, etc., are not preferred). (3) When feasible, blinding of both physician
and patient to the treatment allocation should be accomplished. (Among other
advantages, this defends against co-intervention bias—the selective use of
additional screening, diagnostic, or therapeutic procedures in one group more
than the other.) (4) All patients randomized must be accounted for in the
primary analysis. (5) Outcome measurements should be made by observers
who are blinded to the treatment allocation.

Methodologic standards for the design, conduct, analysis, and reporting of
randomized trials continue to be refined.[13–15]

Precision

Randomized trials are concerned with *estimation* (estimating the size of effect
of treatment) as well as with *hypothesis-testing* (testing whether an effect is
real, rather than due to chance). Although a randomized trial offers the most
powerful design for providing an unbiased estimate of the size of difference
in outcomes of the treatment regimens being compared, the estimate can be
imprecise.

The measure of precision most commonly cited is the 95 per cent confidence
interval. The confidence interval displays the uncertainty in the trial's
estimate of the size of effect by presenting the upper and lower bounds for
the anticipated true treatment difference. The 95 per cent confidence interval
indicates that if the trial were to be repeated 100 times, the true value would
be expected to be included within the calculated confidence interval on 95
occasions.

The confidence interval tends to widen when the data are very variable, or
the sample size small, or both. Thus, imprecision in estimation is a particular
problem in trials which enrol only small numbers of patients. As the number
of patients increases, the confidence interval narrows.

The *clinical* significance of a true treatment effect depends on the size of the treatment effect and on the complications and costs of treatment. Weighing these considerations is a matter of clinical judgement. The determination of *statistical* significance, on the other hand, is a determination that a treatment effect is real—i.e. unlikely to be due to chance. Statistical significance is a function of the size of the observed difference in outcome between the treated and control groups relative to the amount of variability of the outcome within both the treated and control groups. A clinically significant difference may be suggested in a study whose sample size is too small to achieve statistical significance. Alternatively, a difference which is so small that it may be of little clinical importance can be rendered statistically significant if the sample size is very large.

Applicability

The generalizability of the results of a trial—i.e. the appropriateness of generalizing the trial's conclusions to a particular clinical practice or individual patient—depends on the physician's answers to the questions:

1. Were the study patients recognizably similar to his/her own?
2. Is the intervention feasible in practice?
3. Were all clinically relevant outcomes reported?

It is important to acknowledge that the patients who participate in randomized trials are not necessarily representative of all patients with the index disorder. Because strict eligibility criteria must be met, only some patients with the index disorder will be found eligible. Of eligible patients, only a portion will enter the trial; and those that do enter may not be representative of all those who were eligible.[16] Thus, in applying the results of a trial to clinical practice, it is essential to note whether patients to whom the results are being applied would have been eligible for inclusion in the trial and, if so, whether such patients have identifiable characteristics which call into question whether the overall result of the trial is applicable to them. Frequently, guidance can be obtained by noting how subsets of patients with distinguishing clinical or laboratory characteristics at entry fared within the trial.[17] Further guidance may be sought by noting the characteristics of eligible patients who were *not* entered in the trial; but the frequent failure to report such data has been documented.[18]

Thus, the limits of applicability of the results of a randomized trial are determined, in general, by the range of variation among entry characteristics and intervention policies as described in the index trial. The wider these limits, the wider the limits of applicability of the conclusions. It is not warranted, however, to extend the results beyond the limits tested in the trial. A famous example of inappropriate generalization in neonatal practice was the extrapolation of the restricted oxygen policy to the care of all premature infants after the report in 1954 that oxygen restriction greatly reduced the incidence and severity of retrolental fibroplasia. The fact that all infants who entered the trial had to be at least 48 hours old was overlooked in making this extrapolation. It was estimated subsequently[19] that 16 excess deaths (mainly from respiratory disorders in the first days of life) were caused for every case of retrolental fibroplasia prevented, even though the original trial reported no excess mortality due to oxygen restriction. The extension of a study's results to a different patient population, therefore, should first be done under the auspices of a new randomized trial.

Applicability also depends on the range of outcomes that are evaluated in a trial of a new treatment. Although the investigator may assess only a single outcome, many interventions have the capacity to affect more than one outcome of clinical importance. This is especially a problem in neonatology, where many clinical outcomes of interest are interrelated. Before a new therapy is adopted for widespread use we need evidence concerning its effect on all the major outcomes it is likely to influence.

Meta-analysis

There are two general reasons why the results of randomized trials may differ:[20]

1. There may be a failure to control bias in individual trials (systematic error)
2. There may be variation due to chance in the results of individual trials, particularly those of small sample size (random error).

Considering a theoretical population of identical trials of an efficacious drug, if we typically set power for identifying a true treatment effect at 80 per cent (beta=0.20), then one in five such trials incorrectly reports the drug as having no benefit. In fact, many trials have power closer to only 50 per cent, and half of such trials will miss a true treatment effect. Alternatively, in a population of trials of a drug which has no real efficacy, one in 20 (at alpha = 0.05) will incorrectly find a significant treatment effect. Thus, to place the result of an apparently unbiased but small trial in context, the physician needs access to all the relevant (and unbiased) trials which have tested the same intervention.

A formal overview of comparable trials of an intervention, sometimes called a 'meta-analysis',[21] seeks to obtain a summary estimate, in a defined population, of the effect of an intervention on each outcome of interest. A valid overview of randomized trials requires that all relevant and 'groupable' trials be identified, using predefined inclusion and exclusion criteria. Next, the trials are examined for their methodologic quality; those whose methods fail to meet predefined criteria for methodologic quality are excluded. Then the results of the included trials are tabulated, and a summary estimate of treatment effect is calculated. This summary effect (sometimes termed a 'typical' effect) is some form of weighted average across trials; the weights are inversely related to the variance in the estimate of treatment effect provided by each participating trial. The variance in any single trial is a function of the number of patients studied, the homogeneity of the patients on entry to the trial, the homogeneity of the response in untreated (control) patients, and the homogeneity of response in treated patients.

The results of a meta-analysis of randomized trials have several uses: (1) A meta-analysis provides increased statistical power, especially when individual trials are all relatively small; this increased power can resolve uncertainty arising from disagreement between individual trials as to whether a treatment effect is real or due to chance. (2) A meta-analysis provides increased precision in the estimate of effect size; this increased precision can be critical in weighing benefits of a treatment against clinical side-effects, in choosing between alternative treatments when more than one has a true beneficial effect, and in quantitating the cost-effectiveness of the treatment. (3) A meta-analysis can also be useful in exploring the differences between studies in their results and in generating hypotheses (not posed at the start of individual trials) about the source of such differences. (4) A meta-analysis provides an existing structure for the incorporation of new evidence from comparable trials performed in the future.

Systematic reviews of evidence from randomized trials of therapy in perinatology[22] and neonatology[23] have recently been completed. Reviewers employed meta-analyses of comparable trials in order to detect the typical effect of treatment and to increase precision in the estimate of effect of treatment. The results, published in the form of textbooks entitled *Effective care in pregnancy and childbirth* and *Effective care of the newborn infant*, constitute comprehensive summaries of the best available evidence concerning the likely effects of therapeutic interventions in perinatology/neonatology.

PREFERENCES

Decision-making under uncertainty

The decision whether or not to intervene with a particular patient involves the simultaneous consideration of a range of possible outcomes, and their estimated probabilities of occurrence in this situation. Taking such decisions is known as decision-making under uncertainty, and can be usefully depicted by a graphical device, the decision tree. Figure 5.2 shows a simple decision tree for an intervention decision. Alternative 1 represents a particular intervention, while alternative 2 represents the decision not to intervene. The square symbol indicates a decision node, while the circles indicate chance nodes. Each alternative leads to a chance node that displays the possible outcomes and their probabilities.

Even in a simple decision problem like the one show in Fig. 5.2, with only two alternatives, one stage of uncertainty, and a limited number of outcomes, the decision problem can be exceedingly complex. The decision-maker must consider the probabilities, some of which may be quite small, and must consider the imprecision of these probability estimates. Depending upon

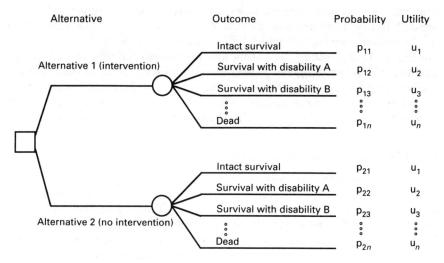

Alternative	Outcome	Probability	Utility

Alternative 1 (intervention)

Intact survival — p_{11} — u_1

Survival with disability A — p_{12} — u_2

Survival with disability B — p_{13} — u_3

Dead — p_{1n} — u_n

Intact survival — p_{21} — u_1

Survival with disability A — p_{22} — u_2

Survival with disability B — p_{23} — u_3

Alternative 2 (no intervention)

Dead — p_{2n} — u_n

Fig. 5.2 A simple decision tree for an intervention.

the viewpoint adopted (see below), the following data may or may not be relevant: the impact of the various outcomes on the life of the index patient; the impact of the various outcomes on the life of all others affected, including family, relatives, friends, acquaintances, and non-acquaintenances; the monetary costs and benefits for the patient and all others affected; and the time costs and benefits for the patient and all others affected. Given all these considerations, the decision-maker must determine preferences for the various outcomes and combine these with the probabilities in such a way as to reach a decision regarding the relative desirability of the alternatives.

Who is the decision-maker?

Under normal circumstances, for example in situations involving a competent adult patient, the patient is the ultimate decision-maker. The patient may very well receive assistance from a number of individuals, including family, friends, and the physician. However, there are a number of situations where the patient is not competent to make the decision: for example, in neonates and young children, in cognitively impaired individuals, and perhaps in emotionally disturbed individuals. The general approach in these cases is that an appropriate proxy should make the decision on behalf of the individual.

In general, the proxy should be an individual who has the best interests of the patient at heart, and does not have any conflict of interest in the case. However, in the instance of perinatal decision-making, the parents have the most obvious claim on the role of proxy, despite the fact that they can be viewed as having a conflict of interest. This claim is based on the view that not only do the parents have the interests of the index patient at heart, but that they are also an integral part of, and a major stakeholder in, the patient–family unit which will be intimately affected by the decision. For example, in a study comparing two procedures for prenatal diagnosis, chorionic villus sampling and genetic amniocentesis, parents in the trial were used as the primary source for the measurement of preferences for the various outcomes.[24] The outcomes included not only consequences for the parents, but also important consequences for the fetus, and for other family members.

Providing help in decision-making

Even in the simple case depicted in Fig. 5.2, reaching a decision can be exceedingly complex. Moreover, most real-world problems are much more complicated than the one shown in Fig. 5.2. Often there are many more alternatives and a wide variety of outcomes to be considered. Given the limited cognitive processing ability of the human brain, it is not surprising that individuals need help in dealing with these kinds of problems. Help can be provided in a variety of ways.

No doubt the most widespread form of help is that provided by the physician who describes the range of alternatives, the possible outcomes, and their likelihoods. The physician is often also in a position to help the patient think about the impact of the various outcomes on the life of the patient and family. However, it is not easy for every physician to be fully aware of all the ramifications of various treatments for every condition or disease. One alternative, currently being tested in prostate surgery, is to develop a video that describes the treatment alternatives and the impact of the various outcomes. The prostate surgery video shows a patient who selected surgery and one who did not. Each patient describes his reasons for making his particular decision. The attempt is to provide the new patient with balanced information on the pros and cons of the surgical intervention to help the patient reach his own decision.

Although the video approach helps the patient better understand the alternatives and the outcomes, it does not address the issue of how to deal with probabilities. Many people do not have a good intuitive sense of probabilities. It has been demonstrated, for example, that individuals consistently over-weight low probabilities and under-weight high ones.[26] As an attempt to overcome this problem, along with providing information on the alternatives and outcomes, Levine and Gafni have devised a breast-cancer decision instrument.[27] This instrument uses visual aids to help the patient better appreciate the probabilities of the various outcomes, and thereby reach a more informed decision. However, the breast-cancer treatment decision depicted in the instrument has a simple structure, with only a few outcome states. The approach may not be generalizable to more complex decision-situations.   Utility theory, on the other hand, is a general approach to the provision of help in decision-making under uncertainty, which is applicable in all problems, no matter how complex.

Utility theory

Utility theory for decision-making under uncertainty was developed by von Neumann and Morgenstern in 1944.[28] It is unfortunate that von Neumann and Morgenstern chose the word utility to refer to their concept. The problem is that the term utility had been in use for several centuries to refer to a variety of concepts, all of which differed from the new use by von Neumann and Morgenstern. Previous utility concepts included utilitarian ethics from the field of philosophy, and ordinal and cardinal utilities from the field of economics. To differentiate the von Neumann and Morgenstern type of utility appropriately, it should properly be referred to as vNM utility. However, most authors fail to make this distinction, and to this day there remains a considerable amount of confusion, with researchers from various disciplines talking past each other.

vNM utility theory is put forward as a normative theory.[29] That is, it is promulgated as a theory of how one should make decisions under uncertainty, if one wishes to be rational in a specifically defined sense. The rationality here refers to adherence to the basic axioms of vNM utility theory. The axioms can be stated in a variety of ways, and will not be repeated here. A three-axiom version is available in Torrance and Feeny.[30] The appeal of vNM utility theory is twofold. First, the axioms are compelling in the sense that most people upon reflection feel that the axioms are sensible and are axioms that a rational decision-maker would wish to follow. Second, vNM utility theory provides a simple 'divide and conquer' procedure that allows one to simplify and solve even the most complex decision-problems in a way that is entirely consistent with the basic axioms.

The procedure for applying vNM utility theory begins with the assignment of utility scores to the outcomes at the end of the decision tree. The most preferred outcome is given a score of 1.0, and the least preferred a score of 0.0. All other outcomes are assigned utility scores relative to these two. Using the probabilities of the outcomes, the expected utility of each alternative is calculated. For example, in Fig. 5.2 the expected utility of alternative 1 is $p_{11} u_1 + p_{12} u_2 + p_{13} u_3 + \ldots + p_{1n} u_n$. The alternative with the greater expected utility is the one that should be selected. This is the alternative that would be preferred by an individual who subscribes to the axioms of vNM utility theory and whose preferences for the outcomes are given by the utility scores. Further details on the methods as applied in health care are available in two textbooks.[31, 32] Reviews of applications in health are also available.[33, 34, 35]

Although vNM utility theory was developed as a normative theory of how decisions ought to be made, not a descriptive theory of how decisions are in fact made, nevertheless it has been thoroughly investigated as a possible descriptive model. Not surprisingly, it generally fails to describe the way in which individuals actually make decisions. Not only is this not surprising, but indeed, if individuals naturally made decisions following vNM utility theory, there would be no need for such a theory. One could simply give individuals complex problems and they would consistently solve them in a rational manner.

In decision theory, the normative and descriptive approaches are polar positions. The normative approach defines how a perfectly rational individual who subscribed to the vNM axioms would make decisions. The descriptive approach describes how actual individuals do in fact make decisions. Some researchers now have suggested a middle ground, the prescriptive approach.[36] The prescriptive approach attempts to help real individuals wrestle with their particular decision. It is based heavily on the normative approach, but attempts to be more sensitive to the individual and places more emphasis on helping the individual to reach a decision with which he/she is comfortable. Not all researchers agree that this middle prescriptive ground even exists.[36] Indeed, it could be seen as merely a sensitive and sensible application of the normative approach to the specifics of the individual and his/her decision.

Von Neumann–Morgenstern utility theory is not the only normative model available for decision-making under uncertainty. A variety of other models have been suggested but, to date, none have replaced the vNM approach.[37] Von Neumann–Morgenstern utility theory remains the dominant normative paradigm for decision-making under uncertainty even half a century after its development.

Measuring patients' preferences

Suppose a patient is asked for preferences regarding three possible outcomes: A, B, and C. One can measure ordinal preferences; this is a simple ranking of the preference order for the three outcomes. Alternatively, one can measure cardinal preferences; this is a numeric score with interval scale properties. Within cardinal preferences, one can use instruments that do not involve probabilities, in which case the resulting scores are called values. Alternatively, instruments that do involve probabilities produce scores that are called utilities. Utilities are the appropriate measure of preference for use in decision-making under uncertainty.

The standard gamble is the classical method for measuring vNM utilities. The method is derived directly from one of the underlying axioms of vNM utility theory. The standard gamble measurement for a chronic health state preferred to death is depicted in Fig. 5.3. The individual is asked to choose between two alternatives. Alternative 1 is the health state A for the rest of the individual's life, a specific number of years, t. Alternative 2 is an uncertain prospect which has a probability p of making the individual healthy for the rest of life, the same t years, and a complementary probability of $1-p$ of causing immediate death. The individual is asked to choose either alternative 1 or alternative 2, or to indicate that the two alternatives are equally preferred. Based on the response, the probabilities are changed, in a systematic way designed to minimize measurement biases, until the indifference probability is determined. The indifference probability is that probability p at which

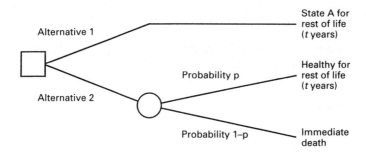

Fig. 5.3 Standard gamble for a chronic health state preferred to death.

the individual is indifferent between alternative 1 and alternative 2. The indifference probability is the von Neumann–Morgenstern utility for state A for the rest of life, t years, on a scale where the utility of 'healthy for the rest of life', t years, is 1.0 and the utility of immediate death is 0.

The standard gamble is a complex question to ask of an individual. Elaborate visual aids and careful interviewer procedures have been developed to make the interview more user-friendly. The measurement procedures are described in greater detail elsewhere.[30, 38–43]

Two other preference-measurement approaches that are widely used are the visual analogue scale and the time trade-off technique. Because these methods do not incorporate probabilities, they measure values as opposed to utilities. In the visual analogue scale, the respondent marks a line or indicates on a thermometer-like scale where his/her preference for the state lies relative to the end-points of the scale. The ends of the scale are identified with two other health states, one good and one bad. The visual analogue scale is a widely used instrument because it is relatively quick.

In the time trade-off approach the subject is asked to choose between two alternatives. Figure 5.4 shows the time trade-off question for a chronic health state preferred to death. Here, alternative 1 consists of health state A for the rest of life, t years. Alternative 2 consists of being healthy for a shorter time, x years, followed by death. The subject is asked to choose between alternative 1 and alternative 2, or to indicate that they are equally preferred. On the basis of this choice, the value x is changed systematically until the individual is indifferent between the two alternatives. The time trade-off score for health state A is the indifference value of x divided by t.

Much is known about the measurement characteristics of these three approaches (standard gamble, visual analogue scale, time trade-off), and their relationships to each other. Interested readers can refer to the references cited above. Several characteristics that are particularly relevant to this paper are the applicability, the precision, and stability over time.

The instruments described above require the subject to read, understand, and choose. Thus, they are applicable only to those who can read in the

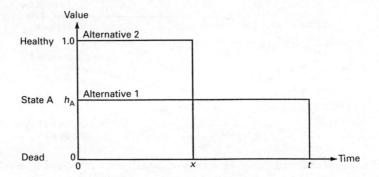

Fig. 5.4 Time trade-off for a chronic health state preferred to death.

language of the instrument. This provides a lower limit on age, which is a function of the instrument-maker's ability to simplify the wording. It also requires people who are able to handle the cognitive task. This can be a problem particularly amongst the very elderly, where a cognitive screening test can be used to precede the use of these instruments. Thus the instruments are not universally applicable in measuring preferences—that is, there are many patients whose preferences cannot be measured directly with such instruments.

With regard to precision, both the standard gamble and the time trade-off have a standard error of a single measurement of 0.13 on a scale where 'healthy for the rest of life' is 1.0 and immediate death is 0. Thus, the 95 per cent confidence interval on a single measurement of utility or value is ± 0.26 on a scale of 0 to 1.

Preferences for health states are not necessarily stable over time. For example, Christensen-Szalanski measured the preferences for women for natural childbirth as opposed to having an anaesthetic, and repeated the measures periodically during the birthing process.[44] He found that their marked preference for natural childbirth reversed at the actual time of delivery, but returned again afterwards. On the other hand, Llewellyn-Thomas and colleagues found that women's preferences for health states associated with cancer were stable between an initial measurement when the state was hypothetical and a later measurement when the woman was experiencing the particular health state.[45] Other empirical work has investigated the stability over time by re-measuring the preferences for the same health states at a later time. Such measurements would correlate perfectly (correlation coefficient of 1.0) if there were perfect stability over time. In fact, the 1-week test–retest correlation coefficient in standard gamble scores has been reported as 0.80,[46] and the 4-week test-retest in time trade-off scores is 0.81.[47] In summary, the limited empirical evidence suggests that preferences are often stable, but not necessarily.

The three measurement instruments (standard gamble, time trade-off, and visual analogue scale) have known relationships to each other. Standard gamble scores are greater than time trade-off scores, which, in turn, exceed those from a visual analogue scale.[30,48] The relationship between any two of the three instruments can be expressed as a power function.[49,50]

In addition to measuring patients' preferences for the health-status outcomes, one needs to measure the economic and time costs and benefits that will fall on the patient and family. The patients' preferences for incurring such costs or receiving such benefits also enter into the decision-making process. In addition, the economic costs and benefits that do not fall on the patient should be determined. These may or may not enter into the decision, depending upon the viewpoint adopted, as is discussed below.

Application in deciding whether or not to intervene

A single measurement of a health-state preference is inadequate for use in patient decision-making; multiple measures may be required. The situation is similar to the measurement of blood pressure where a single measure is insufficient to use for clinical decision-making. In the measurement of blood pressure, multiple measurements are required for a number of reasons: the underlying truth (blood pressure) is not stable but changes with circumstances, and the measurement process contains both random error and systematic error (bias). An example of the latter is the anticipation bias, in which the clinician is influenced by the anticipated results.

In the measurement of health-state preferences the same reasons exist for needing multiple measurements. The underlying preferences may not be stable; they may be changing, especially if the subject has not previously thought hard about the particular health states and her/his preferences. In this case, the interview may be as much about helping the subject to develop preferences as measuring them. The preference-measurement process contains random error, as described above, and may contain systematic error. An example of systematic error would be interviewer effect, which is always a potential problem in any interviewer-administered measurement of subjective phenomena. An additional problem in undertaking multiple measurements of preference, unlike blood pressure, is the difficulty in blinding the subjects to their previous answers. One approach might be to use alternative instruments, such as the standard gamble, visual analogue scale, and time trade-off. This would have several advantages. It would allow the subject to think of the situation from a number of different perspectives, thus providing a more broadly based set of preference responses. It would enable repeat measures to be taken without reusing the same instrument. And finally, it would allow all the measurements to be converted into utilities using the power function relationships that link the different instruments. The simplest approach would be to use the known relationships that apply to populations, although, ideally, individual-specific power function relationships would be best. Such relationships could be developed for each individual by measuring preferences in that individual for a sufficient number of additional states using all three instruments.

In addition to preferences for health states, costs should also enter into the decision analysis. Certainly, the monetary and time costs and benefits to the patient and family will enter. In addition, an argument can be made that a patient should also be sensitive to costs that fall on others. For example, if treatment involves the use of large amounts of a scarce resource, the opportunity cost would be the foregone benefit to those other patients denied access. Certainly some patients may want to consider this broader definition of cost.

The decision analysis by (or for) the patient could take a cost-effectiveness approach or a pure utility-theory approach. In the cost-effectiveness approach, the costs of the alternative interventions would be compared to the effectiveness of the interventions as measured through the patient's preferences for the outcomes, using traditional cost-effectiveness analysis.[51] In the pure utility-theory approach, the utility for the net economic cost or benefit and net time cost or benefit would be combined with the utility of the health outcomes to give the expected overall utility of each alternative. This could be approached in a number of ways, including the use of multi-attribute utility theory.[52]

The above discussion describes the application of utility theory to an individual patient making a specific treatment decision. There are many problems in attempting to use utility theory in this way, including the needs to gather systematically a great deal of information regarding the disease and its treatments, to convey this information to the patient or the proxy, to measure preferences with sufficient precision, and to help to interpret the results. An alternative approach is to use utility theory to establish practice policies.[53] These in turn can be used as guidelines to facilitate the decision-making for a particular patient.

Finally, it should be emphasized that utility theory, on the basis of its normative nature, should not be used blindly as an automatic decision-making device. It is simply an aid to inform the decision-making process. Other considerations, not captured by utility theory, should quite appropriately enter into the decision. It is important for users to appreciate this point, and not to follow the quantitative results blindly.

Application in program evaluation

Health-state preferences can also be used in program evaluation.[38,51] Indeed, this currently is the most common purpose for measuring health-state preferences in health care. It involves the aggregation of individual preferences into a group preference, a procedure that is not without controversy.[54] It also raises the question of whose preferences should count. Generally, the contenders are the preferences of patients who have the condition, or those of the general public. The latter group is justified on the basis that they are potential patients at risk for the condition as well as being tax-payers or insurance-premium-payers who are partially funding the system. In program evaluation, there is no question about the appropriateness of costs entering into the decision. At this level, costs are definitely relevant, although, depending upon the viewpoint of the analysis, different costs may be required.[51] For example, in an economic evaluation of neonatal intensive care of very-low-birthweight infants carried out from a societal perspective, a wide variety of costs were analyzed, including health-care costs (hospital, medical, dental, and drugs), other costs (institutional costs, special services, appliances, and special education), and the costs of lost productivity (lost earnings).[55]

In program evaluation, aggregate health-state preferences, often utilities, are used as quality-adjustment weights to determine quality-adjusted life years (QALY) gained. Programs are then compared on their incremental cost per QALY gained.[56] Although a utility-weighted QALY is not itself a utility except under very special circumstances, it may be a reasonable approximation to a utility. Empirical work is under way to investigate this point. On the other hand, there is an alternative justification for QALYs which argues that the objective of health care is to maximize health, and QALYs measure health.[57] This is known as the 'extra-welfare' argument for QALYs, because it is not based on utility theory and welfare economics.

Summary

In deciding whether or not to intervene, it is clear that the preferences of the patient, or his/her representative, for the alternative outcomes matter. Utility theory provides a formal method for measuring these preferences and incorporating them into the decision. Techniques exist to measure preferences, but they require special instruments and great care. Moreover, single individual measurements are not particularly precise.

To date, preference measurements have been used fairly extensively in program evaluation, but not a great deal in individual clinical decision-making. More work is required to explore their applicability in this latter domain.

CONCLUSION

The following elements required for use of epidemiologic data for prognostication and decision-making are now in hand:

(1) methodologic standards for studies of prognosis and evaluation of treatment effectiveness;
(2) up-to-date, systematic reviews and summaries of evidence regarding effectiveness from randomized trials of therapy in perinatology and neonatology; and
(3) methods for health-state preference measurements, including measurement of both utilities and values.

To date, research in the field of perinatology/neonatology has focused almost exclusively on health outcomes defined in biomedical terms. The challenge for the future is to expand the concept of 'effect' to include preference. Short-term objectives might include description of the range and stability of parents' preferences as measured in the perinatal period and beyond. Ultimately, perinatologists/neonatologists must consider facing up to the challenge posed by Malcontent,[58] who argues for an experimental test of perinatal decision-making that incorporates parental preference: 'For a start, we might ask, do *arbitrary* decisions at the time of impending birth of the smallest babies (presumption to initiate all-out treatment in most cases) result in improved long-term social outcomes in affected families, as compared with *discretionary* decisions (after discussion with parents, and based on their wishes, initiate either all-out treatment or non-invasive supportive care)?" The decision regarding the policy of care of a baby born at the threshold of viability is only one example of the opportunity to test the incorporation of preferences into perinatal decision-making. More common (if less dramatic) clinical scenarios abound in which valid evidence of effect defined in terms of perinatal mortality and neonatal morbidity is lacking, and where parental preference, if it were allowed to operate as discussed above, could well be pivotal in identifying the preferred treatment alternative. Such situations include, among others, whether or not to transfer a high-risk pregnant woman to a tertiary care facility which may separate her from the support of family and friends, whether or not to use tocolytic drugs (with their attendant maternal side-effects) in women who go into pre-term labor at 28 weeks' gestation and beyond, induction of labor versus serial fetal monitoring in post-term pregnancy, and alternative policies, some of which require prolonged hospitalization of the baby, in the management of neonatal jaundice.

In summary, methods exist to enable individual treatment decisions to be based simultaneously on the best epidemiological evidence of effectiveness from experimental studies, and on the actual measured preferences for the alternative outcomes of those to be affected. This new approach to perinatal decision-making should itself be implemented in a carefully controlled experimental manner in order to test the approach scientifically.

REFERENCES

1. Venn, J. *The logic of chance*, 4th edn, p.5. Chelsea Publishing Company, New York, 1962.
2. Silverman, W. A. Foreword. *In Effective care of the newborn infant*, (ed., J. C. Sinclair and M. B. Bracken). Oxford University Press, 1992.
3. Department of Clinical Epidemiology and Biostatistics, McMaster University Health Sciences Centre. How to read clinical journals: II To learn the clinical course and prognosis of disease. Can. Med. Assoc. J. 1981; **124**: 869–72.
4. Ozminkowski, R. J., Wortman, P. M., and Roloff, D. W. Inborn/outborn status

and neonatal survival: a meta-analysis of non-randomized studies. *Statistics in Med.* 1988; **7**: 1207–21.

5. Saigal, S., Rosenbaum, P., Stoskopf, B., and Sinclair, J.C. Outcome in infants 501–1000 gram birth weight delivered to residents of the McMaster health region. *J. Pediatr.* 1984; **105**: 969–76.

6. Escobar, G. J., Littenberg, B., and Petitti, D. B. Outcome among surviving very low birthweight infants: a meta-analysis. *Arch. Dis. Child.* 1991; **66**: 204–11.

7. Von Bernuth, H., Von Harnack, G. A., and Vogelsang, U. Organisatorische Probleme bei der Betreuung von Risikokindern. *Monatschr. Kinderh.* 1970; **118**: 570–1.

8. Ashton, B., Piper, M. C., Warren, S., Stewin, L., and Byrne, P. Influence of medical history on assessment of at-risk infants. *Dev. Med. Child. Neurol.* 1991; **33**: 412–18.

9. Ng, Y. K., Fielder, A. R., Shaw, D. E., and Levene, M. I. Epidemiology of retinopathy of prematurity. *Lancet* 1988; **2**: 1235–8.

10. Office of Technology Assessment. Congress of the United States. Neonatal intensive care for low birthweight infants: costs and effectiveness. *Health Technology Case Study* 38, December 1987.

11. Stanley, F. J. Survival and cerebral palsy in low birthweight infants: implications for perinatal care. *Paediatr. Perinat. Epidemiol.* 1992; **6**: 298–310.

12. Sackett, D. L. Bias in analytic research. *J. Chron. Dis.* 1979; **32**: 51–63.

13. Chalmers, T. C., Smith, H., Blackburn, B., *et al.* A method for assessing the quality of a randomized controlled trial. *Controlled Clin. Trials* 1981; **2**: 31–49.

14. Department of Clinical Epidemiology and Biostatistics, McMaster University Health Sciences Centre. How to read clinical journals: VI. To learn about the quality of clinical care. *Can. Med. Assoc. J.* 1984; **130**: 377–81.

15. Reisch, J. S., Tyson, J. E., and Mize, S. G. Aid to the evaluation of therapeutic studies. *Pediatrics* 1989; **84**: 815–27.

16. Harth S. C., and Thong Y. H. Sociodemographic and motivational characteristics of parents who volunteer their children for clinical research: a controlled study. *Br. Med. J.* 1990; **300**: 1372–5.

17. Sackett, D. L. Inference and decision at the bedside. *J. Clin. Epidemiol.* 1989; **42**: 309–16.

18. Charlson, M. E. and Horwitz, R. Applying results of randomised trials to clinical practice: impact of losses before randomisation. *Br. Med. J.* 1984; **289**: 1281–4.

19. Cross, K. W. Cost of preventing retrolental fibroplasia. *Lancet* 1973; **2**: 954–6.

20. Horwitz, R. I. Complexity and contradiction in clinical trial research. *Am. J. Med.* 1987; **82**: 498–510.

21. Sacks, H. S., Berrier, J., Reitman, D. *et al.* Meta-analysis of randomized controlled trials. *New Engl. J. Med.* 1987; **316**: 450–5.

22. *Effective care in pregnancy and childbirth*, (ed. I. Chalmers, M. Enkin, and M. J. N. C. Keirse). Oxford University Press, 1989.

23. *Effective care of the newborn infant*, (ed. J. C. Sinclair and M. B. Bracken), Oxford University Press, 1992.

24. Feeny, D. H. and Torrance, G. W. Incorporating utility-based quality-of-life assessment measures in clinical trials: two examples. *Med. Care* 1989; **27**, No. 3, Suppl:S190–S204.
25. Wennberg, J. E. On the status of the prostate disease assessment team. *Health Services Research* 1990; **25**: 709–16.
26. Tversky, A. and Kahnemann, D. The framing of decisions and the psychology of choice. *Science* 1981; **211**: 453–8.
27. Levine, M. N., Gafni, A., Markham, B., and MacFarlane, D. A bedside decision instrument to elicit a patient's preference concerning adjuvant chemotherapy for breast cancer. *Ann. Int. Med.* 1992; **117**: 53–8.
28. von Neumann, J. and Morgenstern, O. *Theory of games and economic behaviour.* Princeton University Press, 1944.
29. Howard, R. A. Decision analysis: practice and promise. *Mgmt Sci.* 1988; **34**: 679–95.
30. Torrance, G. W. and Feeny, D. Utilities and quality-adjusted life years. *Intl J. Technol. Assess. Hlth Care* 1989; **5**: 559–75.
31. Weinstein, M. C., Fineberg, H. C., *et al. Clinical decision analysis.* Saunders, Philadelphia, 1980.
32. Sox, H. C., Blatt, M. A., Higgins, M. C., and Marton, K. I. *Medical decision making,* Butterworth, Boston, 1988.
33. Kassirer, J. P., Moskowitz ,A. J., Lau, J., and Pauker, S. G. Decision analysis: a progress report. *Ann. Int. Med.* 1987; **106**: 275–91.
34. Lusted, L. B. The clearing 'haze': a view from my window. *Med. Decs. Making* 1991; **11**: 76–87.
35. Beck, J. R. Decision-making studies in patient management: twenty years later. *Med. Decis. Making* 1991; **11**: 112–15.
36. Bell, D.E., Raiffa, H., and Tversky, A. Descriptive, normative, and prescriptive interactions in decision making. In *Decision making: descriptive, normative and prescriptive interactions* (ed. D. E. Bel, H. Raiffa, and A. Tversky, pp. 9–30. Cambridge University Press, 1988.
37. Fishburn, P. C. Expected utility: an anniversary and a new era. *J. Risk Uncert.* 1988; **1**: 267–83.
38. Torrance, G. W. Measurement of health-state utilities for economic appraisal: a review. *J. Hlth Econ.* 1986; **5**: 1–30.
39. Froberg, D. G., and Kane, R. L. Methodology for measuring health-state preferences. I: Measurement strategies. *J. Clin. Epidemiol.* 1989; **42a**: 345–4.
40. Froberg, D. G. and Kane, R. L. Methodology for measuring health-state preferences. II: Scaling methods. *J. Clin. Epidemiol.* 1989; **42b**: 459–71.
41. Froberg, D. G. and Kane, R. L. Methodology for measuring health-state preferences. III: Population and context effects. *J. Clin. Epidemiol.* 1989; **42c**: 585–92.
42. Froberg, D. G. and Kane, R. L. Methodology for measuring health-state preferences. IV: Progress and a research agenda. *J. Clin. Epidemiol.* 1989; **42d**: 675–85.
43. Furlong, W., Feeny, D., Torrance, G., Barr, R., and Horsman, J. *Guide to design and development of health-state utility instrumentation,* CHEPA Working Paper 1990;9. McMaster University, Hamilton, Ontario, Canada.
44. Christensen-Szalanski, J. J. J. Discount functions and the measurement of

patients' values: women's decisions during childbirth. *Med. Decis. Making* 1984; **4**: 47–58.

45. Llewellyn-Thomas, H. A., Sutherland, H. J., and Thiel, E. C. Do patients' evaluations of a future health state change when they actually enter that state? *Med. Decis. Making* 1991; **11**: 323.
46. O'Connor, A. M., Boyd, N. F., and Till, J. E. Influence of elicitation technique, position order and test–retest error on preferences for alternative cancer drug therapy. In *Nursing research: science for quality care. Proceedings of the 10th National Nursing Research Conference*, pp. 49–5 University of Toronto, 1985.
47. Churchill, D. N., Torrance, G. W., Taylor, D. W., *et al.* Measurement of quality of life in end-stage renal disease: the time trade-off approach. *Clin. Invest. Med.* 1987; **10**: 14–20.
48. Read, J. L., Quinn, R. J., Berwick, D. M., Fineberg, H. V., and Weinstein, M. C. Preferences for health outcomes: comparisons of assessment methods. *Med. Dec. Making* 1985; **4**: 315–29.
49. Torrance, G. W. Social preferences for health states: an empirical evaluation of three measurement techniques. *Socio-Economic Planning Sciences* 1976; **10**: 129–36.
50. Torrance, G .W., Zhang, Y., Feeny, D. H., Furlong, W. J., and Barr, R. *Multi-attribute preference functions for a comprehensive health status classification system*, Working Paper No. 92–18. McMaster University, Center for Health Economics and Policy Analysis, 1992.
51. Drummond, M. F., Stoddart, G. L., and Torrance, G. W. *Methods for the economic evaluation of health care programmes*. Oxford University Press, Oxford, 1987.
52. Keeney, R. L., and Raiffa, H. *Decisions with multiple objectives: preferences and value tradeoffs*. Wiley, New York, 1976.
53. Eddy, D. M. Clinical decision making: from theory to practice—Practice policies—guidelines for methods. *JAMA* 1990; **263**: 1839–41.
54. Torrance, G. W., Boyle, M. H., and Horwood, S. P. Application of multi-attribute utility theory to measure social preferences for health states. *Oper. Res.* 1982; **30**: 1043–69.
55. Boyle, M. H., Torrance, G. W., Sinclair, J. C., and Horwood, S. P. Economic evaluation of neonatal intensive care of very-low-birthweight infants. *New Engl. J. Med.* 1983; **308**: 1330–7.
56. Weinstein, M. C. Principles of cost-effective resource allocation in health care organizations. *Int. J. Tech. Assmt Hlth Care.* 1990; **6**: 93–103.
57. Culyer, A. J. The normative economics of health care finance and provision. *Oxford Review of Economic Policy* 1989; **5**: 34–58.
58. Malcontent. Fumes from the spleen. *Paediatr. Perinat. Epidemiol.* 1990; **4**: 402–4.

5B ABSTRACT MEDICAL KNOWLEDGE, NEWBORNS, AND UNCERTAINTY: A CHALLENGE TO PHILOSOPHY OF MEDICINE

David C. Thomasma

INTRODUCTION

The art of medical decision making often masks an enormous range of science. The subjective act of decisional closure seems, on the surface, impervious to objective analysis, until one reads a thorough sketch of the complexity of objective criteria like that presented by Drs Sinclair and Torrance. The sheer difficulty and range of considerations they examine would seem to banish forever the hunch, the 'gut feeling', the secret tilts in one treatment direction over another, that to outside observers seem to govern decisions in perinatology, indeed, in all of medicine.

Yet a gnawing doubt remains that, despite the best of decision analysis, the major difficulty of applying abstract data to individuals still remains. Rejecting the 'elusive ideal of wholly objective, impersonal, and detached instrumental analysis' as 'not only unobtainable but destructive', Tribe has called for a 'subtler ... and more complex style of problem solving'.[1] This style, others have argued, ought to mirror more directly the way physicians and patients actually make decisions together, both of them facing similar risks and benefits. If this were not done within the context of trust within the doctor–patient relationship, if people did not trust one another, then they would flee into the abstract and mathematical, presuming to run away from the risk that is involved in every problem of daily living. Yet this flight would bring them no comfort. As Bursztajn *et al.* note, 'Decision analysis, designed to help people free themselves from the dead rituals of medicine, came in S.'s view to look like a dead ritual itself. It was at once unconvincingly abstract and forbiddingly detailed'.[2]

The criticism is evoked by reading the Sinclair and Torrance article. Yet their argument confirms, rather than denies, the criticism. Anyone trying to employ decision analysis to help in perinatology or any other branch of medicine faces a formidable task. As Hilary Putnam notes, the knowledge involved in modern medicine includes both abstract and probabilistic reasoning as well as practical and value-laden reasoning. He argues that the difference between the two has occupied every major thinker in the past two centuries:

The difference between these two ways of understanding events—the difference between controlling objects and relating to subjects, between 'objectifying reason' and human (or humane) understanding, if you like—has exercised thinkers in every generation in the last two hundred years.[3]

Thus, physicians and patients face a crisis about what it means to be 'scientific' in medicine; should patients be tested to death in order to apply with greater certitude the knowledge we have gained from others, or should they receive healthy doses of compassion, care, and personal attention? If too much attention is paid to decision analysis, its sheer complexity would overwhelm us. As Sinclair and Torrance note: 'Even in a simple decision problem with . . . only two alternatives, one stage of uncertainty, and a limited number of outcomes, the decision problem can be exceedingly complex.'[4]

Rather than duplicate their examination of difficulties inherent in the processes of decision analysis, in this complementary piece I want to explore the following three questions:

1. Is it justifiable to apply abstract, epidemiological data to individuals?
2. If so, how is this accomplished? What assumptions are made?
3. Are there specific problems when applying epidemiological data in medical decisions to any patients, particularly in perinatology?

I will take the disjunction between the abstract and the individual and analyze it in terms of inductive cautions. Rather than cover ground already explored by Sinclair and Torrance on decision analysis and logical studies on inductive reasoning in medicine,[5] my focus will be on the data used to help the physician's decision-making and the problems associated with this in clinical judgment about both competent and incompetent patients. To complement Sinclair and Torrance properly, I would like to explore the philosophical ramifications of their thorough study.

IS APPLYING ABSTRACT DATA TO INDIVIDUALS JUSTIFIABLE?

The problem of applying general or abstract knowledge to individuals is a central problem in making clinical judgments. This philosophical problem lies at the heart of differential diagnosis, confirmed diagnosis, prognosis, and the construction of a rational treatment plan. In each of these instances, abstract data and knowledge must be adjusted to fit the particular circumstances of the individual's body and functions, and the course of the disease, as well as the person's values.

Sinclair and Torrance note the many ways that abstract knowledge applied to individuals may not work—as a result of poor decision-analysis skills; because some individuals are outliers; because the collective universal embodied in the data may not have covered the set of individuals to which the knowledge is being applied; because the analogy does not fit the patient precisely enough; and, I would finally add, because of the mystery of life itself. So the question of applying such knowledge to individuals becomes one of utility—how many failures will we tolerate to justify the application of general data? If one baby dies per year because it does not "fit" the abstract data, but thousands of others are saved because they do, is this justifiable?

First and foremost a clinician reasons analogously, fitting the individual case at hand into the outlines of a paradigmatic case that represent the 'classic' instance of the disease or injury. The latter is developed from many sources, the chief among them being the natural history of the disease, the experience of other clinicians who have helped design the standards of care as defined in the literature, and the individual clinician's own experience with the disease and treatment outcomes. No matter how solid the data, the interpretative filter will always be the physician's clinical judgment. At the bedside, for example, one hears discussions of the 'classic case', a review of the literature, appeals to leading authorities and educators, past experience with similar cases, and the like. This process of weeding through analogous experience and cases is not unlike the clinical ethics methodology of casuistry.[6, 7]

As the physician addresses the problems of the newborn with the family, medical values appear most prominently. Among these are probabilities regarding treatment plans and outcomes. The use of probabilities is actually predicated on an assumed value: that the family wants the patient to live as long as possible. But families often possess a complex of values, only one of which is longevity. It is important to consider these other values in any dialogue with the physician about experimental therapy and other, less experimental, but risky, medical procedures. The possibility of the treatment plan's having a negative impact on other values besides longevity should be thoroughly discussed before proceeding.

Decisions about medical treatments are sometimes made in the midst of heart-rending uncertainty. The risks and benefits are difficult to determine with any degree of certainty, but are most often measured in terms of longevity. Longevity may not always be the most important value to be preserved when patients face either death from no intervention, or possible long-term negative effects should interventions be 'successful'. A good example would be decisions to be made about a premature baby born of a mother who abandoned it several days after birth to continue her drug habit. Before court-ordered custody hearings, physicians must make decisions in the best interests of the baby on medical grounds alone. But if the baby's lungs might not ever develop properly, the earlier interventions to save her life will make no sense. Greater reliance on data and less fear about legal consequences will aid in treatment decisions.

Suppose, instead, that it is unclear about whether the baby's lungs will develop properly. Surely we must try to save her life, then, using all the technology and care at the disposal of the staff. Should this effort be measured against the almost certain brain damage that will have occurred from hypoxia? If the child's life is saved after a three- or four-month intensive course in the newborn intensive care unit, what will count as 'graduation' from the unit? Just being alive with a host of ancillary lifetime health-management problems? Who will care for the baby? Does it matter if that question has not yet been settled?

Another example, this time less heart-rending, may be helpful. Suppose a pregnant woman wishes to have her child at home, and consults her physician about this. He notes that there is small risk for both the mother and child dying in any birth. Further, the doctor states that there is no evidence that having the baby at home is riskier for a low-risk mother than having it at the hospital. But, he also notes, if she is the one for whom high-risk eventualities do occur, having the baby in the hospital rather than at home may mean the difference between life and death. She might respond that she knows the risk, but does not think she will be 'the one'.

At this point, the future mother, her husband, and the doctor, must move to the realm of values rather than objective data, to interpret these values in light of the risks and benefits they foresee.[8] Among the risks must be the possibility of human error as well as of some physiological or genetic mishap. Recall Sinclair's and Torrance's data about the risks against survival of low birthweight infants in their area.[9] Among the benefits might be control of the birthing environment as far as possible, returning once more to the more human processes of giving birth in a family environment rather than medicalizing that process in the hospital. Data alone do not supply us with sufficient means by which to make decisions. These must be accompanied by our value-interpretants of the data, or at the very least, by the values embedded in the biography of the family, should the patient be incompetent like all newborns.

APPLYING DATA TO NEWBORNS

The values in medical decisions are supplied in obstetric/gynaecological and pediatric cases by the family, who are usually the father and mother. Both of them are at risk at the time of the decision-making as well, since the problems their child experiences are not 'normal' for birth and delivery.[10] This further complicates an already difficult ethical situation. For normally, the major method by which application of general knowledge to individuals takes place is by tailoring such knowledge to the individual's assessment of risks and benefits in the light of that individual's values and life-plans. That cannot occur in the case of incompetent patients, such as newborns.[11]

We then turn to more 'solid' objective data, usually called 'medically indicated treatment'. Yet the epistemological status of medical indications as a basis for treatment is also at issue in this application. Are such indications merely an application of standard and objective data to individuals, or are they themselves partially composed of subjective, evaluative aspects?[12] Current thinking about medical futility is appropriate here. There are few objective data in the final analysis of medically futile treatment. That judgment of futility lies in the clinical context, in conjunction with medical data, the goals of therapy, the values of the patient, the physician, the social environment, and the like. An analogy can be made with medical indications, or in fact, with all medical treatment.

When I asked above if it is justifiable to apply abstract data to concrete individuals, I also meant by 'justifiable', morally so. Clearly, it is done. In fact the whole point of developing an epidemiological database is to help us make decisions in individual cases, to define the borders of good or probable outcomes versus bad or unnecessary or even futile treatment.

The moral sense in medicine predominates at the moment scientific data is applied to individuals possessing values. The moral sense interprets the objective standard as a *norm* governing what is good for the patient. The physician must make a clinical judgment which aims at making a good decision with and for the patient.[13] According to the moral sense, then, a treatment plan is not only one which deals with scientific data, medical agreements about appropriate treatment, and the individual characteristics of the patient, but is also about the values of the patient. Further, it interprets all these data and values from the point of view of what is 'good for the patient'.[14] For this reason, the values of the patient determine what the patient considers to be his or her 'good'. Beneficence is thereby the overriding value of medical care.[15, 16]

But what of caring for newborns? Since they do not have a biography as yet—a history of choices made in which values are the precipitate— and therefore are only just acquiring an identity, would the benefit be determined only on the basis of objective, medically indicated criteria, even if these be somewhat uncertain? At the heart of the moral sense is a judgment of proportion between burdens and benefits. The calculus of burdens and benefits is not a utilitarian exercise in which burdens of continued treatment are weighted against the value of a patient's life as judged from a social perspective. Rather the calculus represents a normative judgment in which one decides how beneficial the treatment would be for the bodily condition of the patient, in the absence of the patient's wishes or preferences.[17] Actually this constitutes the morality of parenting and caring for a handicapped infant.[18]

It seems difficult, if not impossible, to avoid an affirmative answer to the question about the moral justification of applying abstract knowledge to individuals. If the proper cautions are met, it is unavoidable to accept generalized knowledge and apply it to the present instance. Thus, it is morally justifiable, since we have no other place to turn. It is the best possible choice in an ethical dilemma about continued treatment of an infant, or the transfer of a low-birthweight infant to a tertiary-care setting, or the decision to withdraw treatment from a newborn with bilateral hemorrhages in the brain.[19] Since we do not have the patient's values when treating incompetent patients, we can presume the value of continued life itself, unless the family and physician jointly determine that we are doing damage to the individual newborn, that we are cruelly prolonging a life that has been assaulted by nature itself.[20]

This is why the 'Baby Doe' regulations require continued treatment of handicapped infants, such that their rights as individuals do not suffer as a result of their handicap alone.[21] Treatment, fluids and nutrition, and pain-control medication can only be withheld or withdrawn if the infant is terminally ill and dying. Because a clear prognosis is often lacking, and the definition of 'dying' is difficult to determine in a high-technology environment, physicians early on who, like Duff and Campbell, proposed a subsequent quality of life index for withdrawal of care,[22] under the Baby Doe regulations could be seen as child abusers.[23] Furthermore, should the infant be judged to be dying, and a proper infant-care review committee hearing be conducted, withholding and withdrawing care still contains many ethical pitfalls.[24] Thus Helga Kuhse can argue that withdrawal or withholding of feeding to bring about the death of a handicapped newborn is not in the baby's best interests, a value that must predominate in the care of such newborns. While death itself might be in the baby's interests, a method of slow and sometimes painful dying by dehydration and starvation cannot be said to be in the baby's best interests.[25]

This moral presumption of the value of continued life to the individual neonate[26] depends upon general knowledge applied to an individual to improve that individual's lot. To make that judgment is a moral enterprise, because one must interpret a range of values, including the value of continued life, against projected outcomes that derive from collected experience. If the interventions will not improve the chances of a meaningful life, they should not be considered appropriate to the level of function the newborn enjoys. If the outcome is uncertain, interventions should be ordered with the caution that they or their consequences must be reconsidered later when the outcomes are clearer.

THE PSYCHOLOGY OF CHOICE AND THE BELL-SHAPED CURVE

Much of the machinery of modern medicine supports an impressive armamentarium of surgical, chemical, and biological interventions. All of these are the products of extensive research and the registration of patient data on computers. Faced with these possibilities, especially difficult decisions arise for newborns and their parents, since any such decisions are compounded in complexity by the illnesses newborns face at the beginning of life. This is raised in order to demonstrate more poignantly the difficulties associated with making concrete decisions with abstract data. This approach also helps locate the value dimensions of these dilemmas. The data support surgical, chemical, and biological interventions. All of these are posed for patient choices.

Among the many surgical interventions are repair of esophageal malformations, making stomachs out of intestines, realigning the spine, and placing feeding tubes directly into the stomach to support nutrition. Among the chemical interventions are a wide variety of drugs to control both the electrical and plumbing malfunctions of the heart, drugs that improve mental function, some that improve cardiac output, pills to control blood pressure and oxygenation, and the chemicals used in kidney dialysis to replace failed kidney function. Among the biological interventions are proposed genetic manipulations, eventual germ-line therapy, artificially created antibiotics, and the newer forms of cancer therapy, especially Interleukin 2.

All have their own side-effects. For example, a patient with spreading liver cancer may require experimental therapy that, coupled with radiation, will most certainly shut down one kidney. Parents may be concerned that they would not want their child to live life with just one kidney. Yet she may have only months to live anyway. In addition, most people can live with only one kidney for the rest of their lives. All of these are value considerations.

Every time a new procedure or experimental therapy is announced, the range of choice available for parents expands. This choice is complicated by the fact that the procedure or experimental therapy has been found to be effective but its effectiveness is in part a consequence of an abstraction from the concrete circumstances each patient experienced. This raises some of the ethical dilemmas so prominent today. But it also raises important epistemological issues. In the past, the physician was expected to choose the best treatment for the patient, and recommend it. Partly because of experimental therapies, this sort of traditional medical paternalism is fading. In its place, increasing emphasis is put on parental or patient decision-making and autonomy.[27]

These two dramatic alterations in medicine—its technological capacity and ethical challenges—create special difficulties for parents faced with decisions about serious illness. Experimental therapy is, by definition, investigation. It is experimental therapy accepted over standard therapy on the basis that it will be better.[28] It may not be. Rather the recommendation is based on a negative judgment—that previous therapy has not worked well. Further, the physician cannot tell parents what to do in this regard. They must grapple with their own values, and the test this offer makes for their philosophy of parenthood and their courage.

Choices are influenced by values and goals. Choosing among therapies starts by being a no-win situation. Typically, families face the following facts: their newborn has a serious disease that will cause the baby to die; standard therapies have not been successful in either stemming the disease or prolonging life; experimental therapy is available; this therapy is based on generalized conclusions of previous experimental studies, as well as the experience of other patients in similar but not exactly the same circumstances; this therapy presents a greater risk that standard therapy; and a choice between standard therapies and experimental therapies is possible.

But what is the choice? The choice is between probabilities. The probability is high that one's baby will die soon. On the one hand, standard therapies offer little hope of increasing the probability of survival. On the other hand, experimental therapies are untried, and may or may not increase survival. In fact, they may lessen it. Or worse, they may increase survival but at greater expense to the comfort and well-being of the infant. Many families judge, after a while, that their child 'has suffered enough'. This judgment arises from the totality of interventions tried, and the loss of a sense that progress is being made.

Many parents reason that taking the best shot means increasing the risk at present by consenting to the study, on the chance that they may be able to provide a better life for a longer time in the future. Experimental therapy in some areas may not offer a greater chance at longevity, but rather a better quality of life during the time remaining. Therefore some families may choose the risk in favour of a greater quality of life. Still others decide that, in a no-win situation, they would rather not put their child at greater risk. Rather than longevity, this group of parents seems to value quality of life. Further still, others factor into the decision helping medical research and future generations. These parents want to make the best out of a terrible situation. None the less, this is usually a secondary consideration for most.

Of major importance in making choices is how they are framed. Here the parents' values can sometimes run headlong into those of the physician. If the physician puts the possibilities for cure, remission, or improved function in the most positive light, then the parents will tend to choose in favour of the research protocol (some studies suggest 70 per cent of persons will do this consistently). If exactly the same possibilities are cast in a negative light, about the same percentage of parents would choose not to participate.[29] Drs Sinclair and Torrance deal with this question very well.

The reasons for this phenomenon are not hard to find. Neonatal parents, like patients themselves, honor and respect their physicians. Their physicians' advice is very important. Many physicians 'pre-judge' the clinical trial, and would not offer it for their patients unless their suspicion is that it will improve upon the standard of care.[30] How much greater the incidence of this respect in the newborn intensive care unit, when families that must make decisions, have to do so about very vulnerable, tiny persons, who do not yet have a value history? But the problem with experimental medicine is, of course, that the physicians' past experience and clinical hunches do not count. The study is designed to compare therapies scientifically. A central feature of the study is that previous research using animals or laboratory results suggests one therapy may be better than another. But here is the rub. We do not know in advance that this is the case when it is used in human beings. Further, we do not know if the data from previous studies will exactly fit the concrete circumstances of this particular patient.

This point is only slightly different when considering risky medical procedures rather than experimental therapies. In such cases, physicians can describe the risks and benefits for the parents, but they cannot predict how the child might react. If there is a 10 per cent chance that the baby might die from the procedure, that 'percentage' only describes past experience with patients like him. The population to which the infant might be compared in this risk might instead be more favorable than this. He might be a bit more developed than the others in the previous study, or in a more advanced newborn intensive-care environment, or under the care of more skillful physicians. Or the comparison might be unfavorable. The baby might be less developed than others, be hypoxemic, be weakened by other concomitant problems from prematurity, while others in the comparison population did not have those complications. The physician then must weigh all the variables and still make a suggestion about proceeding. His or her clinical hunches are only that. They cannot accurately predict how patients will do after the procedure is finished. However, such 'hunches' do play a role in deciding about treatment, even if such treatment plans are objectively based on real data.

Further, experimental studies themselves often compare therapies by assigning one or the other intervention by lot to the patient. Neither the patient nor the physician knows which therapy is being given. This is a 'double-blind' study—both the patient and the physician are in the dark. It is the preferred method for rooting out bias and the placebo effect.[31]

Finally, many therapeutic studies use historical controls. This means that the current therapy is initially judged to have such promise compared to past (historical) therapy, that it will be studied against reports of progress in the past. It will not be compared to another treatment in the study itself. The problem with historical controls, of course, is that the control over the fit between current patients and others is abandoned. The increased risk is that this analogous fit will not be coextensive enough to make an impact on healing or stemming the tide of the disease.

Given the risky business of advising parents in the presence of so much uncertainly, some physicians help them decide by describing 'the bell-shaped curve'. This is a curve drawn on a graph of a population of patients' experience with survival from the disease in question. A number only make it a few days or weeks. Gradually more patients live several months to one and one-half years. Then the number of patients who live longer falls off dramatically. Perhaps only one or two make it five years. The shape of the number of patients, the population curve, looks like an inverted bell.

Using this method, the physician can remain 'value neutral' about the possibilities (and not unduly persuade the parents to accept or reject therapies) by saying that some babies die in a matter of weeks, more last from several months to a year, and a very small number survive beyond one year. The physician would point out that the patient may fall anywhere along that path. Then possible treatments may be discussed, the results of which also represent bell-shaped curves. Within this discussion the value of prolonging life and the problem of quality of life can also be addressed. The proper way to frame the discussion is to caution that therapy carries its own risks of reduced survival and a probability of only extremely modest gains. The gains might be represented by shifting the bell-shaped curve a few months forward towards longevity. That is to say, rather than inadvertently holding out hope that a patient will gain some survival by being placed on an experimental treatment plan, the physician would only promise a possible improvement in the bell-shaped curve.

This is a sophisticated point. But it can be explained this way. No one knows where the patient falls on the curve; no one knows if that placement will be affected by a new experimental therapy. The baby may die earlier than anticipated. Or the infant may die earlier than he or she would have had they not been placed on the study. Depending on the disease (fortunately not all are intractable to treatment), the percentage of probability of moving the curve forward, not just the patient's own survival within the curves, should also be discussed. Is it high or low? This is another way of stating the overall risks of the procedure for all patients who have entered the study in the past.

HOW ARE ABSTRACT DATA APPLIED TO INDIVIDUALS?

The greater the abstraction, the less appropriate its application to concrete, individual instances. This theorem holds true unless the inductive product contains a set coextensive with the individual's characteristics, or at least analogously so. It is only on the basis of this 'set' that valid inferences can be made.

Any attempt to apply general computerized records to individuals will result in confronting the same problem. Epidemiological data culled from some groups in society may not apply directly to others. In this instance, social as well as individual judgments will be made, with the opportunity for error correspondingly expanded beyond individuals to social groups. Thus clinical judgment represents a micro version of the macro instance of the problem occasioned by epidemiology and past experience in medical care.

Research and practice are logically distinct activities. 'Research' refers to a class of activities designed to produce generalizable knowledge, whereas 'therapy' describes a class of activities meant to benefit individual patients or a distinct group of patients. The distinction is important, as research data are often applied to individuals who were not part of the original set. Typically such an appeal is made at the bedside by a phrase like: 'A recent study showed that . . .'. This appeal is made without either much attention to the limiting parameters of the original research, or much awareness of the limits of any application of general knowledge to individuals.

Some inferential cautions are required.

Inference from inductively gathered data can only be validly applied to an individual if: (1) the individual's relevant characteristics are part of the set; (2) the individual falls into a statistically secure field; (3) some common notes of all possible individuals are found in the inductive product (or a 'nature' of all the individuals is discovered and collated in the inductive product); and (4) the value assumptions of the abstract data are *de facto* values of the individuals to whom the data are to be applied.

What do these points mean for clinical judgment, however?

It is important that an attempt is made to fit the patient clinically into the data-pool of the research or epidemiological studies. There is a tremendous problem of applying abstracted, computerized data to individuals who may not fit the class from which the data set has been extrapolated. Is there not an assumption of a common human nature involved in such extrapolation? And is that assumption accurate in this instance?

The fit between the population studied and the population to which the data might apply is often not accurate enough to warrant any kind of scientific certitude. Undoubtably, further research will help gain a better fit. If this fit is not equivocal, at least it can become more analogically accurate. Many ethical issues are related to a lack of fit. Most ethics consults arise when the prognosis seems grim, and there is no objective way to decide about outcomes, either resulting from the disease or from proposed treatment plans.

THE POSSIBILITY OF A SCIENCE OF INDIVIDUALS

MacIntyre and Gorovitz suggested some time ago that medicine might be a science of individuals, in much the same way that environmental scientists have discovered ways to predicate general statements of individual hurricanes.[32] I think that such a science is an impossibility. Rather it should be called a *techne*, a discipline that combines science with the art of dealing with the concrete.[33] The problem of the abstract and the concrete is an ancient one. As is well known, the problem of Ideas in Plato, the universals in Aristotle, the medieval debates about abstraction from nature, the late-medieval reaction to substances, and the modern disclaimer of any knowledge of real world essences, are only part of the picture.

William Desmond has studied this problem in detail. As he argues, many philosophers since Hegel have been concerned about the charge that philosophy (indeed, all abstract disciplines, including epidemiology) inevitably favors sameness over otherness, identity over difference, the abstract over the concrete. The Hegelian dialectic, for example, subordinates difference to identity—not to speak of its materialistic cousin, the Marxist dialectic. Desmond argues that philosophy should also be concerned with the 'metaxological', a term he coins to describe the betweenness in the dialectic, the active will to be both unique and other.[34] A discourse about this intermediate realm is important precisely because it involves the fit required between the individual and the abstract.

Pellegrino and I have argued that philosophy of medicine must concern itself with relationships, a fuzzy area of contemporary philosophy to be sure, but essential if one were to examine the relation between the doctor and the patient.[35] The epistemological question of applying generalized data to individuals is certainly part of this needed exploration. It might take the following lines.

Oliver Sacks quotes Ivy McKenzie as saying 'The physician is concerned (unlike the naturalist) ... with a single organism, the human subject, striving to preserve its identity in adverse circumstances.[36] What is crucial about this point is that the identity of the individual must be helped to be preserved by the application of abstract knowledge. But this identity is not only physical. It is also constructed over time through value-based choices, the values eventually coming to stand for the individual's unique identity.

Clinical judgment, then, is an art of making that analogous fit. If the data is bad, the fit cannot take place. Sinclair and Torrance cite the famous example of inappropriate generalization in neonatal practice of restricted oxygen policy.[37] Since neonates were involved, the values of the patients were not, and neither were issues of their identity, since they had not yet constructed them. But a further problem of analogous fit lies in that very realm of subjectivity. If particularities of values and circumstances are ignored in the abstraction of the data, the same particularities are ignored in the application to the individual. This latter point refers back to the fourth caution. The individual's particular value-system is essential—something lacking in newborns of course.

The paradigmatic and the abstract can cloud the importance of the narrative and the concrete for healing patients. Sacks argues later in his book that 'The concrete is readily imbued with feeling and meaning—more readily, perhaps, than any abstract conception. It readily moves into the aesthetic, the dramatic, the comic, the symbolic, the whole wide deep world of art and spirit'.[38] It is hard to imagine that dealing with this realm could be called a science of individuals. Nevertheless, the importance of fitting the data to the individual cannot be gainsaid.

Naturally, physicians, nurses, and other health professionals are concerned about the well-being and values of their patients. But these quality-of-life factors are less amenable to measurement than longevity is. Yet quality of life is an important consideration for most patients. It is often left out of the discussion of chemotherapeutic trials. As noted earlier, however, it is a centerpiece of other research medicine, when only an improved function, rather than increased lifespan, can be offered.

Suppose one newborn on a study lived five and one-half years, but during that time, entered the hospital a total of ten times, spending over half of those years confined in a bed. During that time, the patient's family spent innumerable hours at the bedside in the hospital, and the economic burden on the family was dramatically increased. On the same study, another patient lived only 2 years and three months, but had to be hospitalized only twice. She died at home, and her family was not unduly stressed.

How can these two outcomes compare? In terms of longevity, the five-year survival rate, the second person fared much worse than the first. Yet in terms of values, family and economic values, the second child might have had a more successful result from the therapy than the first. This cannot be measured scientifically. Nor can it be presented by discussion of probabilities of survival.

Such problems of longevity and quality-life years come to bear on decisions to treat defective newborns as well. If a premature child is born to a mother, newly divorced, who already has other children and a full-time job, and the infant suffers before birth from bilateral hemorrhages to the brain, along with poorly developed lungs, treatment decisions are often dictated, not by the mother's wishes about the child, but by epidemiological data suggesting that such infants improve slightly and may possibly 'go home'. After months of newborn intensive-care therapy, the infant is stable. It is still too early to judge the level of profound retardation. The mother, at the end of her rope, may ask that nothing further be done to preserve the child's life. The physicians, on the other hand, are proud that their technology, technique, and care have been successful.

The mother and the physicians are judging success from two entirely different perspectives. Should the baby be brought home, she would have to quit work, by which she supports the other children, in order to care for the new baby full-time. She would very probably need some home-based nursing assistance as well. The child will grow up profoundly retarded, unable to care for himself for all the years he may continue to live as a result of the masterful care of the physicians. Thus, longevity for the family members can be seen as a threat to their security, while it is simultaneously seen by physicians as a value towards which their science and art strive.

CONCLUSIONS

Research medicine is an important part of modern health care. Parents should be encouraged to participate in this effort by minimizing their child's risks and by public support, so that the economic burdens can also be decreased. But in the end, a choice for a better or longer life for the child rests on the degree of risks the family chooses. Weighing probabilities about treatment under the advice of their physicians, parents need support and guidance for their most profound values. More than their lives are at risk. Their history and circumstances are also in danger of being neglected in the application of the general to the specific.

Further, philosophy of medicine should explore the problematic 'metaxological realm' along the lines suggested in this paper. Not only the doctor–patient relationship, but also the relationship between abstract data and particular individuals should be examined much more thoroughly than it has been in the past.[39]

I have made several claims and defended them:

1. The epistemological problems of the general and the individual cannot be encapsulated in the notion of a science of individuals, nor are they readily resolved through decision-analysis theory, as Sinclair and Torrance demonstrate. Instead, the adjustments between data and individuals must take into account the personal value history of the patients, their own need to preserve their identity, and the circumstances from which the

data themselves were abstracted. This adjustment appears to be a *techne*, a discipline aimed at doing right.

2. These epistemological and ethical problems are compounded when one considers decision-making for defective newborns. Here the families of such newborns must trust the physician's judgment in ways that are not part of the normal doctor–patient relationship, since decisions are to be made about a very vulnerable individual who has not yet constructed a value-history. This trust must occur in the midst of experimental designs and/or abstract data, that may or may not apply to the newborn, and may not have yet been demonstrated sufficiently for the physician to recommend one treatment over another on a purely objective basis.

3. When patients, or families, are asked to make a choice, it is most proper to discuss the movement on the bell-shaped curve when discussing risks and benefits.

4. Abstract data may give a false impression of scientific certitude. If they result from too much abstraction from one individual population, they may not apply so readily to another population.

5. The abstraction from the concrete may tantalize everyone involved into neglecting the rich and important realm of the particular. This concern does not apply so much to the scientists interested in gathering general data, but to the practicing physician who employs it. This employment can sometimes be dangerously inattentive to the concrete, and, most especially, to the concrete value system of the family.

NOTES AND REFERENCES

1. L. H. Tribe, Policy Science: Analysis or Ideology. *Philosophy and Public Affairs*, **2** (1972), pp. 66–110.
2. Harold J. Bursztajn, Richard I. Feinbloom, Robert M. Hamm, and Archie Brodsky, *Medical choices, medical chances: how patients, families, and physicians can cope with uncertainty.* p. 172. Routledge, New York/London, 1990.
3. Hilary Putnam, Preface. In Bursztajn *et al.*, pp. ix.–x.
4. Sinclair and Torrance, this volume, p. 000.
5. For example, see E. A. Murphy, E. M. Rosell, and M. I. Rosell, Deduction, inference and illation, *Theoretical Medicine* **7** (1986), 329–54.
6. Albert Jonsen, Casuistry as methodology in clinical ethics, *Theoretical Medicine* **12** (1991), 298–302.
7. Albert Jonsen and Stephen Toulmin, *The abuse of casuistry.* University of California Press, Berkeley, 1988.
8. Bursztajn *et al.*, pp. 351–5.
9. Sinclair and Torrance, this volume, p. 000.
10. Warren Reich, Caring for life in the first of it: moral paradigms for perinatal and neonatal ethics. *Seminars in Perinatology* **11** (9) (July, 1987), 279–87.
11. E. D. Pellegrino, The anatomy of clinical-ethical judgments in perinatology and neonatology: a substantive and procedural framework. *Seminars in Perinatology* **11** (3) (July, 1987), 202–9.

160 DAVID C. THOMASMA

12. D. C. Thomasma, Philosophical reflections on a rational treatment plan. *Journal of Medicine and Philosophy* **11** (1986), 157–66.
13. Edmund D. Pellegrino and David C. Thomasma, *A philosophical basis of medical practice*. Oxford University Press, New York, Chapter 7. 1981.
14. Edmund D. Pellegrino and David C. Thomasma, *For the patient's good: the restoration of beneficence in health care*. Oxford University Press, New York, 1988.
15. Erich Cassell, Healing, *Hospital Physician* **12** (1976), 28–9.
16. Jay Katz, *The silent world of doctor and patient*. The Free Press, New York, 1984.
17. D. D. Raphael, Handicapped infants: medical ethics and the law. *Journal of Medical Ethics* **14** (1988), 5–10.
18. J. Blustein, Morality and parenting: an ethical framework for decisions about the treatment of impaired newborns. *Theoretical Medicine* **9** (1988), 23–32.
19. Angela Holder, The deformed infant: medical aspects. In *Medical ethics*, (ed. N. Abrams and M. Buckner), pp. 368–73. MIT Press, Cambridge, Mass., 1988.
20. David C. Thomasma and Susan Braithwaite. New guidelines on foregoing life-sustaining treatment in incompetent patients: an anti-cruelty policy. *Annals of Internal Medicine* **104** (1986), 711–15.
21. Federal Register, Part VI: Department of Health and Human Services, *Child abuse and neglect prevention and treatment program; final rule and model guidelines for health care providers to establish Infant Care Review Committee*. pp. 14878–14901. US Government Printing Office, Washington DC., Monday, April 15, 1985.
22. Raymond D. Duff and A. G. M. Campbell, Moral and ethical dilemmas in the special care nursery. *New England Journal of Medicine* **289** (1973), 890–4.
23. George J. Annas, Baby Doe redux: doctors as child abusers. *Hastings Center Report* **13** (Oct., 1983), 26–7.
24. I. M. Kopelman, T. G. Irons, and A. E. Kopelman, Neonatologists judge the 'Baby Doe' regulations. *New England Journal of Medicine* **318** (1988), 677–83.
25. Helga Kuhse, Death by non-feeding: not in the baby's best interests. *The Journal of Medical Humanities and Bioethics* **7**(2) (Fall/Winter, 1986), 79–90.
26. David C. Thomasma, Looking to quality of life instead of length of life. *Medical Ethics* **3**, no. 4 (Oct., 1988), 6, 10.
27. H. T. Engelhardt, jr., *The foundations of bioethics*. Oxford University Press, New York, 1986.
28. K. Schaffner, (ed. Ethical issues in the use of clinical control. *Journal of Medicine and Philosophy* **11** (1986).
29. A. Tversky and D. Kahneman, The framing of decisions and the psychology of choice. *Science* **211** (1981), 453-8.
30. D. Marquis, An argument that all prerandomized clinical trials are unethical. *Journal of Medicine and Philosophy* **11** (1986), 367–84.
31. H. Brody, *Placebos and the philosophy of medicine: clinical, conceptual, and ethical issues*. University of Chicago Press, 1980.
32. S. Gorovitz, and A. Macintyre, Toward a theory of medical fallibility. *Journal of Medicine and Philosophy* **1** (1976), 51–71.

33. E. Loewy, *Ethical dilemmas in modern medicine.* Edwin Mellen Press, Lewiston/Queenston, 1986, pp. 6–8, discusses the notion of medicine as a *techne*, a skill aimed at a moral end, rather than merely a skill. This is an important understanding for the fourth caution noted in the text.
34. W. Desmond, *Desire, dialectic, and otherness.* Yale University Press, New Haven, 1987.
35. E. D. Pellegrino, and D. C. Thomasma, *A philosophical basis of medical practice*, pp. 39–57.
36. As quoted on the frontispiece of O. Sacks, *The man who mistook his wife for a hat and other stories.* Summit Books, New York, 1986.
37. Sinclair and Torrance, this volume.
38. Sacks, p. 166.
39. See E. Cassell, Moral thought in clinical practice: applying the abstract to the usual. In H. T. Engelhardt, Jr., and D. Callahan (eds), *Science, ethics, and medicine*, pp. 147–60. Hastings Center, New York, 1976.

6

Withholding and withdrawing therapy and actively hastening death

6A WITHHOLDING AND WITHDRAWING THERAPY AND ACTIVELY HASTENING DEATH I

Mildred Stahlman

The heading of this chapter encompasses three separate decision-making processes, each with separate arguments for and against each act; and therefore initially they will be discussed separately. Since they are considered by some to be steps in the same decision-making process, they will also be discussed in this context.

THE DILEMMA

The decision-making for the perinatologist (I include obstetricians and neonatologists in this term) regarding the withholding of therapy or actively hastening death begins with the previable fetus whose life is threatened, either by fetal or maternal disease or by malformations which are potentially correctable *in utero*. Modern technology, such as ultrasound, fetal blood-sampling, and placental biopsy has changed the medical model of the maternal–fetal relationships, shifting the emphasis from consideration of a single unit to one in which the fetus can be regarded as a distinct patient in its own right.[1] This consideration of mother and fetus as separate patients has occurred, not because of any change in the maternal–fetal relationship, but because of a change in how physicians think about and relate to their patients during pregnancy. If there is a treatable condition which is life-threatening to the fetus, but not to the mother, at a fetal age before extra-uterine life is reasonably possible, physician and parents must agree on the best plan of action (for example fetal transfusion or fetal surgery), with the mother fully informed and aware of the degree of risk to her life and health which fetal therapy entails, and this must be weighed against the potential benefits to her fetus. In most instances pregnant women will request treatment to promote fetal health, authorizing physicians to proceed with fetal therapy. Mattingly points out 'a woman's failure to volunteer for fetal therapy may seriously violate her fiduciary responsibilities to the fetus, this disqualifying her as proxy, but the physician's duties to her remain intact.[1] Consent must be competent, informed, uncoerced, and harmless to third parties. I believe pre-viable fetal survival is a secondary consideration to that of the mother, as one has no past and an unknown future, the other, a known past and reasonable prediction of a future. However, if the fetus is at a gestational age which is potentially viable *ex utero*, and both the fetus and mother are in mortal jeopardy, the decision-making becomes much more difficult, and the maternal (and paternal) wishes have to be weighed heavily. We are reminded of the Sixteenth-century English ballad about Jane Seymour, the third wife of Henry VIII, who desperately wanted a male heir to the throne. It begins 'Queen Jane lay in labour for nine days or more'. As it becomes obvious to all that either mother or baby, or both, are going to die if labor is further prolonged, Jane cries out in anguish 'cut my side open and take my babee'. This doomed woman sacrificed her own life for that of her son, the future Edward VI. In this instance, politics may have played a role in the decision-making; and who can guess what the outcome might have been had the baby also died?

In contrast to the obstetrician's dilemmas of fetus and mother, the neonatologist's decision-making on withholding life-sustaining treatment usually begins in the delivery room with the birth of a very low-birthweight pre-term infant. At the present state of our medical skill and technology, less than 24 completed weeks' gestation and less than 500 grams birthweight in a normally grown (not small-for-dates) infant are considered to be the lower limits of *ex utero* viability. As biologists, we recognize that organ systems of these extremes of immaturity have virtually no chance of sustaining prolonged life, even with the best intensive care and technology. However, decision-making on the basis of these criteria in the delivery room is often made with only partial or erroneous information, and to give the fetus the benefit of the doubt is to sustain life until accurate information (for example weight, measurements, blood gases, and, especially, response to intervention) can be evaluated. This approach leads up to the next and more difficult dilemma, that of withdrawing therapy that is considered futile. This decision-making often becomes repetitive in the newborn intensive care unit, as a critically ill infant's prognosis is reevaluated from minute to minute and hour to hour. The decision to withhold additional therapy may then be interwined with or substituted for active withdrawal of life-sustaining therapy. In addition, maternal, paternal, and, perhaps, other familial hopes have been raised, and multiple members of the care-giving team become emotionally as well as medically involved. Often the medical burden falls upon a house officer, perhaps new to neonatology, new to decision-making about life-and-death matters, and reluctant to take this ultimate responsibility. We ill-prepare our medical students in many instances, and as young house officers they are dismayed by their role. In addition, nursing personnel readily identify with their tiny, helpless patients, and may falsely encourage families to hope for a sanguine outcome despite all objective evidence to the contrary. An experienced, objective, and at the same time, caring senior person must be involved in continuity in these matters, and must be able to offer factual outcome information, understand options, and truly act as the baby's advocate, with parents, with nurses, and with less experienced colleagues.

When are we tempted to actually hasten death? Obstetricians may be forced to destroy a fetus in order to save the mother's life or, in such instances as extreme hydrocephalus, in order to deliver the fetus and end the pregnancy when all else fails. The neonatologist, on the other hand, is rarely faced with the dilemma of active euthanasia. It might be argued that the withholding or withdrawing of necessities for survival, such as nutrition, ventilation, oxygen, or antibiotics in specific instances, regardless of the future quality of life, is the moral equivalent of active euthanasia. If these treatments prolong and sustain life with some hope and some future, however painful and unpleasant, this would be true. If, however, these modalities only prolong suffering in a doomed patient who has already begun the dying process, however slow, the opposite is true, and the physician is fulfilling his or her obligation to relieve the patient's suffering, and has no moral obligation to prolong dying; indeed the opposite is true. In the case of infants who cannot express their own wishes, active euthanasia is not an option the physician should consider, regardless of pressures from family or others who honestly seek to do what is best for their infant, if long-term survival is a possible alternative.

The dilemma becomes profound, however, when the withdrawal or withholding of life-sustaining modalities is considered in patients who are sure to have limited lifespans, and whose continued lives may be considered hopeless and intolerable to patients, parents, and caregivers alike, but for whom the dying process has not yet begun. What of the patient with short-gut syndrome who does remarkably well for months on Total Parenteral Nutrition (TPN), a growing and developing little 'person', and no longer a newborn infant before a distinct personality develops? When *should* or *may* TPN be discontinued and certain death hastened thereby? When may the respirator be withdrawn from the spina bifida patient with Type II Chiari defect (i.e. brain-stem damage with central apnea) whose prolonged life is totally dependent on this technology? In neither situation has the process of dying commenced. These are among the most gut-wrenching dilemmas faced by parents and caregivers, and no easy generalization comes to mind. This 'slippery slope' decision-making may require a legal acceptance before parents or physicians can take steps actively to hasten death in such instances. The spectre of Nazi selection of the mentally retarded, the handicapped and the deformed for extermination before racial genocide became a policy should caution all of us to be extremely wary of accepting active euthanasia as policy in any set of circumstances. If it is to be condoned under any circumstances, they must be extraordinarily carefully regulated, and highly individualized.

THE RESOLUTION

At the present time, in the United States, one is not legally bound to initiate or continue 'extraordinary' care if it is considered virtually 'futile' according to the 'Baby Doe' regulations.[2] However, these same regulations and the President's Commission for the Study of Ethical Problems in Biomedical and Behavioral Research[3] strongly suggest that hospital infant-care committees be available to assist physicians in the difficult task of decision-making which will ultimately result in death, as opposed to survival with severe, and often painful, and limiting handicap. The regulations suggest that these committees be made up of individuals from a wide spectrum of backgrounds, bringing diverse approaches to the decision-making process. Membership on such committees may consist of such individuals as nurses (not necessarily neonatal or perinatal nurses), hospital administrators, medical ethicists, lawyers, lay representatives of handicapped persons, and physicians (not necessarily neonatologists, or specialists in the area of the patient's medical problems).

The decision to withhold or to withdraw life-sustaining treatment can be justified only if one has a set of medical (not social or emotional) circumstances whose outcome can be predicted with accuracy. This accuracy has been significantly increased by certain types of modern technology, and by long-term follow-up studies on medical and behavorial outcomes of a wide variety of neonatal conditions, including extreme prematurity, chronic lung disease, and many congenital abnormalities. Prevention or termination of prolongation of the inevitable process of dying is a humane medical act which is part of the responsibility of the physician–patient relationship. The physician's first responsibility is to act in his or her patient's best behalf, especially in the case of minors or those who cannot decide for themselves. We *are* our patients' advocates. Secondly, our responsibility is to act in the family's best behalf; and finally, to act in society's best behalf. If all these interests overlap, decision-making is infinitely easier than when they are desparate. However, neither the law nor a committee can abrogate the responsibility of the physician for his patient. The law is governed by blind justice, and mercy is added only by those humans administering it. In medicine, it is the caregivers who must act on objective information, tempered by compassion. We all need all the advice, judgment, and help we can get from committees on infant care, from other caregivers, and, especially, from families; however, in the final decision-making, it is the physician's responsibility to explain the harsh medical realities, present a plan of action, seek agreement, and remove the sense of guilt from the family and to bear it her or himself. As Cambell states, 'Unless we are to apply modern treatments indiscriminately, and this in my view would be irresponsible, it is difficult to see how a "child advocate", an ethics committee or the courts could do any better.'[4] There are those who accuse physicians of 'playing God'. It is not the physician at the bedside who plays 'God', but the lawmakers or committee members who may assume a rigid stance against withholding or withdrawing *any* treatment, which then must be used or continued, simply because it *can be* used. It is those caregivers who stand helpless at the bedside, suffer grief with the family, but recognize the medical implications of continued hopeless treatment in changing the inevitability of the outcome that are playing, not 'God', but man, human, fallible, suffering man who, along with his medical training, has assumed his ultimate responsibility as a physician. This is the difference between what Dr Raymond Duff calls 'close-up ethics' and 'distant ethics'.[5] Distant ethics is infinitely easier, as absolute principles can be decreed without any real or active participation in the decision-making involving a patient, whose circumstances are not only different from those of every other patient, but are constantly changing. I submit that the physician who practices close-up ethics based on the best medical knowledge available will make fewer mistakes in judgment than those who retreat to the position of distant ethics where responsibility is diffused to a wide variety of people, who may or may not have the best medical information, and, importantly, have no personal identification with the patients, their families, and their plights.

Is there an ethical difference between withholding medical treatment or intervention and withdrawing life-sustaining treatment already instituted? To suggest that there is an ethical difference between withholding medical treatment/intervention and withdrawing life-sustaining treatment or intervention already instituted implies that the principles on which such decisions are made have different informational bases, and that the interpretation of this information into prognosis is equally accurate in both circumstances. The decision to withhold treatment in the delivery room is often impossible because information is incomplete, and therapy that may later be withdrawn will be instituted until the prognosis is clear. I submit that, once the futility of the treatment or intervention is decided, based on sound and accurate medical information, the prolongation of dying is only rarely justified, and withholding or discontinuing futile treatment to maintain bodily functions becomes the same decision. Rarely, exceptions may lie in cases of the brain-dead or permanently comatose dying patient whose organ donation can be a life-saving act of love for another dying patient, or in short-term prolongation of bodily functions until families can be present to understand and accept the inevitability of death. Once death is inevitable, or what we usually refer to as 'once the patient is unsalvageable', then the process of dying should be allowed to proceed with its own natural history. One of the hard and bitter lessons physicians have to learn is that they cannot save *all* their patients, that they *cannot* play God and cheat death, even for those they love. What, however, has been given the physician, instead, is the ability to alleviate physical pain, and under many circumstances, mental anguish and fear. I believe that every person has the right to die without fear or pain, and with the preservation of as much human dignity as is possible. Our modern technology tends to make objects out of people, and the last vestiges of human dignity are easily destroyed.

One positive side of modern ICU technology is the improvement in accuracy of diagnosis and prognosis which it affords. However, a reliance on technology also changes the care-taker's attitude toward the humanness of the patient. This is particularly true of newborn infants who cannot communicate to express their own wishes. They are restrained, helpless, usually ventilated by artifical means, fed by artifical means, and so surrounded by machinery and monitors that handling, except to inflict more pain, is limited. Mothers cannot caress their babies, hold them, and soothe away their pain and fear. These hopeless babies' lives become quickly regimented into the needs of a busy intensive-care environment, and the less acute and the more chronic their problems, the less daily attention they demand. Caregivers often pass by their beds quickly during rounds with few comments, as nothing further seems relevant to a successful outcome of their hospitalization, and the daily recognition of one's failure as a healing physician is painful and to be avoided. As one organ system after another gradually deteriorates and finally fails, how much more pain, suffering, anxiety, and fear must our patients be asked to endure? How long should loving parents, when faced with the inevitability of losing their child, be expected to watch this process proceed slowly, and in an unnaturally prolonged way, with *life-sustaining* functions maintained long after *life-saving* measures are possible? What would you wish if it were your child? Is hastening death ever a proper option for the caregivers and the family? I think not, as this decision would impact on all concerned in important and undefined ways in their future behaviour. I do not believe in half-way measures, in discontinuing a ventilator but providing oxygen, in keeping a glucose drip going but omitting oral or parenteral feeding. These truly prolong dying. One might argue that they prevent suffering; but that prevention can and should be done by other means, such as sedation and analgesics. Starvation, dehydration, and suffocation are not to be substituted for responsible and caring management of the dying patient.

What effect could active euthanasia have on caregivers or family? Once accepted, future acceptance of euthanasia, perhaps of an elderly relative, or even easier, of someone unknown to the decision-maker and considered useless to society, becomes one step easier, and the same respect for life and one's role as a preserver of life and health is placed in future jeopardy. In addition, parents, whether they want this baby or not, should never be asked to participate actively in its death. Parental guilt feelings and self-blame are all too common with every abnormal pregnancy and every disasterous outcome, and the future relationships of parents to each other and to other children are fragile and strained, often to the breaking-point. Only the most solid of marital bonds are able to survive with renewed strength following the loss of a child.

What role should parents play in decision-making concerning discontinuing life-support systems for their offspring? Most parents truly want what is best for their baby, and their decision-making will be dominated by this caring attitude. Many parents (and, unfortunately, the public in general), however, have been led by the press, by television, and, sadly, by the egos of doctors, to believe in medical miracles which seldom happen, and they refuse to accept that *their* infant will not be the recipient of such a miracle. Denial is the first stage of grieving, and is very strong in many parents facing the unhappy reality of their baby's fate as described by the neonatologist. Parents, all too frequently young parents, who have never dealt with a seriously handicapped child or a dying baby, are woefully unprepared to listen to and understand the medical situation and the proposed plan of action. Over ten years ago I wrote in a similar context.

We are in an age of abnormal fear of dying. When we were born at home and died at home, death was often looked upon as a release from suffering, a deliverance to be welcomed, a friend to be accepted, if not loved. In rural societies, birth and death of animals were understood as natural events and man interpreted his own life and death in the same natural terms. Death was not only considered inevitable, but familiar. Today we are born in "sterile" delivery rooms, cared for in "sterile" nurseries, rarely fed from our mother's breast, and raised to look upon death as the worst and most fearful of outcomes. Most nonmedical people have never seen a person die, except violently on TV, and the prolongation of death in terminal illnesses in most hospitals lends them no comfort when considering their own mortality. We have, strangely, lost our humanity in trying to prolong human life without regard to its quality or its cost in human suffering. We have forgotten that a most important sentence in the Hippocratic oath is the pledge that the physician will do what he thinks is in the best interest for this patient.[6]

Often it is the grandparents of these infants who must eventually help make the hard decisions. Neonatologists must patiently explain and explain again the hopelessness of the situation, and not hurry the process of understanding, acceptance, and grieving. We must keep foremost in mind that we, the physicians, do not have to live continuously with these decisions; only parents do. Most neonatal ICUs offer a private room for grieving, where parents are given their dying child from whom life-support systems have been withdrawn, to hold in their arms and cradle as life slips away. At this point, I often suggest that the infant be named, if this has not already been done, as this makes the infant not only a person, but a family member, and grieving can proceed more normally.

These parents are the easy ones to deal with when compared with parents of an unwanted baby. In these tragic circumstances, parents may request life-support systems withdrawn from a potentially salvageable infant, whose future will predictably be one of severe handicap. The physician, as always, must act as the baby's advocate and, using all the social services available, try to salvage a caring relationship between parent and baby. *All* children need caring parents who will support them in good times and bad. Even the best of children sometimes try their parents to the breaking-point. Severely handicapped infants try their parents every hour of every day, and it requires generosity of spirit, patience, love, understanding, and great strength to manage these babies on a day-to-day basis. In addition it requires great resources, including financial, which may be severely depleted by prolonged hospitalization. It is the salvageable infants, regardless of handicap, that demands the most of their parents, who may not want them, and of society, which may not pay for them.

What consideration should be given the costs to society? These are just as real as the costs in pain and suffering to the patient, the costs in grief, sorrow, guilt, blame, family disruption, and, all too often, bankruptcy to the family. Today's medical technology is enormously over-priced in most instances, driven in part by industries seeking to make a profit in their manufacture of technology or drugs, in part by hospitals seeking to make a profit in their use, partly by the insurance industry's acceptance of inflated charges, partly in physicians' tendency to rely upon technology instead of their own skills in diagnosis and treatment, and partly by the physician's desire to avoid litigation. In the care of the uninsured, society will eventually pay the bill for prolonged dying. The cost–benefit ratio of certain types of procedures and of resuscitation considered futile in infants with extreme immaturity (for example of 23 weeks or less) is seriously being considered in a number of state legislatures. The United States, the most affluent country in the world, has faced the hard fact that resources for medical care *are* limited, and health-care planners are now making decisions as to who will live and who will die. Physicians should find this development in our society totally unacceptable. Veach states 'Human life and dollar profits just cannot always fit on the same scale. We are in a dangerous situation when society can hold that any one individual, infant, child, or adult, is too useless, too non-productive or too costly to protect with full civil and moral rights. The physician always has been aware of this.'[7] Resources are always limited, more so in most other countries than in our own. The availability of resources for the preservation of salvageable life is simply a matter of setting national priorities. The decision to withhold or withdraw medical care from newborn infants who are unsalvageable, just like the decision to continue treatment, however costly, to those who are salvageable, must be made without the consideration of societal costs. We must work to change our priorities instead and strive to live in a humane society as well as in a just society if we are to be called 'civilized'.

The management of unsalvageable infants, and the decision-making regarding the termination of their care, has been an evolving process in the United States and in other Western countries. Twenty years ago, before newborn intensive care was so well developed, before *fetal* medicine was a sub-speciality of obstetrics, and before many of the technical innovations made 'survival of the unfit' possible, physicians—pediatricians, obstetricians, surgeons—took a fatalistic, and often bluntly realistic view of attempts to salvage either very-low-birthweight, severly malformed, or genetically handicapped infants, such as those with Down syndrome, especially if the handicap were complicated by additional malformations. Laws protecting the handicapped were rarely interpreted as relating to newborn infants, and a cloak of silence surrounded the common practice of failing to resuscitate the malformed or very-low-birthweight baby in the delivery room, or of placing a grossly deformed infant behind a curtain, to be treated with benign neglect. As outcomes improved, accepted practices changed, and gradually, with education of both the professionals and of the public, general awareness of changes in salvageability demanded rethinking of long-held dogmas. Even less than ten years ago, active euthanasia of severely malformed infants was under consideration in Australia, where Kuhse and Singer[8] made a cogent analysis of the proposition that *all* human life is not of infinite value. These values were actively questioned in Britain and in the United States, by physicians and by the public.[9,10] Should the quality of a given life, the life of the family, and the burdens placed on society play a role in decision-making? Obviously, in certain specific instances, each of these considerations is consciously or unconsciously added into the equation, for example in the case of the anencephalic infant, or the trisomy 13 or 18 with a predictable short-lived irreversible future. However, we had already begun to question our old ethical values of life with handicaps by the time of the 'Baby Doe' case. The fact that unrealistic and rather naive regulations arose from this case did not change the positive effects on public education about the potential future development of Down syndrome children and other infants with mental and physical handicaps. Public debate of these regulations, the court challenges, and attempts to tie the right to medical treatment to civil rights contributed to a wider and more factual understanding of the problems faced by the survivors, by their families, and by the society in which they lived and on which they depended for support. This gradual acceptance of the rights of the handicapped, including those of newborns, has happened throughout Western societies, perhaps precipitated and hastened by the 'Baby Doe' crisis.

More recently, increased public awareness of the wide spectrum of severity of these handicaps and the increased potential for mainstreaming these children into society, albeit in a protected ambit, has been highlighted by the inclusion of Down syndrome, mentally retarded, and autistic individuals as sympathetic characters in movies and in television series. Not all infants with potentially severe mental or physical handicaps can be accurately evaluated for their level of future potential in their first weeks or months of life. Many will continue to remain institutionalized for their entire lives, a great cost to themselves, to their families, and to society; but I perceive a more understanding society, both professionally and publically, than existed twenty years ago. Additionally, we are on the threshold of a new and exciting scientific era of genetic engineering, and tissue and organ transplantation research. Hearts, livers, kidneys, thymuses, and bone marrow are being transplanted into infants previously considered unsalvageable. Lungs will be next, as is now possible in adults, followed by gut, pancreas, and other organs. The possibility of single-gene transfer, even *in utero*, is rapidly developing. New techniques in plastic and reconstructive surgery for severe and deforming malformations are producing extraordinary results, both cosmetically and functionally. Conditions once considered hopeless may, in the future, become treatable, even curable. Each of these new treatment modalities will have their costs and their successes and failures, and will present new ethical dilemmas. But they will change our way of thinking about salvageability, and will give us great hope for the future of our profession, of our patients, and of the humane society in which we choose to live.

REFERENCES

1. Mattingly, S. S. The maternal–fetal dyad. Exploring the two-patient obstetric model. *Hastings Center Report* **22**, 13–18 (1992).
2. Department of Health and Human Services. Child abuse and neglect prevention and treatment program; final rule model guidelines for health care providers to establish infant care review committees. *Federal Register*, Part VI, April 15 (1985).
3. President's Commission for the Study of Ethical Problems in Medicine and Biomedical and Behavioral Research. *Seriously ill newborns. Deciding to forego life-sustaining treatment.* A report on the ethical, medical and legal issues in treatment decisions. (1983).
4. Campbell, A. G. M. Which infants should not receive intensive care? *Arch. Dis. Child.* **57**, 569–71 (1982).
5. Duff, R. S. 'Close-up' versus 'distant' ethics: deciding the care of infants with poor prognosis. *Sem. Perinatol.* **11**, 244–53 (1987).
6. Stahlman, M. T. Ethical dilemmas in perinatal medicine. *J. Pediatr.* **94**, 516–20 (1979).
7. Veach, R. Ethical dilemmas in current obstetrics and newborn care. *Sixty-Fifth Ross Conference on Pediatric Research*, Duck Key, Florida, May 13–15 (1972).
8. Kuhse, H. and Singer, P. Should the baby live? *The problem of handicapped infants*. Oxford University Press (1985).
9. Emery, J. L. Attitudes of parents and paediatricians to a baby's death. *J. Royal. Soc. Med.* **83**, 423–4 (1990).
10. The Gallup Report. *Public evenly divided on whether deformed infants should be kept alive or allowed to die.* Report 13, June (1983).

6B WITHHOLDING AND WITHDRAWING THERAPY AND ACTIVELY HASTENING DEATH II

Robert Weir

In the first part of this chapter, Mildred Stahlman sets the stage for an analysis of some of the ethical problems connected with perinatology. In particular, she places current ethical problems in maternal–fetal medicine and neonatology in a historical and social context that helps to explain the difficulty of the problems, the multiple parties involved in problematic cases, and the ways in which some of the problems have changed over the last two decades.

In terms of historical context, she points out that many of the ethical problems in these two subspecialities of obstetrics and pediatrics did not exist twenty years ago. Before technological innovations made fetuses directly accessible as patients and the development of neonatal intensive care made the 'survival of the unfit' possible after birth, the ethical problems now regularly present in maternal–fetal medicine and neonatology had either not yet emerged or at least had not yet developed the magnitude they now have. In addition, the 'Baby Doe' and subsequent Child Abuse regulations, State laws on child abuse, and evolving societal standards regarding normalcy had not yet begun to change mainstream attitudes in the United States toward individuals with disabilities. Likewise, government panels, national policies, the media, and occasional court cases in Britain, Australia, and other industrialized countries had not begun to have much effect on the medical mangement of obstetrical cases involving maternal—fetal conflicts or neonatal cases involving non-dying infants with severe neurologic impairments.

In terms of social context, Dr Stahlman concentrates on the various parties frequently caught up in the dynamics and difficulties of a decision in a neonatal intensive care unit (NICU) to withhold or withdraw life-sustaining treatment from an infant who was born too small, too young, or too disabled to be 'salvaged' with the best medical care possible. The parents in such a case, she correctly observes, are often young, inexperienced, and 'woefully unprepared' to understand the infant's medical condition and the plan of medical care proposed by the physician(s) in the case. Some of the medical team is also unprepared for such a case. with residents sometimes being new to neonatology, reluctant to assume appropriate responsibility, and dismayed by their role in a life-and-death situation fraught with medical and moral uncertainty. Nurses may complicate matters by holding out false hope for families expecting a medical miracle, and members of pediatric ethics committees, while offering instructive advice, may not really be helpful through their 'distant ethics' to the attending physician, who must seek agreement from the parents to a plan of medical management that will result either in their child's death or their child's remaining alive with severe to profound disabilities.

In addition, the first part of the chapter contains a descriptive account of numerous ethical aspects of decisions to withhold or withdraw therapy and, possibly, of decisions actively to hasten some patients' deaths. Reflecting her years of experience practicing 'close-up ethics' in pediatric settings, Dr Stahlman communicates views that would be shared by many neonatologists regarding the suffering, salvageability, and dying of neonates, the benefits and limitations of medical treatment, the roles of parents and physicians, the escalating costs of intensive care, and the changing medical and societal attitudes toward children with developmental disabilities.

We now turn to a critical analysis of some of the ethical issues raised in the first part of the chapter. Many of the issues we will address are specific to neonatology; some of them also pertain to obstetrics; and a few of them have application to other clinical settings as well.

1. *Do human fetuses and neonates differ from each other—or from older humans—in terms of ontological and moral status?* The relevance and importance of this question is clear from Dr Stahlman's earlier comments. At one point she indicates that, in her view, the ontological and moral status of fetuses changes with fetal viability. At another point she describes a young pediatric patient with short-gut syndrome, maintained for months with TPN, as being a little 'person' rather than being a neonate lacking a distinct personality.

Put in a general way, this question about ontological status asks, 'What kind of entity is it whose life or death is at stake in the decisions made by pregnant women regarding abortion, or in the decisions made by neonatologists and/or parents in an NICU?' Put more specifically, the question concerns personhood: 'Do any, or do all, fetuses and neonates count as persons, in the sense that most children and adults count as persons?'

To make some sense out of these questions, it is necessary to describe a consensus philosophical view about the concept of personhood. That consensus, to the degree that it exists, focuses on the intrinsic rather than the extrinsic qualities of persons. Most philosophers agree on at least the core properties or traits of personhood, if not on all of their applications. The resulting consensus view holds that for a human being (or non-human being of some sort) to count as a person requires the possession of three necessary and jointly sufficient properties: consciousness, self-awareness, and at least minimum rationality.[1]

The possession of personhood, therefore, has to do with neurological development and, at least among human beings, the absence of profound neurological dysfunction or impairment. The answer to the question of whether fetuses and/or neonates are to be counted as persons depends on three interrelated factors: (a) how much neurological development is required for personhood; (b) how much neurological impairment is necessary to rule out personhood; and (c) whether any significance is to be placed on the principle of potentiality as it applies to personhood.

When applied to the debate regarding the ontological status of fetuses and neonates, these factors contribute to the identification of three distinguishable positions. The first position holds that *all fetuses and neonates*, whether normal or neurologically impaired, *are non-persons*. Individuals holding this view tend to make four related claims:

(1) personhood is a moral category attaching to beings (of any species) with certain characteristics, principally cognitive capacities;
(2) fetuses and neonates lack the cognitive qualities that make a human into a person;
(3) being a *potential* person does not count; and
(4) only *actual* persons are entitled to the moral benefits of personhood, including the right not to be killed.[2]

The second position stands at the other end of a philosophical and political spectrum and represents a very common view of neonates (but not of fetuses) held by many persons. This position, which holds that *all neonates are actual persons*, can also be presented in terms of four related claims:

(1) personhood is a moral and legal category attaching to human beings at a chronological point determined by social consensus, with conception, viability, and birth as three alternatives for such a point;
(2) neonates count as *actual* persons, as do all other human beings who are past the chosen chronological point;
(3) being a *potential* person does not signify very much; and
(4) neonates and all other *actual* persons are entitled to the moral and legal benefits of personhood, including the right not to be killed.

The third position stands between the other positions, differing from the first position's insufficient claims and the second position's excessive claims regarding the personhood of human newborns. This position, which holds that *most neonates (and many fetuses) are potential persons*, can be compared with the alternative views on the basis of its four claims:

1. personhood is a moral category attaching to beings (of any species) with certain characteristics, principally cognitive capacities;
2. neonates lack the intrinsic qualities that make a human into a person, as do fetuses;
3. having the potential to become a person through the normal course of development does count, and neonates without severe neurological impairment (and fetuses having exhibited brain activity) have this potential; and
4. all *potential* persons have a *prima facie* claim to the moral benefits of personhood, including the right not to be killed, because they will subsequently acquire an *actual* person's moral and legal right to life.[3]

The last of these positions is the preferable way of describing the ontological and moral status of neonates (and many fetuses). This position is better than the neonates-are-not-persons view because it grants more than a species value to human newborns—and avoids the major weakness of having to allow, in principle, for the indiscriminate termination of an indeterminate number of neonatal lives, whether these lives are cognitively impaired, physically disabled, or normal. The third position is also better than the neonates-are-actual-persons view because it takes the philosophical and psychological concept of personhood seriously—and avoids the major weakness of having to say, in principle, that a baby has no more claim to the moral benefits of personhood than an early human embryo does.[4]

2. *Who should make the decisions that will lead to the deaths of some fetuses and neonates, and what standard(s) should be used for these decisions?* The answer to these questions is reasonably clear in obstetric cases, especially in terms of the law. Although under continuing challenge from 'pro–life' groups, the 1973 *Roe v. Wade* decision is still the law of the land.[5] According to that US Supreme Court decision, the appropriate decision-maker in abortion cases is the woman who is pregnant. However, the decision she makes, if made during the second trimester, may be subject to State regulations (for example, spousal notification, a mandatory waiting period). If made during the third trimester, her decision may be restricted in many States by consensus medical views or State laws related to fetal viability.

The ethical and legal standard for pregnancy-termination decisions, subject to medical and legal restrictions in various States, is the autonomy of the pregnant woman. The same standard governs decisions by pregnant women who refuse diagnostic procedures, medical therapies, or surgical procedures (for example, a cesarean delivery for fetal distress) that might promote fetal well-being or even save the life of the fetus. In such situations, recent case law and the ethical position taken by the American College of Obstetrics and Gynecology (ACOG) indicate that the pregnant woman's autonomous decision should prevail over fetus-related medical concerns.

The most significant appellate-level court decision is the decision of the District of Columbia Court of Appeals in the case *In re* A. C., a case that involved an earlier court-mandated cesarean section at 26 weeks' gestation for a woman dying of cancer—even though she, her family, and her attending physicians had agreed that the delivery of the baby was secondary in importance to keeping her comfortable as she died. The court's decision emphasized the importance of the pregnant woman's autonomy: 'we hold that in virtually all cases the question of what is to be done is to be decided by the patient—the pregnant woman—on behalf of herself and the fetus.[6]

In a similar fashion, ACOG has addressed the issue of maternal–fetal conflicts on two occasions. In 1987 the ACOG policy stated that 'the use of the courts to resolve these conflicts is almost never warranted'.[7] Two years later the policy was repeated and reinforced in an ACOG bulletin: 'The obstetrician should make an effort, through discussion and consultation, to make the woman aware of the implications of her actions for the health of the fetus ... no other party, including the state, should override her autonomy in order to enforce [her] obligations.[8]

In the context of neonatology, the procedural and substantive questions asked above do not have answers that are quite as clear. In fact, the questions themselves are frequently conflated, with resulting answers being somewhat more clear, at least in the United States, about the appropriate standard for decision-making than about the persons who should make the decision.

In terms of an appropriate substantive standard, decision-makers in NICUs have two major alternatives. The more conservative standard is the ethical and legal standard put forth by the US government in the 1985 Child Abuse regulations. These regulations, drafted as revised rules to succeed the invalidated 1983 'Baby Doe' regulations, mandate the provision of life-sustaining treatment for all neonates who are not permanently unconscious or dying. Decision-makers adhering to these regulations choose to sustain the lives of all neonates, no matter how small, premature, or severely disabled, unless an infant fits one of three exceptional circumstances specified by the regulations: (a) 'the infant is chronically and irreversibly comatose; (b) the provision of [medical treatment] would merely prolong dying ... or otherwise be futile in terms of the survival of the infant; or (c) the provision of such treatment would be virtually futile in terms of the survival of the infant and the treatment itself under such circumstances would be inhumane'.[9]

Controversial from the start, the Child Abuse regulations are now widely ignored by neonatologists, for a variety of reasons. The regulations are ignored, in part, because they have become recognized as a regulatory equivalent of a 'toothless tiger': health professionals are usually reluctant, except in the most egregious cases, to report parents of extremely premature or severely disabled infants to State authorities when they refuse life-sustaining treatment for their children; State departments of human services do not have sufficient funding or personnel to investigate reported instances of child abuse in NICUs; State legal authorities are disinclined to prosecute any reported cases; and the financial penalties ostensibly imposed by the federal government on non-compliant hospitals are trivial to non-existent. In addition, the regulations are ignored because of their substance: their wording is inherently vague, they were drafted primarily to fit fairly simple neonatal cases (Down syndrome and myelomeningocele cases, not cases of extreme prematurity), and they seem to call for life-sustaining treatment in some cases that many neonatologists think would be contrary to the best interests of the infants whose lives and futures are at stake.[10]

The result is that the Child Abuse regulations, while still in place as federal policy, now represent an ethical standard for decisions to withhold or withdraw treatment that is followed somewhat reluctantly by neonatologists and parents in only a minority of cases. Most cases involving decisions to initiate, continue, or abate life-sustaining treatment are governed by another, less conservative standard. The patient's-best-interests (PBI) standard focuses neither on the narrow questions of whether an infant is permanently unconscious or dying nor on the question of whether the technological intervention in a given case is futile, although such considerations can be important to a determination in some cases that life-sustaining treatment is or is not in an infant's best interests. Rather, the PBI standard represents an ethical norm for decision-making in a wide range of cases, including cases in which an infant is neither unconscious nor dying and the medical treatment is not futile, at least in any statistical sense.

As described elsewhere, the PBI standard has several variables that can be used in making decisions to withhold or withdraw treatment in neonatal cases. The variables are as follows: (a) the severity of the patient's medical condition; (b) the availability of curative or corrective treatment; (c) the achievability of important medical goals; (d) the presence of serious neurological impairments; (e) the extent of the patient's suffering; (f) the multiplicity of other serious medical problems; (g) the life expectancy of the child; and (h) the proportionality of treatment-related benefits and burdens to the child.[11]

As to the procedural question raised earlier, there continues to be some disagreement both in theory and in practice. The conventional answer to the question about decision-making authority is that the parents of premature or disabled children are the appropriate persons to make decisions about withholding or withdrawing therapy that could result in the deaths of their children. It is they, Dr Stahlman observes, who have 'to live continuously with these decisions'. It is they, Nancy King argues, who should be given 'transparent' medical information by physicians—and all other information that parents might consider 'significant enough not to want to do without' as they try to make an informed decision regarding the initiation, continuation, or abatement of life-sustaining treatment.[12]

Yet few if any neonatologists are willing to give parents unlimited discretion. On the basis of their specialized medical knowledge, experience with numerous other difficult cases, consultation with appropriate pediatric subspecialists, prognostic skills, tolerance for medical uncertainty, and personal ethical judgments, neonatologists exert enormous influence on parents. The result is that, for some neonatologists, the physician's role in the decision-making process is regarded as central in importance. Dr Stahlman's words ring true for many (but not all) neonatologists: "We all need all the advice, judgment, and help we can get ... however, in the final decision-making, it is the physician's responsibility to explain the harsh medical realities, present a plan of action, seek agreement, and remove the sense of guilt from the family and to bear it her or himself'.

A third alternative is now in place in many US hospitals. As was mentioned earlier in the chapter, both the President's Commission and the Child Abuse regulations (as well as the American Academy of Pediatrics) recommended in the early 1980s that hospitals with NICUs establish pediatric ethics committees to provide multidisciplinary advice on difficult cases.[13] The advantage of such committees is that they, working together over time, can bring relevant knowledge and information, impartiality, emotional stability, and consistency to a case discussion in a way that may prove helpful to both the parent(s) and the physician(s) in an ethically problematic case.[14] Such committees do not make decisions to withhold or withdraw treatment, but serve in an advisory capacity to help the attending physician in a case to determine whether the initiation, continuation, or abatement of life-sustaining treatment is in the patient's best interests.

3. *Is there any difference between withholding life-sustaining medical treatment and withdrawing life-sustaining treatment?* In terms of ethics and the law, the answer is no: there is no morally significant or legally significant difference between withholding and withdrawing treatment, if the reason for the decisions made at different points in time is the same.

A decision by parents and/or physicians not to attempt to sustain a neonate's life can be (but need not be) morally blameworthy and punishable by law; likewise, a decision by parents and/or physicians to stop trying to sustain a critically infant's life can be (but need not be) morally blameworthy and punishable by law. The morality of either decision that results in an infant's death, as well as the legal liability connected with the patient's death, depends on the facts of a particular case. However, if the reason for either decision is that the treatment that could be used/is being used is medically futile or contrary to the infant's best interests, then the two decisions are morally and legally equivalent.

In spite of this moral equivalence, a number of neonatologists, other physicians, and nurses continue to think, mistakenly, that withdrawing life-sustaining treatment is morally more significant and certainly more legally serious than withholding treatment. Several reasons contribute to this view. First, there are psychological reasons. The process of initiating treatment, regularly checking on the patient undergoing treatment, and monitoring the effectiveness of the treatment unquestionably creates expectations in the minds of the neonatologists, nurses, other pediatric specialists, and parents that the treatment will work, and that the patient will be better off for having had the treatment. When the treatment does not work as expected or hoped, a decision to stop the treatment can contribute to feelings of disappointment, guilt, and failure on the part of the physicians and nurses. Moreover, when an infant dies subsequently to the withdrawal of treatment, some physicians and nurses feel that they somehow had a role in bringing about the death (through a faulty diagnosis, delayed intervention, and the inability to manage the symptoms of illness), in a way they would not feel in regard to an infant's death when no life-sustaining treatment was initiated because of the severity of the patient's condition.

A second set of reasons are philosophical in nature. Neonatologists, like other physicians, are trained to treat diseases and cure patients of their medical problems. Given this 'bias to treat' some neonatologists adhere to what they regard as the technological imperative, and become convinced that anything less than 'going all out' to prolong infants' lives is tantamount to 'giving up' or abandoning patients. The urgency and importance of 'going all out' gains increased psychological and moral weight in cases in which treatment has been initiated and continued for some time, but without the expected success. To stop the process—and admit that even technological medicine has limits—is difficult.

Third, there are legal concerns, whether legitimate or not. Many physicians believe, often without sound reasoning, that the distinction between actions and omissions has relevance to clinical cases involving the deaths of patients. For them, withholding life-sustaining treatment is less serious morally and legally because a physician merely omits to do something that may prevent a patient's death, rather than actually engaging in an action (stopping antibiotics, removing a ventilator, or removing a feeding tube) that may lead to a patient's death. When informed of the philosophical weakness of the act–omission distinction, some physicians are still unduly concerned about the legal implications of withdrawing (as opposed to withholding) life-sustaining treatment.

In an important sense, the concern some neonatologists have about withdrawing life-sustaining treatment from their patients can lead to morally irresponsible care of patients. Whether for psychological, philosophical, or ostensible legal reasons, neonatologists who think they cannot withdraw life-sustaining treatment once they have started it may simply decide not to start it in selected cases.

A preferable alternative in some cases, for neonatologists and their patients, is the use of time-limited trials. By initiating a form of life-sustaining treatment for a specific time-period, several benefits can be achieved. The physician(s) can establish whether the treatment is beneficial in the case at hand, the nurses can observe improvement or the lack of it in a patient, and the infant's parents can have a temporal milestone that will proclaim either the improvement of the patient's condition or the ineffectiveness of the treatment being used. Even if a subsequent decision is to withdraw the treatment, and thereby possibly to hasten the patient's death, the withdrawal of a life-sustaining treatment that proves futile or contrary to a patient's best interests is morally preferable to not having tried the treatment at all.

4. *What if the treatment to be withdrawn is a nasogastric tube or a gastrostomy tube?* The issue of stopping technologically supplied nutrition and hydration is as controversial in pediatric cases as it is in adult cases, as is reflected by Dr Stahlman's comments in the first part of the chapter. If anything, this issue is even more difficult in neonatal and other pediatric cases, because of the increased emotional attachment to young lives (especially on the part of parents and nurses), the symbolic importance of feeding (for some people), and the never-autonomous status of the patients whose lives are being sustained, perhaps at a minimal biological level, by medically administered nutrition and hydration.

The mainstream ethical postion that has emerged on this issue in the United States, especially concerning adult cases, regards technological nutrition and hydration as a form of life-sustaining treatment that is morally equivalent to mechanical ventilation and other life-sustaining technologies. The reasons for this judgment are several: 'artificial' feeding and hydration initially requires skilled medical and nursing care, involves some medical

risks and complications for patients, necessitates surgical intervention in
some cases, is used to combat or cope with a disease process that inhibits a
patient's normal ability to swallow, and is primarily intended to supplement
nutritional intake or support nutritional and fluid needs for a limited period
of time until a patient's underlying pathological condition improves.

Although the provision of technological nutrition and hydration is beneficial on balance for the great majority of adult and pediatric patients who
receive this medical treatment (like the child on TPN mentioned earlier),
the circumstances in at least some cases (for example, cases of persistent
vegetative state) are such that this treatment is contrary to the best interests
of the patients. Even the Child Abuse regulations acknowledge a moral
and legal limit on technological feeding by stating that effective medical
treatment includes 'appropriate nutrition, hydration, and medication'.[15]

Anne Fletcher, a neonatologist at the Children's Hospital in Washington,
DC, agrees. Writing with John Paris, an ethicist, she emphasizes that the
language of 'appropriate nutrition, hydration, and medication' allows for
the kind of discretionary decision-making that is required by complex NICU
cases. For illustrative purposes, they describe three clinical cases in which
parents and physicians decided against the continuation of technological
feedings: a premature baby with necrotizing enterocolitis; a neonate with
severe birth asphyxia; and a three-month-old girl dying with multiple medical
complications incompatible with long-term survival. In each of these cases,
Fletcher and Paris think that the abatement of technologically supplied
nutrition and hydration was medically and ethically appropriate.[16]

Joel Frader, a pediatrician at the University of Pittsburgh, is another
advocate of this view. He argues that the same kind of reasoning about
the provision of technological feeding 'should apply equally well to infants
and older persons, even though feeding babies has special social significance'.
He suggests that, in at least a few instances (for example, hydranencephaly
or renal agenesis), the provision of fluids and nutrition to neonates will only
prolong their dying or extend their suffering. In these rare cases, he says that
'good medical practice, that is, palliation, could require allowing dehydration
and malnutrition'.[17]

5. *What about the morality of actively hastening death in neonatal cases?*
For Dr Stahlman, this question is both unthinkable and unavoidable in some
of the 'gut-wrenching' cases that occur in NICUs. On the one hand, she holds
that the intentional killing of infants 'is not an option the physician should
consider', at least in cases where long-term survival of an infant is possible.
On the other hand, in (a) cases of suffering, 'doomed' infants who are dying
and (b) cases of non-dying infants with 'limited lifespans' who have a quality
of life that is 'considered hopeless and intolerable' by parents and physicians,
she suggests that a 'carefully regulated' legalization of euthanasia might be
acceptable.

To address the question of euthanasia with neonatal patients is not easy to
do, even for non-physicians who do not work in NICUs. For most persons, it
seems, any serious consideration of killing babies is high on the intuitive list

of actions that would be intrinsically immoral to perform. Yet at least some neonatologists, some other pediatric specialists, and some other informed persons cannot avoid asking the question, because they are aware of the severe, prolonged suffering that at least some infants experience in NICUs, PICUs, and a few other pediatric clinical settings.

For anyone raising the question, it is important to distinguish between (a) acts of withholding or withdrawing life-sustaining treatment and (b) acts of euthanasia. The distinction is not always clear, either in hypothetical or real cases; but the mainstream ethical position on this issue in the United States is perhaps best articulated in the words of a Hastings Center task-force report on the termination of life-sustaining treatment in adult cases: 'These Guidelines have been formulated in the belief that *a reasonable, if not unambiguous, line* can be drawn between forgoing life-sustaining treatment on the one hand, and active euthanasia or assisted suicide on the other'.[18]

The line that distinguishes most acts of withholding/withdrawing treatment from most acts of euthanasia is even more difficult to draw in neonatal cases, given that any acts of euthanasia with neonates or other young pediatric patients are acts of *non-voluntary* euthanasia. Nevertheless, the 'not unambiguous' line is usually characterized by five differences between these two sets of actions. First, the intention of the physician is usually different in these two actions, with the physician's intention of bringing about the patient's death being most clear whenever the physician gives the patient a lethal dose or injection. In acts of abating life-sustaining treatment, by contrast, the physician's intention is less clear: it *can* be aimed at bringing about the patient's death, or it is more commonly aimed primarily at relieving the patient's suffering or stopping futile treatment. Second, the cause of death is different. As is commonly recognized in adult cases, the primary cause of a patient's death when life-sustaining treatment is withheld/withdrawn is usually not the physician's act of abating treatment (assuming a morally responsible physician), but the patient's underlying medical condition. Third, acts of abating treatment, such as deciding against a surgical intervention in a severe case of myelomeningocele, do not always result in the patient's immediate death. Fourth, acts of withholding/withdrawing treatment generally provide opportunities for additional forms of care by physicians and nurses prior to a patient's death. Fifth, especially when contrasted with acts of non-voluntary euthanasia, acts of abating treatment do not present long-term problems of abuse as they become recognized as general practices in the care of critically and terminally ill patients, whether in adult or pediatric settings.[19]

Should any neonatologist decide actively to hasten a neonate's death, even with the known illegality of the action, he or she would have two alternative ways of carrying out the act of intentional killing. The alternative that would most clearly, undeniably be an act of non-voluntary euthanasia would be some kind of direct action (for example, intravenous postassium chloride) that would quickly kill the child. Another, much more ambiguous alternative would be planned inaction (for example, a decision not to provide beneficial surgery or nutritional support for a neonate with an intestinal obstruction known to be lethal in the absence of surgery) that would have the infant's death as its intended consequence.

The point is simple, but important: although acts of abating life-sustaining treatment are not usually acts of euthanasia, they *can* be, depending on the facts in a case. If a child is denied life-sustaining treatment that is clearly in the child's best interests, based on the PBI standard, then one can reasonably conclude that the child's death was intentionally (or negligently) caused by the physician(s) and other responsible parties in the case.

Are neonatal cases of non-voluntary euthanasia ever morally justifiable, perhaps as a moral option of last resort, even though they are illegal? The correct answer, difficult as it is, is affirmative, if three necessary and jointly sufficient conditions are in place. First, the withholding or withdrawing of treatment shall have been done on the basis of a careful, thoughtful determination (perhaps involving a pediatric ethics committee) that life-sustaining treatment is not in the best interests of the child. Second, having made the decision to allow the child to die, it becomes clear to the decision-makers that the child is not going to die quickly and is going to *endure prolonged suffering* in the absence of treatment. Third, the decision to cause the child's death is carried out in a manner that will quickly and painlessly end the child's life.[20]

Are there any cases that actually fit these criteria? That's hard to say. Fortunately, the number of cases of intense, prolonged suffering by patients in NICUs seems to have diminished in recent years as neonatologists, pediatric anesthesiologists, pediatric critical-care nurses, and pediatric neurologists have begun to give more attention to the recognition of patient suffering and effective pain-management with neonates. Of course it remains to be seen whether their combined efforts can actually remove the need, even on rare occasions, to raise the question of actively hastening the deaths of some neonates. We hope they succeed, as do our medical and nursing colleagues who regularly provide care for suffering infants in NICUs who are on the borderline between life and death.

REFERENCES

1. Joel Feinberg, Abortion. In Tom Regan (ed.), *Matters of life and death*, 2nd edn, pp. 256–92. Random House, New York, 1986.
2. Thomas H. Murray, Why solutions continue to elude us. *Social Science and Medicine* **20** (June 1985): 1102–7.
3. Robert F. Weir, Selective nontreatment—one year later: reflections and a response. *Social Science and Medicine* **20** (June 1985): 1109–17.
4. Robert F. Weir, Life-and-death decisions in the midst of uncertainty. In Arthur L. Caplan, Robert H. Blank, and Janna C. Merrick (eds), *Compelled compassion*, pp. 1–33. Humana Press, Totowa NJ, 1992.
5. *Roe* v.*Wade*, 410 US 113 (1973).

6. *In re* A. C., 573 A. 2d 1235, 1237 (D. C. App. 1990).
7. American College of Obstetricians and Gynecologists Committee on Ethics, Patient choice: Maternal–Fetal conflict (October 1987), p. 2. Reprinted in Association of Professors of Gynecology and Obstetrics, *Exploring issues in obstetric and gynecologic medical ethics*, p. 75. APGO, Washington, DC, 1990.
8. American College of Obstetricians and Gynecologists. *Technical Bulletin: ethical decision-making in obstetrics and gynecology*, November 1989, p. 4. Reprinted in APGO, *Exploring issues*, p. 98.
9. Department of Health and Human Services, Child abuse and neglect prevention and treatment program, *Federal Register* **50** (1985): 14878–901.
10. Loretta Kopelman, Thomas G. Irons, and Arthur Kopelman, Neonatologists judge the 'Baby Doe' Regulations. *New England Journal of Medicine* **318** (1988): 677–83.
11. Robert F. Weir and James F. Bale, Jr., Selective nontreatment of neurologically impaired neonates. *Neurologic Clinics* **7** (1989): 807–22.
12. Nancy M. P. King, Transparency in neonatal intensive care. *Hastings Center Report* **22** (May–June 1992): 24.
13. Robert F. Weir, Pediatric ethics committees: ethical advisers or legal watchdogs? *Law, Medicine, and Health Care* **15** (Fall 1987): 99–108.
14. Robert F. Weir, *Selective nontreatment of handicapped newborns*, pp. 255–7. Oxford University Press, New York, 1984.
15. DHHS, Child abuse, pp. Y 14878–901; emphasis added.
16. John Paris and Anne B. Fletcher, Withholding of nutrition and fluids in the hopelessly ill patient. *Clinics in Perinatology* **14** (1987): 367–77.
17. Joel Frader, Forgoing life-sustaining food and water: newborns. In Joanne Lynn (ed.), *By no extraordinary means*, pp. 180–5. Indiana University Press, Bloomington, IN, 1986.
18. Hastings Center project, *Guidelines on the termination of life-sustaining treatment and the care of the dying*, p. 6 (emphasis added). The Hastings Center, Briarcliff Manor, NY, 1987.
19. Robert F. Weir, *Abating treatment with critically ill patients*, pp. 300–19. Oxford University Press, New York, 1989.
20. Weir, *Selective nontreatment*, pp. 220–1.

7

Organ transplantation

7A ORGAN TRANSPLANTATION I
Joyce L. Peabody

BABIES IN NEED

Case 1: Baby J. was born at term to a Gravida 2, Para 1, Ab 0, 24-year-old white female. The pregnancy was uneventful and labor and delivery proceeded well. Apgars were 9 and 9 at 1 and 5 minutes respectively. The baby was admitted to the normal newborn nursery of a small community hospital. Routine care was administered and the infant began breast-feeding shortly after birth. Mother, father, and a two-year-old brother were all ecstatic regarding the new addition to their family. Both sets of grandparents were notified of the new arrival and immediately booked plane reservations to visit and to begin spoiling their new granddaughter. Two days following the delivery, the obstetrician and pediatrician discharged the mother and newborn to home, with follow-up appointments at one week for routine post-partum and pediatric care. However, on the morning of the planned discharge, Baby J. demonstrated perioral cyanosis during breast-feeding. The nursing staff reassured the mother that this was not uncommon and notified the pediatrician. The pediatrician decided to keep the infant in the hospital for an additional day of observation. Throughout the day, episodes of central cyanosis developed, and a chest radiograph demonstrated an enlarged heart. By evening, the infant was refusing all feedings and had developed a metabolic acidosis. The pediatrician requested transfer of the infant to the nearby tertiary-care medical center for further evaluation. Soon after admission, an echocardiogram demonstrated the findings of hypoplastic left-heart syndrome. The cardiologist and neonatologist called the family and scheduled an appointment to discuss their findings and the options for treatment. One hour later the neonatologist was informed that the parents and both sets of grandparents were anxiously awaiting the physicians in the family waiting-room.

Any physician who lived through a similar scenario prior to 1980 can well remember the agonizing task of telling a family that their infant had a lethal congenital heart defect and that absolutely nothing could be offered to save their baby's life. Unlike the extremely premature infant who, from the moment of the early onset of labor, gives warnings of a life-threatening condition, infants with hypoplastic left-heart syndrome typically appear normal and healthy at birth, and only become distressed as the ductus arteriosus begins to close. Many such infants may go home before showing any sign that something is wrong. The shock to the family upon learning that their child will die before reaching his or her first birthday is one that eludes description. The sense of helplessness and failure experienced by the physician upon making this diagnosis is also indescribable. Similar comments can be made for the experience of families and physicians when a baby is found to have life-threatening liver, kidney, or other major organ disease. It is, therefore, of no great surprise that the development of orthotopic organ transplantation as a medical option for babies with life-threatening organ impairment has been met with tremendous excitement from the lay and medical communities alike. It is estimated that perhaps 6000 babies annually in the United States alone could benefit from heart, liver, or kidney replacement.[1-3]

Three major medical advances are responsible for the development of orthotopic organ transplantation as a medical option for young infants. The first is modification of cardiopulmonary bypass for the special needs of pediatric patients, the second is the discovery of the immunosuppressive effects of cyclosporin,[4] and the third is development of surgical techniques specially designed for transplantation of small organs.[5] By 1992, over 130 orthotopic heart-transplantation procedures had been performed at Loma Linda University Medical Center by the team under the direction of Dr Leonard Bailey on infants of less than 6 month of age. Actuarial survival statistics at 1 year of age hover around 85 per cent, with very few late deaths. By 1992, approximately 50 centers in the United States had developed infant heart transplantation programs. Liver transplantation has been an accepted modality for use in infants since the 1980s, and, currently, approximately 80 centers in the United States offer this surgical option for infants. Survival at 1 year after liver transplantation is approximately 80 per cent.[6] Renal transplantation has also been shown to be feasible and life-saving in small pediatric patients.[3]

The feasibility of orthotopic organ transplantation in the 1990s has clearly changed the role of the physician in dealing with cases such as that of Baby J. The physician can now offer some hope, and the walk to the waiting-room to inform the parents of a diagnosis such as hypoplastic left-heart syndrome is now considerably less burdensome. However, it is not unusual for medical procedures to become available before the social conscience has had time to consider the 'whys and wherefores', the 'shoulds and should nots', and the 'rights and wrongs' of the procedures, as well as whether the procedures 'are or are not' financially affordable. Therefore, while the burden of giving parents a prognosis with no hope has been lifted, it has been replaced by an even more complex responsibility, which is to consider the ethical intricacies relating to orthotopic organ transplantation.

Who should receive?

One of the ethical controversies surrounding orthotopic organ transplantation is the registration criteria for recipients. The inclusion and exclusion criteria for recipients of orthotopic organ transplantation have long been a controversial area in adult transplantation programs. At various times and in various centers, adult candidacy has been based on medical need, psychological willingness and ability to cooperate, likelihood of success, life expectancy following transplantation, and even social contributions and ability to pay. In the mid-1980s, organ transplantation in newborns was clearly experimental. Inclusion criteria for recipients were established by the investigating team. These early inclusion criteria included such things as a definitive diagnosis of a lethal anomaly or disease of a major solid organ, informed consent from one, and preferably two, parents, and absence of factors that would significantly increase the risk of transplantation and immunosuppression, such as active infection or prematurity. Other non-medical or more qualitative criteria for *exclusion* were considered, but were found to be controversial and unacceptable to the lay community and difficult, if not impossible, to enforce consistently. Some of these factors included psychosocial issues regarding the stability of the home environment, the presence of other congenital malformations, or guarded neurodevelopmental prognosis. Once the transition from experimental to innovative or standard therapy was made by third-party payers' recognition of orthotopic organ transplantation, none but purely medical inclusion criteria seemed appropriate and acceptable.

Can we or should we ever say no?

Despite recipient criteria based primarily on medical need, several specific questions have arisen regarding recipient candidacy. A major group of infants under consideration for heart transplantation are those infants who have suffered a severe hypoxic/acidotic insult in the perinatal period. For some, the developmental prognosis is guarded, and questions have arisen regarding their candidacy in view of the scarcity of donor organs. Currently, however, orthotopic heart transplantation is generally managed as is any other medical modality in which fully informed consent is sought from the parents, including an explanation of the additional risks and concerns regarding the child's prognosis. If the infant is considered likely to benefit from orthotopic cardiac transplantation, even if the neurodevelopmental prognosis is guarded or other complications add risk to the procedure, the procedure is offered to the family.

Questions have also arisen regarding the inclusion of infants with significant chromosomal anomalies. Here again, infants with Down syndrome are considered for registration pending the parent's informed consent. The agonizing ethical struggles surrounding the Baby Doe regulations in the 1980s have been revisited many times in the consideration of children with major anomalies for orthotopic organ transplantation. In fact, they have even been magnified by the additional condition of limited organ supply. While the practice of most centers involved in organ transplantation in infants is to maintain an approach consistent with the value system of beneficence—what is best for the individual—the utilitarian argument—what is best for the greatest number—surfaces frequently. The opinions regarding selection factors for recipients are as diverse as the pluralism of our society would suggest. However, any attempt to include factors other than medical need has been reminiscent of the attitude of the biased and judgemental selection committees summarized in the early years of adult transplantation as 'no place for a Henry David Thoreau with bad kidneys'.[7]

Should parents be allowed to say no?

A provocative and current question is should *parents* be allowed to say no to orthotopic organ transplantation once the physicians have determined that this procedure would be of potential benefit for a life-threatening condition in the child? Clearly, just as with adults, informed consent is necessary for any major surgical procedure on a minor. In babies consent is typically sought from the parents. However, parental autonomy is not absolute. Precedent does exist for prohibiting parents to dissent to life-saving treatments. The State has expressed a countervailing interest in both the preservation of life and the protection of innocent third parties. The most obvious example is the regular practice of healthcare providers of obtaining court orders to allow potentially life-saving blood transfusions in minors whose parents dissent on the basis of religious convictions. Arguing that the benefits of transplantation are as clear as other court-enforced treatments, some have pointed out the irony of refusing to permit parents to decline intensive care for a 700-gram premature infant while continuing to allow the no-treatment option for ortho-topic heart transplantation for a baby with hypoplastic left-heart syndrome. Survival to discharge is currently 50 per cent for the first treatment and 80 per cent for the second. Despite this apparent inconsistency, at the time of preparation of this manuscript, Loma Linda University Medical Center and, to my knowledge, other centers offering heart transplantation do continue to allow the parents the option of no surgical intervention. The rationale behind this practice is based on[1] the still-uncertain long-term prognosis for these infants; (2) the scarcity of organ resources; and (3) the current lack of universal acceptance of this as a standard of care. This practice results, in some instances, in a disturbing experience for physicians, as they are told that the 'Baby Doe regulations' prohibit them from limiting intensive care on a 500-gram infant with a grade III intraventricular hemorrhage because such limitation of care would be based on quality-of-life judgements, and, yet have to watch an otherwise completely healthy term infant with hypoplastic left-heart syndrome die untreated. There are also occasions when a financially destitute single parent will opt for heart transplantation for a neurologically impaired newborn, while an upper-middle-class family with many more apparent resources to support a chronically immunosuppressed child will decide to allow that child to die. Often, the couple may prefer to conceive again and go for a more 'perfect offspring'. Such instances cause the health-care provider to question the fairness of allowing parental preference to be such a powerful determinant.

ORGANS IN DEMAND

Case II: Baby V. was born at term to a Gravida 4, Para 0, Ab 3, 35-year-old-white female. Soon after birth, the baby became cyanotic and a diagnosis of complex congenital heart disease was made. No palliative procedures could be offered and orthotopic cardiac transplantation was the only treatment option available to the family. Baby V.'s parents had been struggling for the past 10 years with problems of infertility, and this was the first time they had successfully conceived and carried a baby to term. Because of the high premium the parents placed on this birth, it took them little time to agree to have Baby V. registered for heart transplantation with a local procurement center. Complete evaluation of the infant revealed no additional risk factors; however, the parents were informed that the average wait for a size and blood-type appropriate organ was 46 days, with some infants waiting as long as 3 months. Baby V. was transported to the transplantation center, where she received supportive care to maintain her in the best condition for surgery. Her parents relocated to the area surrounding the transplantation center, a move of more than 2000 miles. Her father quit his job and applied for work in the new locality. The family carried a beeper which would notify them the moment an appropriate donor was found. Unfortunately, the beeper never sounded. Despite all aggressive medical interventions to keep Baby V. alive, complications of her low systemic blood flow and high pulmonary blood flow culminated in death due to a massive thrombosis in the descending aorta, with superimposed severe necrotizing enterocolitis and systemic infection.

Unfortunately, cases similar to Baby V. are not uncommon. Nationally, 30–60 per cent of children less than 2 years of age who are registered for organ transplantation die before a suitable donor is found.[8–10] In addition, of those infants surviving the wait for a donor, there is increasing morbidity with increasing time until transplantation. Often, somatic, as well as head, growth is delayed;[11] complications of low blood-flow states and congestive heart failure become more difficult to manage; maintenance of central venous lines and prostaglandid infusions becomes more hazardous; and an increased incidence of pulmonary hypertension is found.[12,13]

Why is the organ pool so small?

An ironic twist for pediatricians and pediatric intensivists is that the very advances that have decreased infant and childhood mortality have increased the waiting time and thus the mortality and morbidity of infants in need of donor organs. Advances in prenatal care of high-risk pregnancies, improved intensive care for newborns with problems of cardiopulmonary adaptation, enhanced emergency medical care responses to pediatric victims of drowning and trauma, and heightened awareness and early intervention in cases of child abuse, along with car-seat and speed-limit laws, have all dramatically reduced the number of early childhood deaths in the last two decades. Still, approximately 110 infants of less than 1 year of age die each day in this country. One must ask why, then, is the pool of donor organs so small? One obvious and perhaps permanent limitation to the donor pool is that many infants die of cardiopulmonary insufficiency, and thus have hearts and livers which have suffered irreversible ischemic insults. Practically, only those infants who are declared brain-dead and have persistent and adequate circulatory function can be considered as donors. Causes of brain death vary, but include metabolic abnormalities such as hypoxic/ischemic encephalopathy, trauma, and sudden infant death syndrome. However, the percentage of infants who meet even these criteria that are referred as potential organ donors is estimated to be less than 10 per cent. Why?

Is encouraged volunteerism working?

Recognizing the shortage of donor organs for both adult and pediatric recipients, several initiatives have been proposed in the past decades to encourage organ donation. The Uniform Anatomical Gift Act, passed in the late 1960s and early 1970s in all 50 states and Washington, DC, urged voluntary donation while respecting the individuals' rights to determine the use of their organs. This Act allows an individual to express his or her desire to donate organs after death via an organ donor card or, in many states, a driver's license. In the case of a minor, families or next of kin may consent to the donation of organs.

As a continuation of the response to the organ shortage, the 1984 National Organ Transplant Act (PL 98-507) expanded and centralized the nationwide network for procuring and distributing organs. The United Network for Organ Sharing (UNOS) based in Richmond, Virginia, received the federal contract to establish a nationwide Organ Procurement and Transplantation Network (OPTN) to obtain organs and match them with recipients. It was intended that the OPTN work closely with the local organ-procurement organizations to improve the effectiveness and efficiency of donor-organ identification and procurement. An additional initiative to increase the supply of organs was the passage of 'required request' laws in 1986. The Department of Health and Human Services regulations to implement this statute, which went into effect on 31 March 1988, made the existence of protocols for informing families of the option of organ donation a prerequisite for hospitals to establish Medicare reimbursement eligibility. As of September 1990, 44 states and Washington, DC had passed legislation requiring hospital personnel to ask family members of potential donors about organ donation. Despite these initiatives as well as nationwide and governmental support for organ donation, far more than 75 per cent of potentially usable infant organs continue to be buried each year. Reasons include lack of awareness by young couples of the possibility of organ donation, stress from the unexpected death of an infant, reluctance of health-care providers to discuss death and organ donation with a grieving family, and restrictions arising from a still encumbered system of organ referral and procurement. It has been estimated by the Loma Linda University transplant team that no less than 6 hours of medical providers' time is required to obtain the necessary informed consent for organ donation and to arrange for procurement of a donor organ. Many providers either do not have the time to or choose not to get involved with such a cumbersome process.

How can the donor pool be expanded?

Two clear and necessary steps must be taken to expand the small organ donor pool. These include education and heightening the awareness of both lay and medical communities. In addition, continuing attempts to reduce the inefficiency and frustrations encountered by families and physicians involved in organ donation are vital. Another step which has been taken, by necessity, by transplant surgeons is the relaxation of the criteria for acceptable donor organs and the prolongation of acceptable ischemic times. Cardiac transplant surgeons have demonstrated that a documented cardiac arrest as long as 30 minutes and an arterial pH as low as 6.5 have been recorded in donors of successfully functioning grafts.[14] Donor inotropic support with catecholamines, initially a relative contraindication to organ donation, has been proven compatible with successful cardiac function following transplantation. Cardiac grafts procured from distant locations having ischemic times exceeding 8 hours have also demonstrated successful function following transplantation. While worrisome, the longer ischemic times associated with distant procurement have resulted in no known adverse effects on the graft when properly handled.[14] The size-match requirement has also been liberalized to include successful donor–recipient dyads who varied in size by more than 200 per cent.[15]

Should we relax the 'dead-donor' rule?

In addition to the steps described above for expansion of the donor pool within the current Uniform Determination of Death Act, some have argued that there is a need to relax the 'dead-donor' rule and consider some other populations of infants for organ donation. Clearly, the most commonly considered and controversial group at this time is anencephalic infants. For years, infants with anencephaly have been considered as a potential source of solid organs.[16–18] In fact in June 1966, almost 18 months before Christian Barnard, MD, performed the world's first human-to-human heart transplant, Adrian Knatrowitz, MD, planned what would have been the first such transplant from an anencephalic newborn to a two-month-old infant. Once asystole occurred, resuscitation of the graft was attempted, albeit unsuccessfully. Soon after Dr Barnard's operation, Dr Kantrowitz performed successfully the first human-to-human heart transplant in the United States. However, the Uniform Determination of Death Act, along with the heightened medical, legal, and moral sensitivities regarding the rights of disabled infants, have placed such early uses of organs from anencephalic infants under strict scrutiny.

While experience with these infants as organ donors has recently been reported in Europe,[19] currently in the United States anencephalic infants who receive customary care are no longer routinely considered acceptable as heart or liver donors. By the time naturally occurring cardiorespiratory arrest occurs, the heart and liver have suffered, presumably, sufficient ischemic injury no longer to qualify as acceptable grafts. Furthermore, since the current cardiorespiratory legal definition of death includes the word 'irreversible', many have felt that waiting for cessation of heart function, declaring the anencephalic infant dead, and then restarting cardiac function in the donor or recipient could be considered cause to discredit the original declaration of death. Moreover, because brain-stem function is initially demonstrable in live-born anencephalic infants, they do not automatically meet the current legal requirements for total and irreversible cessation of whole-brain function called for in the Uniform Determination of Death Act.[20]

Some advocates of the use of the organs of anencephalic infants have supported efforts to change the law to allow the organs of liveborn anencephalic infants to be used without a requirement of total brain death.[21-26] One such effort was California Senate Bill, #2018, introduced in 1986 by Senator Marks and subsequently withdrawn because of adverse public opinion. The most recent effort to change the law to recognize anencephalic infants as a unique population who may donate organs once the diagnosis of anencephaly is confirmed was in progress in the Florida Supreme Court (the case of Baby Theresa) at the time of this manuscript's preparation. Such efforts either propose to make anencephalic infants dead by definition at birth or suggest that anencephalic infants should be an exception to the 'dead-donor' rule and that death should not be necessary in order for their parents to donate organs from their anencephalic infant. Both lines of reasoning, no matter how well-intended, are ethically and practically problematic. If all anencephalic infants were declared dead at birth, what would happen to those infants whose parents did not desire to donate organs? Would we discharge a 'dead' infant home? Would we bury an infant who was anencephalic but not a potential organ donor, because, in the eyes of the law, he was 'dead', while in the eyes of the parents he was still breathing, kicking, crying, and sucking? Even more problematic are questions such as: Would the infant have a birth certificate and a death certificate signed simultaneously? Would the infant count as a live birth for the purpose of tax deductions? Would his care in the hospital be covered by insurance if he were legally dead? If the infant is considered a live birth, at what stage would he be considered dead? The second consideration which would allow anencephalic infants to donate organs outside of the 'dead-donor' rule is equally problematic. All three of the critical factors in the tradition of organ donation: (1) informed consent; (2) the 'dead-donor' rule; and (3) the benefit of giving to a living relative, would be absent. The anencephalic infant would neither give informed consent, nor be dead, nor benefit a relative by the donation.

Others have explored techniques to modify the customary care rendered to anencephalic infants in order to maintain the function of organs which might be donated while waiting to determine whether death within current legal

definitions would occur. While the experience of Canadian physician, Calvin
Stiller, MD, with baby Gabriella has documented that such attempts can
possibly lead to organ donation, the study of twelve infants treated in this
fashion at Loma Linda University Medical Center strongly suggests that it
is not feasible to utilize this technique for organ procurement routinely.[27]
Furthermore, numerous ethical concerns arise out of such experiences. These
have been discussed elsewhere.[28–33]

The media, as one might readily imagine, have not remained silent on these
issues. Instead, the combination of newsworthy ingredients, including organ
transplantation, gross deformities, and babies' deaths, along with medical
and legal controversy, have made the media's involvement in the issues
surrounding anencephalic infants as organ donors even more complex, and
often inflammatory. For example, on 16 April 1992, an article in the *Los
Angeles Times* described the case of Baby Theresa as 'both an ethical enigma
and a cause celebre'. The article went on to question 'but was Baby Theresa
a person, was she ever really alive?'[34] In some ways it is as if the questioning
which began in the 1960s, resurfaced in the 1970s, rose again in the early
1980s, and was finally studied systematically in the late 1980s, had never
taken place. The same questions are being asked, and the same insensitive
and/or designed-to-shock comments are being made, including a statement
from the director of organ procurement for the University of Miami: 'She
[referring to Baby Theresa] better fit the category of benign tumor, rather
than human being. She was a ball of tissue. The question is whether she
existed at all.[34] Another example of such comments is a statement from
Robert Levine, MD, a Yale University Professor of Medical Ethics, that [a
baby like Theresa] 'has more in common with a fish than a person'.[35]

Thus the issue of considering anencephalic infants as organ donors often
resembles a most ferocious tug-of-war. Despite the complexity of the issues,
our society is being drawn to one or the other of two diametrically opposed
viewpoints, and the two parties appear to be compelled to defend those two
viewpoints with all their strength. I find myself wondering why society cannot
admit the complexity of the issues and enter into an intelligent, fact-grounded
discussion at all levels, rather than persisting in the generation of inflammatory rhetoric and passionate debate. Whatever decisions are made or actions
are taken from such impassioned debates, I would predict that they will be
both misguided and destructive, not only to the future of organ transplantation in infancy, but also to the integrity of patient–physician trust.

I have also worried about the long-term effects on the infants' families
of attempts to donate organs from anencephalic infants. Once again, the
worrisome issue of rationalizing a practice on the grounds that 'the ends
justify the means' surfaces. Are we, in our effort to respond to the parents'
wishes, robbing them of their normal grieving process? The *Los Angeles
Times* reported that Susan Clark, the grandmother of Baby Theresa, 'lifted
the 3 pound baby from its casket during the funeral and held it to her breast
saying, "This was my time, I never had a chance to hold her."'[34]

A final alternative method of procuring organs from the anencephalic infant whose parents want to donate organs would be to declare the infant a 'legal fiction'. To non-lawyers, this seems a contradiction in terms. We have been raised to believe that if anything is objectively real, it is the law. What therefore can constitute a legal fiction? Apparently, legal fiction would allow anencephalic infants whose parents want to donate their organs to be recognized by the law as dead *for the sole purpose of organ donation*. This concept goes against the traditional view that death is a fact, and not an opinion, recently reiterated by the judge reviewing Baby Theresa's parents' plea to allow them to donate their infant's organs in spite of the normal legal prerequisite of death.[34] The concept also suggests the idea of bypassing a law that governs something as serious as the life and death of one infant solely for the benefit of another infant.

What other sources have been considered for donor organs?

Other sources for the expansion of the donor pool for infants needing major solid organs include infants in a persistent vegetative state—a group with problems even more legally and ethically complex than those just described for anencephalic infants. Still another group under consideration are infants receiving intensive care for whom continued support has been judged futile by treating physicians. In these instances, once the parents have agreed on the essentially futile prognosis of their baby, it is customary for mechanical ventilation to be withdrawn and for the infant to die a cardiorespiratory death. Included in this group are prematurely born infants who are suffering severe chronic lung disease, severe intraventricular hemorrhage, or other complications of their prematurity and newborn period that have resulted in a judgment by the treating physicians that continued aggressive care is no longer in the baby's best interest. Many, including leaders in organ transplantation in children, have argued that burying the heart, liver, and kidneys of these patients when they might save another infant's life is immoral and unfair. And therefore many have held that once cardiac asystole has occurred a legal declaration of death might be made, and the organ could be removed and 'jumpstarted' in the recipient's body. This line of argument has clear ethical problems. Practically speaking, it is likely that infants for whom a decision has been made to discontinue life-support may be housed in the same institution where organ transplantation would occur. This potentially places physicians in a conflict-of-interests position where they would be attempting to advocate for two patients, prognosticating futility for treatment of one, declaring death in that individual, and then facilitating organ donation to another needy recipient. In such instances, the risk of the 'slippery slope', no matter how vigorously avoided, is real.

What about non-human organ sources?

Other sources of organs for babies in need which have been considered throughout the last several decades are of non-human origin. The Baby

Fae operation in 1985, conducted by Leonard Bailey, MD, at Loma Linda
University Medical Center, represents the result of one of these considerations.[36] An attractive feature of non-human primate sources for infant
organs is that they completely avoid the 'use' of one human to benefit
another human. They would also bypass the need for parents to consent
to the donation of organs from their children. Furthermore, studies suggest
that more careful and specific tissue-matching could occur if non-human
primate sources were used. However, concerns regarding HIV-type viruses
carried by several of the primate species, as well as opposition from groups
of citizens vehemently opposed to animal experimentation, have blunted
enthusiasm for this source of organs. Artificial organs have been considered
as a bridge option; however, any bridge, whether xenograft or artificial
organ, risks merely delaying the problem of organ shortage and will only
tend to increase the number of infants in need of organs by prolonging
the life of those waiting for organs. This practice could lead ultimately to
greater recipient mortality and morbidity in infant-organ transplantation.
It could also lead to even stiffer decisions regarding donor organ allocation
and possibly even to the sale of organs. The introduction of this utilitarian
approach is foreign to American pediatric practice. Pediatric practice in the
United States has clearly been based on the ethics of beneficence, and there
will need to be considerable adjustment should one begin injecting purely
utilitarian principles into medical practice.

PARENTS IN SEARCH

Case III: Mr. and Mrs. G. were Canadian parents expecting their first child.
Both parents were devout Catholics, and rejected maternal serum alpha-fetal
protein (MSAFP) testing early in pregnancy because of their anti-abortion beliefs.
However, in the eighth month the mother became concerned because the fetus
had stopped kicking. Ultrasonography revealed that the infant had anencephaly.
The mother's obstetrician offered her induction, cesarean section, or continuation
of the pregnancy to term. The parents chose to continue the pregnancy to term
and to donate their baby's organs. Baby G. was born at term in a community
hospital in Canada. For the first 24 hours, the infant required no aggressive
support. However, on the second day of life, the infant, at the parents' request,
was transferred to an intensive-care center and placed on mechanical ventilation
for the purpose of preserving the infant's organs for donation while allowing
the baby to die. After several days, the infant met the criteria for total brain
death, and was confirmed dead by two Canadian physicians. On the first day
following death, a search for an age-matched, blood-type appropriate recipient
was unsuccessful. On the following day, Baby G. was matched with a registered
recipient still *in utero*. Baby P. had been diagnosed *in utero* as having hypoplastic
left-heart syndrome, and the parents, after considerable discussion, chose to
register the infant at 34 weeks' gestational age for heart transplantation. A
decision was made by Baby P.'s obstetrician to deliver the baby by repeat
cesarean two weeks prematurely to take advantage of the available organ.
Baby G. was flown to Loma Linda University Medical Center, where her heart

was transplanted into Baby P.'s chest when Baby P. was 4 hours of age. At the time of writing Baby P. is approaching 5 years of age and is thriving.

Searching is a common activity in transplantation medicine. Searching for the ideal immunosuppressant drug, searching for new and improved techniques of cardiopulmonary bypass, searching for donors, and searching for improved ways to diagnose rejection are but a few examples. The case of Baby G. represents searching for good out of such a tragic outcome of pregnancy. Those who have not personally met families who want to donate organs from their anencephalic infants listen to the anecdotal stories of the persistence of these families pushing to donate organs with some degree of scepticism, attributing the accounts to a conflict of interest and the exuberance of the transplant team members. Having spoken personally with well over one hundred families of anencephalic infants, I can attest to the perseverance that these families demonstrate in searching for a way to bring the gift of life out of their tragedy. The ethicist, Annas, has also addressed the issue of searching. He referred to the case of Gabriella as 'not a case of a dying child in search of an organ, but a dying organ in search of a child'.[37] In truth, the case of Gabriella was a case of parents in search of meaning. Further, when the mother, Mrs W., contacted over one hundred hospitals during the third trimester of her pregnancy, she was in search of a group of physicians who would help her realize her greatest wish, that of donating the organs from her anencephalic infant.

Why such a persistent and determined search?

The answer is relatively simple. Before the introduction of the concept of donation, all the focus on a pregnancy involving an anencephalic infant is on the deformity of the child and the hopelessness of the child's prognosis. When considering organ donation, however, the focus changes to what is normal and healthy in the child, typically, the heart, liver, and kidneys. Also, the parents want to contribute to a life, if not their own child's, then maybe another child's. There are some ethical concerns which arise from this change of focus. Examples include: (1) Are the parents shifting their advocacy from their deformed child to that of another child, although it is a stranger, with a more optimistic prognosis?; (2) Do parents have the right to consent to intervention such as mechanical ventilation when there is no clear benefit to their child?; (3) Do such actions indeed help the family through their tragedy, or do they distort the normal grieving process?; and (4) Do such acts of apparent generosity put undue pressure on other families of anencephalic babies to donate their child's organs against the parent's own beliefs?

How do parents search for donors?

The parents of Baby P. were unusually lucky in that an organ became available even before their child's birth. As was mentioned earlier, the

average waiting time for a heart is 47 days, and the average waiting time
for a liver is similar. This is a desperate time for families, as they often
watch their infant struggle to stay alive, face the complications of the delay,
and, in at least 30 per cent of the instances, die while waiting. The stress on
families frequently forces them into an active participant role in the organ
search. Many families chose to go to the public media with pleas for organ
donation. In some instances, this has resulted in a family's 'jumping the
queue' and having a donor organ made available to them because of their
personal appearance on television or radio. Ethical concerns have been raised
regarding these instances, since the tradition of donation has held that the
donor should be free of direct knowledge of a specific individual's need. Still, it
is difficult, if not impossible, to persuade a donating family to give to the child
next in line instead of to the person with whom they have already identified.
Another even more graphic and active participation in the search for organs
is illustrated by the number of recent cases in which couples have conceived
children for the sole purpose of abortion in order to donate fetal tissue, such as
pancreas or adrenal glands. Also, couples have conceived children in order to
donate bone-marrow tissue to a relative. Finally, there are a growing number
of living donors, such as mothers, donating portions of organs, such as liver,
to one of their children in need. These cases, although well-intended, also
deviate from the traditional model of organ donation, which ethically should
be free of conflict of interest.

SOCIETY IN DISTRESS

Case IV:

Dear Dr. Peabody,

I have been following your efforts at Loma Linda to procure organs from
anencephalic infants. I have been very supportive of your activities and have
felt that you were doing the right thing. However, you blew it, when you allowed
one of your colleagues to say over national television that these infants are not
persons but are worm-like creatures and primitive life-forms! These children
are, after all, children. Furthermore, the persistent use of the word "harvest" is
inappropriate. Harvesting is for crops, not people. Please teach your colleagues
greater sensitivity regarding their choice of words in this most difficult and
sensitive area of pursuit.

Sincerely, [name withheld to respect privacy].

In 1988, during the Loma Linda University Medical Center's study to
determine whether organs could be procured from anencephalic infants by
modifying the infant's care to maintain organ function, voluminous mail
was received from members of society commenting on the program. One
such piece of mail came from a lady in the Mid-West. Upon very delicate,
lace-edged, pink stationery, the letter above was written. Other opinions
ranged from support of the idea of using anencephalic infants as organ

donors to outrage and expressions of concern. One newspaper described this pluralism of societal views as: 'Some say it could lead to treating human beings as commodities, blurring lines on when and how it is appropriate to take someone's organs. Others label the program too cautious. In it's effort to respect life, good organs have withered away in dying bodies, they say.'[38]

Other correspondence came to Loma Linda University Medical Center from families of children who they believed had the condition of anencephaly, but who were stated to be nine years old or older and thriving. Such instances have not been confirmed in the medical literature, but point to the fact that some members of our society are uneasy about this means of expanding the donor pool. In addition, families who had infants hospitalized in the intensive-care nursery with conditions distinctly different from anencephaly, such as prematurity and suspected sepsis, called frantically, seeking reassurance that *their infants* were not being considered for organ donation.

What does all this correspondence and opinion-sharing tell us? One insight derived from the study was that society may not be ready for a third definition of death. Considerations of expanding the legal definition of death to include a diagnosis of anencephaly or to include absence of neocortical activity have been seriously undertaken in several states. However, upon reflection, it has only been a little over a decade since a *second* definition of death has existed. Most still think of death as cessation of heart function: that is how our grandparents died, that is how our pets died, and that is how most people still anticipate dying. Clearly, the experience at Loma Linda University Medical Center during the study of anencephalic infants as potential organ donors demonstrated that even the medical community is somewhat unclear and confused regarding the legal criteria for organ donation. For example, well over twenty cases of infants with conditions quite different from anencephaly, some of which were not fatal, such as polycstic kidney disease and hydrocephalus, were referred by physicians and families to the protocol at Loma Linda University Medical Center, despite the explicit inclusion criteria that allowed only infants with a confirmed diagnosis of anencephaly to be considered.

Clearly, society is distressed, and needs a very focused educational program about organ donation and transplantation. Yet what might set the progress of transplantation back further than anything else is placing too much pressure on society to intellectualize such emotional issues as death and dying. Society needs time for dialogue, discussion, and emotional adjustment regarding such matters. In my opinion, this process should not be hurried. A Gallup Poll, taken in 1988, documented that only 42 per cent of those surveyed had considered donating their own organs after death. Moreover, most proclaimed potential donors do not carry donor cards, suggesting some ambivalence in their decision. In another survey, this one conducted by Arthur Caplan, Ph. D., of the Center for Biomedical Ethics at the University of Minnesota, two hundred hospital administrators and four hundred health-care professionals from five Mid-Western states were interviewed regarding attitudes affecting organ donation. Results of the survey showed that despite the legally mandated requirement of request mandate, 60–70 per cent of health-care professionals are simply not complying with the law.[39]

Attitudes regarding the possible implementation of a policy of 'presumed consent' were also polled. 'Presumed consent' would reverse the burden of notification of desire to the individual who does not want to donate organs. Except for cases of active dissent, organs could be legally removed for donation after death was declared. Despite the recognition that presumed consent could increase expected organ availability by a factor of 30–40 per cent, most Americans surveyed expressed general distaste for such non-voluntary systems of organ procurement. Furthermore, most Americans found both the buying and selling, as well as a generalized taking of organs, offensive. Dr Caplan has emphasized the importance of trust as a key issue in the gap between the donor organ pool and the need for organs, and has warned that aggressive steps to expand the donor pool may effectively shrink the organ supply if such steps threaten trust. Other major concerns related to the fairness issues expressed by health-care providers in the survey included (1) that the allocation of resources is too closely related to the ability to pay; (2) that attention by the media brings donor organs to specific recipients ahead of other more medically needy recipients; and (3) that minority groups who use a disproportionate number of organs are under-represented as donors.[39]

MEDICAL RESOURCES IN SHORTAGE

Case V: Early in my involvement with cardiac transplantation for infants in the first weeks of life, I was bothered by an ambivalence which arose from the tremendous excitement surrounding saving the lives of infants who just a year before would have certainly died and my recognition that this costly program was proceeding in the face of persistent homelessness, hunger, and inadequate medical care for other American children. My own ambivalence was magnified by criticism from others that such a costly experimental program had no place until the community of health-care professionals had addressed the facts that more than 30 per cent of pregnant women are denied access to prenatal care, that more than 30 per cent of this country's children under 5 years of age do not have health-care insurance, and that more than 30 per cent of infants go without even the basics of health-care maintenance, including immunizations. When discussing these concerns with a colleague, an analogy was drawn to medieval times, when large populations accepted a life of poverty in order to build enormous cathedrals. The cathedral was said to be the statement of belief in the future and the belief in the grandeur of creation, even in the face of present famine and need. The analogy has been of consistent concern to me for the past five years. One wonders whether it is true that current poverty and lack of medical resources for the poor are irrelevant considerations in the progress of organ transplantation and whether it is true, as many have stated, that refusal to spend dollars on organ transplantation would not insure transfer of those dollars to feeding, sheltering, or providing health care for our poor children.

At the beginning of this chapter I asked the question, 'Can we ever say no?' I now ask the question, 'Should we ever say yes?' Ironically, a review of our country's statistics on health care only aggravates the ambivalence. R. W. Evans, Ph. D., Senior Research Scientist from Battelle Seattle Research Center in Seattle, Washington addressed this controversy.[40] While sentimentality and even a sense of worship of our children prevail in middle-class and upper-middle-class America, society's support for *all* of its children is embarrassingly lacking. The number of reported child-abuse cases and the number of deaths resulting from abuse are increasing annually, as are the rates of suicides and homicides of children. In 1981 there were 1.2 million cases of child abuse reported in the United States, and in 1985, 1.9 million such cases were reported, an increase of more than 54 per cent.[41] Although figures vary, during 1987 between 1100 and 4000 children in the United States died of causes attributed to abuse. Shockingly, the three leading causes of death among children and young adults between the ages of 15 and 24 years are accidents, homicides, and suicides. Between 1950 and 1987, the homicide rate among persons of 15 to 24 years increased 122 per cent. Taken together, in 1988 homicides, suicides, and accidents accounted for more than 76 per cent of all the deaths occurring in those between 15 and 24 years of age.[41] Furthermore, in 1987 more than 12 million children in America had no health insurance.[42] A similar number of children have not received even standard childhood immunizations. Considering the societal problems of our youth, one ponders the following questions: Can society, in fact, ever afford to say yes to heart or liver transplantation for newborns? Is transplantation like a cathedral that society is building out of respect for our belief in creation and, as some have said, our belief that 'children are God's message that life should go on?' Or is it, as many have worried, that society is more prone to place dollars into spectacular, sensational feats of technology than into the basic needs of our country's youth? Until these ethical questions are answered, it is unlikely that the real issues of organ procurement will ever be effectively addressed.

Acknowledgement

I want to express my sincere appreciation to my Administrative Assistant, Sandy Misen, without whom this work and this manuscript could not have been completed.

REFERENCES

1. Bailey, L., Assaad, A., Trimm, R., *et al.* Orthotopic transplantation during early infancy as therapy for incurable congenital heart disease, *Ann. Surg.* **208** (1988).
2. Kalayoglu, M., Stratta R., Sollinger, H., *et al.* Liver transplantation in infants and children, *J. Pediatr. Surg.* **24:** 70–6 (1989).
3. Trompeter, R., Bewick, M., Haycock, G., *et al.* Renal transplantation in very young children, *Lancet* **1:** 373–5 (1983).

4. Borel, J. Immunosuppressive properties of cyclosporine A (CyA.) *Transplant Proc.* **12**: 233 (1980).
5. Allard, M., Assaad, A., Bailey, L., *et al.* Session IV, Surgical techniques in pediatric heart transplantation, Proceedings of the Loma Linda International Conference on Pediatric Heart Transplantation, *The Journal of Heart and Lung Transplantation*, Suppl. **10**, 5:2, 808–27 (9/10-91).
6. Busuttil, R., Seu, P., Millis, J., *et al.* Liver transplantation in children, *Ann. Surg.* **213**: 1, 48–57 (1-91).
7. Sanders, Dukeminier. Medical advance and legal lag: hemodialysis and kidney transplantation, *UCLA L. Rev.* **15**: 357 (1968).
8. Starnes, V., Stinson E., Oyer, P., *et al.* Cardiac transplantation in children and adolescents, *Circulation* **76**: Suppl:V-43-V-47, (1987).
9. Zitelli, B., Malatak, J., Gartner, J. *et al.* Evaluation of the pediatric patient for liver transplantation, *Pediatr.* **78**, 559–65 (1986).
10. Malatak J., Schaid, D., Urbach, A., *et al.* Choosing a pediatric recipient for orthotopic liver transplantation, *J. Pediatr.* **111**, 479–89 (1987).
11. Baum, M., Cutler, D., Fricker, F., *et al.* Session VII: Physiologic and psychological growth and development in pediatric heart transplant recipients, Proceedings of the Loma Linda International Conference on Pediatric Heart Transplantation, *The Journal of Heart and Lung Transplantation*, Suppl. Vol. **10**, 5: 2 848–56 (9/10-91).
12. Dajnowicz, A., Emery, J., Nystrom, G., *et al.* Time to cardiac transplantation delays neonatal head growth, *Pediatric Research*, Vol. **31**, 4: 2, 10A-#44, (4-92).
13. Emery, J., Johnston, J., Murphy, J., *et al.* Session III: Initiating the pediatric heart transplantation process, Proceedings of the Loma Linda International Conference on Pediatric Heart Transplantation, *The Journal of Heart and Lung Transplantation*, Suppl. Vol. **10**, 5: 2, 802–7 (9/10-91).
14. Boucek, M., Kanakriyeh, M., Mathis, C., *et al.* Cardiac transplantation in infancy: donors and recipients, *J.Pediatr.* 171–6 (2-90).
15. Fullerton, D., Gundry, S., de Bogona, J., *et al.* The effects of donor–recipient size disparity in infant and pediatric heart transplantation, *J.Thoracic and Cardiovascular Surgery*, accepted for publication.
16. Goodwin, W., Kaufman, J., Mims, M., *et al.* Human renal transplantation. I. Clinical experience with six cases of renal homotransplantation, *J. Urol.* **89**: 13–24 (1963).
17. Martin, L., Gonzalez, L., West, C., *et al.* Homotransplantation of both kidneys from an anencephalic monster to a 17-pound boy with Eagle–Barrett syndrome, *Surgery*, **66**: 603–7, (1969).
18. Iitaka K., Martin, L., Cox, J., *et al.* Transplantation of cadaver kidneys from anencephalic donors, *J. Pediatr.* **93**: 216–20 (1978).
19. Holzgreve, W., Beller, F., Buchholz, B., *et al.* Kidney transplantation from anencephalic donors, *NEJM*, **316**: 1069–70 (1987).
20. Uniform determination of death act #7180 of the Health and Safety Code, *Uniform Law Annot.* **12**: 310–13 (1980).
21. The anencephalic newborn as organ donor. *Hastings Cent. Rep.* **16**(2): 21–3 (1986).
22. Caplan, A. Ethical issues in the use of anencephalic infants as a source

of organs and tissues for transplantation, *Transplant Proc.* **20**(Suppl.5): 42–9 (1988).

23. Walters, J. and Ashwal, S. Organ prolongation in anencephalic infants: ethical and medical issues, *Hastings Cent. Rep.* **18**(5): 19–27 (1988).

24. Harrison, M. The anencephalic newborn as organ donor, *Hastings Cent. Rep.*. **16**: 2(4-86).

25. Caplan, A. Ethical issues in the use of anencephalic infants as a source of organs and tissues for transplantation, *Transplant Proc.* **20**(Suppl. 5):1-82, (1988).

26. Truog, R. and Fletcher, J. Anencephalic newborns. Can organs be transplanted before brain death? *NEJM*, **321**: 388–91, (1989).

27. Peabody, J., Emery, J., and Ashwal, S. Experience with anencephalic infants as prospective organ donors, *NEJM*, **321**: 6 344–50 (1989).

28. Peabody, J. The use of anencephalic infants as organ donors, Bioethics Consultation Group, *Clinical Ethics Report*, Vol. 3, 1,2 (1992).

29. Botkin, J. Anencephalic infants as organ donors, *Pediatr.* **82**: 2, 250–6 (8-88).

30. Arras, J. and Shinnar, S. Anencephalic newborns as organ donors: a critique, *JAMA*, **259**: 15, 2284–5, (4-88).

31. Churchill, L. and Pinkus, R. The use of anencephalic organs: historical and ethical dimensions, *The Milbank Quarterly*, **68**: 2 (1990).

32. Landwirth, J. Should anencephalic infants be used as organ donors?, *Pediatr*, **82**: 2, 257–8, (8-88).

33. Campbell. C. *Hastings Center Report*, **18**: 5 (10/11-88).

34. Clary, M. Baby Theresa's gift: debate over organ-harvesting laws, *Los Angeles Times*, (16-4-92).

35. Chartrand, S. Donation of living baby's organs raises debate, *The Sun*, (28-3-92).

36. Bailey, L., Nehlsen-Cannarella, S., Concepcion, W., *et al.* Baboon to human cardiac xenotransplantation in a neonate, *JAMA* **254**: 3321–9 (1985).

37. Annas, G. From Canada with love: anencephalic newborns as organ donors?, *Hastings Center Report*, **36–38**, (12-87).

38. Baby hope, *Knoxville News-Sentinel*, Sunday, P. 4, (3-7-88).

39. Priester, R. Unfolding issues for organ transplantation, *Organ Transplantation*, The Center for Biomedical Ethics, (1-88).

40. Evans, R. Can society afford pediatric heart transplantations? Proceedings of the Loma Linda International Conference on Pediatric Heart Transplantation, *The Journal of Heart and Lung Transplantation*, Suppl. Vol. 10, 5:2, 867, (9/10-91).

41. Grant, J., *The state of the world's children 1988. Oxford University Press, New York*, (1988).

42. Short, P., Monheit A., and Beauregard, K. Uninsured Americans: a 1987 profile, *presented at the Annual Meetings of the American Public Health Association*, Boston, Mass. (11-88).

7B ORGAN TRANSPLANTATION II

Albert R. Jonsen

Dr Joyce Peabody's essay provides a fine overview of the ethical questions that surround organ transplantation in the perinatal period. Her survey manifests the ethical sensitivity and sophistication that many physicians have developed in recent years. She not only speaks from her own experience, but also from her absorption of the ethical literature and the debates that have been prompted by the practice of pediatric organ transplantation. She poses many of the right questions, and suggests answers where answers seem reasonable. I shall focus on only one question, 'Should the "dead-donor" rule be relaxed?' That one question, however, must be posed within the context of the values and assumptions that underline common ethical views of organ transplantation. I shall first describe that context, using two other questions that Dr Peabody raises, namely, 'Who should give organs?' and 'Who should receive organs?', and then address the specific question about the relaxation of the 'dead-donor' rule.

THE ETHICAL CONTEXT OF ORGAN TRANSPLANTATION

Transplantation is the only medical technological that intrinsically requires the removal of a physical part or substance from one individual and its placement in the body of another solely for the therapy of the recipient. The immunological barrier that separates individuals radically from each other had to be broken before such an action could succeed as therapy. This barrier began to fall only fifty years ago, and was penetrated in a major way only in the last twenty or thirty years. Thus before this time the idea that the bodily part of one person could be medicine for another was unthinkable or, at most, miraculous. The legend of Saints Cosmas and Damien, brother physicians of the fourth century, tells that they transplanted the leg of one man to the body of another, but attributed the success to the power of God.

When this miraculous therapy becomes standard and accepted practice an unprecedented relationship between humans comes into being. Some persons need the organs of others. They need them because without them they will die. Through human history, people have needed each other in manifold ways, but they have never before needed a part of another's body in order to live. The idea of such an exchange was fantastic: the vampire legend told of the need of the 'undead' for the lifeblood of innocent persons, but that was horrible fantasy. With transplantation, the need for another's bodily part or substance moves from myth, miracle, and fantasy to actual reality.

Human relationships, diverse as they are, are woven around the reciprocity of giving and receiving. Communicating, contracting, conceiving, while wholly different in form and content, are essentially reciprocities of giving and receiving. Much of the ethical life involves problems about when, what, and to whom one should give or take, withhold and grant, offer and refuse. The 'golden rule', described in many traditions as the sum of morality, describes a reciprocity: do unto others as you would have them do unto you. Moral systems consist largely of values placed on various facets of human reciprocity and rules and principles governing the exchanges. Philosophers have divided these systems in many ways; but often they have distinguished broadly between exchanges that are obligatory and those that are voluntary.

At the beginning of the transplant era, authors commented perceptively on the unprecedented relationship that organ transplantation has brought to human life. Almost always, they placed the exchange of organs between humans into the class of voluntary reciprocities, and used the language of gift and donation to describe it.[1,2,3] The early reluctance of Catholic moral theologians to approve of organ transplantation was softened by the thesis that the use of one person's organs for the good of another fell into the moral category, not of mutilation, as they had formerly thought, but of charity.[4] The law also conceived of transplantation in terms of a voluntary giving. The Anatomical Gift Act was legislated in every state; several legal cases have denied one person's claim on the organ or bodily substance needed from another. Public policy has been reluctant to move very far beyond the voluntary donation of an organ; required request was as far as it would go. Even 'presumed consent' has not been favored. Involuntary harvesting of organs from the recently dead or the dying has been repudiated by almost all who have considered it. We have also reinforced the donation concept by looking unfavorably upon indeed outlawing, any commodification of organs.

This view must, of course, be stretched a bit. The Anatomical Gift Act allows relatives to make a gift of their deceased member's organs, even if the descedent has not explicitly offered them. Pediatric transplantation depends completely on 'proxy' donation, in which parents are the gift-givers from the bodies of their dead children. We even allow them to make donation from their living children, if the child source will not undergo 'undue' risk and may receive some benefit. Despite these extensions of donation to proxy donation, the donative framework around transplantation remains strong.

Our common view of gift-giving is very open: the nature and value of the gift is determined only by the generosity of the giver and some general social conventions about propriety. However, giving the gift of a vital organ does have limits: an individual who donates is not permitted to injure or damage him-or herself or another by the donation. The donative viewpoint permits only a limited altruism: it does not go as far as 'giving one's life for another'. In particular, the donation of a single organ whose removal would terminate

the life of the donor has been prohibited. It was for this reason that the legal
and medical determinations of death by neurological criteria were devised in
the 1970s and 1980s. Thus, the donative viewpoint is narrowed: single organs
necessary for life, donated during life or after death by appropriate proxies,
can only be taken once the source is dead. This is what Dr Peabody calls 'the
dead-donor rule'.

Thus, in American society and in most of the world, the new relationship
between persons that emerges from the new reality of organ transplantation
has been conceptualized and legalized as a relationship of voluntary donation,
charity, or supererogation. In other words, we have maintained that no one
has an absolute right, or even a qualified right, to the organs of another,
no matter how desperately needed. We could have done otherwise, deeming
organs a public resource or making them a market commodity, but we have
not done so (although someday we might). Up to now, we have attempted to
develop our philosophy and policy of organ transplantation under the guiding
principle of donation: organs are never taken, they are freely given and gladly
received. We shall call this the donative viewpoint.

The donative viewpoint says nothing explicit about the destination of
donated organs. It does, however, say something implicit, namely, that no
one, regardless of need, has a moral claim on the organs of another. If organs
become available only by the free choice of the source's surrogate, no duty
to give nor any right to receive is involved. The practical consequence, then,
of taking the donative viewpoint, is that the supply of organs will probably
always fall short of need. Only when as many people are persuaded to
donate as many organs as are needed by patients, and only when this
persuasion is effective, and only when systems are established to bring
the organs to the recipients, will the supply meet the need. This is in the
far, probably unattainable, future. In the meanwhile, the donative view will
preserve the autonomy and integrity of the givers, but leave many potential
receivers bereft.

Although Renee Fox and Judith Swazey have perceptively described the
'alterations in the theme of gift' that have taken place in recent years,
the donative view prevails.[5] It is rarely suggested that the entire sphere
of the transplantation reciprocity be seen as a matter of justice or utility.
Under a justice viewpoint, such a proposal would link givers and receivers
by obligations and moral claims. The patient who needed an organ would
also have a right to one; society would be under an obligation to be sure
that the requisite supply was available, even if this meant overriding the
desires of potential givers (though probably not the obligation to do no harm).
Under a utilitarian viewpoint, organs would be harvested and implanted
under formulae that would effect the greatest good of the greatest number
of persons (on the utilitiarian condition, of course, that the greater number
would be satisfied by such a distribution.)

The donative viewpoint, then, covers only one side of the relationship. The
receivers, dependent upon donation, must often wait, and must sometimes
go without. They are essentially mendicants in the shadow of affluent, but

often uninterested, possessors of useful organs. On the side of those in need, considerations of justice or utility, quite different from the donative viewpoint, are brought to bear.[6] However, the conditions of justice do not establish any rights in the needy. They have only to do with fairness or efficiency in doling out the donated organs. Since the earliest days of transplantation, the problem of distribution of scare resources has been debated. Various proposals, some based on theories of justice, some on utility, have been proposed. However, these proposals touch only the recipients. Ironically, this mimics the social situation that prevailed in Western culture for many centuries: the rich were told that they should care for the poor out of charity; the poor were told that they had no right to the possessions of the rich; gifts of the rich to the poor, when given, should be fairly distributed.

Our ethical view of transplantation is bifocal: when we consider the source of organs we take the donative viewpoint, which is steeped in voluntarism and altruism; when we consider the destination of organs we shift to justice or utilitarian viewpoints, which parcel out organs according to rule. It is unlikely that our cultural values will accommodate the radical change to a comprehensive justice or utility view which would replace the donative view with policies for involuntary retrieval of organs. Thus, we are likely to continue to suffer a radical disparity between needed and available organs.

Within the donative viewpoint, the question, 'Who should give?' is directly answered. Those who choose to do so, either for themselves or for others over whose bodies they have legitimate authority. The question, 'Who should receive?' is much more difficult to answer, since no individual has a moral claim on the organs of another. Their moral claim is much more general, namely, it is the claim that the sick have on the services and assistance of others who can help them.

THE 'DEAD-DONOR' RULE

These very general considerations about the ethics of organ transplantation bring us to Dr Peabody's question, 'Should the dead-donor rule be relaxed?' She narrows this broad question to another that is pertinent to perinatal transplantation, namely, "Should organs be retrieved from anencephalic infants." She reviews the clinical experience, noting that such transplantation has been attempted, and then comments that current law, defining death in terms of irreversible loss of whole-brain function, excludes living anencephalics as sources of organs. She then notes that some have advocated changing the law, either by declaring anencephalics death by definition at birth or declaring them exceptions to the dead-donor rule. 'Both lines of reasoning', she says, 'no matter how well intentioned, are ethically and practically problematic.' She then comments 'the issue of considering anencephalic infants as organ donors often resembles a most ferocious tug of war. Despite the complexity of the issues, our society is being drawn toward one or the other of two diametrically opposed viewpoints'. Dr Peabody does not mention that she herself initiated a bold, but largely unsuccessful experiment to salvage organs from anencephalic infants under the conditions of our present law.[7]

The arguments pro and con these 'diametrically opposed viewpoints' are drawn from a considerable literature generated in the late 1980s. Very capable ethicists line up on both sides of the question. For example, Englehardt, Fletcher, Zaner argue in favor; Capron, Churchill, Arras argue to the contrary. Their arguments are plausible in both directions. A plausible case can be made in favor of procurement of anencephalic organs by rethinking the concept of person or by providing exception to the brain criteria for death.[8,9] A case almost as plausible can be made against such procurement by upholding the current definition of death for public policy reasons and by pointing to the dangers of taking the first step on the slippery slope that would gradually include other hopeless and useless, but not dead, individuals as sources of viable organs.

I shall not review these arguments in detail. The literature is open to those who wish to ponder the pros and cons. I will attend to only one feature of the argument, namely, what ought to be done when reasonable arguments made by learned commentators seem to support both sides of an argument, not conclusively but plausibly.

This is a complex philosophical problem. However, rather than launching a head on philosophical attack to crack its complexities, I will relate a personal experience. Sometime during 1985, Dr Michael Harrison, the talented pediatric surgeon who had pioneered fetal surgery, visited my office. We were at that time colleagues on the faculty of the Medical School, University of California, San Francisco. He was excited by an innovative idea. The State of California had recently passed the Uniform Definition of Death Act, whereby legal determination of death could be made on clinical evidence of 'irreversible cessation of all functions of the entire brain, including the brain stem'. The Uniform Statute had been developed in 1981 by the President's Commission for the study of Ethical Problems in Medicine and in Biomedical and Behavioral Research, and had been endorsed by the American Medical Association, the American Bar Association and the National Conference of Commissioners on Uniform State Laws.

Dr Harrison's innovative idea was that the recently passed statute might be amended in such a way as to allow the salvage of organs from anencephalics. He was aware that several transplantation attempts using anencephalics organs had been reported. Anencephalics could, he proposed, be considered 'brain absent', rather than 'brain dead'. These infants, as distinguished from other individuals of the human species, had never developed the neurological structure we call 'brain'. The primary purpose of the new 'brain death' statute was to protect brain-injured individuals, who might possibly recover, from exploitation. This is irrelevant for individuals who had never had a brain.

In addition, the anencephalic cannot survive longer than a few days, and thus should be considered a dying individual whose death is soon expected. In such a situation, as he wrote in a later article, an approach that would allow salvage of organs from the still living anencephalic would 'give us the chance to recognize the contribution of this doomed fetus to manking'.[14]

I used to call my friend Dr Harrison 'ethicogenic', a causer of ethical problems. His imaginative and compassionate surgical innovations raised many ethical issues, which he took very seriously.[15] His enthusiasm for the possibility of increasing the supply of organs for pediatric transplant created just such problems, as I pointed out to him. I could not share his enthusiasim. I had been a member of the President's Commission that had crafted the Uniform Statute that he wanted to change. I felt that the Statute was in itself an important advance, that its formulation had been based on sound considerations, and that its adoption by almost all State legislatures and in many courts was a significant achievement. It was not the time, I thought, to advocate a change, even if the arguments in favor of change were plausible. Dr Harrison petitioned the Chancellor of the University to convene a committee to consider the issue. He did so, appointing me chair, and (as might be suspected), the committee concluded that it would not be prudent to advocate a change in the statute. Dr Harrison, on his own initiative as a private citizen, convinced the influential state legislator, Senator Milton Marks, to draft Senate Bill 2018 (1986), amending the statute to allow anencephalic transplantation; but public response was not favorable, and the bill was never submitted to the California legislature.

PHILOSOPHICAL AND PRACTICAL ARGUMENTS

An asymmetry should be noticed between my position and that of Dr Harrison. He was presenting considerations that looked like an 'ethical argument'. I was countering with prudential, policy considerations that were only remotely ethical. His ethical argument was that it would be a good thing to redeem some benefit from the tragedy of anencephaly, bringing the gift of life to another threatened child while not harming the anencephalic, whose life was doomed under any circumstances. Nothing was to be gained by anyone in permitting useful organs to be lost. The brain death criterion protected the majority of individuals from exploitation or misdiagnosis, but not the anencephalic.

My arguments did not dispute these points. Rather, I argued that the whole-brain criteria had significant advantages. The Commission's Report had noted these: it saw death as a single phenomenon, not defining it differently for different purposes; it underlined the idea of death as deterioration of the organism as a whole; it represented an incremental, not a radical, change in the public and legal conception of death, and was uniform among peoples and situations.[16] These were practical considerations, based on considerations about what constitutes sound reform of law and practice in a certain society and culture. In addition, I suggested that the exemption of the 'brain absent' from the statutory requirements was not immune from the slippery-slope problem. It was not a strong enough concept, I thought, to resist erosion into wider and wider exceptions, and as it did so it would slide from the probably acceptable into the dubiously accep⁺able and then into the unacceptable; but, as it did, people would lose thei ⸳ sensitivity to the distinctions, and slip along almost absentmindedly into reprehensible practices. This familiar argument is 'remotely ethical', in that it usually presumes that the first step is ethically acceptable, or at least plausibly so, but that the later steps that people are very likely to take are not. The slippery-slope metaphor almost implies that once the first step is taken, the others cannot but follow, because the social mind, like waxed skis on an icy slope, will slide, willy-nilly. The ethical argument is remote, because the ethically problematic case is not at the beginning, but at the bottom of the slope, where the trees and rocks are.[17]

Such an argument, as many have pointed out, rests on presumptions and prejudices rather than on science and fact. We can point to past examples of such catastrophic slides, but we can neither demonstrate their exact causality nor predict with assurance that the instant case will career downhill in similar fashion. Nevertheless, the argument appears to have persuasive power for many folk. It favors a conservative view of social change. Finally, many philosophers disdain such arguments. One acute philosopher, Richard Zaner, uses the criteria of classical logic to condemn:'Such purported arguments seem quite fallacious: they either deny the antecedent, affirm the consequent, or are a form of *ignoratio elenchi.*'[18]

During the 1980s, after the publication and almost universal adoption of the Uniform Determination of Death statute, some competent philosophers expressed skepticism about the Commission's choice of the whole-brain criteria. They usually did so because they judged that a much more persuasive philosophical case could be made to demonstrate that a person should be considered dead after the irreversible loss of cognitive function. They thus favored a 'higher brain' definition. In so doing, they cast speculative doubt on the philosophical soundness of the conception that was now almost universally the law of the land. While I found myself in sympathy with these philosopher's critique of the whole-brain criterion, I maintained my allegiance to the Commission's definition, a position some might call 'irrational' or 'illogical'.

Another line of philosophical argument, closely related to the former, militated against the whole-brain criteria and implicity strengthened the argument in favor of the use of anencephalic organs. The former argument proposes that a human body no longer capable or, by logical extension, never capable of cognitive activity should be considered dead. The second argument claims that 'personhood' should be defined in terms of actual or potential rationality. By implication, a human individual with no such capability should not be called a person, and thus should not be accorded the rights associated with personhood. Further, the important moral maxim, 'treat persons as ends, not merely as means', does not apply.[22] Not everyone who favored use of anencephalic organs espoused such an argument: Harrison, for example, was willing to attribute personhood to the anencephalic, but, at the same time, to see it as equivalently 'dead', or, somewhat inconsistently, as 'imminently dying'.

The argument about personhood reflects one of the deepest quandaries of Western philosophy. Since Socrates ironically suggested that 'human being' could be defined as a 'featherless biped', thinkers have wondered what were the essential, defining characteristics of the human being and the human person. It is difficult to sort out of the roiling debate any definitive answer: those who argue for potential rationality can be questioned about what potentiality means, those who support actual rationality may draw the circle of human personhood so close as to exclude the sleeping and the senile, those who favor species identity open it wide enough to include the zygote, those who propose a social attribution of personhood can be charged with opening the way to prejudicial arbitrariness. The interminable debate over the morality of abortion bears witness to this. However, given this disagreement, the case in favor of including anencephalics within the realm of human personhood is, in my judgment, not quite as strong as the case for excluding them.

Where does all this leave us? At the level of speculative argument about the appropriate definition of death and the nature of personhood, the debate is, in my view, close to, but not quite, a draw. There are plausible arguments that tend toward the higher-brain criteria for death and the rationality criteria for personhood; there are plausible arguments against both. Yet, in my judgment, the arguments in favor are the more convincing. If we were all always philosophers we might sit in suspended animation over these issues, saying neither yes nor no, waiting for the final conclusive argument to be announced, as the ancient skeptics were said to do. But we do not have that luxury: we must formulate an answer that can shape our actions and our policies. Under this constraint, we might decide that, even when arguments are inconclusive, we should follow the more persuasive lines: we should follow our philosophical consciences. However, this choice plunges us into the moral turmoil of what we now call a 'pluralistic society'.[23] It is not as if, in each person, the arguments pro and con played a duet. Rather, in this society, some persons espouse the pro arguments with vehemence; others are just as devoted to the con side. We end up with what Dr Peabody called, 'a most ferocious tug-of-war.'

Faced with this prospect, we might take another course: namely, to look away from the speculative arguments and ask about the practical issues and implications. These questions are, as I mentioned above, pragmatic and only remotely ethical, as in the 'slippery slope'.

Centuries ago, moral theologians debated the now incredible question whether a nobleman could kill someone who insulted him. Many moralists were convinced that plausible arguments could be marshalled in favor of the affirmative. One who so believed, a certain Cardinal de Lugo, commented, 'this conclusion is speculatively probable, but should not be allowed in practice'.[24] Immanuel Kant hated this distinction, which he called 'an old saw',[25] nevertheless, pace the old philosopher, the old saw deserves consideration. Can it be that mundane, pragmatic considerations might override plausible speculative arguments, and a right course of action should be prohibited?

One article on the con side illustrates this approach. Shewmon *et. al.* state, 'suggestions to include anencephaly within the definition of "death" pose many problems, including further expansion to other categories of patients with severe neurological impairments, damage to public confidence in death determinations and adverse impact on families that do not wish to regard their anencephalic child as dead'.[10] The authors go on to cite certain empirical problems regarding the misdiagnosis of anencephaly, suggesting that many different conditions, some of them considerably less devastating than complete anencephaly, can be mistaken for that condition. They propose that rationales for the inclusion of a category of anencephaly or brain-absence in the statute 'are broad enough to define other categories of dying, neurologically impaired patients as equally "dead", especially persons in persistent vegetative state.' They note that such an amendment would subjugate the important social determination of death to the need for organ transplantation, undermining 'the public's already tenuous confidence in brain-based determinations of death' and resulting in a decline of donations. Finally, some parents who suffer the tragedy of the birth of an anencephalic and may wish (as many do) to offer it cherishing comfort during its short life will be informed that, despite its movement and spontaneous reactions, it is 'dead'. They will be dismayed.

These reasons are primarily practical, not ethical. Yet, like the objection of the long-dead de Lugo to revenge killings, they suggest that the relaxation of the 'dead-donor' rule 'ought not to be allowed in practice'. He cited, as his reasons, his estimation that the practice of revenge killing, even if justifiable ethically, would bring about confusion, distrust, and pitched battles in the streets. Shewmon *et. al.* do not believe that anencephalic organ salvage would instigate pitched battles, but they estimate that it would effect confusion and distrust. People would never be certain whether their death would be 'their own' or 'for others'. They would be unsure whether an individual was really dead, or whether that individual should be counted live for this purpose and dead for another. Individuals would enjoy the rights and privileges of personhood at one time and not at another, depending on social needs and utility. Such social effects are enough, in their view (and in mine), to hold the line, or as certain authors say, 'place the wedge' at the whole-brain definition.[11] Confusion and distrust are social states in which even plausible ethical practices cannot be soundly and successfully implemented. Clarity and trust are, in a sense, the moral matrix in which ethical arguments and conclusions can be devised and rendered real as practice and policy.

If there are sound reasons to expect that an ethically justifiable revision of practice would result in some concrete and specifiable form of 'confusion and distrust' such a revision should be postponed or abandoned. There is, however, one crucial proviso: the practice or policy proposed for reform must be 'ethically neutral'. An unethical practice must cede to ethical reform, even at the price of confusion and distrust for the injustice and actual harm is a worse evil than the difficulties of implementing the reform in a social matrix of confusion and distrust: indeed, the presence of unjust social practices have probably already generated such a matrix.

The arguments in favor of the use of anencephalic organs show, at best, that such a use is permissible. That is, all things being equal, it is a policy that should not be prohibited as ethically wrong. The arguments do not show that use of such organs is ethically obligatory. The words 'all things being equal' now become significant: the 'all things' are the other mundane, practical, or, as the philosophers sometimes confusingly say, 'non-moral' considerations that attend any action or policy. Should these advise against the permissible, the permissible 'ought not be allowed in practice'.

THE MORAL VIEWPOINTS AS CONTEXT

Here we return to our prefatory remarks about the 'donative' and 'justice' viewpoints that govern our ethical thinking about transplantation. If the sick had a moral claim in justice on the organs of others, a much stronger case could be made in favor of mandatory efforts to increase the supply of organs. However, we have proposed that this case has not been made, and cannot be made without erosion of the dominant donative viewpoint. It is not the case, at least on the basis of current arguments, that 'burying the heart, liver, and kidneys of these patients when they might save another infant's life is immoral and unfair', as Dr Peabody cites some 'leaders in organ transplantation' as saying. It is indeed unfortunate and tragic that some should die when a life-saving resource might be obtained; but it cannot be condemned as immoral and unjust unless the donative–justice framework is restructured. In the absence of restructuring these moral viewpoints, the pragmatic, mundane considerations associated with confusion and distrust, if not with pitched battles, should guide the adoption of policy.

A reconstruction of the moral framework for organ transplantation must accommodate our cultural presuppositions about the relationships between individuals. Unquestionably, in different cultures, the relationship would be differently described. Professor Rihito Kimura, for example, says 'Japanese bioethical principles require a more subtle sense of the ways in which all living things are related to one another, based on the Buddhist notion of *En* (relatedness). A sharing-of-life principle would be more appropriate in a Japanese social context than a right-to-life principle, because it affirms the values of dependent life and togetherness.[26] (Ironically, even with this cultural value, the Japanese have not been enthusiastic about organ transplantation for other reasons.) The donative principle with which we work flourishes in a culture where the individual as such is supreme, and where individual inviolability, privacy, and rights dominate moral reflection. By two means alone, contracting and charity, do individuals reach out beyond themselves; and, of these, only contracting has a strong sense of obligation.

Often enough we hear John Donne's famous line, 'no man is an island, entire unto itself ... every man's death diminishes me, because I am involved in mankind'. We may be moved by this sentiment; but we have not built our philosophies and ethics upon it.

Strangely enough, the science of immunology, on which transplantation depends, once maintained that each man was an island, entire unto itself. The body of each individual would reject the pieces and parts of any stranger. The discovery of blood groups and then human leukocyte antigens revealed compatibility between individuals, and now we know that the more compatible the HLA antigens between donor and recipient, the less likely it is that transplanted tissue will be rejected. We now know more: the great bulk of the human genome is shared between all human individuals; each single person owns only a tiny fraction of uniqueness. While immunological barriers remain high, they are not impenetrable. We are each deeply 'involved in mankind' in a physical, bodily sense.

Does knowing this have any relevance for our philosophical understanding of the moral relationship between humans? Thus far, the revelation of genetic and immunological identity has not overcome the strong currents in our culture toward autonomy and individuality. Whether it will do so, and whether it would be a human benefit should such a philosophical and psychological revolution take place, are open questions.

REFERENCES

1. Fox, R. and Swazey, J. *The courage to fail: a social view of transplantation and dialysis.* University of Chicago Press (1974).
2. Titmuss, R. *The gift relationship.* Pantheon, New York (1971).
3. Ramsey, P. *The patient as person.* Yale University Press, New Haven (1971).
4. Kelley, G. *Medico-moral problems.* Catholic Hospital Association St. Louis (1958).
5. Fox. R. and Swazey, J. *Spare parts: organ replacement in American society.* Oxford University Press (1992).
6. Childress, J. Ethical criteria for procuring and distributing organs for transplantation. In James Blumstein and Frank Sloan (eds.) *Organ transplantation policy, Issues and prospects.* Duke University Press, Durham and London (1989).
7. Peabody, J., Emery, J., and Ashwal, S. Experience with anencephalic infants as prospective organ donors. *New Engl. J. Med.* 321: 344–50 (1989).
8. Englehardt, H. T. (ed.) Harvesting cells, tissues, and organs from fetuses and anencephalic newborns. *J. Med. Phil* 14 (1) (1989).
9. Fletcher, J., Robertson, J., and Harrison, M.. Primates and anencephalics as sources for pediatric organ transplants. *Fetal Therapy* 1: 150–64 (1986).
10. Shewmon, D., Capron, A., Peacock, W., and Schulman, B. The use of anencephalic infants as organ sources: a critique. *JAMA* 261: 1773–81 (1989).

11. Churchill, L. and Pinkus, R. The use of anencephalic organs: historical and ethical dimensions. *Milbank Quarterly* **68** (2): 147–69 (1990).
12. Arras, J. and Shinnar, S. Anencephalic newborns as organ donors: a critique *JAMA* **259**: 2284–5 (1988).
13. Capron, A. Anencephalic donors: separate the dead from the dying. *Hastings Cent. Rep.* February 5–9 (1987).
14. Harrison, M. Organ procurement for children: the anencephalic fetus as donor. *The Lancet* **2**: 1383–6 (1986).
15. Harrison, M., Golbus, M., and Jonsen, A. Fetal surgery for congenital hydronephrosis. *New Engl. J. Med.* **306**: 591–3 (1982).
16. President's Commission for the Study of Ethical Problems in Medicine and in Biomedical and Behavioral Research. *Defining death* U.S. Government Printing Office Washington, DC (1981).
17. Schauer F. Slippery slopes. *Harvard Law Review* **50** (2): 361–83, (1985).
18. Zaner, R. Anencephalics as organ donors. *J. Phil. Med.* **14**: 61–78 (1989).
19. Green, M. and Wikler D. Brain death and personal identity. *Phil. Pub.Aff.* **9**: 105–33 (1980).
20. Youngner, S. and Bartlett, E. Human death and high technology: the failure of the whole-brain formulations.*Ann. Intern. Med.* **99**: 252–8 (1983)
21. Zaner R. M. (ed.) *Beyond whole-brain criteria* Kluwer, Dordrecht (1988).
22. Cefalo, R. and Engelhardt, H. Anencephalic tissue for transplantation. *J. Phil. Med.* **14**: 25–43 (1989).
23. Cutter, M. Moral pluralism and the use of anencephalic tissue and organs. *J. Phil. Med.* **14**: 89–96 (1989).
24. De Lugo, J. *Responsorium morale* (1651). In Jonsen, A. and Toulmin, S. *The abuse of casuistry*. University of California Press, Berkeley (1988).
25. Kant, I. *On the old saw, It may be right, but it won't work in practice* E. Ashton (trans.), Philadelphia (1974).
26. Kimura, R. Anencephalic organ donation: a Japanese case *J. Med. Phil.* **14** (1): 97–102 (1989).

8

The boundary between therapeutic and non-therapeutic research

8A DUBIOUS DISTINCTIONS BETWEEN RESEARCH AND CLINICAL PRACTICE USING EXPERIMENTAL THERAPIES: HAVE PATIENTS BEEN WELL SERVED?

Jon Tyson

The obstetric faculty in a large perinatal center decide to order a cord blood pH determination at birth routinely. This decision was made partly to help assess the quality of obstetric and neonatal care, partly to understand better the problems of individual infants, partly to increase knowledge about the physiology of birth asphyxia and the relationship of cord blood pH to perinatal outcome, and partly to avoid unjustified malpractice litigation. (A normal pH value indicates that severe asphyxia was not present at birth.) Cord blood pH determinations are part of 'standard care' in many teaching hospitals, and a low pH value may prompt immediate therapy of the infant for acidosis. Yet it is unclear whether such treatment would improve, worsen, or have no effect on outcome. No special effort will be made to obtain and report the pH determinations as quickly as possible.

Should routine determination of cord blood pH as described above be classified as clinical practice, therapeutic research, or non-therapeutic research? How should the classification influence whether informed consent and the approval of the institutional review board (IRB) are required?

The neonatologists in the same center decide to institute stricter indications for phototherapy and exchange transfusion, and to require a higher serum bilirubin value than previously required. While these therapies have been used in neonatal care for decades, their value and proper indications are controversial.[1] The neonatologists do not attempt a randomized trial to resolve this uncertainty, largely because an extended period of study and a major commitment of personnel time and effort would be required. However, the proportion of infants who are found at autopsy to have kernicterus (brain damage from bilirubin toxicity) will be carefully monitored. The neonatologists intend to improve the care of individual infants (by avoiding unnecessary use of therapies which have potential hazards) and to gain knowledge that may help in the care of other infants (verification that the new treatment regimen does not result in an obvious increase in autopsy-identified kernicterus). No data will be collected that are not already available in clinical or autopsy records. IRB approval and informed consent are not required and will not be sought. However, any serious unanticipated hazards of the new treatment regimen are less likely to be promptly identified than if a randomized trial of this regimen were conducted.

Are these neonatologists simply practicing medicine (with prudent attention to autopsy findings) or are they really conducting research (albeit of low quality)? Is this question a matter of whether the revised treatment regimen is considered experimental, how the treatment regimen is allocated and evaluated, or whether the physicians intend to increase knowledge? Should treatment regimens of uncertain value be considered experimental even if they are commonly or routinely used? Are infants and their parents well served by regulations requiring more careful monitoring when a new and unproven treatment regimen is used in a proper controlled trial than in uncontrolled clinical practice?

These anecdotes describe examples of a wide variety of activities in the author's center which prompt questions like those noted above. Such questions can be asked frequently in other perinatal centers and in all areas of medicine. The answers given by physicians are often uncertain, and sometimes conflict with those of ethicists or IRB members. Yet current regulations rest on an assumption that research and clinical practice have been clearly defined and distinguished and appropriately regulated.

In this chapter, I will present the perspective of a neonatologist who believes that fundamental problems remain in distinguishing clinical investigation and clinical practice, and that these problems compromise the ethical and scientific integrity of both medical research and medical care. Current regulations and policies have undoubtedly done much to protect the welfare and autonomy of patients in research. The likelihood of disgraceful abuses like those which have occurred in the past[2] seems to have been considerably reduced. However, I will argue that the welfare and autonomy of patients in general have not been well served by widely-used definitions of research and clinical practice and by more stringent regulations for use of an unproven therapy in a proper controlled trial than in uncontrolled clinical practice.

In addressing these issues, terms commonly used to define, categorize, and distinguish research and clinical practice will first be described. Questions about the proper definition and use of these terms will then be presented citing examples which have arisen in my perinatal center. Finally, strategies that might be used to improve the way that research and clinical practice are regulated will be suggested for formal evaluation.

COMMONLY USED TERMS AND CONCEPTS

Therapeutic and non-therapeutic research. In 1975 the National Commission for the Protection of Human Subjects of Biomedical and Behavioral Research[3] (referred to as the Commission in the rest of the chapter) stated that:

Research refers to the systematic collection of data or observations in accordance with a designed protocol.

Therapeutic research refers to research designed to improve the health or condition of the research subject by prophylactic, diagnostic or treatment methods that depart from standard medical practice . . .

Nontherapeutic research refers to research not designed to improve the health condition of the research subject by prophylactic, diagnostic or treatment methods.

However, the term 'therapeutic research' has been criticized as a contradiction in terms, in that research is performed to advance knowledge, not to benefit the patient.[4] Levine[5] asserts that therapeutic research as defined by the Commission does not exist, and that 'all ethical codes, regulations, and commentaries relying on the distinction . . . contained serious errors'. Partly for this reason, the Commission has abandoned the use of the term 'therapeutic research'.

In this chapter 'therapeutic research' is defined as research to evaluate interventions intended to benefit individual patients. The term 'non-therapeutic research' refers to other clinical research, usually to address physiologic questions, for example, the changes in blood glucose during the first postnatal week. A specific research project may contain both therapeutic and non-therapeutic components.

The difference between therapeutic and non-therapeutic research has at times been considered highly important. Indeed, some attempts have been made to ban all non-therapeutic research in children. Yet, the basic issue is whether there is an ethically acceptable relationship of risks to benefits— given all that is known or can be reasonably anticipated about the risks and benefits. There may be no discernible increase in risk in a non-therapeutic study, for example a study of heart rate in healthy newborns. Moreover, therapeutic studies may entail unacceptable risk—for example, a study in which the available evidence indicates that the hazards of treatment are very likely to exceed the benefits.

Thus, the difference between therapeutic and non-therapeutic research is *not* a fundamental ethical distinction, and the regulations governing research quite properly focus on the risk/benefit ratio to participants, rather than on the 'type of research' question.

Innovative and non-validated therapies. The Commission has described innovative therapies as 'novel procedures' which are 'deviations from common practice in drug administration or in surgical, medical, or behavioral therapies . . . tried in the course of rendering treatment'.[3] Like innovative therapies, many 'standard' therapies have uncertain value, and may be ineffective or even harmful. The Commission and a number of writers have used the term non-validated therapies to refer to all therapies of questionable value, whether or not they are frequently used.[5]

Most definitions of such therapies have not been accompanied by criteria to distinguish validated from non-validated therapies. Such criteria are not easily defined. Even in large, well-performed randomized clinical trials, it may be difficult to determine whether a therapy is truly beneficial. Less rigorous studies are a notorious source of misleading data, and a cause of unjustified treatment recommendations and widespread iatrogenic disease.

For the purposes of this chapter, the term 'non-validated therapy' will refer to a therapy which has either not been tested in a well-conducted randomized trial or benefit is not identified in one or more trial and there is no published meta-analysis to show an overall benefit. These criteria minimize, but do not eliminate, the possibility that a truly ineffective or hazardous therapy would be classified as validated. However, the above criteria are more stringent than many observers might use.

Experimentation. The Committee on Drugs of the American Academy of Pediatrics[6] has defined experimentation as 'the use of unproven methods, medications, or doses'. By this definition, 'unproven therapies, while they may be called "innovative treatment" are actually experimentation' whether or not research is being performed.[6] This definition is similar to other commonly used definitions. There is increasing recognition that many, if not most, therapies have unproven value, and that informal experimentation is commonplace in clinical practice.[5, 6]

Medical practice vs. medical research. In the *Belmont Report*[7] the Commission stated: 'For the most part, the term 'practice' refers to interventions that are designed solely to enhance the well-being of an individual patient or client and that have a reasonable expectation of success . . . By contrast the term "research" designates an activity designed to test a hypothesis, permit conclusions to be drawn, and thereby to develop or contribute to generalizable knowledge'. Yet the likelihood of success in clinical practice cannot always be estimated, and research may be conducted to generate rather than test hypotheses.

For these reasons, definitions like the following may be used: 'The term, research, refers to a class of activities designed to develop or contribute to generalizable knowledge . . . The practice of medicine . . . refers to a class of activities designed solely to enhance the well-being of an individual patient.'[6]

The words 'designed to' may be understood to mean 'intended to' or 'for the purpose of'. Current thinking generally differentiates clinical practice from research in terms of physician intent. For this reason, the Commission specifically states that 'service' programs may be included under research. Read and practice might be defined in terms of the physician's methods—for example, whether a proper research protocol was written. However, IRBs responsible for regulating research would lose jurisdiction over experiments performed without a protocol—the kind of experiments in which patient welfare and autonomy may be at greatest jeopardy. Many who write about the ethics of research believe that physician intent allows medical research and practice to be separated into mutually exclusive activities. This view is challenged below.

SHOULD CLINICAL PRACTICE AND RESEARCH BE CONSIDERED SEPARATE AND DISTINCT ACTIVITIES DISTINGUISHED SOLELY BY PHYSICIAN INTENT?

Current definitions to distinguish research and practice based on physician intent can be challenged on multiple grounds:

(1) *Physician intent cannot be objectively determined.* This basic problem has received surprisingly little discussion.

(2) *Clinical practice is not necessarily designed solely to improve patient well-being.*
To build or maintain a practice, the physician may accede to patient demands for unnecessary medications. To avoid violating hospital policies, the physician may discharge patients earlier than may be best for them. To minimize unreimbursed costs, the physician may not order expensive though possibly beneficial tests. In attempting to avoid malpractice litigation, the physician may perform unnecessary tests.

(3) *Obtaining generalizable knowledge—a better understanding of disease and its proper treatment—is a desirable and inextricable component of clinical practice.*
Patients benefit from what their physician has learned from other patients. Astute physicians learn the most, and their patients benefit the most. The important issue is not whether physicians should intend or do intend to gain generalizable knowledge, but how it is most ethically, accurately, and fully obtained.

(4) *An intent to increase generalizable knowledge is particularly desirable and common in the area of clinical practice which is most difficult to distinguish from research—the use of unproven and therefore experimental interventions.*
When such interventions are used, patient welfare is particularly dependent on the physician's attention to detecting unanticipated side-effects as well as hoped-for benefits. This fact is well known to physicians. It may be unusual or even rare to begin using 'innovative' therapies *solely* for the patient's benefit. 'I'll try it,' clinicians say, 'and see if it works.' Although the assessment may be only anecdotal, the physician intends to gain generalizable knowledge—whether the therapy is likely to benefit not only the patient being treated, but other similar patients as well.

(5) *Physician intent to benefit the individual patient may be greater, not less, in controlled studies than in uncontrolled clinical use of non-validated therapies.*
The use of therapeutic regimens in controlled studies is scrutinized not

only by IRBs but also by funding agencies, data-monitoring committees, peer reviewers, and the critical audience of physicians and scientists who read medical journals. This weighty net of supervision and monitoring is a potent incentive to investigators to use non-validated therapies in the safest and most effective way possible, on the basis of a careful assessment of the best available evidence. The practicing physician is not subject to such monitoring, and may have little time to be as painstaking.

(6) *The importance of physician intent* per se *is doubtful*, particularly when non-validated therapies are used.

The regulation of research is based on the ethical principles of beneficence and respect for persons. Under these principles, the central issue is patient welfare and autonomy, not physician intent. The history of perinatal medicine demonstrates the disasters that can occur when well-meaning physicians use non-validated treatment regimens. Noting these problems, Silverman[8] contends 'The time has come to examine the high moral status accorded to an individual doctor's treatment preference, particularly when that choice is backed by weak evidence.' Freedman[9] notes 'The ethics of medical practice grants no ethical or normative meaning to a treatment preference, however powerful, that is based on a hunch or anything less than evidence publicly presented and convincing to the clinical community. Persons are licensed as physicians after they demonstrate the acquisition of professionally validated knowledge, not after they reveal a superior capacity for guessing.'

Thus, current regulations are based on dubious assumptions and a misunderstanding of the nature and importance of physician intent in research and practice.

Nevertheless, advocates of current regulations may contend that the procedures for regulating research in the US work well in practice and should not be altered. However, the feasibility and benefits of this approach are challenged in the next two sections.

IS IT FEASIBLE TO REGULATE AS RESEARCH ALL ACTIVITIES THAT INCLUDE AN INTENT TO INCREASE GENERALIZABLE KNOWLEDGE?

An enormous number of clinical activities would be included in any serious attempt to regulate all activities intended to increase generalizable knowledge. In neonatal units, for example, these activities occur daily in scrutinizing the care of each patient during attending rounds, in discussing perinatal care during conferences, in conducting quality-assurance programs, in routinely collecting data to assess the care and outcome of high-risk newborns, and in evaluating the health and developmental status of infants assessed in the follow-up clinic. Such activities are advocated by the American Academy of Pediatrics as a standard part of perinatal practice.[10]

The activities in rounds, teaching conferences, and quality-assurance programs might be exempted from IRB approval and informed consent. Nevertheless, the regulation of the remaining activities classified as research as defined above would remain a staggering and unmanageable burden for physicians and IRBs.

IRB members and ethicists may not appreciate this point, in part because IRB approval is not sought for the vast majority of these activities. To make this point clear, the following anecdotes describing activities in our perinatal center are provided to indicate the spectrum of clinical activities that include an intent to increase generalizable knowledge:

1. A neonatal resuscitation team is organized and specially trained to care for all high-risk infants at birth. The intent is not only to benefit the infants, but also to improve the documentation of care given in the delivery room and to make observations that may result in improved methods of care. Similar motives underlie many other routine practices in neonatal units.

2. Additional incubators need to be purchased. Two commercially available models, both used in many neonatal units, are being considered. Some babies are randomly assigned to one model, and some to the other. To assess the function and reliability of the incubators, temperature is more intensively monitored. Risk is not increased. With all the equipment used in neonatal units (for example, monitors, ventilators, oximeters, catheters, endotracheal tubes, etc.) and the frequency with which aging equipment needs replacement, testing of this sort occurs frequently in neonatal units, as in many other hospital areas.

3. One of the neonatologists decides to administer vitamin A supplements to high-risk newborns in the hope of preventing bronchopulmonary dysplasia. For a limited period, he will order blood levels of vitamin A, a test which is not ordinarily performed. This testing is intended to benefit the involved infants by allowing intake to be adjusted to achieve desirable blood levels. However, it is also intended to produce generalizable knowledge—a regimen of vitamin A supplementation which will safely achieve desirable blood levels in most infants.

   Vitamin A supplementation may be considered to be non-validated therapy, although its use is supported by one published and one unpublished clinical trial. However, use of the 'standard' regimen for administering vitamin A is supported by weaker evidence and can be considered to be equally or more experimental than the administration of the vitamin A supplements. This situation is similar to many situations in which the better of alternative approaches to care is unclear.

4. A desperately ill infant with pulmonary hypoplasia does not respond to conventional ventilator therapy. The neonatologist systematically manipulates the ventilator settings to assess the effect of different airway pressures and wave-forms. He intends to identify the optimal settings for the infant in the shortest possible time. However, as in other

instances when physicians experiment to find the best therapy for a specific patient, there is also an intent to identify how similar patients might also be best treated.

5. An outbreak of severe infections due to bacteria resistant to multiple antibiotics occurs in the neonatal unit. The usual measures to combat such outbreaks fail. The application of 'triple dye' to the umbilical cord is considered as a strategy to prevent colonization with pathogenic bacteria. This agent is routinely used in some centers. Yet neither its effectiveness nor its toxicity have been carefully studied, and there is reluctance to institute routine use of triple dye unless it is shown to prevent colonization with the resistant bacteria.

The hospital's infection-control committee has the responsibility and authority to institute measures to halt the outbreak. The committee decides that during a trial period triple dye will be applied to alternate infants on admission to the neonatal unit. In this way, chance will determine which infants receive the uncertain benefits and hazards of triple dye. Moreover, the application of triple dye to half the infants may be sufficient to control the outbreak. However, the primary reason for using this procedure is assess the effect of triple dye on colonization with resistant organisms. The findings will be used to determine whether to use this agent routinely. A moderate effect is identified, and later published in the medical literature.[11]

6. The best body position—prone or supine—for premature infants after they have recovered from any initial illness is unclear. Body position may have an important effect on the risk of death due to sudden infant death syndrome (SIDS).[12] The neonatal faculty agree that this issue is not resolvable by a randomized trial in their center. The time required to complete such a trial—perhaps 10 years—would be too long, and the current requirements for informed consent are likely to be insurmountable.

An arbitrary decision might be made to place all infants in one position. However, if the wrong position is selected, the number of infants who died might be substantially increased.

To avoid this problem, the neonatal faculty are considering using a strategy known as 'play-the-winner'. All premature infants would initially be nursed in a specific position (for example, prone). When a death occurred, all succeeding premature infants would then be placed in the opposite position (for example, supine). After the next infant died, infant position would then be reversed again.

To the extent that body position has an important effect on mortality, this strategy would minimize overall mortality and the number of infants given care in the less desirable position. If body position has no effect on mortality, risk of death would be unaffected. Although originally developed as a research tool, 'play-the-winner' (or various modified versions) can be used clinically as a method for physicians to modify their treatment practices according to their clinical experience.

Each of the above anecdotes, like the two at the beginning of the chapter, involve situations in which the best treatment regimen is unknown and experimentation is therefore unavoidable. The risk to individual patients does not appear to be increased by the activities in these anecdotes; in fact, risk may be reduced.

Yet, because there is the intent to gain knowledge in altering the patient care, IRB review would be required for these and all similar activities under current regulations. However, most clinicians—and I suspect many IRB members—would regard such supervision as unnecessary and unreasonable. In some cases, time constraints would preclude obtaining either informed consent (anecdote 1) or IRB approval (anecdote 4).

Above and beyond the question of feasibility, there is also a serious question about potential harm from the current use of physician intent to define and regulate medical experimentation.

DO CURRENT REGULATIONS AND PROCEDURES CAUSE HARM BY DISCOURAGING CONTROLLED STUDIES AND ENCOURAGING HAPHAZARD CLINICAL USE OF EXPERIMENTAL THERAPIES? A PERINATAL EXAMPLE.

Noting that IRB approval and written informed consent for non-validated therapies are required only in formal research, Smithells[13] has quipped 'I need permission to give a new drug to half my patients but not to give it to all of them.'

The effect of this double standard is difficult to determine. The number of studies submitted to IRBs is carefully tabulated. However, there is no way to determine how many clinical trials are *not* proposed and how many patients are treated with poorly evaluated therapies because of this double standard.

Nevertheless, this double standard can be expected to discourage proper testing and encourage routine clinical use of non-validated therapies, [8] particularly in emergencies. The care of asphyxiated newborns, for example, has been assessed in very few clinical trials.[14] This problem is not attributable to an absence of controversy. Indeed, the value of sodium bicarbonate infusion has been disputed for decades. Although widely recommended, this therapy may increase the risk of intracranial hemorrhage and reperfusion injury. Whether the risk of death or cerebral palsy among severely asphyxiated infants is increased, decreased, or unaffected by this therapy remains to be determined.[14, 15]

For this reason, a clinical trial of sodium bicarbonate administration was proposed in our center. This proposal is discussed in some detail to indicate the problems in investigating emergency therapies and the effect of more stringent requirements for the use of non-validated therapies in research than in practice.

For the following reasons, the trial was proposed with a request to waive the requirement for informed consent when it could not be reasonably obtained:

1. *The research question could not otherwise be answered in the author's center or in virtually any center in the US.*

   A very large number of infants must be studied to assess the effect of sodium bicarbonate on death or cerebral palsy. Although the study hospital has the third largest delivery service in the country, the study would require at least 3 years if 90 per cent of severely asphyxiated infants were enrolled. Longer clinical trials are very difficult to complete successfully.

   Moreover, requiring informed consent would produce a major selection bias and perhaps misleading results. Mothers of infants most likely to fare poorly are least likely to receive prenatal care and most likely to present in advanced labor or have complications, medications, or procedures that would prevent valid consent. Performing a multi-center trial would increase enrollment but would not avoid this bias.

2. *Consent would often have questionable validity.* It would be necessary to obtain consent in labor because the need for immediate care of asphyxiated infants precludes consent following birth and because it would not be feasible to obtain consent in prenatal clinics, given the number and location of these community clinics. Consent usually could not be obtained from the father because the great majority of our mothers are unmarried or not accompanied by their husband. Given the excruciating pain of many women in labor, it is doubtful valid consent can be obtained, even in the absence of blood loss, potent medications, traumatic procedures, etc. This is one reason that informed consent for tubal ligation can not be legally obtained during labor. While 'informed consent' has been obtained during labor in many studies, there appear to be no data to show that such consent is valid.

3. *Chance would determine if an asphyxiated infant would receive sodium bicarbonate whether or not the trial were performed.*

   Informed consent is often considered mandatory whenever therapy is randomly assigned, i.e., determined by chance. Yet, to no lesser extent, chance determines which asphyxiated infants receive sodium bicarbonate in clinical practice. Some clinicians administer sodium bicarbonate to asphyxiated infants; others do not. Chance determines which physician is on call when an infant is born. Moreover, for many physicians, especially those most knowledgeable and uncertain about this therapy, the decision to administer or forgo sodium bicarbonate is in essence a mental flip of the coin.

4. *Infant risk would not be increased by the study procedures for treatment and evaluation.*

   Infant care would be unaffected except that resuscitation would be more carefully regulated and neurodevelopmental outcome more carefully assessed. The study might, in fact, reduce risk.

5. *Seeking informed consent during labor might harm the fetus.*
The anxiety of some mothers would be increased by informing them that
their baby's treatment might increase the risk of death or cerebral
palsy. There is strong experimental and human evidence that increased
anxiety during labor increases the risk of birth asphyxia and maternal
complications.[16–20] Increased maternal anxiety would be most likely to
precipitate fetal distress in medically unstable mothers, the group from
whom valid consent would also be most difficult to obtain and whose
infants it is most important to study. Requiring informed consent from
these mothers might increase the number of severely asphyxiated infants
two-or threefold above the usual low rate (1 per cent) in the study hospital. The investigator argued that well-meaning and usually appropriate
requirements could produce serous harm in this circumstance.

Nevertheless, the IRB ruled that consent must be obtained for all patients
enrolled. This ruling precluded a successful trial, and for this reason, it was
never initiated. The trial was proposed in 1977. To date, no trial has been
performed to resolve whether sodium bicarbonate administration increases
or decreases the number of asphyxiated infants who die or develop severe
neurologic handicap. Haphazard use of sodium bicarbonate continues.

This proposal would not be noteworthy if effective ways had been developed to encourage proper testing and discourage routine clinical use of
non-validated therapies. IRBs seem quite reluctant to waive consent for
proposals in circumstances where consent might be ethically and legally
waived. Under Sections 46, 116D and 46.117C or the Code of Federal
Regulations 45 CFR 46, an IRB may waive some or all requirements for
informed consent when the research could not otherwise practicably be
performed, the rights and welfare of the subjects would not be adversely
affected, the research involves no more than minimal risk, and no procedures
are performed for which written consent is required outside the research
context.

Judging from published clinical trials, this waiver has been rarely granted,
despite the pressing need for clinical trials of therapies used in emergencies
and other circumstances where valid consent is unlikely to be obtained.
Unfortunately, these are precisely the circumstances when the unanticipated or unrecognized hazards of unproven therapies are likely to be most
devastating. As Eisenberg reminds us [21] 'Impeding research, no less than
performing it, has ethical consequences.'

SHOULD THE REGULATION OF MEDICAL EXPERIMENTATION BE AS STRINGENT IN CLINICAL PRACTICE AS IN RESEARCH?

The total number of patients who receive experimental therapies in clinical
practice is undoubtedly orders of magnitude greater than that of those who

receive them in research. Data about patient risk in research are limited, but suggest that risk to individual patients is not greater than in clinical practice.[22] Thus the total number of patients who have suffered adverse consequences from the use of experimental therapies may also be orders of magnitude greater in clinical practice. In perinatal medicine alone, thousands of infants have died or been left handicapped by well-meaning but poorly-tested regimens of oxygen, sulfonamide, chloramphenicol, thalidomide, diethylstilbestrol, benzyl alcohol, E-ferol, or other agents.[23]

The double standard for the use of experimental therapies in clinical practice and research has been increasingly criticized on grounds of patient autonomy as well as patient welfare.[24, 25] At a recent consensus conference, three-fourths of participants agreed that there should be no fundamental difference between the information given to obtain informed consent for a controlled trial and that given in daily practice.[26] Gillon[27] contends that 'Doctors are no less morally obliged to respect the autonomy of their patients than that of their research subjects.'

Chalmers[28] has called for equally stringent procedures for informed consent in clinical practice and randomized trials when unproven therapies are used. In principle, I support this recommendation. However, current procedures should be reconsidered for clinical research as well as clinical practice.

NEED FOR RESEARCH ON THE REGULATION AND EFFECTS OF MEDICAL EXPERIMENTATION.

As Pellegrino[29] notes 'The patient must decide how much autonomy he or she wishes to exercise . . .' There is increasing evidence that some, if not many, patients do not desire detailed risk disclosure or participation in medical decisions.[30–32] More research is needed to assess the wants and needs of patients and the risks and benefits of detailed risk disclosure and seeking written consent.[33–35] Elsewhere in this book, Silverman has argued persuasively for the need for such research.

The effects of participating in research on patient risk and outcome warrant considerable study. Patient risk may be reduced not only by receiving a new and improved therapy, but also from increased attention to patient care and monitoring or from the Hawthorne effect, the effect of being under study upon the persons being studied.[36, 37] These effects may have important effects on patient outcome. During the Dublin fetal heart-rate monitoring trial, the stillbirth rate was lower than that during the year before or the year after the trial.[38]

Formal study of the Hawthorne effect and other mechanisms by which research may affect outcome is needed. Specific strategies to improve the ethical quality of medical experimentation in medicine should also be studied. Some potential strategies are noted below.

POTENTIAL METHODS TO IMPROVE THE ETHICAL QUALITY OF MEDICAL EXPERIMENTATION

1. Experimentation in clinical practice

The following measures are directed toward circumstances in which the use of a non-validated therapy may be most harmful.

A. *Require written informed consent when a non-validated (experimental) therapy is used in lieu of a validated therapy.*

Non-validated or experimental therapies might be defined as interventions that have not been reported to be beneficial in all clinical trials to date (one or more) or in a meta-analysis of all the trials. A listing of published clinical trials for all therapies in obstetrics and neonatology is provided, with meta-analyses, through the Oxford Registry of Perinatal Trials and in textbooks based on this registry.[39, 40]

This approach could be implemented most simply if physicians—without monitoring or supervision from a clinical practice committee or IRB—were fully responsible for recognizing whether validated or non-validated therapies were used and for providing adequate written information and obtaining valid consent. The motivation for the physician to comply would be a desire to inform his patients and to protect himself from censure or litigation if the therapy had untoward effects.

B. *Require specific written consent for new non-validated therapies (whether or not a validated therapy is available).*

Serious hazards are most likely to be unrecognized when the therapy is relatively new. Non-validated therapies may be considered new if they have not been recommended in peer-reviewed journals for more than 10 years.

C. *Evaluate a policy of reimbursement for new and non-validated therapies only when they are used in proper studies to assess their value.*

Third-party payment is now withheld for use of therapies designated as experimental. However, the definition of 'experimental therapies' is unclear, and reimbursement is now provided for clinical use of many therapies that meet the above definition of a non-validated and therefore experimental therapy.

Curtailing reimbursement for non-validated therapies that have been widely used is not likely to be feasible. However, at a time when there is great pressure to reduce health-care costs, the withholding of reimbursement for new and unproven therapies is a strategy that might have considerable appeal. The principle that patients do not have the right to demand therapies of questionable value has already been endorsed by our society in establishing the Food and Drug Administration.

Private insurers are unlikely to pay for therapies not eligible for Medicaid or Medicare reimbursement. If governmental funding agencies were to withhold reimbursement for all new therapies until their value was demonstrated, third-party expenditures for health care might be greatly reduced. Some of the monies saved could be used to pay for use of non-validated therapies in studies employing the most rigorous design feasible—ordinarily, a randomized clinical trial. (Cohort studies could be acceptable for evaluating the treatment of disorders which are rare or virtually always fatal.) Linking payment for the use of non-validated therapies to their use in a way which allows their value to be assessed would encourage prompt, rigorous testing of promising therapies. It would also greatly reduce the likelihood that treatment methods would be widely used before being recognized to be ineffective or even hazardous.

2. Experimentation in medical research

A. *Redefine the term 'minimal risk'.*
This term is of major importance, in part because studies which impose minimal risk are eligible for expedited review and a simplified consent procedure. Minimal risk, as defined in the federal regulations, [41] 'means that the risks of harm anticipated in the proposed research are not greater, considering probability and magnitude, than those ordinarily encountered in daily life or during the performance of routine physical or psychological examinations or tests'.

As has been discussed in detail by Kopelman, [42] this definition is unsatisfactory, for a number of reasons. A major problem is that it is unclear whether it is the total risk to research subjects or the risk imposed by the research that is at issue. The term minimal risk would be better defined as minimal differential risk[43] a minimum level of risk imposed by the research above the risk experienced clinically by the kind of patients eligible for study.

B. *Recognize that randomization is a procedure that does not in itself increase risk.*
Randomization is simply a tool to assure comparability of treatment groups. The issue is how the procedures used to treat or evaluate the patients influence their risk of an adverse outcome.

C. *Classify alternative therapies as having equivalent risk (or risk–benefit ratio) when the most desirable therapy has not been determined in proper clinical trials.*
Under this approach, randomized assignment to alternative treatment methods for which there is 'clinical equipoise' would not be considered to increase patient risk.[9]

D. *When patient risk is not increased by any research procedures, exempt investigators from obtaining informed consent when allowed under the Code of Federal Regulations.*
As was noted above, this Code allows IRBs to waive some or all requirements for informed consent when the research could not otherwise practicably be performed, the rights and welfare of the subjects would not be adversely affected, the research involves no more than minimal risk, and no procedures are performed for which written consent is required outside the research context. Providing risk is interpreted as

discussed above, consent might not be required in clinical scenarios like the anecdotes described in this chapter. Consent of course could be required for any procedures that increase risk even minimally, for example, blood sampling not required clinically. Nevertheless, the proper evaluation of emergency therapies could be greatly enhanced if IRBs granted this exemption whenever appropriate.

E. *Consider requiring a signature only to refuse consent—rather than to grant consent—for studies which in the opinion of the IRB do not increase patient risk.*

We have experienced as high as a 30 per cent refusal rate in a randomized trial in which indigent high-risk infants are assigned a highly experienced primary care nurse who is available in a clinic 40 hours per week and by telephone at all other hours. Transportation is provided as needed. The control group receives conventional follow-up care. The intervention is known to reduce both loss of infants to follow-up and inconvenience to the mothers. The study is being conducted to determine whether the intervention is a cost-effective approach to follow-up care which reduces mortality and need for pediatric intensive care in high-risk populations.

Current procedures discourage enrollment in such studies. In our society, a signature is ordinarily required only when extra risk is incurred or extra expense or responsibility is accepted. It is misleading to require a signature when risk is not increased, particularly if inconvenience, expense, or discernible risk is reduced. Requiring a signature to refuse rather than to grant consent would be a more accurate way to convey the advantages and disadvantages of participation. As has been shown by Mutch and King,[44] enrollment is likely to be increased when a signature is required to 'opt out' than to 'opt in' to such a study.

In conclusion, limitations in medical knowledge make experimentation using unproven therapies both common and unavoidable. Attempts to draw a clear boundary between research and clinical care using unproven therapies are futile. Neither patient welfare nor autonomy are well served by the double standard requiring institutional review and written informed consent for experimentation in research but not for experimentation in clinical practice. High priority should be given to developing and evaluating better methods to meet the needs and wants of patients and their families whenever experimentation occurs.

REFERENCES

1. Newman, T. B. and Maisels, M. J. (1992). Response to commentaries *re*: evaluation and treatment of jaundice. *Pediatrics* **89**, 831.
2. Rothman, D. (1987), Ethics and human experimentation. Henry Beecher revisited. *New Engl.J.Med.* **387**, 1195.

3. The National Commission for the Protection of Human Subjects of Biomedical and Behavioral Research: *Research on the fetus: report and recommendations*. DHEW Publications No. (OS) 76-128, Washington, 1975.
4. Rolleston, F. and Miller J. (1981). Therapy or research, a need for precision. *IRB. Rev Human Subjects Res*, Aug. Sep. 1.
5. Levine, R. J. (1986). *Ethics and regulation of clinical research*, 2nd. ed. Urban and Schwarzenberg, Baltimore.
6. American Academy of Pediatrics Committee on Drugs (1977). Guidelines for the ethical conduct of studies to evaluate drugs in pediatric populations. *Pediatrics* **60**, 1977.
7. The National Commission for the Protection of Human subjects of Biomedical and Behavioral Research: *The Belmont Report. Ethical principles and guidelines for the protection of human subjects of research*. DHEW Publication No (OS) 78-0013, Appendix II, DHEW Publication (OS) 78-0014, Washington, 1978.
8. Silverman, W. (1988). SSPR Mini-symposium. Methodologic controversies in clinical research: consent for experimentation involving neonates *AM. Jr. Med. Sci.* **296**, 354.
9. Freedman, B. (1987). Equipoise and the ethics of clinical research. *New Engl.J. Med.* **317**, 141–5.
10. American Academy of Pediatrics and American College of obstetrics and Gynecology. *Guidelines for perinatal care, 3rd* edn. Elk Grove Village, Ill, 1992, pp. 191–6.
11. Rosenfeld, C.R. , Laptook, A. R., and Jaishree, J. (1990). Limited effectiveness of triple dye in preventing colonization with methicillin-resistant *Staphylococcus aureus* in a special care nursery. *Pediatr. Infect. Dis.J..* **9**, 290.
12. Guntheroth, W. G. and Spiers, P. S. (1992). Sleeping prone and the risk of sudden infant death syndrome. *JAMA* **267**, 2359.
13. Smithells, R. (1975). Iatrogenic hazards and their effects. *Postgrad.Med. J. 51* (Suppl 2), 39.
14. Tyson, J. (1992). Immediate management of the newborn infant. In *Effective care of the newborn infant* (ed. J. C. Sinclair and M. B. Bracken), p. 22. Oxford University Press, New York, 1992.
15. Volpe, J. (1981). Neonatal intraventricular hemorrhage. *New Engl. J. Med.* **304**: 886.
16. Kennel, J., Klaus, M., McGrath, S., Robertson, S., and Hinkley, C. (1991). Continuous emotional support during labor in a US hospital. A randomized controlled trial. *JAMA* **265**, 2197.
17. Sosa, R., Kennell, J., Klaus, M., Robertson, S., and Urrutia, J. (1980). The effect of a supportive companion on perinatal problems, length of labor, and mother–infant interaction. *New Engl. J. Med.* **303**, 597.
18. Copher, D. and Huber, C. (1967). Heart rate response of the human fetus to induced maternal hypoxia. *Amer. J. Obstet. Gynecol.* **122**, 47.
19. Haverkamp, A., Thompson, H., McFee, J., and Cetrulo, C. (1976). The evaluation of continuous fetal heart rate monitoring in high-risk pregnancy. *Am. J. Obstet. Gynecol.* **125**, 310.
20. Myers, R. (1975). Maternal psychological stress and fetal asphyxia: a study in the monkey. *Am. J. Obstet. Gynecol.* **122**, 47.

21. Eisenberg, L. (1977). The social imperatives of medical research. *Science* **198**, 1105.
22. Cardon, P. V. , Dommell, F. W., and Trumble, R. R. (1976). Injuries to research subjects. *New. Engl.J. Med. 295*, 650.
23. Silverman, W. (1987). Human experimentation in perinatology. *Clin. Perinatol.* **14**, 403.
24. Chalmers, I. and Silverman, W. (1987). Professional and public double standards on clinical experimentation. *Controlled Clin. Trials*, **8**, 388.
25. King, J. (1986). Informed consent. *IME Bull.*, Suppl. No. 3, p. 2.
26. Blum, A. L., Chalmers, T. C., Deutsch, E., Koch-Weser, J., Rosen, A., Tygstrup, N., and Zentgraf, R. (1987). The Lugano statement on controlled clinical trials. *J. Int. Med. Res.* **15**, 2.
27. Gillon, R. (1985). Beneficence: doing good for others. *Brit. Med. J.* **21**, 56.
28. Chalmers, T., Frank, C. S., and Reitman, D. (1990). Minimizing the three stages of publication bias. *JAMA* **263**, 1392.
29. Pelligrino, E. D. (1992). Is truth telling to the patient a cultural artifact? *JAMA* **268**, 1734.
30. Strull, W., Lo, B., and Charles, G. (1984). Do patients want to participate in medical decision making? *JAMA* **252**, 2990.
31. Sherlock, R. (1986). Reasonable men and sick human beings. *Amer. J. Med.* 80: 2–4.
32. Lankton, J., Batchelder, B., and Ominsky, A. (1977). Emotional responses to detailed risk disclosure for anesthesia, a prospective randomized study. *Anesthesiology* **46**, 294.
33. Thomas, K. (1987). General practice consultations: Is there any point in being positive? *Brit. Med. J..* **284**, 1200.
34. Loftus, E. and Fries, J. (1979). Informed consent may be hazardous to your health. *Science* **204**, 9.
35. Simes, R., Tattersall, M., *et al.* (1986). Randomised comparison of procedures for obtaining consent in clinical trials of cancer. *Brit. Med. J.* **293**, 1065.
36. Wyte, W. F. (1961). *Men at work*. Dorsey Press, Homewood, Illinois.
37. Malcontent. (1991). Fumes from the spleen. *Paediatr. Perinatol. Epidemiol.* 5: 4.
38. Grant, A. (1989). Monitoring the fetus during labour. In *Effective care in pregnancy and childbirth* (ed. I. Chalmers, M. Enkin, and M. J. N. C. Keirse), Oxford University Press, 1989. p. 846.
39. Chalmers, I., Enkin, M., and Keirse, M. J. N. C. (1989). *Effective Care in pregnancy and childbirth*. Oxford University Press, New York.
40. Sinclair, J. C. and Bracken, M. B. (1992). *Effective care of the newborn infant*. Oxford University Press, New York.
41. Department of Health and Human Services. *Code of Federal Regulations. 45 CFR 46. Protection of human subjects*. OPRR Reports, 1981.
42. Kopelman, L. (1981). Estimating risk in human research. *Clin. Res.* 29: 1–8.
43. Abramson, N. S., Meisel; A., and Safar, P. (1986). Deferred consent. A new approach for resuscitation research on comatose patients. *JAMA* **255**, 2466.
44. Mutch, L. and Kind, R. (1985) Obtaining parental consent—opting in or opting out? *Arch.D. Child.* 60: 979–80.

8B THE INTERSECTION OF RESEARCH AND PRACTICE

Tom L. Beauchamp

Research involving human subjects is a worthy social undertaking, but it is also morally perilous when subjects are exposed to some level of risk for the advancement of science. Clinical practice is no less praiseworthy, and presumably less perilous because patients are exposed to risk only in their interests, not for the advancement of science. The research scientist and the clinical practitioner both seek to benefit the ill and injured; but scientific activity is primarily directed at unknown future patients, whereas clinical activity is designed for the benefit of known, current patients.

So described, the boundaries of research and practice seem well defined. However, as Dr Tyson points out, we have difficulty in classifying a wide variety of activities into these categories. The research–practice distinction is serviceable but untidy. I will begin my treatment of the distinction with a conceptual analysis, noting any disagreements with Dr Tyson. Then progressively I will move beyond conceptual questions to related moral problems about clinical trials and other forms of research involving patient populations.

KEY CONCEPTS

Consider first the terms *therapy* and *research*. Therapy refers to a set of activities designed solely to benefit an identifiable individual or class of persons. A therapeutic activity is not necessarily a treatment, however, because it may be a diagnostic procedure or even a preventive intervention. Research, by contrast, refers to scientific activity designed to produce general knowledge. These two concepts are not inconsistent or mutually exclusive: research is united with therapy when there is an attempt to discover better methods of treating or preventing illness. This form of investigation is commonly called *clinical research*; but this term is systematically ambiguous, because it refers to attempts to provide therapy both for identifiable current patient–subjects and for unidentifiable future patients. Of course, biomedical research also can be far removed from research into the treatment or prevention of illness or injury. There is no widely acknowledged term to refer to the many forms of *non-clinical biomedical research*, but they can be consolidated for our purposes as research that is not specifically designed to provide a therapeutic benefit.

This framework of distinctions becomes still more untidy when we include additional concepts that have frequently been used in our classification system. *Non-therapeutic (clinical) research,* by definition, offers no demonstrable prospect of medical benefit to current subjects of the research, whereas *therapeutic (clinical) research,* by definition, does offer some prospect of medical benefit to current patient–subjects, at least by evaluating interventions proposed for their treatment. This use of the term 'therapeutic' requires caution, however, because it can lead us to ignore the fact that it is *research,* and therefore is not designed exclusively for the benefit of subjects of the research. As a systematic effort to generate scientific knowledge, therapeutic research should be distinguished from both *routine therapy (standard care)* and *innovative or non-validated therapy,* which are all directed at the treatment of particular patients (even though at times physicians may piggyback an attempt at generalized knowledge during the treatment of patients).

Dr Tyson proposes to understand these terms in a slightly different way than I have suggested. He holds that therapeutic research evaluates interventions that are intended to benefit individual patients, and that non-therapeutic research is all other clinical research. A non-validated therapy is one that has not been shown to be beneficial in a randomized clinical trial (perhaps because a trial was inconclusive). I believe he also means to use 'experimental therapy' as synonymous with both 'non-validated therapy' and 'innovative treatment'. This usage invites an analysis of the terms 'experimental' and 'experimentation', to which I will turn momentarily.

Part of the untidiness in our classification scheme comes from the fact that many complex activities in biomedicine cluster together in ways that cut across several of these categories. Many sequences of events do not fall cleanly into (1) practicing medicine, (2) doing therapeutic research, or (3) doing non-therapeutic research. A complex series of steps involving collection of data can involve clinical practice, therapeutic research, and non-therapeutic research. The problem is not whether the three can occur together in the same sequence of events, but whether our concepts are sufficiently sharp that we can analytically distinguish in this sequence of events between the components that constitute clinical practice and those that constitute one of the two forms of research.

I believe that we can use these distinctions with conceptual clarity to classify our various activities, but I am not convinced that we can do so through what Dr Tyson lands on as the central concept: physician intent.

PHYSICIAN INTENT

Dr Tyson's paper features physician intent because he believes that 'Current thinking generally differentiates clinical practice from research in terms of physician intent.' He does not document this claim, and I believe it cannot be documented. Physician intent, so far as I can see, plays virtually no role in current thinking about how to differentiate clinical practice from research. It is not the intention of the clinician or investigator, but the design of the inquiry and its scientific or non-scientific structure that makes the difference.

Dr Tyson's thesis leads him to argue that whenever there is an intent to gain generalizable knowledge, as occurs in several of his very interesting anecdotes, this circumstance is by definition research (or approximates to research, or at least shows how close practice often comes to research). This, in turn, shows how 'dubious' many of these distinctions are. The matter is important, he thinks, because almost all clinicians in his examples would not consider what they are doing to be research, but only therapy. Following Dr Tyson's analysis, it would be wrong to say that these physicians are unwarrantably confused; rather, he thinks the lack of clear differences in our dubious distinctions causes the confusion.

Although I disagree with Dr Tyson about the role of physician intent, I agree that 'the importance of physician intent *per se* is doubtful, particularly when non-validated therapies are used' and that 'physician intent to benefit the individual patient may be greater, not less, in controlled studies than in uncontrolled clinical use of non-validated therapies'. True on both counts; but these conclusions are irrelevant if physician intent is irrelevant to the distinction between clinical practice and research.

TWO FORMS OF GENERALIZABLE 'KNOWLEDGE'

Dr Tyson argues both that (1) 'obtaining generalizable knowledge—a better understanding of disease and its proper treatment—is a desirable and inextricable component of clinical practice' and that (2) a therapy that has not been shown scientifically to be beneficial is a non-validated therapy. I accept both claims, but I resist some of his arguments that build on these claims. He apparently wants to argue that in clinical practice physicians commonly seek to obtain generalizable knowledge about non-validated therapies, and that this fact makes it very difficult to distinguish research from practice. This argument works, however, only if 'generalizable knowledge' is used equivocally to refer to both knowledge gained by non-scientific inductive techniques (knowledge that cannot validate) and knowledge gained by scientific techniques (knowledge that succeeds in turning a hypothesized therapy into a validated therapy). It would be conceptually tidier and more faithful to the standard uses of these notions to say that in research (by definition) we seek to generalize to scientific conclusions (knowledge), and that in testing an innovative therapy and in other approaches that use non-scientific inductive generalizations we cannot claim to reach scientific conclusions (and so, at best, obtain a more tentative claim to knowledge and do not validate a 'therapy').

Research is not research unless it is driven by a scientific protocol; the science behind the research is what allows us to validate the hypothesis that an intervention is therapeutic. I do not want to limit biomedical science to randomized clinical trials, as Dr Tyson seems to want to do; but I also do not want to allow all inductive techniques used by physicians to test innovative therapies to amount to science. I do not deny that the nature of science is a much disputed subject in the philosophy of science; but I do want to deny that, as Dr Tyson puts it, the intent to reach generalizable knowledge in clinical practice makes it difficult to distinguish practice from research. The key problem, then, is how to distinguish a scientific methodology in biomedicine from an inductive technique that amounts to less than biomedical science.

Some of Dr Tyson's arguments similarly rely on an ambiguity in the words 'experimental' and 'experimentation', although the ambiguity does not originate with him. Dr Tyson seems to hold that whatever is scientifically unproven is therefore experimental and counts as mere experimentation. This might mean one of two very different things: (1) an experiment is a scientific strategy resting on unproven hypotheses that, once proven, advance the hypothesis to position as a scientifically validated conclusion; or it might mean that (2) an experiment is not a scientific undertaking, and so can never on its own generate a scientific conclusion. On the first understanding, an experiment is serious scientific work of testing hypotheses; on the second, it is on the order of the pursuit of guesswork or hunches.

I prefer to say, more simply, that scientific experimentation is scientific research. These terms are synonymous, and that to which they refer is identical. In several classic works in early modern science the term *experimentum crucis* or 'crucial experiment' (more literally, an 'experiment of the *crux*') was used to point to a decisive research situation—i.e., a decisive experimental condition—indicating that one hypothesis is shown to be better supported in a competition with other hypotheses.[1] From that day to this there has never been any sharp boundary to be drawn between research and experimentation in science.

However, because of a connotation of conjecture without adequate controls that is sometimes attached to 'experimentation',[2] we would probably be better off simply to drop the word 'experimental'. The National Commission took exactly this route: it adopted 'research' and abandoned 'experimental' and 'experimentation'. I am suggesting the same strategy, and at the same time proposing that 'research' be confined to 'scientific research' and never given some in-between status so that it applies to both scientific and non-scientific techniques that reach for generalizable knowledge.

THE REGULATION OF RESEARCH AND PRACTICE

One possible conclusion from this line of argument is that Dr Tyson is off the target in raising the question, 'Is it feasible to regulate as research all activities that include an intent to increase generalizable knowledge.' Ideally, what should be regulated *as research* is simply scientific research, not all those other activities that look something like research, are called

THE INTERSECTION OF RESEARCH AND PRACTICE

'research' in journals, or have some physician intent to increase generalizable knowledge. Perhaps these other activities should be regulated, but not because they are research involving human subjects. Research is scientific research, not something else.

Dr Tyson would rightly be dissatisfied with this conclusion, because we would still have to debate both (1) what constitutes real science and how it is to be distinguished from pseudo-science and (2) whether pseudo-science should be regulated in the same way research is regulated. Some of Dr Tyson's interesting examples function to this end by showing how a spectrum of inductive techniques used in clinical activities in his perinatal center raise questions about the nature of science and about unfairness in regulation. He is quite right to point out that the intent to gain knowledge by use of low-grade or low-quality 'science' often triggers IRB review in today's regulatory climate.

I agree with him that these are not trivial problems. But, setting aside the important question of how to define science (as well as how to distinguish good science from inferior science), we should not have to debate what constitutes research. Research is the systematic investigation of hypotheses and theories that is controlled by sound scientific techniques and designed to develop or contribute to generalizable knowledge. Research is not merely the systematic pursuit of hunches or the use of inductive reasoning to reach general conclusions.

At first glance it seems to follow from this argument that we should only regulate *research*—meaning scientific research—through the IRB system, not activities that look in certain respects like research. Perhaps the latter activities should be reviewed or regulated for other reasons, but not because they are instances of research. I am unconvinced, however, that we should move to this conclusion.

The IRB system derives from the public policy process, which includes specific regulations and guidelines promulgated by government agencies. Public policies that protect subjects of biomedical research have never been developed from a careful understanding of the difference between good science and inferior science. They were almost always motivated by moral problems in the protection of human subjects who might be exploited or treated poorly. Scientifically inferior forms of investigation are certainly not likely to produce fewer moral problems. Some of the most important historical examples leading to regulatory activity involved poor science or non-scientific activities. Regulations, then, were never intended to protect human subjects involved in science while ignoring inferior forms of investigation.

I am, then, not convinced that the IRB system should be tailored to review only research (in the sense I have defined it). Although paradoxical and no doubt unsatisfactory to Dr Tyson, the best public policy may be to have the conceptually untidy policy we currently have. This policy leaves the IRB with some discretion about the activities in its institution that closely resemble scientific activity and that involve the use of patients. Surely the most basic question that confronts contemporary biomedical ethics is which investigatory activities should be reviewed, not whether the activities constitute research, practice, or some in-between territory. Any attempt to draw precise limits in public policy for IRBs may do less to protect persons rather than more.

This conclusion is consistent with Dr Tyson's quite convincing thesis that some current supervision of the activities of clinicians is improper. Nevertheless, we will want to avoid setting up a body of rules in which it is easy to skirt the system by declaring that what one does is not scientific, and therefore not research, and therefore not reviewable. A major problem in the past has been not submitting a protocol to the IRB simply to avoid review. As Dr Tyson rightly puts it, we would want a policy that helped us avoid situations in which harm was caused to patients because controlled studies were made unattractive and haphazard clinical strategies made correspondingly more attractive.

We may also want to regulate activities such as clinical practice and behavioral therapy for reasons having nothing to do with attempts to reach generalizable knowledge. This objective would lead to requirements that are not applied through the IRB system. For example, we might require that informed consent be obtained for all interventions that carry a certain level of risk. This requirement would presumably apply equally to clinical and research settings.

FUNDAMENTAL ETHICAL DISTINCTIONS

Dr Tyson argues that 'the difference between therapeutic and non-therapeutic research is *not* a fundamental ethical distinction', because the core ethical problem about protecting human subjects is the relationship of risks to benefits. His point is sound, but needs qualification. First, the therapeutic–non-therapeutic distinction is not an ethical distinction at all, let alone a fundamental one. Correct labelling of a set of research events as 'therapeutic' or as 'non-therapeutic' does not determine whether one form of action is better or worse, or more or less justified, than the other. Some particular instance of therapeutic research may be worse than some particular instance of non-therapeutic research; but the converse is also true. Rightness and wrongness depend on principled justification of the action, not on the *type* of action it is.

None the less, we may need to be more cautious about the conduct of non-therapeutic research—for example, by requiring more careful and thorough review of non-therapeutic activities. It is appropriate for public policy and review committees to look more carefully at contexts in which research is aimed at benefits for future patients and in which risks are not balanced by compensating benefits for current patients. If the distinction between the therapeutic and the non-therapeutic were to indicate an appropriate place to raise or lower moral requirements, then it would play a legitimate moral role.

Second, the conclusion that regulations governing biomedical investigations should properly focus on risks and benefits to subjects, not on the type of research under review, does not entail that risk–benefit ratios should be the exclusive focus. Ethically justified investigations must satisfy several conditions, including the pursuit of important knowledge, a reasonable prospect that the research will generate the knowledge that is sought, fair selection of subjects, and the necessity of using human subjects— as well as a favorable balance of benefits over risks.[2] Only after each of these conditions has been met, as certified by investigators and by an institutional review board, is it appropriate to request persons to participate in the investigation.

RANDOMIZED CLINICAL TRIALS

In pursuit of his views about the importance of risk, Dr Tyson argues that 'randomization is a procedure that does not in itself increase risk'. He believes that as long as true clinical uncertainty prevails, randomized assignment in clinical trials is justified. Although he does not examine a number of problems about randomized clinical trials, there is a strong argument to be made on behalf of his conclusions. I want to examine the attractiveness of his position before turning to some subtleties in this controversy that should lead to second thoughts about or at least qualifications of his conclusions.

Controlled trials protect against unwarranted enthusiasm for and guesswork about therapies, replacing them with scientifically warranted conclusions. To assign group members *randomly* helps eliminate bias in assignments as well as distortions of study results that would weaken or discredit the conclusions of the research. Defenders of these trials, such as Dr Tyson, argue, quite reasonably, that the trials are to be used only if genuine uncertainty prevails about the worthiness of standard or untested therapies. This 'null hypothesis' leaves reasonable and attentive clinicians in a circumstance of 'clinical equipoise'.[3] That is, available evidence indicates that the relevant expert medical community is undecided about the relative merits of and finds equally acceptable any one of the treatment strategies to be tested in the randomized clinical trial. No patient, under this conception, receives a treatment believed to be less safe or more effective than an alternative, and therefore no person is asked to make a sacrifice. Ineded, patients may actually benefit from sound results achieved through the research. These trials therefore do not seem unjustifiable for current patients, and are strongly supported by their promise for future patients.[4]

None the less, we should ask whether this pure ideal of a clinical trial squares with the reality of the impure circumstances under which clinical trials are conducted. Before the beginning of a randomized clinical trial, many physicians believe that certain forms of evidence about a treatment's safety, side-effects, invasiveness, etc. make the treatment more or less preferable, by comparison to another treatment being tested. The trial demands that such beliefs be waived as unproven and undeserving of recognition; yet it is not entirely satisfactory to maintain that trials confirm or correct physician's preliminary but unproven beliefs. This response avoids moral problems about the physician's obligations to inform the patient by disclosing all relevant information. Surely every physician has an obligation to discuss honestly his or her beliefs about risks, benefits, and appropriate strategies or recommended treatments. This is the bare minimum that a patient expects from his or her physician. To conceal beliefs relevant to the patient's decision about participation is nothing less than deception. It is only a rationalization to argue that the available evidence indicates before the research that treatments are not distinguishable in safety and efficacy. Once apprised of the known facts and physician beliefs, patients themselves often turn out to have definite preferences for one treatment for personal reasons having nothing to do with a scientific outcome. These reasons cannot be anticipated by their physicians.

It is also sometimes difficult in a randomized clinical trial to ascertain whether the research should be terminated when some but not all physician-researchers indicate their satisfaction with the preliminary evidence and apparent trends. One procedural way to resolve this situation is to distinguish roles: individual physicians make disclosures and help their patients reach a conclusion about participation, whereas a data-monitoring committee decides to end a trial when it has determined that equipoise has shifted and equal uncertainty is no longer present. This strategy, however, only relocates the problems. Now the committee must determine whether to ask patients to assume risks and whether clinical equipoise has been eliminated. This committee will ask whether equipoise has been disturbed in the relevant expert medical community; but individual physicians and their patients will often be primarily interested in whether uncertainty has been eliminated for them, not whether the expert community has modified its views.

Finally, consent forms typically inform subjects that they may withdraw from the research at any time, without affecting their care. However, these patients would probably withdraw only if a disclosure of interim data and trends led them to favor one treatment over another. From the scientist's perspective, these trends are misleading, and often turn out to be mere temporary anomalies. They are therefore not reliable bases for a decision about whether to continue participation. Their unreliability has led to the now common rule that no information about trends is to be released before the final stage or early termination of the randomized clinical trial. This rule has been instituted in part because it is well known that trends provide evidence that is decisive for some patients and physicians, and that their decisions to withdraw could ruin the trial.

In the face of these problems, clinical trials are morally justified only if they satisfy several conditions beyond those mentioned by Dr Tyson. The first is that true clinical equipoise—not merely scientific controversy—must prevail in the community of relevant medical experts. The second is that informed consent must be obtained from subjects, where the information includes an explanation of the situation of equipoise, facts about procedures such as randomization, facts about the monitoring and disclosure of trends, etc. In addition, a data-monitoring committee should determine when clinical equipoise has been displaced, and this committee must immediately report this situation to the relevant physicians and patients. I believe that additional conditions must also be satisfied for justified research, but these are the central conditions.

Equipoise is absolutely essential for justified clinical trials. Without it, the favored treatment must be provided. A trend that eliminates equipoise also eliminates the justification for using the patients involved. Such equipoise is no less necessary for all justified clinical research, not merely in the conduct of randomized clinical trials. But is consent of the magnitude I have proposed also an absolutely essential condition of justified research?

INFORMED CONSENT TO TRIALS

A standard premiss about informed consent to research is that the physician must disclose all major alternatives in order that potential subjects be enabled to make an informed decision about participation. Any method used to determine the selection of a particular treatment falls under this rule of disclosure. Some contend that mention of the fact of randomizaton would cause unnecessary distress, and in some cases would cause patients to refuse to participate, and they argue that randomized trials are exempt from normal disclosure requirements because no treatment is preferred and all treatments are equally safe or risky.

I believe, however, that randomized clinical trials provide no basis for exemption to the standard rules of informed consent. Either a physician-researcher playing a dual role or the patient's primary physician has a fiduciary obligation to disclose all items that are materially relevant to a decision about participation. Failure to disclose the method of randomization and the rationale for its use is simply a failure to obtain informed consent. However, if this information is provided, potential subjects should then have an adequate informational base. Adequate disclosure need not be full disclosure, and subjects can be informed that they cannot be told that the purpose of the investigation without damaging the research. Placebos present one variant of this problem, because if subjects are informed that they are receiving a placebo, the strategy in using the placebo is undercut. But the solution is again to disclose that the research uses a placebo whose identity and pattern of distribution must remain undisclosed.

Clinical trials are of massive importance in medicine; but these trials should not be held out as a necessary condition of all acceptable scientific research. Historical controls are sometimes sufficient, and some trials can be conducted without resort to randomization. A partial randomized trial can

occasionally be introduced by using a small group of subjects who consent
to the randomization, while at the same time following the progress of all
patients who refused randomization but who continue to receive one of
the treatments under investigation.[5] Innovation in research design is as
important as innovation in the scientific hypotheses to be tested, for both
moral and scientific reasons.

DUAL ROLES AND CONFLICT OF INTEREST

The roles of research scientist and clinical practitioner present additional
moral problems when a single person assumes both roles. For example,
the dual roles of research scientist and clinical practitioner can produce
an untenable conflict of interest. As an *investigator*, one acts to generate
scientific knowledge, and owes an obligation of fidelity to one's research.
The investigator's reputation, personal well-being, and personal integrity
depend on reliable and methodologially sound research that results in
scientific acceptance of an interesting set of results. As a *clinician*, however,
obligations of care and fidelity require acting in the best interests of current
patients.

Some who have investigated problems of dual roles argue that research
commitments are inconsistent with clinical commitments to serve the
patient's best interests.[6] This problem about dual roles approximates to
the one just examined about randomized clinical trials, and is not the problem
that now concerns me. Rather, the problem is that clinical judgment can be
biased by an investigator's interest in data generated by his or her study;
and, similarly, accurate reporting of study results and implications may be
biased by seeing the subjects as patients. A dual role generates an interest in
interpreting the study to conform to clinical recommendations and an interest
in making clinical recommendations conform to the study. A risk is created of
loss of scientific objectivity through overinterpretation of data, and a related
risk is created for patients of unnecessary or biased treatment in order to
make treatment recommendations conform to the study. Both risks would
be eliminated if the two roles were kept separate.

The boundaries between clinician and investigator become blurred when a
dual role is accepted. Of particular concern is a failure to keep an appropriate
distance from the study in treating patients and an appropriate distance
from patients in interpreting research data. If this dual role is assumed,
clinician–investigators at a minimum have a fiduciary obligation to inform
patient–subjects of every condition directly relevant to their decisions,
including conditions that involve the clinician–investigator in a conflict of
interest.[7]

There should also be disclosure to an appropriate review committee
regarding the financial connections and additional personal or consulting
connections between investigators and a funding source.[8] Neither form of
disclosure has been provided in the cases I have personally seen.

Yet the goals of and relationships involved in such research may be of major personal interest for investigator–physicians. To take a standard example, many trials are financially supported by the pharmaceutical industry. Federal and foundation sources have limited funds for such trials, and often believe that other, less expensive projects will provide a better return on their available monies. The pharmaceutical industry, by contrast, is willing to assume the financial risk because the returns from a successful trial can be extremely high. Many advantages result from these funding arrangements. More research is sponsored, salaries are easier to cover, and money is freed up for other resources. Many institutions are able to provide better facilities, improved salaries, stronger faculty, superior research, desirable technological improvements, growth of physical plants, enhanced reputations, advanced economic development, and the like.[9]

But there are also risks and moral concerns attached to these arrangements. First, in clinical centers located in universities or staffed by university faculty, many physicians involved in research increasingly have significant time to see patients only as their subjects, not as independent patients. Second, tensions of an explosive sort sometimes arise between clinical investigators involved in commercial research and staff members who oppose commercial funding in the institution because they view it as disruptive to the teaching of staff and the care of patients. Third, researchers often appear to have been captured or 'bought' when they settle into a relationship of an easy and consistent flow of funding. Not infrequently a subtle desire is created to cultivate the relationship, with the goal of arranging an even better contract or grant next time by producing research results that are favorable from a funding source's perspective. The possibility of a commercial venture's emerging from the research can skew its conduct and predetermine acceptable outcomes. In a worst-case scenario, the temptation arises to produce fraudulent research in order that the conclusions contain data favorable to commercial interests.

In some cases these problems of conflict are complicated by other personal interests of the physician–investigator. Medical centers, both inside and outside the university, increasingly are staffed with physicians who have a financial interest in the drugs, medical devices, and technologies they prescribe or recommend to patients.[10] For example, these physicians may own the clinics to which they send patients or have stock or stock options in companies that manufacture the products they recommend. In some cases investigators have advance knowledge of a medical device on which they are personally engaged in research, and they purchase stock in the belief its price will rise. This activity is simply a sophisticated form of insider trading if the knowledge is both accurate and non-public.

These financial interests stand to compromise both the quality of the research and the objectivity of recommendations to patients. Having clinician–investigators with an economic interest in products they are investigating for safety and efficacy is more than our system should allow. Yet this arrangement is a largely unchecked and growing phenomenon.

A CASE OF CONFLICT

Sometimes conflicts of interest slip by unnoticed by the various affected parties, and dual roles are assumed without anyone's recognizing that a moral problem exists. On other occasions, the various parties are all aware that a problem of conflict of interest exists. In a case I saw in 1992 and early 1993, meetings were held between several investigators, representatives of the group funding the research, and a union official representing the patients (who were workers possibly affected by a contaminated workplace). It was agreed by all parties that a conflict of interest would be present if the investigators studying the patients were to undertake (follow-up, in this case) evaluation of the subjects or to become involved in an ongoing clinical relationship. However, one week later, the principal investigator called a member of the executive committee of the funding source to notify it that he had reconsidered the matter and had decided to perform the evaluations himself. He expressed his view that there was no *disqualifying* conflict of interest and that he was ethically obligated to see the patients because he knew more about their condition than anyone else.

The principal investigator then offered the following justification for his actions: The advantages of the investigators performing a clinical evaluation and subsequent care [comparability of test results, scientific expertise, familiarity with the patients, and familiarity with their environment] outweigh the disadvantages [potential conflict of interest and perception of the patients that inconsistent messages were being given to them by physicians and by the funding source]; after the evaluation, patients would of course be allowed an entirely free choice whether to continue the relationship or to select another person with whom they would establish an ongoing clinical relationship.

It appears that the investigators believed they could overcome or justify the presence of the conflict of interest on grounds that their superior expertise and information about the study and about the patients warranted undertaking the dual role. Obviously they were *aware* of problems of conflict of interest. However, they did represent the conflict as a *potential* conflict of interest, rather than the *actual* conflict of interest it was—a misrepresentation, in my judgment. They also never disclosed the conflict of interest to the patients (although their union representative was aware of it).[11]

Even if one were to reach the conclusion that, on balance, these investigators had a sustainable argument and therefore an acceptable conflict of interest, moral problems surrounding the dual roles still would not vanish. There is always a threat that a properly conservative and hedged statement of the results of the research (the investigator's main duty and position of trust) will be sacrificed to benefit investigators or their institutions. For example, if an interpretation of the data would generate more patients and thereby more revenues, an incentive to overstate or bias the results of the study is present. I believe the data were in fact overinterpreted in the study in this case, and I suspect that the opportunity for establishing a connection with patients functioned as an undue influence biasing the statement of study results. Even if I am entirely wrong, a suspicion will rightly hang over any research reported under such conditions. By not keeping the dual roles of investigator and clinician appropriately separate, this unnecessary threat is maximized rather than minimized. The problem can be altogether avoided by using another site as the clinical center. For all these reasons, I believe that a rule should be instituted in research/clinical centers that no patients from a study population will be accepted by members of the research team or their associates.

CONCLUSION

To return to earlier threads of argument, some have maintained that an investigator–physician's ordinary moral commitment to a patient provides strong and adequate protection against abuse, negligence, and conflict of interest. I would argue, however, that we should differentiate roles so that physicians cannot be placed in the position of using their own patients in research. The point is not that a person cannot be both an investigator and a clinician, but that a person should not assume both roles for the same patient–subject.[12] The two roles pull in different directions. The boundaries between research and practice are often difficult to draw; but here at least we can and should draw them with a finer precision than we have in the past.

NOTES AND REFERENCES

1. The concept of a crucial experiment seems to have its origins in Francis Bacon's *Novum organum*, where he referred not to an *experimentum crucis*, but to an *instantia crucis*, or a 'crucial instance', which he used with the meaning of a sign-post or finger-post at a crossroads pointing to the correct route. The *instantiae crucis* for Bacon indicated the proper way toward a solution. [See *Novum organum*, in *The works of Francis Bacon*, 14 vols, ed. James Spedding, Robert Leslie Ellis, and Douglas Denon Heath Friedrich Frommann Verlag, (Stuttgart–Bad Cannstatt, 1961–3), I, p. 294, IV, p. 180 (Bk. II, Ch. 36).] Bacon's successors, beginning with Robert Hooke, used the term *experimentum crucis* in a somewhat altered sense. Hooke [*Micrographia* (London, 1665), p. 54] and Isaac Newton adopted the term during a controversy to determine why the colored spectrum produced by the passage of light through a prism was of oblong rather than circular shape [*Papers & letters on natural philosophy*, ed. I. Bernard Cohen Harvard University Press, (Cambridge, Mass., 1958), pp. 50, 88, 101–9]. This experiment became a historic moment in optics and a model for scientists of a decisive, well-constructed piece of research in the most advanced science of the period. (The best-known discussion of Newton's prism experiment occurs in the *Opticks*; but in this work Newton did not use the term *experimentum crucis*.')
2. The Nuremberg Code and the *Belmont report* of the National Commission for

244   TOM L. BEAUCHAMP

the Protection of Human Subjects provide important foundational analyses. See also Alexander M. Capron, 'Human experimentation' in *Medical ethics*, ed. Robert M. Veatch Jones and Bartlett Publishers, (Boston, 1989), Chapter 6; and Veatch, *The patient as partner: a theory of human experimentation ethics* Indiana University Press, (Bloomington, 1987).

3. See Robert J. Levine, *Ethics and regulation of clinical research*, 2nd edn Yale University Press, (New Haven, 1988), pp. 187–9; Benjamin Freedman, 'Equipoise and the ethics of clinical research', *New England Journal of Medicine*, **317** (16 July 1987): 141–5; and Eugene Passamani, 'Clinical Trials—are they ethical?', *New England Journal of Medicine*, **324** (30 May 1991): 1590–1.

4. Several of these issues are explored in essays in the *Journal of Medicine and Philosophy*, **11** (November 1986), devoted to 'Ethical issues in the use of clinical controls'. An oft-cited criticism of clinical trials is found in Charles Fried, *Medical experimentation: personal integrity and social policy* Elsevier, (New York, 1974).

5. Such a 'semi-randomized clinical trial' is proposed in Veatch, *The patient as partner*, Chapter 9.

6. See, for example, Benjamin Freedman, 'Equipoise and the ethics of clinical research', *New England Journal of Medicine*, **317** (16 July 1987): 141–5; Passamani, 'Clinical trials': 1590–1.

7. See American Medical Association, Council on Scientific Affairs and Council on Ethical and Judicial Affairs, 'Conflicts of interest in medical center/industry research relationships', *Journal of the American Medical Association*, **23** (23/30 May 1990): 2790–3.

8. Cf. Stuart E. Lind. 'Fee for service research', *New England Journal of Medicine*, **314** (30 Jan. 1986): 312–15.

9. See David Blumenthal, *et al.* 'University–industry research relationships in biotechnology: implications for the university', *Science*, **232** (13 June 1986): 1361–6.

10. See Constance Holden, 'Research group forswears financial ties to firms whose drugs it tests', *Science*, **244** (21 April 1989): 282; Arnold S. Relman, 'Economic incentives in clinical investigation' [Editorial], *New England Journal of Medicine*, **320** (6 April 1989): 933–4.

11. Some influences clearly distort judgment, others have some reasonable probability of doing so, and others have some distant possibility of doing so. Only in the case of a distant possibility should one speak of *potentially* having a conflict of interest. There is also a difference between having or potentially having a conflict of interest and a *perceived* conflict of interest. In the latter, there is not a conflict of interest but only the appearance of one.

12. See Fried, *Medical experimentation*, pp. 160–1.

9

Informed consent

9A INFORMED CONSENT IN CUSTOMARY PRACTICE AND IN CLINICAL TRIALS

William A. Silverman

> Wisdom is supple: folly keeps to a groove.
> —Theognis of Megara (6th Century BC)

A survey of interventions and outcomes from November 1987 through October 1988 in seven American neonatal centers[1] disclosed wide variation in practices for the care of very-low-birthweight infants. There were, as well, appreciable differences in survival and in morbidity. 'It appears', the survey group concluded, 'that the practice of neonatal medicine remains in part an art rather than an exact science.' Under these conditions of uncertainty about 'best' medical management, a paradoxical duality has flourished. There are opposing attitudes about the need to obtain parental consent for a specific 'customary' treatment, in contrast to the need for consent to use the same treatment when it is 'under study'.

A DOUBLE STANDARD

I can illustrate the inconsistencies in ethical judgment by describing a pair of imaginary, but entirely plausible scenarios played out in each of two modern neonatal intensive care units (NICUs). In the first of these, a well-designed randomized clinical trial is conducted to compare standard antibiotic treatment for septicemia in infants with neutropenia versus a regimen of the standard treatment plus granulocyte transfusions. The physicians in this unit are genuinely uncertain about the relative merits and risks of the two treatment plans[2] (balanced doubt of this kind has been dubbed 'equipoise'[3]. The parents of an eligible infant are fully informed about the trial, and, for example, they refuse to give consent to enroll their critically sick baby. The decision is accepted by the doctors without question because of a specified set of rules governing clinical research: the autonomy of parents must be respected when they decline an invitation to enroll their child in a parallel-comparison treatment trial.

In the other hypothetical NICU, the doctors profess no doubts about proper treatment: granulocyte transfusion is always added to the standard antibiotic treatment of neutrophil-depleted neonates with septicemia. When the parents of an eligible infant in this hospital refuse to consent, citing religious conviction, for example, a court order is obtained to enforce use of what is now labeled 'customary treatment'. Here the judge relies on respect for the principle of beneficence; considerations affecting the child's threatened life now override those of parental autonomy.

EVOLUTION OF INFORMED CONSENT

How have we come to use the moral principles of respect for autonomy and that of concern for beneficence so selectively and with such powerful practical effect? How have we come to make moral judgments that seem so paradoxical? The clues to the duality are to be found in the historical development of informed consent in the setting of clinical research. 'Study consent', as I will call it, evolved quite independently; it was not a direct outgrowth of older ideas about the need to obtain consent in everyday treatment.[4] The latter—I will label it 'customary consent'—evolved slowly in case law (for example in judicial opinions set forth in specific lawsuits, and, later, in defined statutes). It needs to be understood that the format for 'study consent' appeared fairly recently, and it arrived suddenly, by fiat. Modifications have been shaped by federal regulations and by professional codes. In 'study consent' the courts have played a minor role.

'Customary consent'. Truth-telling and consent-seeking for specific interventions (particularly surgical procedures) have long been a part of medical tradition.[5] Moreover, a patient's right of prior consent has long been protected in many countries under laws of assault and battery. However, the doctrine, until relatively recently, was narrowly defined. Doctors were obliged only to disclose the *nature* of a proposed procedure; the patient reserved the right of refusal. In 1767, for example, a British judge noted[6] 'it is reasonable that a patient should be told what is about to be done to him, that he may take courage and put himself in such a situation as to enable him to undergo the operation'. Following the disclosure, a patient 'voted with his/her feet': voluntary submission was taken as proof of consent.

Until about thirty years ago, the extent of disclosure and consent-seeking in Western countries was very much influenced by concern for a patient's physical health. It was generally believed that a physician's primary obligation (greater than respect for patient autonomy), is to provide medical benefits. For example, in 1803, Thomas Percival declared[7] that the first role of the physician is to be 'the minister of hope and comfort'. And he asked 'How far is it justifiable to violate truth for the supposed benefit of the patient?' He concluded that 'the balance of truthfulness yields to beneficence in critical situations.' The physician does not actually 'lie', in actions of deception and falsehood, Percival argued, as long as the objective is to give hope to the dejected or sick patient. Since there was no appreciable dissent from this view, the beneficence model, roughly as outlined by Percival, served, widely and apparently well, as a guide to doctors when they interpreted their responsibility to patients.[8]

'Informed' consent is a recent American invention. The specific term was coined in 1957 and, surprisingly, only in the context of customary medical practice, not clinical research. The term surfaced in a landmark decision at the end of a lawsuit initiated by Martin Salgo, a patient who was permanently paralyzed following translumbar aortography.[9] The physicians at Stanford University, he asserted, were negligent in carrying out the procedure, and they failed to inform him of the risk of paralysis. The court concluded that Mr Salgo's physicians had a duty to disclose 'any facts which are necessary to form the basis of an intelligent consent by the patient to the proposed treatment'. An appellate opinion went on to suggest that this new duty to disclose risks and alternatives of treatment was a logical extension of the already established obligation to reveal a treatment's nature and its consequences. It had been understood, in the traditional relationship, that patients or their surrogates were free to refuse a proffered treatment.

Legal scholars have pointed out[8] that the *Salgo* decision introduced distinctly new elements into relations of trust between doctors and their patients. Unlike previous opinions about consent to medical treatment, the State Court of Appeals' decision focused on the problem of whether or not the consent had been informed when given. The court thus created an 'informed consent' standard; the nature, consequences, harms, benefits, and alternatives of a treatment were now thought to be information needed by patients to know what they were choosing. (Interestingly, the wording of the very sentence in which the term emerged, left room for a broad interpretation: '[I]n discussing the element of risk a *certain amount of discretion* must be employed consistent with full disclosure of the facts necessary to an informed consent' [italics added].[10]

The standard defined in 1957, represented a break with long-standing custom. But the *Salgo* court's words had relatively little practical effect on the time-honored 'silent world'[11] of everyday doctor–patient communication. 'Customary consent' was, and remains to this day, subject to review only retrospectively, if at all. As a result, the everyday consequences have been surprisingly small.

'*Study consent*'. For nine years after *Salgo*, informed consent was not spelled out as a requirement in general guidelines for clinical research in the US. In February 1966 an important memorandum entitled 'Clinical investigations using human subjects' was circulated by the Surgeon-General.[12] For the first time, extra-mural clinical studies (those using federal funds in studies conducted outside the National Institutes of Health [NIH]), were required to carry out prior review. The inspection was to include 'the appropriateness of methods used to secure informed consent'. The new ruling made it clear that what I refer to here as 'study consent' was to be considered separately from 'customary consent', and the major difference turned on the issue of candor about the state of current evidence.

When obtaining 'study consent', a doctor was now required to disclose the justification for the clinical trial by pointing out that there was insufficient existing information for the doctor and patient to make a rational, informed choice in opting for one of the two or more treatments under investigation. In 'customary consent', doctors have always been inclined (even after *Salgo*) to minimize uncertainties about what they believe to be the 'best' treatment extant. Traditionally, they have felt duty-bound to provide the patient with an unequivocal recommendation for action.

The paradoxical duality I referred to above is rooted in the new ground rules spelled out in the Surgeon-General's 1966 memorandum. The important distinction between consent in research settings and in customary clinical situations was now this:[5] in clinical practice doctors were now *exhorted* to solicit consent by an appeal to medical ethics or to legal self-interest; in research, investigators were now *compelled* by regulation to obtain informed consent.

The practical consequences were immediate and dramatic; 'study consent' became a highly visible step in the planning and, most particularly, in the design of controlled clinical trials. Unlike customary medical experience, 'study consent' was reviewed *prospectively*, and it quickly moved to the center stage of concerns in the conduct of studies.

Conduct of pre-1966 neonatal trials. I can testify first-hand to the state of understanding about 'study consent' in American trials involving neonates before 1966. In the 1950s, before *Salgo*, and in the years up to the Surgeon-General's memorandum, we conducted an ongoing series of randomized clinical trials at The Babies Hospital of Columbia University. They were designed to test the efficiency of a number of previously unevaluated treatments then in common use for the management of low-birthweight neonates. Those planned exercises were carried out before the double standard of consent was introduced by the Surgeon-General. In that paternalistic time, responsibility for prior review and permission to carry out the trials rested with one authority: the chairman of the clinical department—not with a not-yet-conceived-of institutional review board, and not with an NIH study section in Bethesda. Individual decisions to enroll babies in trials at The Babies Hospital and other American hospitals were made by doctors providing everyday care, not by the parents.

In 1953, for example, there were fierce arguments in a meeting convened at the NIH about the propriety of a proposal to conduct the first-ever multi-center randomized clinical trial involving neonates: a comparison of two opposing oxygen-treatment policies for infants with birthweights under 1500 grams. The controversy centered on our (pediatricians', ophthalmologists', and epidemiologists') interpretation of the evidence concerning risks and benefits of the long-standing practice of routine administration of high concentrations of oxygen. The loudest and longest arguments focused on the relative analytic power of observation as compared with that of experiment. The only consent under consideration referred to the willingness of the researchers to collaborate in a rigorous test of a newly-proposed policy of oxygen restriction. The debate never mentioned parental consent. This was four years before *Salgo* and thirteen years before the Surgeon-General's memorandum.

It was taken for granted that a decision of whether or not to enroll a premature infant in a randomized trial of oxygen policy was a clear-cut treatment decision. No one questioned the unspoken view that doctors were granted broad power to take whatever action was necessary to safeguard their patients. Faced with large uncertainties about oxygen-treatment policy, we were convinced that the enrollment decision was the only ethically sound way to balance the equally feared and opposing risks of blindness versus those of death or brain damage in small neonates. The decidedly paternalistic attitude of the time held that it would be cruel to place the heavy decision-making burden on the shoulders of frightened parents, if we were to provide them with the confusing and conflicting evidence then available. Parents were spared the full extent of our anxieties, we believed, when they were told, 'We are doing our best to find a way to minimize the risks faced by your child.'

RESPECT FOR PARENTAL AUTONOMY

The arrival of 'study consent', thirteen years after the national oxygen trial, struck down doctors' arguments based on a beneficence model to justify their broad limits of authority in clinical research. The underlying, indeed the controlling idea of the new dictum for complete disclosure in the formal studies involving babies was, as I have said, one of respect for parental autonomy. How then, can we judge the practical consequences of the 'study consent' policy that has now been in effect for more than twenty-five years?

RESPONSE TO PUBLIC CONCERN

Before looking for answers, we can see, in hindsight, that the 1966 decision of the Surgeon-General was political. It was made in response to a public uproar after news reports revealed that in a study of immune responses to cancer, highly-respected researchers injected live malignant cells into a number of elderly patients without obtaining their permission.[13] Public concern was reinforced by Beecher's widely-read paper, published in 1966.[14] He charged that investigators were endangering the health and lives of their subjects (often prisoners, soldiers, and the mentally retarded) without informing them of the risks or obtaining their permission. Twenty-two examples of abuses were cited; they occurred, Beecher alleged, in the years 1950–60.

Rothman has recently looked back at attitudes and practices established during the Second World War,[15] and he argued that the wartime experience helps to explain clinical researchers' behavior in the post-war era reviewed by Beecher. Drafted soldiers were compelled to risk their lives on the battlefield, and, by extension, researchers on the home front were also seen to be engaged in activities of great military importance. According to the prevailing attitude, the clinical investigators did not need to seek the permission of their subjects any more than draft boards or field officers did of draftees. The use of mentally incompetent inmates and prisoners as research subjects during the war, for example, accorded with public opinion about sacrifices necessary on the home front. 'All citizens should be doing their part, even at great personal cost,' was the attitude noted by Rothman, 'a sentiment that helped legitimize experiments on the mentally ill and the retarded.' The Second World War outlook carried over into the continuing war against disease; it helped explain, Rothman posited, the cavalier behavior of the clinical investigators accused by Beecher.

HEDGING STRATEGY LIMITS RISK

Beecher's assessment of the extent of maltreatment in clinical studies has been debated for years. It is worth noting that the post-1966 requirement of formal 'study consent' was not put in place because of any questions about unwarranted hazards to patients, potential or real, uncovered in therapeutic trials using randomized control design. Indeed, before the Surgeon-General's 1966 memorandum, there were encouraging signs that the hedging strategy of random allocation provided important safeguards: hoped-for benefits and unanticipated risks were distributed equitably. Additionally, the concomitant-control design had the potential for reducing the numbers injured in therapeutic disasters.

The lesson of the oxygen-exposure experience was well known after 1954, and this was followed by experience with Gantrisin treatment in 1956,[16] and with Chloromycetin in 1959.[17] Half the babies enrolled in these controlled clinical trials were spared exposure to the completely unexpected lethal effects of these antibiotics used to treat small neonates. And the lessons about risk-limitation were timely: by 1966, it was evident that similar unexpected disasters were occurring with alarming frequency as the intensity of neonatal treatment increased.[18]

IMPACT OF 'STUDY CONSENT'

From a present-day perspective, it is obvious that despite the absence of objective information about social impact, the dogma of informed consent in neonatal clinical trials is deeply entrenched. The stipulation that consent for enrollment must be in writing has presented very little difficulty. However, there is a strong suspicion that it is virtually impossible to comply fully with the intent of the rule. In neonatal medicine, what should or can be done to ensure that parents understand what they have been told in a disclosure ritual? Has 'study consent' succeeded in providing increased protection for babies? Has the new format resulted, in fact, in increased respect for parents' autonomy over the past quarter of a century?

A wide range of opinion about these issues has been voiced in a flood of letters-to-the-editor, news reports, editorials, articles, and books. At a consensus conference several years ago on the general topic of controlled clinical trials[19] more than four-fifths (79/92) of the respondents indicated that obtaining informed consent is problematic because patients or their surrogates do not fully understand the implications of a formal clinical trial. One neonatologist said, bluntly, 'I think informed consent is a farce . . .The information [given to parents] is what I want it to be.' Some of this skepticism is supported by the findings in surveys of public opinion;[20] but the evidence is weak and unique to the circumstances of a given study.

The quality of information provided in a multicenter controlled trial involving adult patients in Sweden was investigated by questioning the participants eighteen months after the end of trial.[21] Most of the enrollees had been informed, the researchers found, but in many instances the information provided did not follow guidelines of the Declaration of Helsinki.[22] Systematic differences in patients' perceptions among the participating centers suggested that certain hospitals were better at informing their patients than others. The between-clinic variations imply, the investigators concluded, that 'deficiencies in perception were caused by informers rather than by participants'.

Modified consent procedure. A randomized trial of a modification of the standard consent procedure (total disclosure vs. an individualized approach based on patients' wishes) involving adult cancer patients has been carried out in Australia.[23] At the completion of the study there were many unanswered questions, but the authors indicated that the issues could not be explored further—Australian rules requiring total disclosure and written consent no longer can be modified. The situation is much the same in the US, and it is complicated by American litigious propensities. Alternative approaches have been proposed (for example, inform only patients [or surrogates] allotted to the experimental arm of a trial;[24] ask only that patients [or surrogates] indicate 'no objection' to enrollment—Fig. 9.1; a process model of informed consent based on the assumption that decision-making is not a singular event that occurs at one point in time, it is an on-going process[4]). However, review boards have been reluctant to allow any departures from inflexible regulations.

Waivers for consent to enroll patients in comparative trials carried out under emergency conditions (for example, treatment used for seriously ill neonates immediately after delivery) have been granted only reluctantly. 'Deferred consent' has been proposed for these situations.[25] For example, in one trial involving emergency treatment of adults after cardiac arrest,[26] the comatose patients were entered into a comparative trial immediately and consent was thereafter requested 'as soon as it [could] be obtained'. But this permissive interpretation of the rule has not been without its critics, who have noted that 'deferred consent is [by definition] not informed consent'.[27,28]

Methodological issues. More than ten years ago, a lawyer and a psychiatrist reviewed empirical studies of the informed consent procedure to determine the factual basis for many criticisms of the requirement.[29] The studies were evaluated with respect to a specified model of the legal doctrine of informed consent:

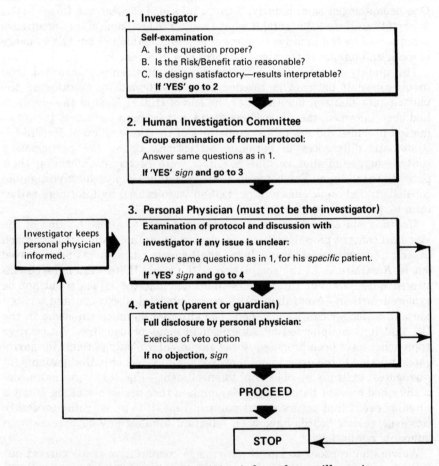

Fig. 9.1 Four formal steps in maintaining informed surveillance in investigations involving human beings. (Reprinted with the permission of W.B. Saunders Co.—copyright assignees of Grune & Stratton, Inc.)

[W]hen *information* is disclosed by a physician to a *competent* person, that person will *understand* the information and *voluntarily* make a *decision* to accept or refuse the recommended medical procedure. [*sic*]

Very few rigorous studies of the consent process have been undertaken, the researchers found; 'there is very little wheat and much chaff'. Given the variety and extent of the deficiencies in published studies, they concluded, 'it would be unwise in the extreme to make law and policy on the basis of the available "facts" '.

A sham 'trial' of two fictitious drugs has been carried out[30] to shed some light on factors that influence patients' decisions to consent to or to refuse to enroll in the comparative test. (In fact, all patients were to receive standard treatment for the relatively minor conditions that brought them to an ambulatory care clinic.) The randomized 'trial' was designed to evaluate the impact of simple quantitative information (the expected speed of action of the two 'drugs') on consent decisions. The results supported the prediction that most, but not all, patients would use quantitative estimates of efficacy provided during the consent process to make a decision to enroll in the fictitious trial. Estimates of the expected effect-size of an innovation are used to determine the dimensions of a trial, the experimenters noted. 'Why not', therefore, 'make this quantitative information available to candidate patients as an important part of the informed consent process?'

Several questions have been asked[31] about this trial, but it is hard to quarrel with the investigators' conclusion that many additional empirical studies need to be conducted to disclose the principal influences that play a role in patients' decisions to participate in treatment trials. In addition, the investigators advise, 'the potentially powerful role played by the physician [in 'study consent'] should be systematically evaluated'.

CONSENT IN PILOT STUDIES

The strictures of prior review and 'study consent' are rarely applied in the initial exploratory stages of a new treatment. Here, since every patient is to be treated, 'customary consent' rules are commonly used. But these pilot studies operate in a gray area of clinical activity. The seeds of duality are often planted at this early stage in the career of a new treatment.[32]

When the first results of exploration seem to be favorable (as compared with past experience), the innovation is quickly baptized as 'standard treatment'—I have called the practice 'bootlegging'.[18] Years go by before the claim is put to a rigorous test, and, as happens too often in neonatal medicine, the exciting treatment is found to have only a minor effect or even to be harmful.

I strongly suspect that a Gresham-like law operates at the exciting, leading edge of clinical research. When anecdotal evidence is readily accepted for publication by prestigious journals, over-eager innovators are tempted to bypass formal trials (for which prior review and 'study consent' are required, relatively large numbers of patients need to be studied, and solid evidence accumulates at a snail's pace). Here (as Gresham, the English financier, demonstrated in the competition between cheap money and expensive currency in the market-place), slapdash study design seems to win out in the short term.

If the suspicion that strict requirements do, in fact, encourage bootleg trials (clues may turn up in the on-going registry of clinical trials in perinatology[33]), the gate-keepers of medical publication (department heads, institutional review boards, and journal editors) will have to face the unhappy implications regarding the protection of patients. The logical solution is suggested by Thomas Chalmers' advice: 'randomize the first patient' in pilot studies.[34] He has called for the same set of rules at every stage in the introduction of untested interventions.

New drugs are not released by the Food and Drug Administration for general use in the US until safety and effectiveness have been tested in controlled clinical trials. (The European Community has adopted similar standards and has provided detailed requirements for informed consent.[35]) Until fairly recently, no similarly effective safeguard has been in place for other untested or poorly tested practices. The strange inconsistency has led directly to the double standard I described in the scenarios involving granulocyte transfusions (see above). The relatively recent introduction and spread of neonatal extracorporeal membrane oxygenation has been pointed out as a striking example of 'how not to assess novel technologies'.[36]

The confused situation is further complicated if, in the first example at the beginning of this chapter, the parents who refuse to allow their neonate to be enrolled in the granulocyte-transfusion trial ask for the new treatment outside the context of the formal trial then under way. The response to this request for transfusion is, I suggest, a powerful test of the authenticity of that trial. If the request is granted, it places a dark cloud over the sincerity of statements made in the 'study consent' ritual to explain the justification for the controlled trial. There is a similar kind of confusion in the second scenario: what is the moral status of the claim of therapeutic privilege by doctors who treat all eligible babies with the as-yet-not-fully-tested treatment?

THE PRECONDITION OF BALANCED DOUBT

The difficulties I have described remind us that there is always an ethical dilemma when a new treatment is proposed to replace the current standard. It is a necessary condition when asking for participation in a parallel-treatment-comparison trial that doctors be in a state of genuine uncertainty.[3] If a neonatologist believes patients in one arm of a planned trial are to be provided with better treatment, he/she usually disqualifies him/herself from participation. The doctor argues that he/she cannot, in good faith, represent to parents that the treatment choices in the granulocyte-transfusion trial, for example, are equal. How can we resolve the apparently irresolvable conflict between the ethical requirement that a patient must always be offered the best treatment known, and the equivocal choice in the comparative trial? The formal exercise is carried out in the sincere hope that the newly-proposed treatment will surpass the accepted regimen.

The paralyzing dilemma can be resolved, however, if we agree that the time has come to examine the high moral status accorded an individual doctor's treatment preference, particularly when that choice is backed by weak evidence. Personal and idiosyncratic decisions about 'best treatment known' cannot be defended, Freedman has pointed out,[3] when there is an honest disagreement among experts about the relative merits of treatment alternatives.

The ethics of medical practice should grant no moral standing to treatment preferences, no matter how strongly asserted, when that opinion is based on anything less than evidence publicly presented and convincing to the clinical community. Freedman reminds us that good medicine is defined not by individual doctors, but by professional consensus.

It follows from these arguments that a doctor with a decided treatment preference may, in good conscience, participate in a controlled trial when he or she acknowledges that there is insufficient evidence to judge 'best action', and when that state of doubt is disclosed, for example, to parents. It also follows that the truthfulness of the request for consent to enroll patients in a comparative trial is tested by the response to parents who refuse. The demands of 'refusers' for the new treatment under test cannot be satisfied in good conscience. It is unfair, I argue, to deny their infants the protection against the unknown risks that is provided by the laws of chance to babies enrolled in the trial.

A dramatic example of this point took place many years ago when we were evaluating adrenocorticotrophin (ACTH) treatment to halt the progression of early retinopathy of prematurity.[18] One doctor refused to allow his patient to take part in our randomized trial because he was convinced that the hormonal treatment 'worked'. He administered ACTH, and the baby died with a fatal infection during the course of this treatment. At the end of the controlled trial, we found that our early enthusiastic hopes for effectiveness in the pilot observations were not confirmed. As compared with untreated controls, there was now convincing evidence that ACTH had not altered the extremely variable course of the early stages of the retinopathy. Moreover, there was a disturbing difference in mortality; more of the treated infants died with serious infections. Before the comparative trial began, we had no hint of the frequency of these serious complications of ACTH treatment.

The rationale for withholding release of new drugs outside the context of a controlled clinical trial reflects the bitter lesson learned at the time of the thalidomide disaster (1957–61).[37] Nothing has happened in perinatal medicine since that time to support the demand that the conservative approach should be repealed. In fact, the fairly recent benzyl alcohol incident (the presumed-to-be-safe agent used as a bacteriostatic agent in bottles of intravenous fluids, was found, belatedly, to increase the risk of kernicterus, intraventricular hemorrhage, and death in small pre-term infants[38]) indicates that iatrogenic disasters continue to occur unabated.

DISTRIBUTIVE JUSTICE IN CLINICAL STUDIES

Another moral principle tested in the present-day 'study consent' requirement is that of distributive justice. Clinical studies have been conducted more frequently among impoverished minorities than among the privileged American classes. The poor were enrolled as subjects in medical investigations because of their convenience (researchers were located in the teaching hospitals used by poor patients) and because of gross insensitivity to the unfairness of the custom. A national commission[39] advised that children who participate in research projects should be selected so that the burdens of participation are distributed justly, that is, among all segments of our society. The recommendation is painfully silent about how this 'just' standard is to be achieved in practice.

In clinical trials, we depend on those who give consent freely.[40] The volunteers-only approach, however, thwarts the basic principle of random sampling that is the only way to assure a reasonable chance for equality of representation. However, it seems unlikely that conscription by lottery will be used to insure against systematic social inequalities in choosing participants for clinical trials.

Social filter effect. We should be ready to question anything done in the recruitment of patients for study that would seem to exaggerate social inequalities. Is it possible, for example, that 'study consent' acts as a social filter? Does it select for refusal those on the upper rungs of the social ladder, the least captive members of the community, those most likely to understand what is requested in the consent ritual? Among consenters, is there a disproportionate representation of those who do not understand, those too frightened to refuse, those who are socially disadvantaged?

The answer to these questions from Australia seems to be, 'Yes, at least some of the time.' Harth and Thong conducted a survey[41] of the sociodemographic and motivational characteristics of a group of a parents who had volunteered their children (age 1–3 years) for a randomized trial of a new drug for asthma, and a comparison group of parents of eligible children who refused permission for the clinical trial. The refusers were better educated, and they were represented more frequently in the occupations associated with higher social class. Parents who gave consent had less social support, consumed more habit-forming substances, and made more visits to the family doctor or clinic than the non-volunteers. The findings suggest, the researchers concluded, that parents who consent to enroll their children in this trial may not only be socially disadvantaged but also emotionally vulnerable. There are important implications of these observations concerning the issue of distributive justice. Similar surveys of consenting and refusing families need to be carried out in other countries and in trials involving children of various ages recruited for a wide range of trials to obtain further estimates of the extent of a maldistribution of the 'burdens of participation' in controlled clinical trials.

One observer has pointed to the possibility of an additional type of informed-consent-related selection bias.[42] It may operate even before the request is made, for example in reluctance on the part of care-takers and researchers to approach, say, Hispanic parents, who one observer thought were less willing to grant consent than Black parents; or a disinclination to ask for consent from the frightened parents of the smallest and sickest infants who are eligible for enrollment in a controlled trial.

'REVERSE CONSENT'

Overblown accounts in the media about neonatal medicine's technical powers seem to have given rise to a new ethical dilemma in NICUs. The predicament involves an issue that might be called, 'reverse consent'. Here, gullible parents with inflated expectations demand that heroic treatment be given to their seriously ill infant, despite advice that desperate measures have virtually no chance of succeeding. Is the doctor obliged to consent to an unrealistic demand for treatment? Is she/he required to yield, on the grounds of respect for parental autonomy?

The scope of autonomy granted to parents by society is broad, but it is not boundless. For example, parents are permitted to refuse to give their consent for customary treatment that merely prolongs their baby's pain and suffering. In the 'reverse' situation, doctors must also be permitted, I argue, to refuse to consent to parents' demand for futile treatment—extreme measures that would subject a baby to needless prolongation of misery. There is a safeguard against arbitrariness in both kinds of mismatch in outlook: parents and doctors are encouraged to seek other opinions. And parents are permitted to change doctors, if necessary, to achieve an improved match in attitude about when to start and when to stop heroic treatment.

A 'transparency' model of customary consent. King has observed a communication problem that may account, in part, for the recent emergence of 'reverse consent' dilemmas in NICUs.[43] Unrealistic optimism may develop, she notes, when a marginally-viable neonate seems to do well in the first day or so after birth, and then begins to decline. As doctors became increasingly convinced by the accumulation of findings indicating a worsening prognosis, a temporal gap may develop between the understanding of the caregiving team and that of the parents. When the implications of technical information collected during the progressive decline are not explained fully, the parents cling to hopes that become increasingly unreal.

Improved informed consent practices, King suggests, may reduce the kinds of disagreements that arise from misunderstanding rather than solely from differences in values between parents and caregivers. Brody's 'transparency model of informed consent',[44] devised for use in primary care, should be considered, King advises, to bridge the gap in understanding that arises in NICUs. The aim of the model is to render the doctor's clinical reasoning transparent to patients as it evolves. 'Essentially', Brody explains, 'the transparency standard requires the physician to engage in the typical patient-management thought process, only to *do it out loud in language understandable to the patient*' [sic].

Although the applicability of the transparency approach to situations found in NICUs has not been demonstrated, the aim, to involve parents more fully in decision-making, is laudable. Moreover (as in study consent), the argument that customary consent should be an ongoing process, rather than a one-time formal ritual, cannot be faulted. King's interesting proposal for a changed approach to parental consent for heroic treatment in NICUs should, as is noted below, be tested formally.

INFORMED CONSENT IN THE FUTURE

Debates about the topic of informed consent will, and should, continue without let-up. It has been impossible, in more than two decades of 'study consent', to devise practices that satisfy the competing moral imperatives of respect for autonomy, concern for beneficence with emphasis on the value of health, and vigilance in the for interests of distributive justice. It has been said[4] that the current doctrine and set of practions compromise all values and satisfy none in their entirety, hence the endless squabbling among doctors and their critics. The uncertainties are particularly intractable when proxy decisions must be made on behalf of very sick young infants in dysfunctional families. For example, a British researcher has asked,[45] 'Do parents who abuse and neglect their children, or who do not seem to understand medical information, have any right to share in making medical decisions for them?'

I will be very surprised if formats are found any time soon that will satisfy parents, doctors, legal experts, bioethicists, and the community-at-large (particularly with the sharp increase in cultural diversity in many Western countries[46]). So long as the arguments remain heavily weighted with opinion and so weakly challenged by concrete evidence, the outlook for progress seems dim.

A way must be found, I suggest, to experiment with various discretionary approaches that would strike a realistic balance among competing interests, that is approaches that would conserve the spirit of informed consent without snuffing out the flame of responsible clinical study. Modern medicine is dedicated to the pursuit of knowledge: the on-going search is seen by the profession as an indispensable goal. Kass has suggested that questions about the use of human beings as means to this end can be resolved, at least in principle.[47] 'By knowingly and freely consenting to serve as an experimental subject, the patient is not serving *merely* as a means; he becomes, as it were, a co-inquirer, Kass notes, and the obligation to secure his consent explicitly acknowledges that he is not to be regarded merely as a means.' (Pappworth has reviewed the long uphill struggle to obtain the medical profession's grudging acceptance of this view: the delicate balance of means and ends in all clinical experimentation.[48])

The double standard of 'study consent' and 'customary consent' will continue as long as we fail to test proposed alternatives to current practice, and as long as we are unable to come to some agreement about the outcomes of importance that will permit a measured comparison of alternatives. (The conceptual dilemmas have been spelled out by Meisel and Roth.[29]

At the Lugano consensus conference,[19] three-quarters of the conferees (70/93) agreed with the statement, 'There should be no fundamental difference between the information given to a patient in order to obtain informed consent in a controlled clinical trail and that given in daily practice.' The issue is particularly relevant in the field of neonatal medicine because of the relatively large number of treatments used in daily practice that have not been subjected to rigorous tests.[1] The consensus is not helpful, however, unless it leads to comparative studies designed to measure the consequences of merging 'study consent' and 'customary consent' in concrete clinical circumstances.

In the immediate newborn period, for example, there are a number of poorly tested treatments that have been accepted widely as customary practice.[49] On the other hand, randomized clinical trials to test some of these measures rigorously (for example sodium bicarbonate intravenously to severely asphyxiated neonates) cannot be undertaken with institutional review board approval in one institution unless informed consent is obtained from the parents before enrollment in the study (Tyson, J. E., personal communication). The studies have been abandoned because of serious questions about the desirability, feasibility, and validity of providing full disclosure and obtaining 'study consent' in the first moments before or after the birth of a seriously compromised baby.

I suspect that it is this kind of impasse that perpetuates the Gresham effect. It encourages informal, poorly designed observational research, carried out without the protective hedge of concurrent controls and random allocation, with no requirement for formal full disclosure, and based on an inadequate number of infants studied.[50] I also suspect that the unsatisfactory situation will continue until current inflexible requirements are compared with formats tempered by common sense.

Applicable limits of the current 'study consent' and 'customary consent' concepts in neonatal studies and in everyday treatment need to be explored systematically. I am mindful here of Lewis Mumford's comments about the endless pursuit for a guide to regulate human behavior. He said[51] 'In so far as ethics provides a sound guide to living, it must have life's own attributes: its pliability, its adaptiveness, its sensitiveness to the occasion.'

(This chapter is adapted from my earlier papers on informed consent published in *Am.J Med Sci* **296** (1988):354–9 and *J.Med Ethics* **15** (1989):6–11.)

WILLIAM A. SILVERMAN

REFERENCES

1. Hack, M, Horbar, J. D., Malloy, M. H., Tyson, J. E., Wright, E., and Wright, L. Very low birth weight outcomes of the National Institute of Child Health and Human Development Neonatal Network. *Pediatrics*, **87**, 587–97 (1991).
2. Cairo, M. S. Granulocyte transfusions in neonates with presumed sepsis. *Pediatrics*, **80**, 738–40 (1987).
3. Freedman, B. Equipoise and the ethics of clinical research. *New Engl. J. Med.*, **317**, 141–5 (1987).
4. Applebaum, P. S., Lidz, C. W., and Meisel, A. *Informed consent: legal theory and clinical practice.* Oxford University Press, New York. (1987).
5. Pernick, M. S. The patient's role in medical decision making: a social history of informed consent. In *President's Commission for the Study of Ethical Problems.* Government Printing Office, Washington, DC (1982).
6. Kirby, M. D. Informed consent: what does it mean? *J. Med. Ethics*, **9**, 69–75 (1983).
7. Percival, T. *Medical ethics; or Code of institutes and precepts, adapted to the professional conduct of physicians and surgeons.* S. Russell, Manchester (1803).
8. Faden, R. and Beauchamp, T. L. *A history and theory of informed consent.* Oxford University Press, New York (1986).
9. *Salgo v. Leland Standford Jr. University*, 317 P2d 170 vol. 54, p.560 (Cal 1957). California Court of Appeals.
10. Katz, J. Informed consent—a fairy tale? Law's vision. *Univ. Pittsburgh Law Review*, **39**, 137–74 (1977).
11. Katz, J. *The silent world of doctor and patient.* Free Press, New York (1984).
12. Stewart, W. H. *'Clinical investigations using human subjects'.* Memorandum (8 February 1966).
13. Katz, J. *Experimentation with human beings.* Russell Sage Foundation, New York (1972).
14. Beecher, H. K. Ethics and clinical research. *New Engl. J. Med.* **274**, 1354–60 (1966).
15. Rothman, D. J. Ethics and human experimentation. Henry Beecher revisited. *New Engl. J. Med.*, **317**, 1195–9 (1987).
16. Silverman, W. A., Andersen, D. H., Blanc W. A., and Crozier, D. N. A difference in mortality rate and incidence of kernicterus among premature infants allotted to two prophylactic antibacterial regimens. *Pediatrics*, **18**, 614–25 (1956).
17. Burns, L. E., Hodgman, J. E., and Cass, A. B. Fatal collapse in premature infants receiving chloramphenicol. *New Engl. J. Med.* **261**, 1318–21 (1959).
18. Silverman, W. A. *Retrolental fibroplasia: a modern parable.* Grune and Stratton, New York (1980).
19. Blum, A. L., Chalmers, T. C., Deutsch, E., Koch-Weser, J., Rosen, A., Tygstrup, N., and Zentgraf, R. The Lugano Statement on controlled clinical trials. *J. Int. Med. Res.*, **15**, 2–22 (1987).
20. King, J. *Informed consent. Institute of Medical Ethics Bulletin* (Supplement No. 3). Luton Ltd, London (1986).

21. Lynoe, N., Sandlund, M., Dahlqvist, L., and Jacobsson, L. Informed consent: study of quality of information given to participants in a clinical trial. *Brit. Med. J.*, **303**, 610–13 (1991).
22. World Medical Association. *Declaration of Helsinki. Recommendations guiding medical doctors in biomedical research involving human subjects*, (Revised by 29th World Medical Assembly). Tokyo (1975).
23. Simes, R. J., Tattersal, M. H. N., Coates, A. S., Raghaven, D., and Solomon, H. J. Randomised comparison of procedures for obtaining informed consent in clinical trials of treatment for cancer. *Brit. Med. J.*, **293**, 1065–8 (1986).
24. Zelen, M. A new design for randomized clinical trials. *New Engl. J. Med.*, **300**, 1242–5 (1979).
25. Abramson, N. S., Meisel, A., and Safar, P. Deferred consent: a new approach for resuscitation research. *J. A. M. A.*, **255**, 2466 (1986).
26. The Brain Resuscitation Clinical Trial II Study Group. A randomized clinical trial of calcium entry blocker administration to comatose survivors of cardiac arrest. *Contr. Clin. Trials*, **12**, 525–45 (1991).
27. Miller, B. L. Philosophical, ethical, and legal aspects of resuscitation medicine. I. Deferred consent and justification of resuscitation research. *Crit. Care Med.*, **16**, 1059–62 (1988).
28. Levine, R. J. commentary. Deferred consent. *Contr. Clin. Trials*, **12**, 546–50 (1991).
29. Meisel, A. and Roth, L. H. What we do and do not know about informed consent. *J. A. M. A.*, **246**, 2473–7 (1981).
30. Simel, D. L. and Feussner, J. R. A randomized controlled trial comparing quantitative informed consent formats. *J. Clin. Epidemiol.*, **44**, 771–7 (1991).
31. Lancet Editorial. Informed consent: how informed? *Lancet*, **338**, 665–6 (1991).
32. McKinlay JB. From "promising report" to "standard procedure": seven stages in the career of a medical innovation. *Milbank Mem. Fund. Quart. Health and Society*, **59**, 374–411 (1981).
33. National Perinatal Epidemiology Unit. *A classified bibliography of controlled trials in perinatal medicine 1940–1984* [and the on-going Oxford Database of Perinatal Trials]. Oxford University Press (1985) [and up-dated electronic publications].
34. Chalmers, T. C. Randomization of the first patient. *Med. Clin. North Am.*, **59**, 1035–8 (1975).
35. Committee on Proprietary Medicinal Products Working Party on Efficacy of Medicinal Products. *European Community Note for Guidance: good clinical practice for trials on medicinal products in the European Community*. EEC Commission, Brussels (1990).
36. Elliott, S. J. Neonatal extracorporeal membrane oxygenation: how not to assess novel technologies. *Lancet*, **337**, 476–8 (1991).
37. Insight Team. *Suffer the children: the story of thalidomide*. Viking, New York (1979).
38. Jardine, D. S. and Rogers, K. Relationship of benzyl alcohol to kernicterus, intraventricular hemorrhage, and mortality in preterm infants. *Pediatrics*, **83**, 153–60 (1989).
39. National Commission for the Protection of Human Subjects of Biomedical and

Behavioral Research. *Research involving children: report and recommendation*, U. S. Dept. of Health Educ. Welfare Publication No. (OS) 77–0004. Govt. Printing Office, Washington, DC (1977).

40. Kauffman, C. L. Informed consent and patient decision making: two decades of research. *Soc. Sci. Med.*, **17**, 1657–64 (1983).
41. Hartn, S. C. and Thong, Y. H. Sociodemographic and motivational characteristics of parents who volunteer their children for clinical research: a controlled study. *Brit. Med. J.*, **300**, 1372–5 (1990).
42. Walterspiel, J. N. Informed consent: influence on patient selection among critically ill premature infants. *Pediatrics*, **85**, 119–21 (1990).
43. King, N. M. P. Transparency in neonatal intensive care. *Hastings Center Report*, (May–June), 18–25 (1992).
44. Brody, H. Transparency: informed consent in primary care. *Hastings Center Report*, (Oct–Nov): 5–9 (1989).

9B STANDARDS OF DISCLOSURE IN INFORMED CONSENT

Amnon Goldworth

INTRODUCTION

In many countries informed consent is now a precondition to customary medical therapies as well as to those which are under experimental study in research settings. Its institutionalization is based on the moral perception that human beings possess a dignity and value which calls for their treatment as ends and disallows their being used solely as means. In addition, it is supported by the recognition that freedom of choice is generally valuable whatever the choice itself may be. This has changed a common perception of the doctor–patient relationship from one in which the doctor decides what to do to one in which the doctor proposes and the patient decides. In most instances, the doctor must no longer judge what to tell the patient nor unilaterally determine what moral values should be assigned to any of the therapeutic options.

Under the best circumstances, the procedure by which informed consent is sought and obtained promotes individual autonomy and encourages rational decision-making. These are achieved when an individual is able to understand the nature, quality, and consequences of a given medical intervention, possesses the information needed to weigh appropriate alternatives, and comes to a reasonable decision which is free from coercion or manipulation.[1]

THE AUTONOMY OF PARENTS

When the patient is an infant and therefore incompetent to decide for himself or herself, informed consent must be secured from a surrogate. Parents are generally recognized by the community and the state as the appropriate proxies for their incompetent children. Various reasons have been offered in support of this parental role.[2] Perhaps the most important concerns the parents in their role as care-takers of the family. It is generally agreed that patient autonomy is of fundamental importance, given the rights of the patient as a human being. When the neonate and his or her rights are concerned, it is the autonomy of the parents which is called for, given their responsibility for the ongoing care of the child. In addition, there is the need to protect the integrity of the family unit. Those of its members who are competent to direct its course should have the freedom to chart its destiny. For instance, when parents are asked to consent to the use of the Norwood Procedure for their child who is suffering from hypoplastic left-heart syndrome, they are being asked to allow their child to undergo a series of surgical interventions which will affect not only the quality of his or her life but also the quality of the entire family's existence for a prolonged period of time. Unless there is evidence of parental incompetence, neglect, or abuse, outside interference in the decisions of parents in such circumstances, whether by a doctor, the community, or the state, is unwarranted.

THE DOUBLE STANDARD

When we attend to the requirements for securing informed consent in the United States, we see that they differ in the clinical and research settings.

Dr Silverman made it clear that these differences in requirements have produced a double standard between the use of 'customary consent' in customary medical treatment and the use of 'study consent' when a specific treatment is under study in a research setting. His example of the research study to determine the effectiveness of adding granulocyte transfusions to the conventional antibiotic treatment for septicemia in infants with neutropenia as compared to the use of granulocyte transfusions as a part of customary treatment in the clinical setting reveals a marked difference in the ability of parents to veto treatments in the two settings.

Another effect, as Silverman points out, is that it encourages potentially dangerous 'bootlegging', in which a new treatment that in early investigations appears promising bypasses the restrictions imposed by study consent entirely by its quick conversion into conventional treatment.

THE QUESTION OF A SINGLE STANDARD

Given the problems caused by the differences in requirements for customary and study consent, should we have the same ones for both? Silverman believes that the same requirements should not be employed until we have studied the consequences of such a change. His call for empirical studies is supported by Alan Meisel and Loren Roth, who observe that 'probably the most important general finding of our review of the studies of informed consent is how little is actually known about how informed consent operates ... and how much doubt there is about the validity of what is thought to be known'.[3]

However, the sorts of investigations that Silverman has in mind can yield significant results only if we have a clear and commonly recognized understanding of what it means for someone to be informed. Conceptual clarity, in this context, will advance us significantly toward resolving the question of the need for a single standard.

THE LAW

As Silverman pointed out, the doctrine of informed consent, and more specifically customary consent, is based on legal opinion. In deciding a 1914 case in which surgery had been performed without the patient's consent, Justice Benjamin Cardozo presented a clear statement of the patient's right to self-determination.

Every human being of adult years and sound mind has a right to determine what shall be done with his own body; and a surgeon who performs an operation without his patient's consent commits an assault, for which he is liable in damages.[4]

However, Cardozo said nothing concerning the requirement for disclosure of information by the doctor. It was not until 1957, in *Salgo* Vs. *Leland Stanford Jr. University Board of Trustees*, that a legal foundation was laid for informed consent.

The suit concerned the questions whether the injection of sodium urokon during a translumbar aortography could have affected the plaintiff's spinal cord and whether the plaintiff, and his wife and son, were informed that an aortography was to be performed. What the court decision established was a requirement that compels disclosure of information on the part of a doctor in order to secure informed consent from his or her patient. The one exception was the possible use of therapeutic privilege which allows a physician to avoid disclosure which she believes is in conflict with her duty to do what is beneficial for her patient. When disclosure takes place, it must satisfy the professional practice standard which holds that what is to be disclosed is determined by what is perceived as reasonable practice by the medical community.[5]

This standard was rejected in 1972 by the court in *Canterbury* vs. *Spence*. At issue in this case was whether a 1 per cent chance of paralysis caused by a laminectomy was sufficient to require informing the patient of this possibility. It was replaced by the reasonable person standard of disclosure, which requires that the consenting party, as a rational agent, is to determine what information is material.[6]

While therapeutic privilege is not significant in the domain of perinatology, there are several other exceptions to disclosure which are worth noting.

One is the emergency exception in which a doctor is permitted to treat without the consent of the parents. What justifies this exception is the fact that there is insufficient time for the doctor to provide the appropriate information and obtain consent. This time constraint must be such that any effort to obtain consent will be perceived to be disadvantageous or threatening to the patient's health.

Another is the incompetence exception. This applies when the parents whose infant needs treatment are unable, by reason of incapacity, to absorb information, and thus are unable to consent. This incapacity may be general, as in the case of someone who is intoxicated, psychotic, severely retarded, or unconscious. Or the incapacity may be specific, as in the case of a woman who is unable to make certain decisions concerning her child's fate while being able to decide to call her husband or drive home.

The third is the waiver exception. Unlike the emergency exception and the incompetency exception, in which external events or internal states prevent the parents from obtaining information, this last exception depends on clear information and understanding. What the parents need to know is that they not only have a right to be informed and the right to decide on the basis of information, but that they also may decide to give up these rights.

A properly obtained waiver is in keeping with the individualistic values promoted by the doctrine of informed consent. The patient [or parent] remains the ultimate decision maker, but the content of the decision is shifted from the decisional level to the metadecisional level.[7]

This exception is related to the issue of trust, which will be discussed in a later portion of this chapter.

THE DEVELOPMENT OF STUDY CONSENT

Unlike the requirements for customary consent, which were established by the law, the requirements for study consent, as Silverman pointed out, were based on political considerations.

Before the Second World War little attention was paid to the conditions in which research was carried on. This changed in 1946, as a result of the Nuremberg trials of Nazi physicians. The Nuremberg Code which followed, and which was recognized in many countries, called for voluntary informed consent. The British Medical Research Council and the 1964 Declaration of Helsinki of the World Medical Association changed parts of this code by distinguishing between research which was likely to benefit the subject and that which would not, and eliminated mandatory consent in the former case.

Notwithstanding the existence of codes and declarations, instances of abuse in research did not result in litigation. Had they 'the rules governing treatment and research would probably have been similar'.[8] Instead, abuse led to the refinement of Federal regulations which affected most research in the United States. The 1966 regulations of the National Institutes of Health required reviews of research protocols by institutional review boards established at universities to determine whether the rights of subjects were protected, whether the methods employed to obtain informed consent from subjects were appropriate, and whether the benefits of the proposed research outweighed the costs to the subjects. These regulations have been in operation ever since.

According to Applebaum, Lidz, and Meisel, 'The most important conceptual difference between the regulations of consent in research and treatment settings is that consent to research is reviewed prospectively, while consent to treatment is ordinarily subject only to retrospective review, if any'.[9]

CRITERIA FOR CONSENT IN DIFFERENT COUNTRIES

The professional practice and reasonable person standards of disclosure are applied in various countries. In the United States and Australia both are used.[10] In Canada the reasonable person standard is used.[11] In Great Britain, it is the professional practice standard.[12].

Both the professional practice and reasonable person standards are perceived to be objective because they claim to appeal to commonly shared evidence which concerns either reasonable professional practice or what a reasonable person needs to know. In contrast is the subjective standard of disclosure, which requires that the doctor provide information which is of material interest to the consenting party as determined by his or her particular values and interests. This standard has been applied in a few court decisions in the United States.[13]. But it is mandated throughout Germany.[14] The following is an interesting example of its use in a German court.

In a recent case the *Oberlandesgericht* (OLG) Karlsruhe went so far as to require a doctor to disclose the 'typical' risks of full anaesthestic to the mother of an eighteen-year-old patient in order to allow her to give an informed consent on his behalf. In reaching this decision the court took into account the woman's low social status which, it was said, precluded the doctor from building the equation 'knowledge that full anaesthetic will be required = knowledge of its risks'. If the objective 'prudent patient' [reasonable person] test had been applied, the plaintiff would not have succeeded, for the prudent patient is assumed, at least in common law jurisdiction, to be aware of the risks of general anaesthesia.[15]

When we turn to study consent, there is no clear indication what standard of disclosure is to be employed.

The existing regulations [in the United States] lay out the types of information that must be communicated to potential subjects. They give no guidance about the specific information that should be conveyed, the emphasis different elements of disclosure should receive, or the method of accomplishing a meaningful explanation.[16]

However, there is no reason to believe that the subjective standard of disclosure is used. What is used in the research, as well as clinical, setting are the professional and reasonable person standards. But both these standards suffer from serious shortcomings.

CRITIQUE OF THE PROFESSIONAL PRACTICE AND REASONABLE PERSON STANDARDS OF DISCLOSURE

Consider the professional practice approach. It operates on the assumption that there is a single standard of practice that applies to all doctors. This assumption was challenged by the court in *Canterbury* v. *Spence*.

There are, in our view, formidable obstacles to acceptance of the notion that the physician's obligation to disclose is either germinated or limited by medical practice. To begin with, the reality of any discernible custom reflecting a professional consensus on communication of option and risk information to patients is open to serious doubt.[17]

But even if a single standard exists, this alone does not guarantee that the information disclosed by the doctor is sufficient for informed consent. In addition, this approach undermines the autonomy of the consenting party, since the information imparted by the doctor may not be of material interest to the consenter, and information which is of material interest to the consenter may not be forthcoming. This is illustrated by the neonatologist who presents information about life-saving procedures for an infant when the parents' chief concern is the quality of their child's life, should she or he survive.

Now consider the reasonable person approach. As John Elster observed

Rational choice is concerned with finding the *best* means to given ends. It is a way of adopting optimally to the circumstances . . . Here we should note that rational choice is not an infallible mechanism, since the rational person can choose only what he *believes* to be the best means.[18]

This characterization of rational choice makes it clear that doctors and parents may differ as to the end to be achieved in treating the infant and may differ in their beliefs concerning the best means by which to achieve the same end. Both the doctor and the parents may be reasonable individuals, and yet differ concerning means and ends. Thus even if the doctor discloses information that could be said to be relevant to some reasonable individual, this does not guarantee that this information is of material interest to the parents of her patient.

In 1983 the President's Commission for the Study of Ethical Problems in Medicine and Biomedical Research said that 'Ethically valid consent is a process of shared decision making based upon mutual respect and participation, not a ritual to be equated with reciting the contents of a form.' Neither the professional practice nor the reasonable person approach necessarily promotes 'a process of shared decision making based on mutual respect and participation', nor does either ensure that information is disclosed which is of particular interest to the consenting party. In addition, neither approach prevents ritualization in the procedure of obtaining consent. In short, both are likely to produce flawed consent.[19]

REASONS FOR THE PREVAILING USE OF OBJECTIVE STANDARDS OF DISCLOSURE

Given the deficiencies of the objective standards, why are they employed? Several factors have combined in support of the prevailing practices. First, the courts and doctors have perceived the need for written consent as a form of protection for doctors against charges of negligence. This is most easily achieved by emphasizing the objective nature of the information imparted by the doctor. Second, the objective approaches are more economical to use than the subjective one. This feature should be understood in the context of institutionalized impediments to doctor–parent interactions. So long as doctors, for whatever reasons, are unenthusiastic about sharing information with parents, the doctor's priorities will reduce the time spent with parents to the minimum required by existing requirements. Third, objective criteria allow the doctor to satisfy requirements for informed consent without having to be overly concerned with the degree of understanding of the parents. It is for this reason that doctors can, at one and the same time, be skeptical of the abilities of parents to understand what they are being told and yet have no serious qualms about using the objective approaches. Fourth, and most important, is the fact that the aforementioned factors were made plausible by an ambiguity in the meaning of the verb 'to inform'.

AN ANALYSIS OF THE VERB 'TO INFORM'

The dictionary definition of this verb is 'to describe', 'to instruct', 'to teach', 'to furnish with knowledge'. One can do each of these and yet fail to be understood by the listener or reader. A simple example supports this point.

At a social gathering following an international conference in London, England, I informed a Japanese professor of my professional background and interests and my views on several of the papers that had been read at the conference. My imparting of information continued until I realized that my smiling and nodding companion did not understand English. This example illustrates two things: (1) one can inform without having communicated anything; and (2) one can believe that one has been understood without such understanding having taken place.

Since informing someone may consist of the conveying of information but not its reception, use of an objective standard of disclosure makes it impossible, without further investigation, to determine whether the individual failed to receive information because of incompetence or because of a lack of sufficient interest in what he or she had been told.

But such investigations either result in the replacement of an objective standard by the subjective standard of disclosure or they prove inconclusive. Suppose that the doctor asks the parents to indicate what they had just been told. If their responses are inaccurate, the doctor must now attempt to discover whether the parents are unable to understand what they were told or whether they are able to understand but lack interest in what they have been told. To determine which alternative is operative will require that the doctor use the subjective approach in place of an objective one. Now suppose that the parents are asked what they remember being told by the doctor some time earlier. If the parents' responses are inaccurate, nothing conclusive follows, because there is no necessary connection between what one remembers later and what one understood before giving consent. Given the stress created by the need to make a decision about a risky procedure, it is quite possible for an individual to forget relevant facts once the decision is made.

THE SUBJECTIVE STANDARD OF DISCLOSURE AND UNDERSTANDING

As was previously suggested, it is possible to satisfy the disclosure requirements using the objective approaches without the consenting party's adequately understanding what has been disclosed. This is not likely in the
use of the subjective approach. In this mode, the doctor needs to know what
the interests and values of the consenting party are. To learn what they are
is not a matter of simply asking 'What are your interests and values?' These
are normally discovered by the consenting party's response to the array of
imparted information concerning technical matters, alternative treatments,
and probable outcomes. Indeed, for the doctor to know that what he is
disclosing is relevant is a function not only of understanding the interests
and values of the consenting party, but also a function of knowing that the
consenting party understands what is being disclosed. For without the latter,
the doctor has no assurance that his disclosure is material.

What gives us good reasons to believe that an individual understands
are certain verbal and nonverbal signs which we interpret as signs of
comprehansion. The therapeutic response of the clinical psychologist or
psychiatrist serves to illustrate this point. During these sessions there is
a verbal and behavioral interplay between therapist and client in which
each utterance or gesture on the part of the one provides the other with
clues about the quality and degree of understanding of the recipient of
the utterance or gesture. There is a constant checking of the verbal and
behavioral signs to assure or reassure each party that the other understands
or does not understand. Lest one believes that it is the special training of the
therapist that allows him or her to determine whether the client understands,
notice that the same process allows the parent to determine that her child
understands arithmetic or allows the college teacher to determine that a
student understands botany.

Unlike the objective approaches, the subjective one forces the doctor to
determine whether the parents understand what she is saying. This process
of discovery has the important feature of helping to overcome obstacles to
comprehension faced by parents under stress who may hear what the doctor
says, but only in the midst of a kind of emotional static generated by fear,
confusion, and a sense of unreality.

THE DOUBLE STANDARD REVISITED AND THE ISSUE OF TRUST

In my summary of the development of study consent, I indicated that the
British Medical Research Council and the Declaration of Helsinki presented
policies based on the difference between experimentation which was likely
to benefit the subject and experimentation which would not. Ranaan Gillon
employs this distinction to support a double standard between customary

consent and study consent when the latter is for non-therapeutic research.[20] Although I do not intend to pursue the matter, it should be noted that the distinction between therapeutic and non-therapeutic research has been questioned by Jon Tyson in this volume and elsewhere.[21]

In customary treatment, the patient assumes that she is not playing the role of subject for the benefit of others. Furthermore, the doctor and patient assume that what the doctor proposes as treatment will benefit the patient. For these reasons, 'it is reasonable for patients to *trust* their doctors to act in their best interests'.[22] This is also true for therapeutic research which is intended to benefit the patient. Thus, consent for customary treatment and therapeutic research are morally equivalent and should be governed by the same norms. In contrast, consent for non-therapeutic treatment should be governed by different standards.

Whether patients or their surrogates trust their doctors is, for our purposes, of less importance than whether doctors should be trusted. In England, patients and parents have no alternative but to trust them, given the legally mandated professional practice standard of disclosure. It is anyone's guess whether doctors would be trusted if the subjective standard were employed.

What are the reasons for the trust relationship other than what is a direct product of the law? One reason is the belief that the doctor is well intentioned: he or she practices medicine in order to benefit sick individuals. A second reason is that the doctor and the patient or parents are in agreement concerning the objectives to be achieved and the appropriate means to be used. A third reason is the belief that the doctor has the requisite skills to achieve medical objectives. If any one of these reasons fails, trust in the doctor is diminished or lost. For instance, the American perception that the doctor is well intentioned could change if the present entrepreneurial trend in the United States intensifies the conflict between the economic interests of the doctor and the best interests of his or her patients.[23]

The ordinary person has good reason to believe that doctors have the requisite medical skills if there are established medical licensing procedures. But the possession of medical skills and being well-intentioned do not guarantee that what the doctor believes should be achieved is in accord with the patient's or parents' view of the matter. Doctors may be convinced that the silence of parents during disclosures is a sign of agreement when, in fact, they are frequently too intimidated by the status and manner of doctors to question them.

Gillon's claim that it is reasonable for individuals to trust their doctors appears to rest on the assumption that the doctor is well intentioned and skilled. However, unless she discovers what is peculiar to her patient or to his or her surrogate in terms of values and interests and how these apply in the medical context, there may be no good reason for the patient or surrogate to trust her.

The concept of shared decision-making is described in the report of the President's Commission on the ethical and legal implications of informed consent. Effective participation calls for

... discussions between professional and patient that bring the knowledge, concerns and perspective of each to the process of every agreement on a course of treatment. Simply put, this means that the physicians or other health professional invites the patient to participate in a dialogue in which the professional seeks to help the patient understand the medical situation and available courses of action, and the patient conveys his or her concerns and wishes.[24]

Shared decision-making is best realized by the application of the subjective standard of disclosure.

SOME PROBLEMS WITH THE SUBJECTIVE STANDARD

The employment of this standard creates legal problems for the medical profession. This is apparent in the German experience. For instance, it does not square with the standards of liability applied in non-medical contexts.[25] In addition, other problems beset the courts by '... tying the issue of causation to the patient's own credibility and allowing the patient to take advantage of hindsight'.[26] Without dismissing the gravity of these legal problems, the law must do what it can to ameliorate them within its own domain, unless it can be shown that the subjective standard is wanting on moral grounds.

MEDICAL VS. PARENTAL AUTHORITY

It is easy for the doctor to see himself as the protector of the infant's best interests. It is also psychologically gratifying when doctor and parents form a therapeutic alliance in which there is an agreement about objectives such as salvaging or prolonging life or providing comfort and minimizing suffering, and the means by which these are achieved. When this occurs, there is a compatibility between the doctor's perception of himself as the infant's benefactor and his duty to protect the parent's right to self-determination.

But whose judgment takes precedence when there is a conflict between the doctor and the parents concerning the best interests of the child? Silverman alludes to one type of conflict in which the parents want their child to be treated despite the doctor's judgment that treatment will be futile. Conflict can also occur when the doctor wants to treat the infant and the parents do not.

Silverman is correct in stating that parent autonomy is not unlimited, and that there is a need for 'reverse consent' in which the doctor can refuse to initiate futile treatment. In the language of individual rights, parental autonomy is a *prima facie* right which can be overruled when parents are incompetent, or neglect or abuse their child. In these circumstances, the infant may suffer either gratuitous harm, injury, or death. Parental autonomy may also be overruled by the implementation of a policy which calls for the allocation of scarce resources.[27]

Although there are clearly recognized instances of incompetence, neglect, and abuse, it is not possible to determine this in all instances. This is due, in large measure, to the lack of clarity or agreement in the use of the concept of futility which serves as a basis for the doctor's refusal to treat. For instance, consider the conflict between the mother of a Baby L, a severely handicapped two-year-old girl, and the child's care-takers.

The mother requested treatment for her child's pneumonia and sepsis, notwithstanding the opinion of the involved doctors and various consultants that 'further intervention would subject the child to additional pain without affecting the underlying condition or ultimate outcome', and that 'unless a reversal or amelioration of the underlying condition could be expected, painful intervention would be futile and inhumane'.[28] Would further treatment, in fact, be futile? Several doctors said no.
One of these, Alan Fleischman, observed

The treating physicians assessed the use of a mechanical ventilator as futile and inhumane in light of the treatment being unable to affect the underlying condition or ultimate outcome. Clearly, the ventilator would not be expected to reverse the neurologic condition of the child, but it should not have been defined as futile in terms of the potential for reversing the intercurrent respiratory illness. We often burden our patients with interventions that have no effect on the ultimate outcome of their chronic illness but do positively affect their acute problem.

Fleischman added

A treatment is futile if it will not succeed in reversing the specific physiologic problem for which it is instituted. It is important not to misuse the language or futility to make quality of life judgments.[29]

Robert Perelman and Norman Fost, who were in accord with Fleischman, added

The central question is whether patients who cannot experience the richness of normal life have experiences that make continued experience from their own perspective better than no life at all. With aggressive treatment, the child survived and continued to require the extensive but pre-existing home care for her neurodevelopmental disabilities. While a mental status of a 3-month-old is admittedly suboptimal, it is not self-evident that it implies a painful existence.[30]

If Fleischman is correct that a treatment is futile if it fails to reverse the specific problem for which it is instituted, then it would appear that the effective treatment of the pneumonia of a permanently unconscious patient is not futile. This is dismissed by Lawrence Schneiderman, Nancy Jecker, and Albert Jonsen in their claim that 'any treatment that merely preserves permanent unconsciousness or that fails to end total dependence on intensive medical care should be regarded as non-beneficial and therefore futile'.[31]

It appears to be incorrect to say that treatment is futile if it does not end total dependence on intensive medical care. For then, for example, the treatment of a severely affected polio victim would have to be judged as futile.

Schneiderman *et al.* answer this by adding that what is excluded from their concept of futility 'is medical care for patients for whom such care offers the opportunity to achieve 'life goals, however limited'.[32]

The expression life goals' can be understood to mean 'goals for life' or 'goals for one's life.' It is with reference to such goals that one can plot the course of one's life as a whole. So understood, young children do not have life goals because they do not have a conception of their own lives as a whole. But, this is also true for many adults. For some adults life is a fragmented experience with little significance beyond the present. For others, the achievement or abandonment of some life goals has, as yet, not been replaced by other goals. Suppose that our polio patient who is totally dependent on intensive medical care has abandoned some life goal but at present does not have any other. It would appear that Schneiderman *et al.* would judge the treatment of this patient to be futile. Surely, cessation of treatment under this circumstance would be arbitrary. But, if treatment cannot be denied to adults on the grounds that they presently do not have any life goals then it cannot be denied to young children on the same grounds.

However, the expression 'life goals' can also mean 'to have goals' in the sense that one has interests which one consistently pursues over time. Our polio patient, who presently does not have life goals in the first sense, can still have them in the present sense. But this is true not only for adults but for young children as well.

It is not sensible to say that the neonate has life goals since he or she is merely responding to stimuli. But, a two year old with a the mental status of a neonate such as Baby J could have limited interests which she consistently pursues over time. For instance, she could regularly cry for food or her mother's touch.

Given the interpretation of 'life goals' the meaning of futile treatment as it relates to the totally dependent is sufficiently clear. Unfortunately, it appears to have no application to real cases.

As we have seen, judgments about the futility of treatment are controversial. Until there is clarity with respect to the concept of futility, a doctor's effort to employ reverse consent will be open to challenge.

Let us now turn to an example of the sort of conflict that occurs when a doctor wants to treat and the parents do not. One such is the widely publicized Baby Doe case, in which the parents refused to consent to life-saving surgery for their Down syndrome infant because they believed that his continued existence would not be in his best interest. Disagreement with this conclusion was widespread. It was, in part, based on the belief that few Down syndrome children are so severely retarded as to be completely dependent on care-takers. Furthermore, those who are mildly or moderately retarded appear to live satisfying lives. The Federal Government's negative reaction to the parents' conduct and the subsequent death of Baby Doe led to legal enactments at both the Federal and State levels that excluded any reference to the issue of quality of life and required treatment for all viable infants.[33]

Was the decision to withhold treatment by Baby Doe's parents justified or an instance of abuse? It is difficult, if not impossible, to say. For instance, in response to the argument that many Down syndrome children are not severely retarded, Baby Doe's parents could have taken the position that the possible risk of having their child live a seriously retarded life outweighed all other considerations.

This position might be discounted by observing that there are no guarantees in the development of any children, including those who are apparently normal, who, for instance, could become emotional cripples whose dependence on others could be as great as that of severely retarded children. If we are willing to gamble with the normal risks of child development why shouldn't the Baby Doe parents have been willing to gamble with the risks of their baby's development?

In answer to this question, Baby Doe's parents might have responded by pointing out that they knew with certainty that their child would never be able to live a normal life, whereas most individuals begin their parenting in ignorance as to the development of their children. One can only wonder how parents will behave when an increasing number of genetic markers for crippling and death-dealing diseases are discovered.

There are no algorithms for cases such as Baby L and Baby Doe. Perhaps the best that can be recommended is that where there are conflicting judgments in the professional ranks or where there are no arguments which tell against parental reasoning, then the wishes of parents should be respected. In circumstances of this sort, the subjective standard of disclosure is the only appropriate means by which the relevant information can be made available.

CONCLUDING REMARKS

Are there differences between customary treatment and clinical research, whether therapeutic or non-therapeutic, that justify the use of different standards of disclosure for informed consent? One difference is that in customary treatment, unlike what occurs in clinical research, the intervention is not experimental. But this difference is not significant if we note that research must satisfy the precondition of 'balanced doubt' on the part of the researcher between the efficacy of the experimental and conventional treatments. Another difference is that customary treatment and therapeutic research are intended to be beneficial to the individual patients, and non-therapeutic research is not. This difference may possibly alter the content of information imparted by the doctor or elicited by the parents in these different settings, but it does not alter the value of employing the subjective standard of disclosure in all settings.

It should also be noted that use of the subjective rule would reduce, if not entirely eliminate, bootlegging, in which study consent is bypassed by conventionalizing treatment which is still experimental. Clearly bootlegging is discouraged if standards of disclosure are the same for both customary and study consent.

Silverman called for studies to determine the effects of applying the same requirements for study consent and customary consent. Although I have favored this arrangement by promoting the use of the subjective standard of disclosure, this does not eliminate the need for empirical investigations to determine the most effective means by which this standard can be implemented. For any such future studies it is worth incorporating the following suggestions offered by Alan Meisel and Loren H. Roth.

1. We will need to know what the parents were told by the doctor. I would add that we also need to know what the parents told the doctor.
2. We will need to know, in detail, why parents are reluctant to obtain information from the doctor. I have already suggested that the status and manner of the doctor can be intimidating. But this is not the complete answer.
3. We will need to catalog the kinds of premises that affect parent decision-making. My earlier reference to a kind of static generated by fear, confusion, and unreality that can partially or completely cloak what the doctor is saying is only one sort of pressure.
4. We will need to learn how to distinguish between the expressed satisfaction or dissatisfaction with the information parents received from the doctor and their actual level of understanding.
5. We will need to learn the nature and extent of the causal connection between what the parents are told by the physician and what the parents decide.[34]

Silverman's call for empirical studies is also based on the perception of the need 'to devise practices that satisfy competing moral imperatives of respect for autonomy and concern for beneficence with emphasis on the value of health and a vigilance in the interests of distributive justice'.[35]

The existing double standard in customary and study consent will not necessarily produce a violation of the principle of distributive justice as embodied in the notion of like treatment for like condition. But one has reason to suspect that the possibility of such a violation is increased by what parents can or cannot consent to in these two settings. Although the use of any single set of requirements will help avoid this result, it is the subjective approach which is best able to satisfy the other moral imperatives. Beneficence toward the infant is likely to be achieved by taking account of the interests and values of the parents, and thus requires the use of the subjective approach. The one way that we can be certain that individuals are being treated as autonomous beings is by satisfying the conditions for valid informed consent, and this requires the use of the subjective approach.

It is my contention that whatever empirical studies are done to determine the effects of merging customary consent and study consent, we adopt the subjective standard of disclosure. This may increase the burdens already borne by the physician. But there are benefits as well. Shared decision-making based on the genuine participation of parents is likely to have a positive psychological effect not only on the parents but on the physician as well. In addition, the application of the subjective standard of disclosure protects and reinforces the moral integrity of the physician. For it is this standard which offers the only morally defensible approach to obtaining valid informed consent.

REFERENCES

1. Applebaum, P. S., Lidz, C. W., and Meisel, A. (1987). *Informed consent: legal theory and clinical practice.* Oxford University Press, New York.
2. Dworkin, G. (1982). Consent, representation and proxy consent. In *Who speaks for the child* (ed. W. Gaylin and R. Macklin). Plenum Press, New York. Cook, R. E. (1980). *Issues in research with human subjects.* National Institutes of Health Publication, No. 80-1858, Maryland. Magnet, J. E. and Kluge, E. W. (1985). *Withholding treatment from defective newborn children.* Brown Legal Publications, Quebec.
3 . Meisel, A. and Roth, L. H. (1983). Toward an informed discussion of informed consent: a review and critique of the empirical studies. *Arizona Law Review,* **25**, 333.
4. *Schloendorff* v. *Society of New York Hospitals* (1914). NY Supreme Court, Vol. 211, NY, 129–30.
5. *Salgo* v. *Leland Stanford Jr. Board of Trustees* (1957). 317 P. 21 170, **54**, 181. California.
6. *Canterbury* v. *Spence* (1972). US App. DC, 464 F20, 787.
7. Lidz, C. W., *et al.* (1984). *Informed consent: a study of decision making in psychiatry,* p. 18. The Guilford Press, New York.
8. Applebaum *et al.* (1987), p. 215.
9. Applebaum *et al.* (1987), p. 219.
10. Cohen, D., *et al.* (1983). Non-intervention in children with major handicaps: legal and ethical issues. *Australian Pediatric Journal,* **19**, 219. Law Reform Commission of Victoria (1989). Informed decisions about medical procedures. *Report,* **24**, 5.
11. Brown, F. N. (1980). Supreme Court judgment: courts may now enforce stricter standards of disclosure on doctors. *Canadian Medical Association Journal,* **123**, 1167. Gilmore, A. (1985). The nature of informed consent. *Canadian Medical Association Journal,* **132**, 1198–1203. CMA Policy Summary (1986). Informed decision-making. *Canadian Medical Association Journal,* **135**, 1208A.
12. Brahams, D. (1985). Doctor's duty to inform patient of substantial or special risks when offering treatment. *Lancet,* I (8427), 528–530. Schwartz, R. L. and Grubb, A. (1985). Why Britain can't afford informed consent. *Hastings Center Report,* **15** (4), 19–25. Mason, J. K. (1990). *Medico-legal aspects of reproduction and parenthood,* pp. 79–82. Dartmouth Publishing, Hants.
13. Mazur, V. J. (1988). Why the goals of informed consent are not realized. *Journal of General Internal Medicine,* **3**, 370–9.

14. Shaw, G. (1986). Informed consent: a German lesson. *International and Comparative Law Quarterly*, **35**, 864–89.
15. Ibid., p. 878.
16. Applebaum *et al.* (1987), p. 232.
17. *Canterbury* v. *Spence* (1972), 783.
18. Elster, J. (1989). *Nuts and bolts for the social sciences*, pp. 24–5. Cambridge University Press.
19. Mason, J. K. (1990). *Medico–legal Aspects of reproduction and parenthood*, p. 79. Dartmouth Publishing, Hants.
20. Gillon, R. (1989). Medical treatment, medical research and informed consent. *Journal of Medical Ethics*, **15**, 3–5, 11.
21. Tyson, J., this volume, Chapter 8A and Levine, R. J. (1981). *Ethics and regulation of clinical research*, pp. 6–8. Urban and Schwarzenberg, Baltimore.
22. Gillon (1989), p. 4.
23. Relman, A. S. (1992). What market values are doing to medicine. *The Atlantic Monthly*, 99–106.
24. A report on the ethical and legal implications of informed consent in the patient and practitioner relationship (1982). *President's Commission for the Study of Ethical Problems in Medicine, Biomedical and Behavioral Research* **38**.
25. Shaw (1986), p. 879.
26. Shaw (1986), p. 884.
27. Truog, R. D. (1992). Triage in the ICU. *Hastings Center Report*, **22**, No. 3, 13–17.
28. Paris, J. J., Crane, R. K., and Reardon, F. (1990). Physician's refusal of requested treatment: the case of Baby L. *New England Journal of Medicine*, **322**, 1013.
29. Fleischman, A. R. (1990). Point–counterpoint: physicians' refusal of requested treatment: views from the Journal's editorial board. *Journal of Perinatology*, **X**, No. 4, 407–15.
30. Perelman, R. H. and Fost, N. C. (1990). Point-counterpoint: physicians' refusal of requested treatment: views from the Journal's editorial board. *Journal of Perinatology*, X, No. 4, 413.
31. Schneiderman, L. J., Jecker, N.S., and Jonsen, A. R. (1990). Medical futility: its meaning and ethical implications. *Annals of Internal Medicine*, **112**, No. 12, 952.
32. Schneiderman *et al.* (1990), p. 953.
33. Stevenson, D. K. and Goldworth, A. (1989). The appropriateness of intensive care application. In *Fetal and neonatal brain injury: mechanism, management, and the risks of practice*, (ed. D. K. Stevenson and P. Sunshine pp. 264–72 B. C. Decker, Toronto.
34. Meisel and Roth (1983), pp. 275–280, 316.
35. This volume, Chapter 9A, pp. 000–000.

10
Government regulations in the United States

10A   GOVERNMENT REGULATIONS IN THE UNITED STATES

Ronald L. Ariagno

INTRODUCTION

The influence of the US Federal Government on the practice of medicine in the 1990s is felt very clearly by the entire nation. The powerful position of the Food and Drug Administration has been experienced by anyone who has attempted to introduce a new medical device or treatment, such as the high-frequency jet ventilator for infant use, or surfactant replacement therapy for pre-term infants who have respiratory failure due to immature lungs and surfactant deficiency at birth. The government regulation process seems to be an intentionally slow administrative maze which is demanding, difficult, often frustrating, and costly to the individual(s) requesting a review and seeking an approval. Nevertheless, the ultimate goal and purpose of the process is to ensure the ultimate protection of the nation's health and people. In the 1960s the inherent delays associated with this process serendipitously led to saving the American people from exposure to the teratologic fetal affects of thalidomide. This drug, commonly used in Europe for the suppression of nausea in early pregnancy, was later discovered to cause serious malformations of the upper limbs (phocomelia) in human infants, although no problems with limb development had been seen during animal testing of the drug.

One of the most notable events during the 1980s in perinatology was the Baby Doe Regulations, which inspired serious public, professional, and legal debate, ultimately extending to the US Supreme Court. The Baby Doe Regulations arose from the Reagan Administration's concern that there was nation-wide discrimination occurring in the medical care provided to handicapped newborn infants. Although there were landmark cases[1-3] in the literature, there was no factual basis for the Administration's allegation that this was a widespread national problem. Federal Baby Doe investigators (Baby Doe Squads) aggressively pursued any potential charge or complaint brought to their attention. In the case of the Baby Jane Doe from Stony Brook, New York, the right of access of the Federal Government to medical records was tested and overruled[4]. The effect of Government regulation on medical practice and the parents' role in the decisions for their children is potentially far-reaching. The pragmatic experience with the Baby Doe Regulations is mixed, and generally has not emphasized the best interest of the individual infant and family. On the positive side, the Baby Doe Regulations have stimulated national debate and the exploration of important issues associated with neonatal intensive care, and raised the issue of what are reasonable limits of care. The Regulations reveal the obvious: namely, the Federal Government does not have sufficient knowledge or expertise to practice medicine, and furthermore the Regulations are just too simplistic to be a true medical guideline. Nevertheless, the Regulations were broad enough to allow reasonable interpretation by ethical and competent medical practitioners and parents. In association with the Government Regulations the establishment of Ethics committees was recommended, and these are now commonplace in hospitals,[5] The purpose of this chapter is to explore in greater detail the evolution of the Baby Doe Regulations, the scholarly responses which it has fostered, and the effect on clinical neonatal intensive-care practice. In the final analysis medical thinking regarding the ethics of neonatal and perinatal practice has been advanced by the Baby Doe Regulations' sometimes painful stimulus beneath the medical mantle. Additionally, there have been some less favorable effects, such as *unrealistic views of autonomy* which are in conflict with reasonable medical care, *the use of certainty as an end-point for decision-making*, and the dissemination of the view that *the quality of life is irrelevant to medical decision-making*. These latter issues deserve comment and discussion.

THE BABY DOE RULE

A recent review of the Baby Doe Rule provides the salient details of regulation which culminated in the final Child Abuse Amendments which were published and signed by President Reagan in October 1984.[1] The final version of the proposed rule was published in the Federal Register (10 December 1984),[6] with a request that comments regarding the rule should be received by 8 February 1985. By 7 February 1985 there was a response from the Public Policy Council of the American Societies of the Academy of Pediatrics (the American Pediatric Society, the Association of Medical School Pediatric Department Chairmen, and the Society for Pediatric Research) which was sent to the National Center on Child Abuse and Neglect, US Children Bureau, 'to express deep concern regarding the impact of the proposed rules, 45 CFR1340, for implementation of Public Law 98-457, the Child Abuse Amendments of 1984 and accompanying interim model guidelines for establishment of infant-care review committees'. Currently, the proposed rule exists as amendments to the Child Abuse Prevention and Treatment Act (CAPTA), in which Congress set forth a strict standard for the treatment of impaired infants. The statute unified 'Right To Life' groups and certain medical organizations by calling for aggressive treatment of virtually all cases regardless of the degree of suffering imposed, the burdensome risks, or the outcome involved. Underlying the Federal rule-making there was deep distrust of parental decision-making, relegating most parents to a non-participatory bystander role. Congress did not make the rule automatically binding on the States, but made eligibility for the receipt of Federal funds dependent upon the incorporation of the rule into each State's law. Most States accepted this condition, and incorporated the rule into State child-abuse agency regulations. Indiana, California, and Pennsylvania decided not to accept the Federal mandate. The levels for CAPTA funding were extremely low, $45,000 to $680,000 (average amount $152,000), and therefore provided little monetary incentive for these States, who had the following expenditures for 1985 specifically earmarked for massive and ever-increasing problems of child abuse and neglect programs: Indiana $46 million, California $481 million, and Pennsylvania $245 million. The total funding for the entire nation in fiscal year 1987 was $9 million. Therefore, each State initially had the choice of applying for the CAPTA money and conforming their laws to the Federal Baby Doe Standard or making their own Baby Doe law and forfeiting the relatively small amounts of CAPTA funds. Next, it may be important to discuss how the Baby Doe legislation came about, and then to discuss in greater detail what it purports to do and how it might be applied in practice.

It is clear that there have been remarkable advances in neonatal care which have made it possible to save the lives of newborns who one or two decades ago would have died within the first few days of life or weeks after birth. Between 1970 and 1980, the mortality in the first 28 days of life dramatically decreased by 24 per cent, which was the greatest proportional decrease in any decade since 1915, when national birth certificates were first gathered.[7] The outcome of the smallest infants, infants weighing 1000–1500 g, also had a dramatic decrease in the mortality rate, from 50 per cent to 20 per cent or less since 1961. Further, half the live-born infants weighing <1000 g (2.2 lb) survived, compared with <10 per cent twenty years ago. In many intensive-care nurseries, infants ≥ 1000 g have a survival rate ≥ 90 per cent and infants ≥ 750 g have a survival rate of almost 70 per cent.[8] Also marked improvements have been reported in the survival of infants with certain congenital defects, particularly congenital heart malformations. It is recognized that not all seriously ill newborns have improved survival— in particular, some infants with very, very low birthweight (<750–800g.) or severe defects cannot survive for long despite modern neonatal intensive care and aggressive treatment.[9, 10] Further, infants who may recover can have severe impairments, either as part of their presenting condition or often as a result of newborn intensive care itself, and this fact is either unappreciated or underemphasized.[10, 11] Several articles[12–14] in fact have reported that with increasing newborn intensive-care efforts for the very, very low birth weight infant more aggressive treatment has extended the duration of time to death, but has not led to improved survival. Thus it has become important to appreciate the effect of various medical interventions and whether or not they will ultimately be beneficial to the child, the family, and the nation.

The need for testing the limits of medical certainty, diagnosis, and prognosis raises profound ethical issues, and should raise the question of whether medical certainty is ever the appropriate principle to apply. In all other areas of medicine the preferred *modus operandi* is to apply probabilistic reasoning to individual patients.[15] In a seminal report from Drs Duff and Campbell,[16] it was clear that modern newborn intensive-care nurseries do allow some infants to expire. The decision to withhold or withdraw treatment for newborns attracted considerable national attention in the 1980s, when it was learned that some infants who were allowed to die had severe congenital defects. The index case was Baby Doe, who died in Bloomington, Indiana in 1982 after his parents refused corrective surgery for birth defects (tracheoesophageal fistula: abnormal connection of the esophagus to the airway; frequently, the esophagus does not have continuity with the stomach); accompanying Down syndrome served as an impetus for the notification of health-care providers that Section 504 of the Rehabilitation Act of 1973 prohibits discrimination on the basis of handicap, and that this rule included the treatment of infants born with disabilities. On 30 April 1982 President Reagan instructed Richard Schweiker, Secretary of Health and Human Services (HHS), to notify health-care providers of the applicability of section 504 of the Rehabilitation Act of 1973 to the treatment of the handicapped patient (newborns). He also instructed Schweiker to notify health-care providers that Section 504 of the 1973 Rehabilitation Act 'forbids recipients of federal funds from withholding from handicap citizens simply because they are handicapped, any benefit or services that would ordinarily be provided to persons without handicaps'. On 18 May 1982, HHS notified all the nation's 6800 hospitals of the applicability of Section 504, and that they risked losing Federal funds if they withheld treatment or nourishment from handicapped infants. Investigative procedures and 'the Baby Doe hotline' for reporting cases by telephone were established to police non-compliance. The notice referred to the Bloomington case, and stated '. . . it is unlawful . . . to withhold from a handicapped infant nutritional sustenance, medical, or surgical treatment required to correct a life-threatening condition, if:(1) the withholding is based on the fact that the infant is handicapped; and (2) the handicap does not render the treatment or nutritional sustenance medically contraindicated'. By March 1983 HHS issued an interim final rule. The rule was promulgated to prohibit discrimination on the basis of handicap under Section 504 of the Rehabilitation Act of 1973 (see Table 10.1).[1] These Rules were declared invalid by US District Court Judge Gerhardt Geseli on 4 April 1983, since the rules were considered an extraordinary intrusion of the State into medical care.

The Regulations are curious on a number of counts: (1) They were issued

Table 10.1 Summary of events leading up to the 'Baby Doe' rule

9/4/82	'Infant Doe' born with Down syndrome and esophageal atresia with tracheo-esophageal fistula; parents refuse surgery; juvenile court judge upholds parents; baby dies 5 days later
30/4/82	President Reagan instructs the Secretary of Health and Human Services (HHS) to notify health-care providers of the applicability of §504 of the Rehabilitation Act of 1973 to the treatment of handicapped patients (newborns)
18/5/82	HHS notifies hospitals of the applicability of §504 and establishes investigative procedures for non-compliance.
7/3/83	HHS issues an interim final rule.
14/4/83	Interim final rule declared invalid.
5/7/83	HHS issues proposed rules, with 60-day comment period.
11/10/83	Baby 'Jane Doe' born with myelomeningocele, microencephaly, hydrocephalus, and other birth defects.
15/10/83	Lawrence Washburn, a right-to-life attorney, contacts New York Supreme Court Judge Frank DeLuca.
18/10/83	Judge Tanenbaum appoints William Weber as guardian *ad litem* for baby Jane Doe without notice to the hospital or parents.
19/10/83	Hearings commence on the petition before Judge Tanenbaum.
20/10/83	Judge Tanenbaum upholds Washburn's petition
21/10/83	Five justices of the New York Supreme Court, Appellate Division, reverse Judge Tanenbaum's decision.
24/10/83	An appeal is filed in the New York State Court of Appeals.
27/10/83	HHS advises university hospital that it is initiating legal action for non-compliance with §504.
28/10/83	New York Court of Appeals upholds baby Jane Doe's parents' right to withhold surgery.
2/11/83	US Justice Department files a petition in US District Court against university hospital for non-compliance with §504.
4/11/83	Arguments begin in the US District Court.
8/11/83	New York State Attorney General's Office files a brief in US District Court, arguing that the Federal Government does not have jurisdiction in this case.
10/11/83	Six organizations representing the disabled file an *amicus curiae* brief supporting the Federal Government's request to inspect the medical records
17/11/83	Judge Leonard Wexler denies the Federal Government's request
18/11/83	Justice Department files notice of appeal.
12/12/83	US Supreme Court refuses Mr Weber's request that it hear the case of baby Jane Doe.
23/12/83	Washburn initiates a class action suit on behalf of baby Jane Doe and other newborn infants similarly situated.

Table 10.1 (*cont.*)

30/12/83	Washburn files a motion to appoint a new guardian *ad litem* for baby Jane Doe.
12/1/84	HHS issues final rules, effective 13 Feb. 1984, on 'Non-discrimination on the Basis of Handicap: Procedures and Guidelines Relating to Health Care for Handicapped Infants'.
20/1/84	Judge Roger J. Miner refuses Washburn's request.
2/2/84	US House of Representatives passes the Child Abuse Protection Bill (HR 1904).
23/2/84	Second Circuit US Court of Appeals affirms the District Court's ruling in university hospital's favor that the Federal Government be denied access to baby Jane Doe's medical records.
1/3/84	Washburn appeals the decision of 20 Jan. 1984.
8/3/84	Shunt surgery performed on baby Jane Doe.
12/3/84	American Medical Association and American Hospital Association file suit in US District Court seeking to invalidate HHS regulations
28/3/84	Baby Jane Doe discharged from university hospital
19/4/84	Washburn withdraws his appeal to the US Court of Appeals
26/7/84	After negotiation with hospital associations, physician groups, and disability and right-to-life groups, the US Senate passes its version of the Child Abuse Protection Bill (S 1003); unlike HR 1904, S 1003 defines 'withholding medically indicated treatment'.
16/8/84	Justice Department announces it will not continue efforts to obtain baby Jane Doe's medical records.
9/84	Both Houses pass an amended bill.
2/10/84	Justice Department appeals the US District Court's decision in May that invalidated the Baby Doe rules published in January
10/12/84	Proposed rule published in the Federal Register; comments for consideration are to be received by 8 Feb. 1985.
7/2/85	Public Policy Council of the American Societies of Academic Pediatrics (the American Pediatric Society, the Association of Medical School Pediatric Department Chairman, and the Society for Pediatric Research) sends missive to National Center on Child Abuse and Neglect, US Children's Bureau to express deep concern regarding the impact of the proposed rules, 45 CFR Part 1340, for implementation of Public Law 98-457, the Child Abuse Amendments of 1984, and the accompanying interim model guidelines for establishment of infant care review committees'.

by an administration that professed to abhor government regulation and demonstrated little involvement with the welfare of children in other settings. (2) They were promulgated despite formidable expert opposition from the president's own Commission[17] for the Study of Ethical Problems in Medicine and Biomedical and Behavioral Research, and from members of the medical profession who actually live with these difficult problems. Judge Gesell's decision followed from a suit against the Baby Doe legislation which was presented by the American Academy of Pediatrics, the National Association of Children's Hospitals and Related Institutions, and the Children's Hospital National Medical Center, and was supported by the American Medical Association and an *amicus* brief. (3) The Regulation's were based on the premiss that all life, no matter how miserable, should be maintained if technically possible. (4) They attempted a remarkable distinction between medical decisions and decisions concerning the well-being of the patient, the latter of which were felt to be outside a physician's purview and better addressed within the purview of the government. The rules overlooked the parents of the handicapped infants except to exclude them from decisions about life-sustaining treatment for their children. (5) They carried an adversarial tone implying that handicapped newborns require protection from their parents and physicians.[18]

In summary, the initial Baby Doe rules and the final one of 1984 are based on the premiss that *all life, no matter how compromised, must be maintained if it is technically possible.* This is ironic, since the Federal Government had chosen to reduce financial assistance to social programs which would prevent high-risk pregnancies and decrease the number of complicated deliveries and reduce the risk of disabling of infants; aid to programs which may provide life-long care to the disabled people and their families had also been reduced. The Federal decision appeared to have been made in a vacuum, with little awareness or responsibility for the consequences that followed the application of the rule. For the many reasons cited above and in what follows, it would be best if the government distanced itself from medical decision-making as much as possible. Usually medical decision-making in the neonatal intensive-care unit is about what is reasonably probable and beneficial, and less often an ethical decision about what is good or bad. Many consider that the envisioned role for protecting the handicapped infant from moral indiscretion is largely fantasized. The government's role should not be one of specifying which infants should or should not receive treatment, but in providing general guidelines for how such decisions should proceed in practice.

Admittedly, medical decisions by experienced professionals even with the most complete and timely information can be extremely difficult. Rhoden[15] has recommended an individualized probabilistic model for decision-making which will be discussed in greater detail when we consider the Baby Doe rule applied to practice. The aggressive 'treatment until certain' approach suggested by the Baby Doe rule is discordant with this approach.[14]

The Section 504 Final Rule was entitled 'Non discrimination on the basis of handicap; procedures and guidelines relating to health care for handicapped infants from the Office of the Secretary, HHS'.[6] These final rules were issued under the authority of Section 504 of the Rehabilitation Act of 1973, which prohibited discrimination on the basis of handicap and penalized programs by withholding Federal financial assistance for failure to abide by these rules. The rules also required the establishment of an effective mechanism for enforcing Section 504 in connection with health care for handicapped infants. Hospitals were encouraged to establish policies and procedures to implement the principle that treatment decisions for handicapped infants should be based on reasonable medical judgments and beneficial treatment or nourishment should not be withheld solely on the basis of an infant's present or anticipated mental or physical impairments. The rules included a recommendation for the establishment of an Infant Care Review Committee to assist hospitals in their effort, and required the posting of an informational notice in hospitals stating the rights of handicapped infants and a 'hotline' telephone number for reporting 'violations'. They did not require provision of futile treatments, nor did they presume to interfere with reasonable medical judgments. The rules required that the State child protective services have established procedures for applying their own State laws protecting children from medical neglect. The involvement of qualified medical consultants was encouraged, as well as the protection of confidential information. It was stated that 'it was hoped that the rules will foster a new process of cooperative efforts and sensible approaches to advance the principle of life and that medical treatments be based on informed judgments of medical benefits and risks and not on stereotypes and prejudices against handicapped persons'. The new rules for health care for handicapped infants indicated that (1) health-care providers are prohibited from withholding treatment or nourishment from an infant who might benefit medically solely on the basis of anticipated physical or mental impairments; (2) stated that it was acceptable to withhold futile treatment or therapy; (3) stated that reasonable medical judgments would be respected; (4) stated that lack of parental consent does lessen the hospitals' obligation to treat handicapped infants; and (5) gave examples of medical conditions and their correct treatment, although HHS recognized the need to evaluate the cases on their individual medical facts. The child-abuse rule defines withholding medically indicated treatment 'as failure to respond to an infant's life-threatening conditions by providing treatment (including appropriate nutrition, hydration, and medication) which in the treating physician's reasonable medical judgment will be most likely to be effective in ameliorating or correcting all such conditions'. Furthermore, 'exceptions to the requirement to provide treatment (but not the requirement to provide appropriate nutrition, hydration, and medication) can be made only in cases in which: (1) *the infant is chronically and irreversibly comatose*; or (2) *the provision of such treatment would merely prolong dying or not be effective in ameliorating or correcting the infant's life-threatening conditions or otherwise be futile in terms of the survival of the infant*; or (3) *the provision of such treatment would be virtually futile in terms of survival of the infant and the treatment itself under such circumstances would be inhumane*'.[6, 19]

THE BABY DOE RULE APPLIED TO PRACTICE

Neonatologists as a group are usually very proactive about providing intensive care for critically ill pre-term and term newborns. At Stanford University Medical Center, as in most institutions in the nation, the practice has been to initiate full resuscitation and intensive-care support routinely unless there is clear documentation that the infant has a lethal disorder which has either no treatment or treatment of such limited potential benefit for the child (for example, anencephaly) as to make the treatment futile, inhumane, or unreasonable. Therefore those infants who otherwise would have been 'stillborn' before the institution of this proactive intensive-care approach are now alive, and require a thorough and expeditious evaluation to diagnose their problems and to determine potential reasonable treatment(s) and the probability that such treatments are likely to improve survival and lead to an outcome with minimal significant associated morbidity due to treatment. Although morbidity may not be entirely avoidable, the morbidity should not be more severe than the infant's presenting problem, and the burden of the treatment should be offset by a clear benefit at a reasonable risk. Theoretically and practically *most* infants in a high-risk perinatal center can be revived and supported with intensive-care technology. However, it does not follow automatically that there is a reasonable probability that all these infants will survive or have a reasonable outcome, i.e., that the benefit to the infant will be greater than the tragedy of non-survival. For example, a term infant with congenital hypoplastic lungs (minimal lung development inadequate to support the body's oxygen or ventilation requirements) who is placed on chronic cardiopulmonary bypass to support the child's oxygen and ventilation requirements artificially. This condition must be regarded as lethal in the absence of some discovery or experimental treatment, for example lung transplantation, that may have some potential to alter this prognosis. Before we dismiss the notion that it is unthinkable to imagine that an intervention may occur just because we have a technology that has a minimal, potential, or unsubstantiated outcome, be advised that this can and does happen, both for good and for ill-conceived reasons. The admonition that is sometimes offered is to 'do everything', which is frequently interpreted by the neonatologist and the newborn-intensive-care staff as permission to do anything that may have any possibility of benefit, regardless how low or unsubstantiated the probability may be that there will be a significant long-term benefit to the child.

The usual neonatology practice, which encompasses an automatic aggressive provision for resuscitation and intensive technological support of the critically ill infant at the outset, is defensible and justifiable when employed for a reasonable benefit for the infant. However, well-reasoned caution and expertise are required to promote and to serve the best interests of the child, the family, and society. It cannot be over-emphasized that the practice of sustaining the infant's vital function long enough to allow time for evaluation of the possibility (and, more importantly, the probability) that continued intensive-care support will provide reasonable benefit is a relatively new challenge. The fact that intensive-care support can effectively support vital function does not mean that the medical problem(s) will resolve, or that the growth and development of the infant can be supported, or that the serious morbidity inextricably associated with intensive-care support can be minimized or prevented. An example would be the case of a 24–25 weeks gestation infant, who will usually require prolonged mechanical ventilator support for weeks and more often months, and under the best of circumstances will have a ≤10 per cent survival and a 50 per cent risk of handicapping morbidity (retinopathy of prematurity, intracranial hemorrhage, and/or chronic lung disease).[9–11] In the majority of cases these infants born at an early gestation are normally developed fetuses who have insufficient independent function for extrauterine adaptation, and are at significant risk for acquiring disease/morbidity associated with the application of intensive-care support. One interpretation of the Baby Doe rule would be that if there is any chance that this very immature infant might survive then everything must be done irrespective of the morbidity (handicap), the quality of life, or the personal cost and suffering which the infant, in particular, and also the family must endure. As was mentioned above, 'do everything' is not tempered by what is reasonable or in the best interest of the infant, and includes any intensive-care treatment irrespective of whether in this application it has a reasonable probability of success or benefit towards the ultimate recovery of the patient. Furthermore, treatment based on a *possible (not probable)* benefit with disregard for the risk to the patient is reprehensible. In contrast, the full-term infant born with Down syndrome (trisomy 21, i.e., with an extra chromosome 21) with a duodenal atresia (a congenital complete intestinal obstruction in the small intestine) that requires a surgical correction which can alleviate the gastrointestinal problem at a relatively low risk does not face the same intensive-care risks as the 24 weeks' gestation pre-term infant. The morbidity of the Down syndrome infant is more often associated with the chromosome abnormality, and not with the intensive-care, which contrasts significantly with the case of the 24 weeks' gestation infant. A final example to illustrate this point can be made by combining the diagnoses of 24 weeks' gestation and Down syndrome in the same patient. Is the recommended treatment obvious? In most cases any additional significant anomaly in the 24 weeks' gestation infant would make the application of intensive care unreasonable and inappropriate.

Rhoden[15] has described three decision strategies: (1) the *'wait until certain'* approach, which includes continuing aggressive treatment until death or until irreversible coma seems almost certain; (2) *statistical prognostic strategy*, which includes withholding treatment from infants for whom as a group the prognosis is grim; and (3) the *individualized prognostic strategy*, which includes starting treatment and then evaluating and re-evaluating, on the basis of the reasonableness of the treatment plan and the probability of benefitting the recovery of the infant. Both the first and the last approach can be compatible with application of the Baby Doe rule; however, the 'wait until certain' strategy is the least medically defensible when the overwhelming probability is that the likelihood of death or surviving with serious morbidity is great if aggressive intensive care is continued. The rule intends to protect the lives of the infants who are at risk, but ignores their human right to die.[20] The orientation of many neonatologists and intensive-care nurseries is towards aggressive intensive care. In many circumstances the approach of 'doing everything' is inappropriately justified as necessary because of the uncertainty of the outcome and the existence of the Baby Doe rule. The rule facilitates the use of overaggressive and medically indefensible plans, which can then be followed with impunity. Neonatologists have raised the question of whether aggressive intensive care in some circumstances is experimental, as a consequence of minimal or insufficient scientific data.[23] For example, a 24-weeks gestation infant with minimal mechanical ventilation and supplemental oxygen (25 per cent) requirements at 72 hours of life, with a bilateral grade 4 (severe) intracranial hemorrhage, has a significant probability of major acquired abnormalities (brain abnormalities and limitation of development). In order to survive the infant would require a minimum of several months of intensive care, during which additional risk of unavoidable complications must be endured. This infant is not capable of independent function, and simple non-intensive care measures cannot support function. Is aggressive intensive care reasonable? With the Baby Doe rule as a guide it could be and is interpreted as such in many intensive-care units in the nation. Where is the wisdom of this legislation, and what is the evidence that this is in the best interest of the infant? The rule did not deal with the issue of what neonatal intensive care is, and the potential unavoidable adverse effects which are incurred if it is applied aggressively. The result in practice, which may not have been anticipated, is that the rule is often used as the defense for aggressive and medically indefensible intensive care.

THE INFANT CARE REVIEW COMMITTEE

The rule deserves credit for raising our consciousness about ethical issues in perinatology (pregnancy and newborn problems) and for recommending infant care review committees for resolving difficult issues. At Stanford University Medical Center an infant care committee was in place in 1975 before the Baby Doe rules. The following is an outline which summarizes high-risk circumstances which *may* indicate when a formal bioethics review may be helpful:

1. *Conditions or diagnoses present at birth or known prenatally*: (a) very, very low birthweight (≤750gms) or extremely pre-term infant (<28 weeks' gestation);(b) infants with multiple congenital anomalies in which the potentially lethal condition(s) can only be palliated in contrast to corrected, or where other significant aggravating circumstances such as

prematurity are present;(c) hypoplastic ventricle syndrome; (d) inborn errors of metabolism which present in the neonatal period and have only research therapies and palliation available; (e) pulmonary hypoplasia; (f) severe brain injury or central nervous system malformation in infants who are ventilator-dependent; (g) severe congenital musculoskeletal disorders which severely limit or may permanently prevent spontaneous or independent breathing; (h) major congenital malformations consistent with the probability of insufficient gastrointestinal nutrient absorptive surface, which may not provide potential for the development of sufficient intestinal alimentation and independence from parenteral nutrition.

2. *Conditions or diagnoses acquired postnatally*: (a) prolonged ventilator dependence beyond 2–4 weeks; (b) prolonged parenteral (intravenous) alimentation as the primary nutrition over one month; (c) major central nervous system hemorrhage (grades 3–4) with or without accompanying hydrocephalus; (d) prolonged multi-organ failure for 1 week or longer; (e) potentially lethal condition(s) which does not have a definitive therapy or only has a research therapy; (f) conditions where intensive care is the only 'definitive' therapy for 1 month or longer.

3. *Medical/nursing and intensive-care team considerations*: (a)cases where the entire attending medical staff (three or more) of a multi-care team have attended the infant; (b) cases where there is a major disagreement or impasse about the medical care plan except for the intensive care; (c) cases where the only indication or justification for continuing intensive care is parental demand; (d) cases where there is a major disagreement between members of the intensive-care team regarding what is reasonable or appropriate medical and/or surgical therapy; (e) cases where there is a major and substantive disagreement among consultants.

In our practice the bioethics committee has been very useful to infants, families, and our staff when there are complicated issues which cannot be addressed at the bedside. Nevertheless, the committee has always been advisory and not had the responsibility to decide itself; rather it has appropriately left the responsibility for medical decisions to the medical staff who are responsible for the infant's medical care.

THE CASE OF BABY L AND THE RIGHTS OF THE MEDICAL-CARE PROVIDER

In the Baby L case[21] the physicians refused the requested treatment of the parents for their two-year-old daughter who was born at 36 weeks' gestation, weighing 1970 gms, and had fetal hydronephrosis (dilated kidney system due to blockage of urine flow) and oligohydraminos (decreased amniotic fluid) in the last trimester. Her vital function was depressed at birth, and she had aspirated meconium (infant stool passed during distress before birth) at birth, and required resuscitation at birth and mechanical ventilator support. Her respiratory function improved over several weeks; however, her neurologic status remained very abnormal and depressed, with minimal responsiveness except for pain. She also had poor retention of food in her stomach and had recurrent aspiration of food into her lungs, which was apparently not improved by surgical treatments (a gastrostomy-feeding tube inserted into the stomach through the abdominal wall at 3 months; fundoplication— creating an artificial valve function at the top of the stomach—at 4 months; and a tracheotomy at 7 months). She had been discharged home at 14 months with 24 hours nursing care, but was readmitted in 2 weeks for recurrent pneumonia and seizures. At the time of the physicians' refusal of continuing aggressive care she had worsening pneumonia and sepsis that required mechanical ventilator and cardiovascular support.

It is comprehensible that parents should express their love for their child through a request for medical intervention, in the unbridled hope that by some miracle it may alter the tragic situation. On emotional and subjective grounds their position is fairly clear, and their sincerity is unquestioned. Nevertheless, the reality of the child's condition must be addressed responsibly for the child. From the history given it was unlikely under the best of circumstances that the infant would resolve the continuing dysfunction (mostly neurological) which placed her at very high risk for recurrent pneumonia and sepsis. Although the parents and family were suffering, how does that address the more serious problem and concern, viz, the infant's extended suffering, and at what gain or personal benefit? In surrogate decision-making, in my experience, the other's pain is often not appreciated in a realistic way: for example, while it may be possible to have empathy for another's pain, this is not the same as actually feeling it.

The physicians' refusal to continue aggressive intensive care appears reasonable and medically defensible, since the probability of truly benefiting the child was unlikely. The term 'futile' is an appropriate description, in view of the probable outcome. A meeting of the chiefs of service, primary-care physicians, nurses, hospital counsel, and chairpersons of the institutional ethics committee was convened in this case, and they agreed unanimously that further medical intervention was not in the best interests of the child. The judge acceded to the mother's request, and asked the physicians what they would do if they were ordered to continue mechanical ventilation. The physicians and hospital indicated that following such an order would violate their ethical obligation to the patient. A guardian *ad litem* was appointed for the child. The guardian requested another neurologic consultant, who confirmed the neurologic findings, but nevertheless agreed to assume responsibility for the infant's care.

The infant survived the incident, and two years later she remains blind, deaf, and quadriplegic, receives gastrostomy feedings, and has intermittent intractable seizures. Her lung function is better; however, she requires 16 hours of intensive nursing care per day, and developmentally is at a three-month level. From a medical perspective it is honestly extremely difficult to argue that the benefit to this child was greater than the harm. If intensive care was not needed the decision-making would have been entirely different, and the outcome could have been just as unfortunate; however, intensive care in this case was required, and responsible decision-making was warranted. An order to continue mechanical ventilation is simplistic, like the rule, in that it demonstrates *naïveté* about what is involved in responsibility for the complete care of this child. It is treating a very complex situation as if it were simply the decision to put the switch in the on or off position.

Some philosophers and the law overlook or choose not to consider that intensive care, in itself, is potentially adverse, not neutral, even if applied to the entirely healthy individual. If the logic of what is possible must be followed irrespective of the results one can begin to prognosticate adverse outcomes, as seen in this case, with excellent probability and accuracy. Unfortunately, some would argue that, even though the results predicted are miserable, that does not make the use of aggressive intensive care indefensible in this instance.[22]

On the other hand few would care to generalize the approach of medical decision-makers to chose or recommend management and treatment based on the lowest probability of a favourable outcome. Furthermore, few would choose the position that the quality of the outcome is insignificant. Although intensive care is a common event in the news, its prevalence in the care of newborns is relatively rare. It is difficult medically or economically to think of intensive care as routine. Those professionally trained and skilled to administer intensive care to newborns number a few thousand neonatologists in the entire nation. The order to continue mechanical ventilation is revealing in its limited perspective about what is offered and what is involved in the care of the critically ill infant. Maybe it is a confusion about the difference between 'life-support' and 'support of vital function'; the former is imaginary, and the later is temporarily achievable in many, but not in all, circumstances. It is usually better and wiser to address what is medically probable for the individual in most circumstances, rather than launching into some theoretical paradigm which may eclipse important medical data[23] and the value and rights of a person.[24, 25]

In the Report of the President's Commission for the Study of Ethical Problems in Medicine and Biomedical and Behavioral Research *Deciding to forgo life-sustaining treatment* the problem of the seriously ill newborn with a clearly futile therapy was addressed.[17] They concurred that the decision of surrogates and medical providers not to try predictably futile endeavors is ethically and legally justifiable when there is no probability of saving a life for a substantial period. Nevertheless, they recognized that any prolongation of life and any possibility of hope may lead some parents to demand therapy which is believed by the physician to be futile. Surprisingly, they concluded in this instance that the parents' wish should be accepted, as long as this choice does not cause substantial suffering for the child. They recommend that health professionals who find it personally offensive to engage in futile treatment should arrange to be withdrawn from the case. It is difficult to understand how the best interests of the child are served by causing any unnecessary pain and by denying the human right to die. This invitation to overlook *primum non nocere* does not appear justified from the infant's perspective, which should include the need for comfort and respect. For these infants medicine and law provide no real assistance by demanding aggressive medical therapy. Furthermore, prolonging the infant's process of dying by inadequately conceived medical or legal recommendations is usually indefensible from the perspective of insufficient or no evidence for any reasonable potential benefit. The position regarding treatment options for seriously ill newborns—physician's assessment in relation to parent's preference—as presented in Table 10.2[17] raises the question of whether providing treatment *when the assessment is ambiguous or or uncertain* is defensible in most medical circumstances when there is no measurable probability of benefit for the infant. This same bias is conveyed in the Baby Doe rule, which does not address the issue of the possibility vs. the probability that a treatment will be beneficial. In most medical problems the treatment is based upon experience and data which support the probability of the effectiveness of a plan or recommendation. Accepting any possible treatment without regard for effectiveness courts a preponderance of harm over benefit. Furthermore, a subtlety which must be acknowledged is that a therapeutic recommendation which is reported in the literature may not realistically represent the expertise of most health-providers or of the health-provider responsible for the infant's care. For example, a heart operation for a hypoplastic left heart may be described in the literature as attended with a certain level of success; however, this result may represent only one or two cardiac surgeons' experience. The literature may support the contention that the treatment is effective in the experience of the authors—which does not necessarily imply that it will be in the hands of most cardiac surgeons. Hence the position of the literature may not be consonant with the expertise of most practitioners. The need for an individualized prognostic approach to the patient which includes all the factors that can be identified is obvious.

SUMMARY AND CONCLUSIONS

The Baby Doe rules are generally taken seriously throughout the nation, regardless of whether a particular State has incorporated the Child Abuse Amendments into its State laws. A recent report from the US Commission on Civil Rights[26] focused on questions of discrimination and withholding of medical services from individuals with disabilities primarily because of their disabilities; however, they did not propose to '. . . oversee, evaluate, or question the exercise of legitimate medical judgment inherent in decision-making concerning medical treatment'.

Sound medical decisions are best supported with an individualistic probability strategy which allows the use of complete clinical data, clinical experience, consultation, and the available literature, applied for the benefit of an individual infant. The approach of treating until medically certain of

Table 10.2 Treatment options for seriously ill newborns—physician's assessment in relation to parents' preference

Physician's assessment of treatment options*	Parents prefer to accept treatment**	Parents prefer to forgo treatment**
Clearly beneficial	Provide treatment	Provide treatment during review process
Ambiguous or uncertain	Provide treatment	Forgo treatment
Futile	Provide treatment unless provider declines to do so	Forgo treatment

* The assessment of the value to the infant of the treatments available will initially be by the attending physician. Both when this assessment is unclear and when the joint decision between parents and physician is to for go treatment, this assessment would be reviewed by intra-institutional mechanisms and possibly thereafter by-court.
** The choice made by the infant's parents or some other duly authorized surrogate who has adequate decision-making capacity and has been adequately informed, based on his, her, or their assessment of the infant's best interests.

the outcome is difficult to defend with medical data. The wisdom evolving through the Baby Doe rule saga has been to examine neonatal and perinatal practice critically. The rule runs awry when it pretends to guide complicated decision-making in isolation from medical literature and experience.

It is usually better and wiser to address what is medically probable for the individual rather than launching into some theoretical paradigm which may eclipse important medical data and the value and rights of a person. Medical decisions based on uncertainty issues and the possibility (undefined or unsubstantiated) of benefit, without regard for probability, invite poor, expensive, and medically indefensible practices of dubious benefit for the infant, its family, and society at large.

REFERENCES

1. Stevenson, D. K., Ariagno, R. L., Kutner, J. S. Raffin, T. A., and Young, E. W. D.: The 'Baby Doe' rule. *JAMA*, **255**: 1909–12, 1986.
2. Weir R. F.: Sounding board: the government and detective non-treatment of handicapped infants. *N Engl. J. Med.* **309**! 661–3, 1983.
3. Shapiro, A. L. and Rosenberg, P.: The effect of Federal regulations regarding handicapped newborns: a case report. *JAMA*, **252**: 2031–3, 1984.
4. Fox, D. M. Special section on the treatment of handicapped newborns. *Journal of Heath Politics, Policy and Law*, **11**(2): 195–297, 1986.
5. Fleischman, A. R.: Bioethics Review Committees in perinatology. *Clin. Perinatol.* **14**: 379–93, 1987.
6. *Federal Register.* **49**: 1622–54, 1984.
7. Wegman, M. E.: Annual summary of vital statistics—1980. *Pediatrics*, **68**: 755–62, 1981.

8. Avery, M. E.: History and epidemiology. In *Diseases of the newborn*, (ed. H. W. Taeusch, R. A. Ballard, and M. E. Avery), 6th edn, pp. 1–9. W. B. Saunders, Philadelphia, 1991.

9. Praju, N. K.: An epidemiologic study of very and very very low birth weight infants. In *Clinics in Perinatology*, **13**: 233–50, 1986.

10. Young, E. W. D. and Stevenson, D. K.: Limiting treatment for extremely premature, low-birth-weight infants (500 to 750g). *AJDC*, **144**: 549–52, 1990.

11. McCormick, M. C., Brooke-Gann, J., Workman-Daniels, K., Turner, J., and Peckham, G.: The health and developmental status of very low birth weight children at school age. *JAMA*, **267**: 2204–8, 1992.

12. Hack, M. and Fanaroff, A. A.: Changes in the delivery room care of the extremely small infant (<750 gm)—Effects on morbidity and outcome. New Engl.J.Med. **214**: 660–4, 1986.

13. Hack, M. and Fanaroff, A. A.: Outcomes of extremely low birth weight infants between 1982 and 1988. New Engl. J.Med. **321**: 1642–7, 1989.

14. Fischer, A. F. Stevenson, D. K.: The consequences of uncertainty—an empirical approach to medical decision making in neonatal intensive care. *JAMA*, **258**: 1929–31, 1987.

15. Rhoden, N. K.: Treating Baby Doe: the ethics of uncertainty. *Hastings Center Report*, pp. 34–42, August 1986.

16. Duff, R. S. and Campbell, A. G. M.: Moral and ethical dilemmas in the special care nursery. *New Engl. J. Med.* **289**: 890–4, 1973.

17. Seriously III newborns. In *Deciding to for go life sustaining treatment*. President's Commission for the study of ethical problems in medicine and biomedical and behavioral research. March 21, 1983. Superintendent of Documents, US Government Printing Office, Washington, DC 20402, pp. 97–229.

18. Lantos, J.: Sounding board, Baby Doe five years later, implications for child health. *New Engl. J. Med.*, **317**: 444–7, 1987.

19. *Federal Register*: **50**: 14878-901, 1985.

20. Goldworth, A. and Stevenson, D. K.: The real challenge of "Baby Doe": considering the scarcity and quality of life. *Clin. Pediatr.* **28**(3): 119–22, 1989.

21. Paris, J. J., Crone, R. K., Reardon, F.: Physicians' refusal of requested treatment: the case of Baby L. *New Engl. J. Med.*, **332**: 1012–15, 1990.

22. Journal of Perinatology Editorial Board: Point–counterpoint: physicians' refusal of requested treatment. *J. Perinatol.* **10**, 407–15, 1990.

23. Sinclair, J. C.: Assessing evidence concerning treatment and prevention of diseases of the newborn. In *Effective care of the newborn infant*, (ed. J. C. Sinclair and M. B. Brozken MB, pp. 3–12. Oxford University Press, 1992.

24. Goldworth, A. G. and Stevenson, D. K.: The real challenge of "Baby Doe": considering the sanctity and quality of life. *Clin. Pedia.*, **28**: 119–22, 1989.

25. Whitelaw, A.: Death as an option in neonatal care. *Lancet*, August 9: 328–31, 1986.

26. *Medical discrimination against children with disabilities*, A report of the US Commission on Civil Rights, September 1989, pp. 1–513.

10B BABY DOE AND BEYOND: THE PAST AND FUTURE OF GOVERNMENT REGULATION IN THE UNITED STATES

Henry T. Greely

INTRODUCTION

It is not surprising that a doctor and lawyer see issues from a different perspective, even issues as stark as life and death in the neonatal intensive-care unit. The story Dr Ariagno shows us is a familiar one, and a powerful one; but, to legal eyes, it is not a complete one. This commentary will attempt to add a lawyer's vision to the story. It will first examine more closely the Baby Doe case and regulations. It will then look at the possible future course of government regulation of neonatal life and death in the United States.

THE HISTORY OF BABY DOE AND THE CONSEQUENT REGULATION

Like many stories from the neonatal intensive-care unit, the tale of Baby Doe is a tragic story of hope defeated and joyful expectations dashed. The history of the subsequent eponymous regulations tells a tale of different expectations, also ultimately, if less dramatically, defeated. Both stories ultimately raise hard questions, questions that the US Government may have addressed poorly or improperly, but questions that inherently lack easy answers. I believe it is worthwhile to look at the child, the regulations, and the litigation over those regulations in some detail.

On 9, April, 1982, as on most days, several children were born in Bloomington, Indiana. One of these children, however, was born with both Down syndrome and, for apparently unrelated reasons, problems with his or her esophagus, which have been described in the literature as an esophageal atresia, an esophageal obstruction, and a tracheo-esophageal fistula. Whatever the precise nature of the problem, all agreed that it could easily be remedied by fairly standard surgical interventions. If it were not remedied, however, food could not get into the infant's stomach. The child's Down syndrome, on the other hand, could not be remedied. People with Down syndrome, one of the more common causes of mental retardation, are intellectually impaired, although to widely varying degrees. The severity of Baby Doe's impairment could not be clearly foretold.

The child's parents asked the hospital to withold both the corrective surgery and the intravenous feeding that could have nourished the infant. The hospital asked the Indiana courts whether it should comply with the parents' requests. The courts told the hospital to respect the parents' wishes, so the infant was medicated with phenobarbital and morphine for comfort while he or she starved to death. The infant died while attorneys were seeking to persuade the United States Supreme Court to stay the Indiana decision. After the baby's death, the Supreme Court ultimately dismissed the petition as moot.[1]

This case attracted great public attention and controversy. Within five weeks of the infant's death, the Reagan Administration issued a 'Notice to Health Care Providers', warning that withholding services from handicapped infants that would ordinarily be provided to other infants could violate the Federal Rehabilitation Act of 1973 ('the Act').

The Rehabilitation Act seemed an odd vehicle for intervention in neonatal decision-making. It had been passed as a weak effort to alleviate discrimination against the handicapped (the favored term in 1973, since supplanted by the terms 'disabled' or 'persons with disabilities'). The Act prohibited discrimination against the handicapped by the Federal Government in employment or in the provision of services, by most firms that contracted with the Federal Government, and, in Section 504, by entities that received Federal financial assistance. Almost all, if not all, hospitals in the United States qualify under one or more of those categories as a result of receiving substantial Federal financial assistance or Federal compensation. Violation of the Act could lead to the withdrawal of eligibility for Federal funds. For many hospitals, a withdrawal of eligibility for Federal funds, particularly through Medicare, the program providing health care to the elderly, and Medicaid, the joint State–Federal program providing health care to the poor, would be devastating.

In an effort to implement the threat of action under the Rehabilitation Act, the Department of Health and Human Services ('HHS') issued an 'interim final rule' in March 1983. This rule required that hospitals post warning signs in delivery rooms, pediatric wards, nurseries, and neonatal intensive-care units, setting out the hospital's responsibility to provide 'customary medical care' for handicapped infants. The warning signs were to contain a toll-free telephone number to a Federal 'hotline'. The hotline was to be used by parents, hospital staff, or others to report violations of the Act.

Several medical organizations, including notably the American Association of Pediatrics, sued to overturn the regulations. A Federal trial court judge held that the regulations had been adopted in an invalid manner and, in April 1983, enjoined their application.[2] In July, HHS began the process of adopting new regulations while following the proper procedures for providing public notice and allowing an opportunity for public comment. After the comment period, HHS issued the final rules in January 1984. These rules were similar to the first set of regulations, although they required somewhat more limited posting of the warning signs and provided for intra-hospital bioethical review committees.

In the mean time, a Baby Jane Doe had been born on 11 October, 1983 on Long Island, New York. She suffered from multiple birth defects, including spina bifida, myelomeningocele, microencephaly, and hydrocephalus. These problems would, at best, leave her with severe mental, neurological, and physical deficiencies. Her parents refused to give consent to surgical interventions that might prolong her life. A third party, with no relation to the child but with an expressed interest in protecting the rights of disabled children, brought suit in State court. At about the same time, HHS brought suit in Federal court, seeking permission to inspect the hospital's records in order to see if it were complying with the Rehabilitation Act.

Both law suits were eventually dismissed. In the first suit, the State court system rejected the third party's intervention and upheld the parents' right to make the decision.[3] In the second suit, the Federal district court denied that HHS had the right to intervene in parental decisions about the care of their children under the guise of the Rehabilitation Act[4]; the Second Circuit Court of Appeals affirmed.[5] Less than three weeks after this appellate victory, the parents of Baby Jane Doe changed their minds and allowed corrective surgery to be performed.

Although the dispute over that infant disappeared, the fight continued. The logic of the Second Circuit decision was quickly used to invalidate the January 1984 regulations as well; if the Rehabilitation Act was not an adequate basis for HHS's search for documents about the treatment of infants, it clearly could not support the weight of the Baby Doe regulations.[6] The Second Circuit affirmed summarily.[7] In 1986, at the request of the Federal Government, the United States Supreme Court reviewed this case.[8]

The Supreme Court decision was closely contested. The regulations were held invalid, but without a majority of the justices agreeing on a reason. Four justices, a plurality, held that the regulations were invalid because the Rehabilitation Act's limited scope made them irrational. The Act, they held, would not apply when parents made the decision not to intervene because then the child was not being discriminated against on the basis of handicap *by the hospital*—the hospital was only following the parents' instructions, and would, in fact, probably be subject to suit if it disregarded those instructions. The plurality opinion noted that the Act could apply if the parents wanted intervention and the hospital refused, but the Administration had not shown a single instance where that had occurred, nor did the plurality think such cases were likely to arise. As a result, where the regulations were supported by evidence, they were not justified by the Act; where they were justified by the Act, they were not supported by any evidence.

Four justices are not normally a majority of the Supreme Court. Chief Justice Burger agreed that the plurality opinion had reached the correct conclusion, but 'concurred in the judgment[2]', and neither joined their reasoning nor gave any reasons of his own. Three justices dissented, arguing that the regulations, even limited to cases where parents had given consent, were rational. Justice White's dissenting opinion advanced that idea that

the regulations might be justified to prevent doctors from giving discriminatory advice. Justice O'Connor wrote a separate dissenting opinion; Justice
Rehnquist did not participate.

The Supreme Court decision therefore held that the 1984 regulations under
the Rehabilitation Act were invalid, but, because a majority of the justices
did not agree on any reasoning, it did not tell us much more. Under the
American legal conventions governing such matters, the plurality opinion
does not create a precedent for reasoning that could be followed in future
cases. The decision was unusual in another way, which perhaps reflects some
of the tensions these cases create. The two justices most concerned about
individual civil liberties, Justice William Brennan and Justice Thurgood
Marshall, voted on different sides.

While this litigation over the 1984 regulations under the Rehabilitation
Act continued, action was proceeding on another front. During the summer
of 1984, various interested parties, from the 'right to life' and disability rights
groups as well as from some segments of the medical profession, met to try to
reach a compromise. They succeeded, and, in October 1984, their compromise
was enacted into Federal law as the Child Abuse Amendments of 1984. This
statue conditioned States' eligibility for federal grants under the Child Abuse
Prevention and Treatment Act ('CAPTA') on the States' willingness to treat
as 'medical neglect' any 'withholding of medically indicated treatment'
to handicapped infants. HHS then promulgated regulations implementing
that legislation by requiring State child-protective agencies to establish
procedures for investigating Baby Doe cases. These rules were in no way
affected by the litigation over the Rehabilitation Act regulations.

This Federal law governing eligibility for CAPTA funds appears to provide
three exceptions from the prohibition on 'withholding of medically indicated
treatment'. Treatment may be withheld when, in the treating physician's
reasonable judgment—

(a) the infant is chronically and irreversibly comatose;
     the provision of such treatment would—
     (i)   merely prolong dying;
     (ii) not be effective in ameliorating or correcting all the infant's life-
           threatening conditions; or
     (iii) otherwise be futile in terms of the survival of the infant; or
(c) the provision of such treatment would be virtually futile in terms of the
     survival of the infant and the treatment itself under such circumstances
     would be inhumane.[9]

Since the 1985 implementation of regulations for this 1984 statute, the
discussion of the Baby Doe rules has continued, but they have faced few,
if any, amendments or judicial challenges. States that wish to be eligible
for funds under CAPTA must show the Federal government that they
have appropriate Baby Doe enforcement provisions. As for the Baby Doe
regulations under the Rehabilitation Act, the government has not attempted
to resuscitate them since the 1986 Supreme Court decision.

ONE MEANING OF THE BABY DOE STORIES

Dr Ariagno views the story of the Baby Doe regulations principally as the tale of a bad idea that has had some good ancillary results. To me, the story is one of the successful muddling of a complicated issue. By muddling the issue, this process has allowed work to continue in the face of two deeply held, directly conflicting, and politically powerful views.

Let's begin with the complexity of the issue. On the one hand, few people doubt that parents should have the primary role in making decisions about the health care of their children. Our society has long had exceptions from that general rule in special circumstances, where the particular parents are not competent to make decisions for their children or where the public goal to be served, such as vaccination, is too compelling. The exceptions, however, only highlight the importance of the unarticulated general rule.

The issue becomes complicated because even competent parents may make decisions that seem terribly wrong. A rule that left complete discretion with the parents, as advised by health-care providers, would allow parents, for example, to refuse simple surgery to correct a life-threatening problem in a child because she was the 'wrong' sex. If taken far enough, it might even allow the parents to refuse to feed—and to forbid the hospital to feed—a perfectly health child who was, for whatever reason, unwanted. It might be argued that these are absurd hypothetical situations. But given the history of infanticide in many cultures—and its apparent continuing use against female babies in some cultures today—the situations cannot be dismissed as entirely unrealistic. And, in fact, the background to the Baby Doe litigation provides a corollary.

Much of the controversy about the original Baby Doe case from Bloomington, Indiana stemmed from the infant's underlying disability—Down syndrome. Much of the Administration's justification for the Baby Doe regulation was built around similar cases of infants with Down syndrome. People with Down syndrome are not necessarily severely impaired. They constitute a large share of the participants in the Special Olympics, they are often employed, and many of them are loved and loving human beings. Their lives can certainly be difficult, but it is hard to argue that a child born with Down syndrome is necessarily condemned to a life not worth living. The actions of the parents in the Bloomington case in allowing their child to die seem hard to justify; but those parents were among several couples who made similar decisions for infants with Down syndrome. Baby Jane Doe from Long Island, on the other hand, suffered from much more severe disabilities. Her future course was likely to be far more troubled. State intervention seems less justifiable in her case than for the Bloomington child.

Of course, a justification for State intervention in some circumstances does not necessarily justify the actual interventions pursued in any one case. And, in fact, if drawing the line between good and bad interventions is sufficiently difficult, interventions that are justified in theory may not be justified when their practical costs and benefits are weighed. How justified are the existing Baby Doe regulations?

The answer is unclear, but in interesting ways. The 1984 compromise using CAPTA eliminated Federal enforcement of the Baby Doe rules. States could choose to participate or not to participate in the Federal scheme. If States wanted to participate, they had to tell their child-protective services to treat cases of 'withholding of medically indicated treatment' as 'medical neglect'. Participating States also had to maintain procedures to respond to reports of the withholding of such medically indicated treatment. The Child Abuse Amendments authorized grants to States for providing educational and other child-care support services for affected families. Agencies in participating States are required to set up programs to help affected families locate support services. Finally, the statute and its implementing regulations encourage hospitals to set up 'Infant Care Review Committees' to provide education and advice on legal and ethical issues in treating disabled infants. States that refused to participate forfeited a relatively trivial amount of CAPTA funding; three States have refused. All other States have chosen to participate, by enacting statutes or regulations that conform to at least the minimum requirements of the Federal law. Some States have gone farther.

This scheme deserves much of the criticism leveled at it, by Dr Ariagno and others. The definition of 'withholding of medically indicated treatment' makes no allowances for the quality of life the infant could expect. The exceptions apply only in very limited situations: where the infant is irreversibly comatose, where the infant is inevitably dying, or where the infant is almost inevitably dying and the treatment would itself be inhumane. And the promised grants to help parents raise severely impaired infants have run the gamut from tiny to non-existent.

The crucial question, however, should not be 'What do the existing Baby Doe rules say', but rather 'What have these regulations actually *done*?' The answer to that question, though still murky, does not look quite so bad.

First, the 1984 compromise has removed the Federal Government almost entirely from the business of second-guessing neonatal care. It has delegated that duty to the participating States. The Federal Government's only substantial role is to determine whether or not the State is complying with the Federal law so as to be eligible for its tiny grant under the Child Abuse Prevention and Treatment Act. There is no evidence that the Federal Government has taken even that limited role seriously.

Second, the compromise has softened and obscured the enforcement of the regulations. Rather than Federal agents, the rules are now to be enforced by State child-protective services agencies. These agencies typically have to deal with huge caseloads and wrenching problems, which usually take precedence over investigating complicated cases in neonatal intensive-care units. They have no particular expertise in neonatal medicine, and may often not have the resources, human or financial, to develop that expertise.

The issue of expertise is particularly important because of the third effect of the compromise: it vests substantial discretion in the physician. It is the 'reasonable medical judgment' of the treating physician that determines what treatment 'will be most likely to be effective in ameliorating or correcting all such [life-threatening] conditions'. It is also the treating physician's 'reasonable judgment' that determines whether the exceptions apply. Child-protective services agencies may well be reluctant to challenge a physician's judgments in those areas, particularly if the agencies lack substantial medical expertise in the field.

Fourth, while the compromise has not resulted in zealous enforcement, it does hold some possible sanctions through the State child-protection process. These sanctions may give parents and physicians pause in some cases, particularly those where inaction seems most questionable and the public outcry could be the greatest. Those cases could well include Down syndrome cases.

Finally, the rules moved a 'hot' issue to the proverbial 'back burner'. Congress had 'done something', and no additional decision-making was required. One might consider this a disadvantage, because it postpones the debate on the crucial issue of dealing with the quality of life. But no consensus was near on that issue in 1984, nor does a consensus seem imminent in 1994. Whether quality of life should be considered in treating disabled infants remains deeply controversial, particularly among the disabled and their advocates, who fear that the quality of *their* lives could be held against them. If quality of life should be taken into account, the necessary discussion about where and how to draw the lines has scarcely begun. By not forcing the issue, the 1984 resolution has given more time for our views to evolve without bitter conflict.

The regulations have had some negative effects; but those effects are largely symbolic. They have continued to assert the possibility of government intervention in neonatal medical decisions, which, along with the accusatory tone of the discussion, understandably infuriates the neonatal physicians who live constantly with the stress these decisions bring to themselves and to their patients' families. They have also undercut from what had been a consistent increase in the emphasis on patients' autonomy. The regulations permitted—even required—physicians to overrule the parents' wishes, although the extent to which they have actually been used in that way remains unclear. Finally, while encouraging the development of ethics committees, the regulations may have undermined the committees within their hospitals by presenting them as police rather than as helpers.

On balance, it seems to me that the most important effect of the 1984 compromise has been to make the whole issue less visible. Life-and-death decisions about severely disabled newborns continue to be made, of course, and they continue to be emotionally and intellectually taxing. But the law seems to have done very little about them, except to increase the number of ethics committees that can discuss them and, perhaps, to encourage physicians to think about how they would justify non-treatment for some of the less severely disabled infants. There have not been large numbers of prosecutions by State authorities of physicians who have withheld 'medically indicated treatment'. There may not have been any. Nor has there been a Federal or State prescription of 'cookbook' medicine for newborns under the guise of preventing medical neglect. Apart from its boost to ethics committees, it is not clear that, at a *functional* level, the 1984 Act changed the pre-Baby Doe status quo in any substantial way.

But, of course, this statement really raises a set of empirical questions. Do States that have participated in the Federal program show different patterns of neonatal practice from the three States that do not? Do child-protective services agencies intervene actively in neonatal intensive-care units? Have physicians changed their behaviour because of the chance they will be caught violating the statue? Do physicians use the regulations as an excuse to recommend treatments that they would like to undertake anyway, for reasons ranging from personal conviction to financial gain? And, if so, how often does the rule's availability as an excuse actually change what would otherwise happen? Like most empirical questions about public policy, the studies that might answer them have not been done.

Although I think it is likely that the regulations have had only limited effects, I do not know the answer to those empirical questions. But neither, as far as I can tell, does anyone else. If that is the case, one can urge that the regulations are ill-conceived and illogical, but one cannot argue very convincingly that they have had ill effects, particularly when some of their indirect, albeit limited, benefits are weighed. The regulations are a muddle, staking out some strong but vague positions on proper treatment while leaving an enforcement structure that clearly will not often carry them out. But it is a muddle in an area so practically and politically complicated that a good muddle may be the best outcome we can expect. In that very limited sense, the Baby Doe saga might be seen as a case where, after much sound and fury, the political system actually worked.

FUTURE DIRECTIONS IN THE REGULATION OF NEONATAL MEDICINE IN THE UNITED STATES

Predicting is always hazardous, but I do think it may be valuable to mention four areas that could be of growing importance in the regulation of neonatal practice in the United States: the Americans with Disabilities Act, the right-to-life movement, practice guidelines, and health-care financing reform. Each could have substantial implications for medical ethics.

As was discussed above, the Rehabilitation Act of 1973 was an inappropriate statute for intervention in neonatal decisions. The combination of a new set of issues and a new statute may bring disability law to the forefront of these issues once again.

Dr Ariagno raises this new set of issues through his discussion of the case of Baby L. Increasingly, physicians are arguing that futile medical care is bad medical care, and that they should not be required to provide it. In these cases, the parents would like to continue the treatment, but the physicians believe it is inappropriate and refuse. Because the physicians are making the decision not to treat—and not the parents—the argument that led the Supreme Court plurality to find the Rehabilitation Act inapplicable is no longer valid.

The new statute is the Americans with Disabilities Act (the 'ADA'), passed in 1990. This Act expands the Rehabilitation Act in several respects. Perhaps most importantly, it includes physicians along with other health-care providers as 'public accommodations' under the Act, who, subject to a few limitations, have to make services available regardless of a patient's disability. The remedies available can run against the physician as well as the hospital. And while the remedies under the Rehabilitation Act might have been limited to a threat to cut off by administrative action funding to a hospital, under the ADA physicians could be sued in a Federal jury trial for compensatory and, where appropriate, punitive damages.

The ADA's details are numerous and complex, and the process of clarifying litigation has just begun.* Depending on how some of those details are resolved, the ADA may prove to have far-reaching and unforeseen effects in many areas, including medicine. One of those effects may be to short-circuit the debate over the medical ethics of futility as a reason for a physician not to treat a disabled infant.

My prediction about the future activities of the right-to-life movement is less concrete. With the election of a pro-choice Administration, the right-to-life movement may see its goals for limiting abortions recede indefinitely. As abortion becomes an issue where the movement can do less, it may put more attention into other areas.

The issue of euthanasia has become increasingly topical. The States of Washington and California have both recently rejected so-called 'right to die' initiatives by relatively narrow margins. The success of Derek Humphry's book, *Final exit*, and the activities of Dr Kevorkian have also brought aspects of this issue to the forefront of public attention.

Euthanasia is condemned by many of the people and the groups that support the right-to-life movement; but truly voluntary euthanasia for competent and terminally ill adults has significant public support. The right-to-life movement may try to combine some of its strengths by campaigning against 'euthanasia for babies' in the form of withholding medical care. Infants have such great emotional and political appeal that this might prove a successful campaign for the movement, leading to further political intervention in the neonatal intensive-care unit in pursuit of ethical, moral, or religious goals.

Practice guidelines may create an entirely different kind of intervention.

---

* Recently, one hospital sued to stop emergency medical efforts on behalf of an anencephalic infant. The lower court ruled against the hospital, relying on the ADA and the Rehabilitation Act. In February 1994, that decision was affirmed on other grounds. *In the matter of Baby 'K'*, 16 F.3d 590 (4th Cir. 1994).

These guides to 'appropriate' medical practice—known as 'practice guide-lines', 'practice parameters', 'clinical guidelines', and a variety of other names—are being created at a rapid pace throughout the country. Specialty societies, think tanks, State medical regulators, the Federal government, insurers, health maintenance organizations, and even employers are all drafting protocols for delivering certain kinds of medical care. Some of the protocols are extremely long and complicated; others are short and broad. Some are based on detailed scientific research on outcomes; others seem to have little objective basis.

These guidelines could control the practice of perinatal medicine in a manner far more intrusive, though perhaps less offensive, than the Baby Doe regulations. One set of practice guidelines might be adopted by the hospital as its exclusive protocol for treating a certain kind of disabled infant. Alternatively, insurers or HMOs might select some protocols as setting out the only kinds of treatments they will cover. Or a State legislature or court system could use practice guidelines as strong guides to malpractice liability. Under any of those scenarios, the guidelines could control how medicine is practiced in the intensive care unit. After all, the Baby Doe regulations are just one broad, vague form of practice guidelines. The current movement has the potential to spawn many more versions, some in such great detail that avoiding them will prove difficult.*

Practice guidelines are by no means entirely bad. To the extent that they are based on valid studies and provide appropriate room for discretion in special cases, they could substantially improve medical care. On the other hand, in this particular emotionally-charged field, they could easily be controlled by special interest groups, such as insurers, physicians, or disability rights groups. Because of the great expense of some neonatal interventions, practice guidelines created or used by insurers or HMOs might discourage interventions. For exactly the same reasons, guidelines from professional groups, with an economic interest in many of these same interventions, could encourage them. And it is possible that the forces behind the Baby Doe regulations could win another political victory, and a more substantial one, through the guise of Federally-sponsored guidelines that define appropriate practice in treating disabled newborns. Whoever drafts and then adopts practice guidelines *must* be sensitive to the effects of

---

* Practice guidelines, whose intellectual foundations are based in outcomes research, do face a challenge from increasing interest in a so-called preference-based approaches. These approaches reject the idea that medical science can, at least in some situations, determine the right method to treat a particular condition. Instead, it focuses on providing complete and useful information to those involved in the decision and lets their preferences—or the preferences of a representative sample of those decision makers—guide the treatment. See, for example, the discussion by Dr David Eddy in a series of his articles in the Journal of the American Medical Association on clinical decision-making: from theory to practice, especially *JAMA* 1991, **265**: 105 and *JAMA* 1990; **264**: 1737. This approach clearly would raise less concern about regulation of neonatal practice of medicine; whether it will displace the more controlling practice guidelines approach, particularly given budget worries, remains at best unclear.

those guidelines on ethical issues. One could not, for example, honestly determine the 'appropriate' treatment for Baby Jane Doe purely from outcomes research; the ethical issues are too central to that decision.

Finally, the issue of cost is bound up inextricably with the future of government regulation of perinatal medicine in the United States. The eventual outcome of the Clinton Administration's efforts to reform health-care finance remain unclear. It seems clear, however, that unless the burgeoning cost of medical care is brought under control by other means, direct and intrusive regulation of expensive medical devices, drugs, procedures, and physicians is likely to follow. As a source of many stories about high-cost cases, perinatal medicine could not hope to avoid that kind of regulation, which, again, would necessarily have substantial ethical implications.

CONCLUSION

Ethics and perinatology cannot be separated. The start of life and, tragically, for too many, the almost immediate end of life are often moments of high drama, when all the participants are enveloped in the emotional storm. Ethics, perinatology, and government regulation can be separated, but, compared with other countries, that separation is small in the United States and getting smaller. Our open judicial system means that many issues that would, in other countries, be buried as unreviewed decisions by nurses, doctors, or administrators, become court cases and front-page stories. Our political system, which responds strongly to narrow but deeply-held interests, often translates those stories into hearings and legislation. One can deplore these tendencies, but with as much effect on them as one would have by deploring the onrushing tide. The real goals—of physicians, ethicists, and others interested in public policies in this or any other field—must be to understand the political system, to affect its deliberations, to adjust to its decisions, and to survive the process with ethical standards intact.

REFERENCES

1. *Infant Doe* v. *Bloomington Hosp.*, 464 US 961 (1983).
2. *American Academy of Pediatrics* v. *Heckler*, 561 F. Supp. 395 (1983).
3. *Weber* v. *Stony Brook Hospital*, 469 N. Y. S. 2d 63 (Ct. App. 1983), affirming 467 N. Y. S. 2d 685 (N.Y.App. Div.1983).
4. *United States* v. *University Hosp.*, 575 F. Supp. 607 (E. D. N. Y. 1983)
5. *United States* v. *University Hosp.*, 729 F. 2d 144 (2d Cir. 1984).
6. *American Hosp. Ass'n* v. *Heckler*, 585 F. Supp. 541 (S. D. N. Y. 1984).
7. *American Hosp. Ass'n* v. *Heckler*, 694 F. 2d 676 (2d Cir. 1984).
8. *Heckler* v. *American Hospital Ass'n*, 476 US 610 (1986).
9. 42 U. S. C. §5102.

11

Government regulations in the United Kingdom

11A GOVERNMENT REGULATIONS IN THE UNITED KINGDOM

A. G. M. Campbell

Only one rule in medical ethics needs concern you—that action on your part which best conserves the interests of your patient.

Martin H. Fischer, 1879–1962.

INTRODUCTION

In the United Kingdom, the current position can be stated quite simply. There are no Government Regulations that deal specifically with the care of newborn infants. Traditionally, the regulation and control of medical practice has been left to the medical profession, which through the General Medical Council (established by the Medical Act 1858), sets its own guidelines for professional conduct and discipline. Doctors are expected and, to a large extent, still trusted to act according to various principles or codes of medical ethics that have their roots in the Hippocratic Oath, but which have required reappraisal in the light of modern advances in medicine.

For example, the British Medical Association's submission to the 1948 meeting of the World Medical Association in Geneva contained the statement. 'The spirit of the Hippocratic Oath cannot change and enjoins the duty of curing, the greatest crime being co-operation in the destruction of life by murder, suicide and abortion.' Many still believe that it is morally wrong to procure an abortion; but many doctors (and a majority of the public) came to believe that carrying out an abortion in certain circumstances was ethically acceptable, even a moral responsibility; and in 1967 the Abortion Act was passed. Thus the law was eventually brought into harmony with what was deemed to be ethically correct.

It is important to understand that medical ethics and the law may not coincide, a divergence that is at root of some of the difficulties discussed in this volume, and that it may take some time for differences to be resolved.

As indicated in another context (medical research) *'Social interests and expectations, if they are in fact justified, can expect eventually to be reflected in the law'* (Freund 1965). Thus, some aspects of accepted medical practice that are morally repugnant to some doctors may be perfectly permissible within the laws of the land. For others, doing what is morally acceptable, and even imperative, may be viewed as illegal.

The law is generally reluctant to interfere with medical decisions, unless a particularly difficult or contentious issue comes to light. Nevertheless, doctors as citizens, are subject to the law, and, whatever their moral views, they must be careful to practise within the law. Just as ethical codes have required modification, so too has the law, and the past few decades have been noteworthy for a considerable increase in 'medical law', as reflected in the number of 'test cases' brought to the courts for decision. The civil courts are more and more involved with cases brought because of medical negligence, but even here the medical profession plays an important part, as a doctor's conduct is judged by using other doctors as expert witnesses, and they set the legal standard of care by providing evidence as to how a reasonable doctor would behave in similar circumstances. In criminal law, it remains very rare for a doctor to be prosecuted for actions that are thought to be valid by other responsible doctors.

Inevitably, it takes time for the law to catch up with advances in medical practice and changes in moral reasoning that need some kind of legal framework. During that time doctors have to practise uncertainly, in a kind of 'legal vacuum'. The beginning of life is one area where medical advances have required a rapid expansion in legislative involvement in such issues as abortion and *in vitro* fertilization. The law relating to the appropriate care of infants born alive at the margins of 'viability' or those with severely disabling abnormalities or damage remains uncertain, some recent 'test cases' notwithstanding.

VIABILITY AND RESUSCITATION AT BIRTH

Until quite recently doctors generally considered 28 weeks' gestation to be a rough 'legal marker' of viability—an interpretation of the Infant Life (Preservation) Act of 1929 which is not strictly correct. Section 1 of this Act provides for the offence of 'child destruction' if any wilful act causes *a child capable of being born alive* to die before it has an existence independent of its mother (unless the act is done in good faith to preserve the life of the mother). For the purposes of the Act, evidence that the mother had been 'pregnant for a period of 28 weeks or more shall be *prima facie* proof that she was at that time pregnant of a child capable of being born alive'. By many obstetricians it was also mistakenly assumed that 28 weeks was the maximum legal limit under which doctors could terminate a pregnancy under the 1967 Abortion Act. Whereas this Act legalized abortion in certain circumstances, it did not affect the offence of child destruction if a *viable* fetus was destroyed, a point that brought a recent judicial warning to obstetricians who were willing to do late abortions up to 28 weeks, even for very abnormal fetuses (Brahams 1990).

These issues are important to perinatologists, who are well aware that the past few decades have seen major changes in this perception of viability, and that survival under 24 weeks, though rare, is now possible. These changes are reflected in the recent amendments to the 1967 Abortion Act, which specify 24 weeks' gestation, but sensibly remove any upper time limit for cases where severe fetal abnormality is detected or where there is substantial threat to the mother's health. They are also reflected in the Stillbirth Definition Act, which came into force in October 1992. This act reduces from 28 to 24 weeks the minimum gestation age by which a stillbirth (fetal death) is defined. All babies born dead after 24 weeks' gestation now require stillbirth certification.

It should be noted that problems relating to interpretations of the phrase 'capable of being born alive' will still occur. The medico-legal position is peculiar in that, on the one hand, it can be legal for a *probably* normal fetus to be destroyed up to 24 weeks, although it might have been viable if born alive, and legal for a *probably* abnormal fetus to be destroyed even after 24 weeks, though it may be obviously viable. On the other hand, no matter how immature and no matter how severely afflicted, once an infant is born alive it receives the full protection of the law. The lack of logic in this paradox is stretched even further when one considers that similar protection is afforded an infant whose birth has followed botched efforts at carrying out a 'therapeutic' abortion, a situation that has been called 'the new neonatal dilemma' (Rhoden 1984). A doctor who carries out an abortion in circumstances permitted by the Abortion Act of 1967 might be guilty of murder if the infant does not die until after birth. The view has been expressed that *'if the law of homicide could not take cognizance of things done to a child before or during birth which could cause a child to die after it was fully born, there would be a significant and undesirable gap in the law'* (Skegg 1988). Thus, following an abortion, it is only by ensuring that the infant is not born alive that a doctor can be certain that his or her conduct could not amount to the offence of murder!

What are the responsibilities of the doctor at the birth of a tiny infant at the margins of viability or one with obvious gross malformations? Should these babies always be resuscitated with the skills and modern technical resources that are available, or should they sometimes be allowed to die? Strict interpretations of the law relating to the duty of care to a child indicate that the fact that a child has some disability or potential handicap does not mean that the attending doctor is free to allow the child to die, with or without the request or agreement of the parents. Paediatricians acknowledge this, but believe that there are circumstances when it is ethical and morally right to be selective in the use of intensive life-saving and life-sustaining treatment. In other words they may draw the line at vigorously resuscitating and using intensive treatments for a very tiny infant whose prospects of future handicap are very high, or for an infant with obviously severe neurological abnormalities like anencephaly.

It seems that the law too, is prepared to 'draw lines', or at least to accept that these lines may be drawn! In practice, provided that there is supportive testimony from other doctors, most judges would seem to be very reluctant to say anything that would encourage a jury to take the view that the doctor behaved in a way in which no reasonable doctor would behave. For the very tiny infant, the judge may simply take the view that the infant was 'non-viable', although this label may be anything but precise when applied to individual infants in different circumstances. In a 1987 case in Scotland, a Fatal Accidents and Sudden Deaths Inquiry was held into the circumstances of the death of an infant who weighed <700 g at birth but showed signs of life (Brahams 1988). The paediatrician who attended the delivery room decided that the infant was not viable and allowed her to die, without, for example, putting her on a ventilator. The parents were upset by this decision, apparently taken without their knowledge or agreement, and it was alleged that 'the hospital had a practice of not resuscitating babies under 700 g'.

Not surprisingly, the Sheriff made a number of criticisms of the communication between doctors and parents and the process of decision-making revealed by this case, but accepted the decision itself. He concluded that the baby had died of 'extreme prematurity'. *'The paediatrician had no doubt that the infant was not viable; that was a medical decision, and there was no evidence to suggest that he was wrong'*. In this context it is important to distinguish between basic 'care' and intensive treatments like mechanically assisted ventilation, artificial methods of feeding, etc. There are circumstances where withholding vigorous methods of resuscitation is justified at birth, but none in which it is ever justifiable to withhold 'care'. People talk loosely about a 'non-treatment' decision, when what they really mean is a 'non-intensive treatment' decision. One can list examples of congenital abnormalities, like anencephaly, or tiny infants whose lungs would be too immature to support life for more than a few minutes, where resuscitation is inappropriate; but there is so much variation in complexity and prognosis that considerable latitude must be afforded to the doctors and parents in deciding what is best for the infant. As some of the worst congenital abnormalities may now be detected by pre-natal diagnosis, discussions with the parents before birth should include an attempt to determine their views on the care of the baby after birth. It may be agreed that it would be wrong to make vigorous, and probably futile, efforts to prolong life; but whatever the circumstances the infant must receive the cherishing and basic attention given to other normal infants. This means that he or she should not be left to die in some corner of a delivery room, but admitted to the neo-natal unit and given any treatment necessary to relieve apparent discomfort or distress until death, probably in the arms of the parents (Duff and Campbell 1976).

The tiny 'non-viable' infant will sometimes show surprising vigour at birth, and occasionally such an infant, especially if 'small-for-dates', will do remarkably well. For many, however, resuscitation followed by intensive life-support will merely ensure that dying is unnecessarily prolonged or that survival is accompanied by grievous disability. Some of these problems will be discussed later; but it is because of the uncertainty of prognosis in these situations that it may be wrong to withhold intensive treatment *at birth*. The delivery room is no place to make a 'snap judgement' about diagnosis and prognosis, particularly as it is usually junior, and therefore relatively inexperienced, doctors who are present to carry out the initial care of the infant. If judges or juries are to be satisfied that a decision taken was medically and ethically acceptable, and therefore perhaps not to be considered as an offence, they must be satisfied that there was a proper process of decision-making, by which the infant's interests were protected.

Junior doctors should be given clear instructions about their responsibilities. Whatever the gestational age or condition at birth, an infant born alive should receive standard resuscitation, including ventilation if necessary. At this stage, unless by previous agreement with the parents in the circumstances described above, life-saving measures should not be withheld. Any subsequent decision to continue, withhold, withdraw, or introduce intensive treatment will be the responsibility of a senior doctor or doctors after careful consideration of the facts and discussion with the parents, once further information and subsequent developments indicate that death or severe brain damage is a likely outcome.

It has been argued that a birthweight of 750 g (at the appropriate gestational age) should be considered as one criterion in a flexible 'cut-off' below which intensive measures like positive-pressure ventilation should not be continued *routinely* without at least discussing the implications, with or without treatment, with the parents and making sure that they have an appropriate voice in any further decisions (Campbell 1982). Inevitably such crude criteria will change with time, as the experience of neo-natal units is documented and shared; but some apparently harsh decisions will always be necessary. A line must be drawn somewhere, and there must be some process through which it can be drawn in ways that do not conflict with the duties that doctors and parents owe to infants in their care.

In her review of international attitudes, the late Nancy Rhoden preferred the British compromise between the American 'treat until certainty' approach (probably conditioned by the Baby Doe rules) and that current in Sweden, where doctors seemed more willing to withhold treatment, but were reluctant to withdraw it once started. She called the tendency of British paediatricians to give each infant a 'trial of life' the 'individualized prognostic strategy', and concluded that this approach *'both recognizes and reflects the complex nature of these dilemmas. It is not without flaws—but it is probably the best that doctors, parents and society can do'* (Rhoden 1986).

THE ABNORMAL OR DAMAGED INFANT: ALLOWING TO DIE

In contrast to the situation in the United States, 'non-treatment decisions', as they are often called, have received relatively little publicity in the United Kingdom, although the dilemmas posed by severely disabled infants were discussed earlier in the British medical literature (Slater 1971; Lorber 1972). It is also worth recalling that it was in the UK courts that a paediatrician, Dr Leonard Arthur, was tried for murder, (later reduced to attempted murder), but subsequently acquitted, because one of his patients, an infant with Down syndrome, was sedated and allowed to die (Gunn and Smith 1985). The problem has largely been ignored by British legislators, in spite of occasional proddings by 'pro-life' groups as an extension of their campaigns against the 1967 Abortion Act, and by Members of Parliament when such cases come to public attention. There were also calls for legislation, but the American furore over 'Baby Doe' (see below) received relatively little attention in either the UK medical or the popular press. Perhaps many believed, and probably still believe, that legislation is just too blunt an instrument to address specifically these essentially private tragedies that affect individual families; and that the courts remain the best places to resolve the occasional difficult issues of conflict, or to deal with apparent abuses which infringe or are thought to infringe the laws that already exist to protect life.

Following Dr Arthur's trial, Sir Michael Havers, then Attorney General, stated in Parliament:

I am mindful of the desire of many people to understand clearly what the legal position is in relation to cases such as gave rise to the prosecution of Dr Arthur. I therefore say that I am satisfied that the law relating to murder ... is the same now as it was before the trial; that it is the same irrespective of the age of the victim; and that it is the same irrespective of the wishes of the parents or any other person having a duty of care to the victim. I am also satisfied that a person who has a duty of care may be guilty of murder—by omitting to fulfil that duty, as much as by committing any positive act (Hansard 1982).

In the decade since this trial, while there has been no change in the law, there has been some further clarification of the circumstances in which allowing to die may be a legally valid choice.

American legislation

The many references throughout this volume provide ample documentation of the extent of US Federal involvement in medical decision-making. Before examining the current position of these decisions to withhold or withdraw life-prolonging and life-saving treatment vis-à-vis the United Kingdom law, it may help the reader if the background to the American legislation is briefly summarized here, although it is discussed in considerable detail elsewhere (Chapter 10).

From the early 1970s there was a series of publications about the difficult moral dilemmas facing staff and parents when deciding about the care of infants born with severely disabling abnormalities (Duff and Campbell 1973; Shaw 1973; Todres et al. 1977). These stimulated increasing professional debate and controversy, and, in 1982, heightened public interest and concern about the plight of these infants became focused on an apparent abuse of the discretion that had traditionally been afforded doctors and parents in deciding to withhold life-sustaining treatment. The infant involved, known as 'Baby Doe', received massive media exposure, much of it exaggerated and emotive. Nevertheless, this baby became the catalyst for pro-life and disability groups to force a series of legislative actions to limit this discretion. After a controversial and tortuous passage through the judicial system, there emerged (in 1984), a series of amendments to the Child Abuse Prevention and Treatment Act which brought failure to treat a handicapped infant within the meaning of child abuse and neglect, and required that States receiving federal funds for Child Protection include 'medical neglect' as part of their child-abuse programmes.

Medical neglect was defined as 'failure to respond to the infant's life-threatening conditions by providing treatment (including appropriate nutrition, hydration, and medication) which, in the treating physician's judgement, will be most likely to be effective in ameliorating or correcting all such conditions'.

Three exceptions to this general rule were included in the amendments:

A. when the infant is chronically and irreversibly comatose;
B. when the provision of medical treatment would
   (1) merely prolong dying;
   (2) not be effective in ameliorating or correcting all the infant's life-threatening conditions; or
   (3) otherwise be futile in terms of the survival of the infant; and
C. when the provision of such treatment would be virtually futile in terms of the survival of the infant, and the treatment itself under such circumstances would be inhumane.

This legislation became known as the 'Baby Doe rules', an unfortunate label, as 'rules' imply rigidity, and rigidity of interpretation proved to be one of the main consequences of this unique example of Government interference in what amounts to a family bereavement. Since its introduction, much has been written about its impact on pediatricians and parents and on the infants themselves (Angell 1983; Lantos 1987; Kopelman *et al.* 1988; Caplan *et al.* 1992). 'Aggressive posturing by the United States government through a complex regulatory scheme designed to assure protection of handicapped newborns has in fact wreaked havoc on the whole decision-making process and assaulted the integrity and privacy of the family decisional unit' (Smith 1985).

British legislation

One lawyer has described the current position thus:

In so far as the tradition has been for courts in the United Kingdom to allow themselves to be led by the medical profession, it is not necessarily surprising that both appear to pay lip service to the sanctity of life while leaving a vast discretion to the doctor in charge in consultation with the parents' (Wells 1989).

This 'vast discretion' in action is illustrated by some cases that have come to the attention of the courts in the past ten years; but for any individual infant for whom there is a decision to withhold or withdraw life-sustaining treatment, the legal position of the paediatrician, usually a neonatologist, remains uncertain in the absence of any testing of the facts in court. A neonatologist will remain potentially vulnerable to prosecution as long as it is thought unwise and probably impossible to detail all the circumstances in which it is 'legal' to allow a baby to die.

A doctor cannot always rely on a sympathetic judge, or a jury (as in *R.* v. *Arthur*), that is unwilling to convict someone who is obviously acting out of concern for an infant and its family. However, recent court decisions have developed some experience of case law that provides some guidance for doctors, and indicates subtle nuances in definition that have similarities to the exceptions to the Baby Doe rules described earlier, which are themselves open to wide interpretation. For example, there is the apparent acceptability of withholding certain treatments that merely prolong 'dying', or are seen to be 'virtually futile', words that can have different meanings to different people in different circumstances. One emerging difference from the American scene is that, while the drafters of 'Baby Doe', somewhat naïvely, seemed determined to prohibit any consideration of the future quality of life of the infant, the British courts have paid more attention to its importance, and seem to accept that mere prolongation of biological life, without consideration of its quality, is not always in the infant's or in the family's best interests (see also Chapter 4).

Baby B.

In a case (*re* B.) heard by the Court of Appeal in 1981, surgery was authorized to correct congenital intestinal obstruction in an infant with Down syndrome in the face of parental objection because, in the judges' opinion, the infant's life was not 'demonstrably so awful' that surgery should not be authorized (*re* B. 1981). This judgement suggested that there might be circumstances where the likely quality of life of the infant would be so poor that it would be legally acceptable to let the child die.

R. v. Arthur

Dr Arthur, a highly respected paediatrician, was reported to the Director of Public Prosecutions by a pro-life lobbyist following the death of an infant with Down syndrome. In the infant's medical record he wrote, 'Parents do not wish it [sic] to survive. Nursing care only.' He then prescribed large doses of dihydrocodeine, an analgesic, to alleviate distress; and, less than 3 days later, the infant died, death being ascribed to bronchopneumonia. Subsequent pathological analysis showed that the infant had a number of other abnormalities; but these were not known to Dr Arthur at the time he made his decision to let the baby die. Importantly, they were also not known to those acting for the prosecution, whose poorly organized case pretty well collapsed when the abnormalities were revealed by the pathologist acting for the defence. Whatever their reasons, members of the jury had little hesitation in acquitting Dr Arthur—a decision that was inconsistent with the earlier view of the judges of the Court of Appeal in *re* B. Perhaps the members of the jury were simply reflecting public opinion, which, as far as could be judged by a 'vox pop' poll conducted at the time, indicated that a large majority were in favour of leaving these decisions largely to the child's parents and their medical advisers. Many members of the public thought it wrong that a highly respected paediatrician should have had to face such a serious charge in a criminal court for acting out of concern for an infant and the family.

The Arthur case has been widely discussed in the medical, legal, and ethics literature; but experts continue to disagree about the consequences that can be inferred from it. Some believe that it set a precedent for making it all right to allow some infants to die provided that there was agreement for this action between the doctors and the parents. Others believe that the medical particulars of the case were so unusual, and the judge's instructions to the jury so unsatisfactory in law, that no conclusions can be drawn that would make it useful as a 'test case' (Kennedy 1988).

It is worth noting that, while a team of paediatricians and other doctors testified on behalf of Dr Arthur, no paediatrician appeared for the prosecution. This whole unfortunate episode, in the opinion of one legal correspondent, revealed *'an alarming divergence between the law on the one hand, and prevailing medical opinion on the other'*, and provided the impetus for a proposal for a Limitation of Treatment Bill that would *'regulate the conduct of the medical profession and others in the treatment of chronically disabled infants'* (Brahams and Brahams 1983).

Under the provisions of this proposal, but with appropriate safeguards, it would not be an offence to fail to administer or to cease to administer treatment necessary to preserve and/or prolong the life of an infant under 28 days old with severe physical and/or mental disability. Although there was some support for this proposal among both doctors and lawyers, and it was said to be 'informally commended' by the Director of Public Prosecutions, it came to nothing, and calls for any legislation on these matters were strongly opposed (Havard 1983). Paediatricians, while no doubt tempted to welcome legislation that might give them some legal protection, generally were reluctant to see any increased State involvement in these matters either to enforce life or to sanction death. Most felt that there was considerable merit in doctors' and parents' continuing to explore the least detrimental treatment options for the special circumstances of individual infants in an atmosphere of privacy and trust, even if so doing causes much anguish and uncertainty about the possible legal consequences of their actions. As these infants are now treated almost exclusively in public places like large hospitals, and treatment involves many doctors, nurses, and others in their care, it should also be easy to spot an occasional abuse of this trust or any apparent violation of the infant's best interests that should be brought to the attention of the courts.

The trial also renewed calls for the development of guidelines (a more flexible term?) that doctors could follow, rather than leaving to them and the parents, the discretion (and the agonizing responsibility), for making such decisions on a vague criterion like a 'demonstrably awful life'. It was also felt desirable to lessen doctors' vulnerability to prosecution if, like Dr Arthur, they are reported because someone has a strong moral objection to any violation of the sanctity of life.

Baby C.

In 1989 a High Court judge agreed that a very seriously handicapped infant should be allowed to die and that no further attempts should be made to prolong her life (re C. 1989). This case was appealed by the Official Solicitor, who was unhappy with the drafting of the judgement, particularly the judge's use of the phrase 'treat to die', which might be interpreted to give authority for taking positive steps to end the infant's life. In their judgement, the Lords of Appeal agreed that Mr Justice Ward had 'failed to express himself with his usual felicity', and that the original decision had been too restrictive on the exercise of the doctors' 'normal clinical discretion'. They accepted that the goal of any treatment should be directed to ease the baby's suffering rather than to a brief prolongation of her life (Brahams 1989).

This case only came to court because the baby (for reasons unconnected with the infant), had been made a ward of court before birth, and a court must consent to any major step 'in a ward's life'; but it provided further useful insights into how judges view these treatment dilemmas. Mr Justice Ward referred to the case of Baby B noted earlier, and also indicated his agreement with the kinds of criteria that have been used (and published) by neonatologists during the past two decades:

Inasmuch as one judges, as I do, intellectual function to be a hallmark of our humanity, her functioning on that level is negligible if it exists at all. Coupled with her total physical handicap, the quality of her life will be demonstrably awful and intolerable within the B. test.

This judgement seems to imply that doctors should continue to bear their traditional responsibility for deciding, with the patient and family, when treatment should be withdrawn and for implementing such decisions.

It would be undersirable for the courts to usurp the doctor's role and to become routinely involved in a medical decision which is the prerogative of the patient (if capable), family, and doctors in privacy.

Baby J.

For Baby C., the issue was the use of life-prolonging as distinct from life-saving treatments. In other words the judgement was about a baby who was thought to be dying. In a subsequent case, that of Baby J., the Official Solicitor appealed a decision by Mr Justice Scott Baker that doctors should not be required to ventilate and therefore save the life of a 'gravely ill child', should he collapse, on the basis that: 'a court is never justified in withholding consent to treatment which could enable the child to survive a life threatening condition, whatever the quality of life which it would experience thereafter'. This submission was not accepted by the Court of Appeal, which took the view that there can be some circumstances where the quality of life would be so intolerable that treatment, without which death would ensue, could be withheld even though the child was not 'dying'. The case is also important because it referred not to an infant with congenital abnormalities, but to one born prematurely at 27 weeks with a birthweight of 1.1 kg, who, after weeks of intensive care and many complications, was known to have brain damage. This case is typical of the infants with the complications of immaturity that in numbers have largely superseded infants with congenital malformations in causing difficult moral and legal dilemmas for the staff of newborn units. They are infants born at the margins of viability who, with modern skills and equipment, can now be salvaged, but whose future can be devastated by grievous disability from these complications and/or even by the damage that may result from invasive efforts to keep them alive.

The case of Baby J. is also important in that Lord Donaldson emphasized the need to avoid looking at the problem from the point of view of the decider, but instead to look at it from the point of view of the patient. This 'substituted judgement/best interests' approach is one often stressed in the paediatric literature, 'best interests' being essentially a substituted judgement on what most reasonable people would want done to themselves in similar circumstances to ensure an acceptable quality of life.

In a further case of a 16-month-old infant who had been injured in a fall at his home at the age of 6 weeks and was now severely brain-damaged (also, confusingly, called Baby J.), a Consultant Paediatrician recommended that life-saving intensive interventions such as ventilation should be withheld were the infant to suffer a life-threatening event. In the High Court this was supported by the Health Authority and the Official Solicitor, but was challenged by the baby's mother and by the responsible Local Authority. The court made an interim order pending a full hearing that required the Health Authority to apply life-saving measures as needed for as long as they were effective. This order was struck down by the Court of Appeal on 3 June 1992 on the basis that the court would not order a doctor to treat a patient if, in his clinical judgement, to do so would not be in the patient's best interests (*British Medical Journal* 1992).

Guidelines

From these cases, it is possible to gain some idea of how the courts might respond to the facts of an individual case; but this still leaves neonatologists in some uncertainty about where the line of 'demonstrably so awful', 'negligible intellectual function', or 'intolerable quality of life' can be drawn, and who exactly can draw it. Would there be advantages in drawing up rules of conduct or 'guidelines' along the lines of Baby Doe? Would they provide any further protection for infants and at the same time reduce the vulnerability of parents and paediatricians to court exposure of their private discussions and decisions? Kennedy has been particularly critical of doctors' unwillingness to develop rules of conduct.

It is a matter of continuing astonishment to me that doctors resist the notion that there can be rules or guidelines stipulating how they ought to act. For again, whether or not it is realized or admitted, doctors are already invoking them when making their decisions. They do not decide in some ethical or legal vacuum (Kennedy 1988).

In attempts to fill at least the ethical part of that vacuum, some British paediatricians/neonatologists have offered their own 'guidelines' for debate (Campbell 1982; Whitelaw 1986; Walker 1988). From these, from information from other neonatal units, and from data relating to neonatal morbidity and mortality, it seems likely that policies and practices throughout the United Kingdom are reasonably consistent. It is difficult to see how more detailed criteria can be written down and sanctioned legally without being either excessively restrictive or so vague as to be of little use, thus causing additional difficulties in interpretation that might still have to be argued in court. The criteria used by the courts to decide recent cases do seem quite consistent with those currently in operation in neonatal units, but it must be admitted that these cases represent only a fraction, and not necessarily a representative fraction, of the myriad problems encountered by neonatologists.

It may simply not be possible to detail all the circumstances where withholding or withdrawal of life-prolonging or life-saving treatment may be viewed as morally and legally acceptable. It should also be emphasized that the American experience has not provided any evidence either that abuses were widespread before Baby Doe or that they have been eliminated since Baby Doe. Commentators familiar with what is happening in some American neonatal units believe that the current problem may not be abuse by 'medical neglect' but abuse by over-treatment at incalculable cost (human and financial) to babies and families (Engelhardt 1989). The overtreatment of these tragic infants is one consequence of the too-rigid application of the Baby Doe legislation that makes one apprehensive about the possible effect of similar legislation in the UK. Sadly, in some circumstances this overtreatment has occurred for reasons that seem more designed to protect the interests of institutions and staff from possible legal harassment than to protect the interests of the infants.

The views of the parents and 'quality of life'

One major issue on which paediatricians tend to differ from lawyers, and one that could make 'guidelines' too rigid to be of practical help, is the weight that should be given to the views of the parents, and the need for considerable latitude in decision-making when considering the circumstances of individual families. The parents' attitudes cannot be the decisive factor against life-prolonging treatment (or indeed, for the limitless use of such treatment), but they must be weighed' very seriously, particularly when, as a society, it is the parents that we expect to care for the severely handicapped children that are salvaged as a result of modern treatment, yet we provide them with woefully inadequate resources and supports with which to do it. In the United States this point was made forcefully by the President's Commission for the Study of Ethical Problems in Medicine: '. . . to the extent that society fails to ensure that seriously ill newborns have the opportunity for an adequate level of continuing care its moral authority to intervene on behalf of a newborn whose life is in jeopardy is compromised' (US President's Commission 1983).

One interpretation of the Arthur case could be that a joint decision by doctors and parents to let a baby die is not unlawful if it can be demonstrated that the infant was likely to suffer from a significantly reduced quality of life. In other words quality of life is the critical criterion, and the parents and the primarily responsible doctor are charged with making the value judgements on where to draw the line between acceptable or unacceptable quality in the infant's future interests.

There is nothing new in doctors' allowing patients to die; but the basis for the majority of the current dilemmas faced by neonatologists (and specialists in other branches of 'rescue medicine') is the modern ability to sustain life using modern technology for patients once regarded as 'non-viable' or 'hopeless'. When this is coupled with the recognition that a technical triumph in 'saving life' or prolonging it when all or most of what makes a 'life worth living' has been lost, the tragedy is compounded for the individual concerned and the family. Considering the quality of life is not in conflict with the doctor's duty to 'maintain the utmost respect for human life'. Allowing a patient to die in these circumstances enhances rather than diminishes respect for the value of life.

Understandably, there is great reluctance to decide for others, particularly those who, like infants, have had no opportunity to experience their own lives, develop their own values, and make others aware of the kinds of choices they would probably have made for themselves in similar circumstances. Somebody has to choose for them, and, notwithstanding our increased awareness that the abuse and exploitation of children is a problem for every society, it seems to me that the persons still most likely to have an infant's interests at heart are the parents, often in close contact with other family members, and in consultation with the doctor or doctors most familiar with the medical facts of diagnosis and prognosis. A British lawyer has made this point even more forcibly: 'There is a strong argument for keeping the law out of these cases—the decision of the parents should prevail' (Williams 1981). It would be unwise to follow the American precedent and introduce legislation or even 'guidelines' that could merely make these dilemmas even more difficult to resolve, would probably create new ones, and would not necessarily lead to any improvement in the current, admittedly imperfect, process of decision-making.

Infant Bio-ethics Committees

One American innovation that does have some relevance to the UK is the use of an infant Bio-ethics Committee to provide a wider forum for discussing particularly difficult problems and to help the neonatologists in making decisions that are soundly based on medical facts and ethical principles, and are in the spirit, if not the letter, of current interpretations of the law (Fleischman 1986). In their opposition to Baby Doe, the American Academy of Pediatrics promoted the formation of these committees for consultation when decisions are contemplated to withhold or withdraw life-sustaining treatment. The committee:

preserves the responsibility of the pediatrician to act as primary physician. It allows each case to be judged in all its complexity and individuality. It would not preclude any legal actions that are presently available, although it might reduce the need for such action. It is responsive to public demands for a more thorough decision-making process. An institutional ethics committee will not be a panacea for making ethically correct decisions, but it should increase the probability that such decisions are informed and consistent with the broadest moral values of our society (American Academy of Pediatrics 1983).

In the United States, at best these committees have worked well, but occasionally their actions (or inaction) have made matters worse and alienated family members from the hospital and its staff. It was hoped that their role would be advisory, educational, and supportive. It was never intended that these committees should take decisions on individual patients. Some members, however well-intentioned, may be too remote from the realities of neonatal intensive care, and may pay less regard than they should to the needs of the individual infant and family. They may also be unduly influenced by one or more of the more prominent (and domineering) members to take decisions that put other interests, such as those of the Hospital, before those of the baby.

At present there is usually wide but informal consultation in British hospitals with similar advisers to those on American committees. From observations in the United States I have been critical of the way that a committee can complicate, rather than resolve these dilemmas (Campbell 1992). I also do not think that bringing such issues to a formal committee will solve all our problems; but, if properly constituted, a committee and its members, sometimes acting as individuals, should be helpful to the doctors and nurses, and to the parents who need so much understanding and support. Taking this step may also help to mollify the academic lawyers and others who call for 'guidelines' or even legislation; and perhaps it might also reassure members of the public that justice is seen to be done.

If similar committees become established in British hospitals, it would be essential for the neonatologist to remain as the primary decision-maker and to make every effort to avoid the 'pitfall' of abdicating responsibility for individual patient decisions. An infant bio-ethics committee could be established quite easily in British hospitals and given appropriate authority, in the way that the Department of Health has determined the NHS framework within which research projects are reviewed by a Hospital Research Ethics Committee (Department of Health 1991).

USING INFANTS AS SUBJECTS OF RESEARCH

As with matters affecting the clinical care of infants, there are no regulations to control medical research, and a recent Parliamentary answer indicated that there was no intention to introduce any. What controls exist are derived from the recommendations and guidelines of such organizations as the Royal Colleges and, in the case of children, the British Paediatric Association. In 1975 the Department of Health issued a statement on the *'Supervision of the ethics of clinical research investigations and fetal research*, and has recently issued guidelines on local research ethics committees; but these add little to previous recommendations by the specialist organizations, and in other respects the most recent document is disappointing. It pays little attention to the monitoring of research, and ignores contentious issues important to neonatal intensive care, like the use of innovative therapy, which *'should be subject to the same regime of control that attends research properly so-called'* (Kennedy and Grubb 1989). The document hardly mentions the particular difficulties, or the importance of carrying out research using child subjects, except to indicate that *'those acting for the child can only legally give their consent provided that the intervention is for the benefit of the child'*.

It is generally assumed, therefore, that *'therapeutic research'*, i. e. research carried out as part of necessary treatment, is lawful provided that the permission of the parents has been obtained, whereas *'non-therapeutic research'*, where there is no direct benefit to the individual concerned, is unlawful even though the risks of such research are negligible and the parents agree. Although these assumptions seem reasonable, they do not seem to be based on anything more specific than a legal opinion given to the Medical Research Council in 1963, on which they based their guidelines: 'In the strict view of the law, parents and guardians of minors cannot give consent on their behalf to any procedures which are of no particular benefit to them and which may cause some risk of harm' (Medical Research Council 1963).

There does not seem to be any statute or case law which specifically addresses this topic. Paediatric investigators, possibly mistakenly, have assumed that the phrase 'some risk of harm' allows them some discretion to carry out both therapeutic *and* non-therapeutic research provided that the risks are minimal or negligible in relation to the expected benefits, and that parental consent has been obtained. Indeed, the British Paediatric Association guidelines of 1980 specifically stated that: 'research which involves a child and is of no benefit to that child (non-therapeutic research) is not necessarily unethical or illegal', and indicated how the degree of risk from the research should be assessed in relation to the risks of disturbance, discomfort, or pain (British Paediatric Association 1980). Support for this view is implied in the report of a recent Medical Research Council working party which re-examined the 1963 advice and more directly addressed the problems of non-therapeutic research.

We do not seek to argue that a child's participation in non-therapeutic research is in his best interests. But we recognize that there are circumstances in which it is important to gain knowledge which may be of benefit to children in general and which can only be acquired as a result of research which involves children (Medical Research Council 1991).

On that basis the working party considered that there was a 'strong case' for including children in such research provided that the usual safeguards were observed, for example parental consent, approval by an ethics committee, etc., and that *participation places a child at no more than negligible risk of harm*.

The British Paediatric Association has now issued revised guidelines that continue to make the same point, viz.

The attempt to protect children absolutely from the potential harms of research denies any of them the potential benefits. We therefore support the premise that research that is of no intended benefit to the child subject is not necessarily unethical or illegal' (British Paediatric Association 1992).

The guidelines indicate how paediatricians might evaluate potential benefits, harms, and costs of intended research, and how risks can be defined as 'minimal', 'low', or 'high':

It would be unethical to submit child subjects to more than minimal risk when the procedure offers no benefit to them, or only a slight or very uncertain one. Higher risks in research and novel treatments are accepted when children are enduring very harmful disease. Illness and anxiety alone may put pressure on families to assent to heroic experimental procedures. In cases of severe or chronic disease, therefore, the harms to the child of the condition, of the medical treatment, and of the stress through taking part in research need to be assessed so that all avoidable stress may be relieved.

All these encouraging statements notwithstanding, one can only assume that the paediatric investigator's position remains somewhat uncertain if statements in Parliament are any indication of how the courts might react to a 'test case':

'The position in law is that no parent or guardian of tender years [*sic*] is entitled to give consent to any procedure which is not for the benefit of the child.'

and

In the case of children and young persons, the question of whether purported consent is true consent would in each case depend upon facts such as the age, intelligence, situation and character of the subject and nature of the investigations. There can be no question of purported consent in relation to premature babies (Hansard 1986).

To date no doctor has been charged with carrying out 'illegal' research, but investigators have occasionally been accused of unethical research (Forfar and Campbell 1987). Unfortunately, media distortion and ignorance of the facts may stimulate Parliamentary and public concern and result in demands that 'There ought to be a law!'

In spite of all these uncertainties, it is obviously of vital importance that properly organized and supervised 'ethical' research using children should continue. Inevitably the ethics of such research involves value judgements which will depend not only on who is doing the research but also on the prevailing climate of public opinion. It is therefore particularly important for paediatric investigators to earn and maintain parental and public trust, and for their research to be soundly based scientifically and conducted to the highest ethical standards, with the infants' interests fully protected. If the original restrictive statement of the MRC had always been observed, large areas of research important to all children would have been ruled out. For example, the use of controls in research is often essential to the understanding of a disease process; and the current protection of all children from vaccines resulted from research which involved taking blood samples from many normal children. It is absolutely vital that controlled trials are allowed, or history will continue to record the disastrous consequences of introducing new treatments uncritically (Silverman 1985). Research must be seen as an appropriate, even an essential, part of caring for children.

REFERENCES

American Academy of Pediatrics Committee on Bioethics (1983). Treatment of critically ill newborns. *Pediatrics*, **72**: 565–6.

Angell, M. (1983). Handicapped children, Baby Doe and Uncle Sam. *New England Journal of Medicine*, **309**: 659–61.

Brahams, D. (1988). No obligation to resuscitate a non-viable infant. *Lancet*, **1**: 1176.

Brahams, D. (1989). Court of Appeal endorses medical decision to allow baby to die. *Lancet*, **1**: 969–70.

Brahams, D. (1990). Judicial warning on very late abortions. *Medico-Legal Journal*, **58**, (2): 108–10.

Brahams, D. and Brahams, M. (1983). The Arthur case—a proposal for legislation. *Journal of Medical Ethics*, **9**: 12–15.

British Medical Journal (1992). News: Appeal Court supports doctors' decision not to treat, p. 1527.

British Paediatric Association (1980). Guidelines to aid ethical committees considering research involving children. *Archives of Disease in Childhood*, **55**: 75–7.

British Paediatric Association (1992). Guidelines for the ethical conduct of medical research involving children. British Paediatric Association, London.

Campbell, A. G. M. (1982). Which infants should not receive intensive care? *Archives of Disease in Childhood*, **57**: 569–71.

Campbell, A. G. M. (1992). Baby Doe and forgoing life-sustaining treatment. In

324 A. G. M. CAMPBELL

Compelled compassion: Government intervention in the treatment of critically ill newborn (ed. A. L. Caplan, R. H. Blank and J. C. Merrick) *Humana Press, Totowa, New Jersev.*

Caplan, A. L. Blank, R. H. and Merrick, J. C. (eds) (1992). *Compelled compassion: Government intervention in the treatment of critically ill newborns. Humana Press, Totowa, New Jersey.*

Department of Health (1991). Local Research Ethics Committees DoH, *HSG (91) 5. London. DoH.*

Duff, R. S. and Campbell, A. G. M. (1973). Moral and ethical dilemmas in the special care nursery. *New England Journal of Medicine 1973*, **289**: 890–4.

Duff, R. S. and Campbell, A. G. M. (1976). On deciding the care of severely handicapped or dying persons: with particular reference to infants. *Pediatrics*, **57**: 487–93.

Engelhardt, H. T. Jr. (1989). Comments on the recommendations regarding Section 504 of the Rehabilitation Act of 1973 and the Child Abuse amendments of 1984. In US Commission on Civil Rights: *Medical discrimination against children with disabilities.* pp. 158–165. US Commission on Civil Rights Washington DC.

Fleischman, A. R. (1986). An infant bioethical review committee in an urban medical center. *Hastings Center Report*, **16**, (3): 16–18.

Forfar, J. O. and Campbell, A. G. M. (1987). Medicine and the media. *British Medical Journal*, **295**: 659–60.

Freund, P. A. (1965). Ethical problems in human experimentation. *New England Journal of Medicine*, **273**: 687–92.

Gunn, M. J. and Smith, J. C. (1985). Arthur's case and the right to life of a Down's syndrome child. *Criminal Law Review, 705–715.*

Hansard (1982). 19 (6th ser.) 349.

Hansard (1986). 101 (6th ser.) 656–61.

Havard, J. (1983). Legislation is likely to create more difficulties than it resolves. *Journal of Medical Ethics*, **9**: 18–20.

Kennedy, I. (1988). *Treat me right: essays in medical law and ethics.* Clarendon Press, Oxford.

Kennedy, I. and Grubb, A. (1989). Medical Law. Butterworth, London.

Kopelman, L. M. Irons, T. G. and Kopelman, A. E. (1988). Neonatologists judge the "Baby Doe" regulations. *New England Journal of Medicine*, **318**: 677–83.

Lantos, J. (1987). Baby Doe five years later: implications for child health. *New England Journal of Medicine*, **317**: 444–7.

Lorber, J. (1972). Spina bifida cystica. Results of treatment of 270 consecutive cases with criteria for selection for the future. *Archives of Disease in Childhood*, **47**: 854–73.

Medical Research Council (1963). *Responsibility in investigations on human subjects.* HMSO, London.

Medical Research Council (1991). *The ethical conduct of research on children.* HMSO, London.

re B. (1981), 1, WLR 1421, 1424.

re C. (1989). NLJ Law Reports: 613.

Rhoden, N. K. (1984). The new neonatal dilemma: live births from late abortions. *Georgetown Law Journal*, **72**: 1451–1509.

Rhoden, N. K. (1986). Treating Baby Doe: the ethics of uncertainty. *Hastings Center Report*, **16** (4): 34–42.

Shaw, A. (1973). Dilemmas of 'informed consent' in children. *New England Journal of Medicine*, **289**: 885–90.

Silverman, W. A. (1985). Human experimentation: a guided step into the unknown. Oxford University Press.

Skegg, P. D. G. (1988). *Law, Ethics and Medicine*. Clarendon Press, Oxford.

Slater, E. (1971). Health service or sickness service?. *British Medical Journal*, **4**: 734–6.

Smith, G. P. (1985). Defective newborns and government intermeddling. *Medicine, Science and Law*, **25** (1): 44–8.

Todres, D., Krane, D., Howell, M., and Shannon, D. (1977). Pediatricians' attitudes affecting decision-making in defective newborns. *Pediatrics*, **60**: 197–201.

US President's Commission (1983). *The study of ethical problems in medicine and biomedical and behavioral research: deciding to forego life-sustaining treatment: ethical, medical and legal issues in treatment decisions*. U.S. Government Printing Office, Washington DC.

Walker, C. H. M. (1988). Current topic, ". . . officiously to keep alive". *Archives of Disease in Childhood*, **63**: 560-4.

Wells, C. (1989). 'Otherwise kill me': marginal children at the edges of existence. In Birthrights: law and ethics at the beginnings of life (ed. R. Lee and D. Morgan). *Routledge, London*.

Whitelaw, A. (1986). Death as an option in neonatal intensive care. *Lancet*, **2**: 328–31.

Williams, G. (1981). *The Times*, 13 August, cited in Mason, J. K. (1988). *Human life and medical practice*. Edinburgh University Press.

11B   GOVERNMENT REGULATIONS IN THE UNITED KINGDOM: COMMENTARY

Margaret Brazier

INTRODUCTION

The absence of detailed, formal regulations directing British paediatricians as to how they should care for sick newborn infants is to be welcomed. Bureaucrats in Whitehall, however well-intentioned, cannot prescribe solutions to the tragic human dilemmas which arise when parents find that their much-wanted child is far from whole and healthy. None the less, the absence of detailed 'rules' imposes an awesome responsibility on the child's parents, and on the doctors and nurses caring for her. In a significant number of instances that responsibility will initially rest heavily on the health professionals. If the mother has undergone a difficult labour, or been delivered by cesarean section, her ability to participate in the decision-making process regarding her child may be limited. The father, assuming his active involvement in the birth, will be suffering from a double shock. His partner may be at least temporarily ill and incapacitated. His child, he is now told, is seriously handicapped.

The professionals taking the crucial, early decisions about the infant's future do not operate in a legal vacuum. As Professor Campbell has explained, the law in England has intervened on a number of occasions to decide the fate of individual infants. But within English law there remain considerable areas of uncertainty as to when and how, and for how long, you must actively treat a very sick newborn child. The law's uncertainties reflect, I believe, the moral confusion in society both in connection with the specific question of the care of very sick and handicapped babies and in relation to traditional doctrines of the sanctity of life in general. Only a minority of people in the United Kingdom today regularly practise a religious faith which confers absolute moral certainty in matters of life and death. The majority 'muddle through' in traditional British fashion.

However in the United Kingdom, as in the United States, on the extremes of the debate on sanctity of life views have polarized. Fundamentalists from several branches of Christianity, and from other monotheistic religions, seek to re-establish an inviolable right to life from the moment of conception. They contend that abortion should be equated with murder. The vehemence of some 'pro-life' opinion has in this country, as across the Atlantic, led to public disorder in the streets outside abortion facilities. At the opposite end of the spectrum, a group of radical moral philosophers argue that human life of itself commands no right to respect. Only those human animals who are 'persons' have any moral significance and can lay claim to moral rights (Brazier 1992, chap. 2).

I want in this commentary on Professor Campbell's chapter to attempt four tasks. I do not want to repeat his painstaking account of the detailed case law and professional guidance. But (1) I shall assess the impact of the 'personhood' debate on the care of the newborn. (2) I shall explore the effect of disputes relating to abortion on perinatology. (3) I will examine the rights of parents to decide on their babies' fate. (4) I want to consider whether in terms of law and ethics we actually should treat a newborn baby any differently from her older siblings, her parents, or indeed her grandparents. Are there in reality ethical problems of perinatology, or are such problems particular applications of more general issues concerning prolonging life and the euthanasia controversy?

WHEN IS A BABY A PERSON?

The ethical dilemmas surrounding decisions as to when the life of a severely handicapped baby must be prolonged derive at least in part from the assumption that, once born, the baby has moral rights of her own. There can be no doubt that in law birth is a crucial watershed. As was demonstrated in the previous section of this chapter, at birth English law confers full legal personality on the child, and as a result, those caring for the child are exposed to the full rigours of the laws on homicide. A botched unlawful abortion can lead to a prosecution for murder if the infant none the less survives birth, but dies later of its pre-natal injuries. An obstetrician who carries out an entirely lawful abortion from which a live infant is born finds herself obliged to do all that is feasible to preserve the life of an entity she set out to destroy. Her only source of 'comfort' is that where such prosecutions have been brought, confusion relating to gestational age and capacity to survive has generally resulted in aborted trials (Mason 1988; Brazier 1992, Chap. 13; Towers 1979; *R. v. Hamilton* 1983).

A growing number of moral philosophers, in the United Kingdom most notably Jonathan Glover and John Harris, assert that the dilemma about how to treat sick babies is a false dilemma. Humans are simply one species of mammals. The human animal, be it fetus, newborn infant, or grown adult enjoys no rights derived solely from membership of the human species. Ending a human life is no more or less unethical than ending the life of any other animal. What gives a human moral significance over and above other non-human animals is 'personhood'. *Persons*, not human organisms, have a moral right to life. To qualify as a person a human entity must enjoy those capacities which distinguish her from other animals. That is to say, she must have a capacity for self-awareness, and an ability to recognize herself as a functioning reasoning individual capable of relating to other persons in society. She must be able to value her own life (Glover 1977; Harris 1985).

Fetuses are thus clearly not persons; but nor are newborn infants. Neither abortion nor infanticide is intrinsically morally wrong. A wrong is done only if in destroying a fetus or an infant who is not yet a person, the interests of some undoubted person are harmed. Abortion against the mother's will is a wrong against her. Killing an hour-old baby is a wrong against those who will be harmed by that act—against her parents if they wish her to survive. In neither case has the fetus or the child any independent moral claim.

Were such criteria of 'personhood' to be applied to the ethics of perinatology, it might seem that some of the ethical dilemmas thereof would wiped out 'at a stroke'. The fate of the infant would be decided by her parents. There would be no need to evaluate the degree of handicap of the infant or her potential quality of life. In unadulterated form the 'personhood' criteria dictate that, as no baby is a person, parents might be permitted to terminate the existence of a perfectly healthy infant just because, for example, she looked too much like a hated aunt. Parents dissatisfied with a less than perfect infant could reject a colour-blind child, an infant with a finger missing, and so on, at any time up until he acquired the necessary self-awareness. Harris however contends that in such cases, if persons other than the parents are ready and willing to take on the rejected child, killing the child may contravene those persons' interests. The parents would have no right to kill a child who could be placed for adoption.

The crux of the personhood argument remains however that the infant herself is of no moral significance. She has no claim on society to preserve her life. It is no more unethical to terminate her life directly than it would be were she still *in utero*. Indeed as causing pain to any animal capable of experiencing pain is unethical, killing the rejected infant swiftly and painlessly is a moral imperative. Allowing her to die slowly, perhaps of starvation, would be manifestly unethical.

Implementing philosophical theories of 'personhood' in effect sanctions infanticide on demand. Such a policy would be likely to be regarded with revulsion by the majority of the population in both the United Kingdom and the United States. Legal implementation of 'personhood' criteria is highly unlikely on two grounds. First, public outrage might well threaten public disorder on a scale which would make the 'abortion riots' look tame. Second, translating the ethical debate into legal principle would be to say the least problematic. At what stage in her development does a baby develop the required capacity for self-awareness? When does she become a person? Is it six months, a year, or more? The sicker and more handicapped the child, the later that day will come. The law needs precision. A rule setting the threshold at some particular number of months or years will be random. Attempting to formulate statutory criteria applicable to each individual case will promise endless litigation. Retaining birth as the crucial legal watershed is, if nothing else, the most pragmatic solution. The event is indisputable. The infant, however sick she may be, has, from then on, an existence independent of her mother. There is no longer any direct conflict between the infant's interests in life and health and those of her mother.

Despite the unlikelihood of legislation embodying 'personhood' criteria, the influence of the debate on the ethics of perinatology should not be underestimated. However unpalatable at first sight active infanticide might appear to some, the writings of Harris, Glover, and others force us to recognize some harsh realities and reassess muddled thinking. Changing *mores* on abortion cannot logically be disassociated from the ethical and legal debate on the care of the newly delivered child. What logic dictates than an entity may at 39$^{1/2}$ weeks' gestation be destroyed, but that that same entity, perhaps just 24 hours later, once delivered into the world is entitled to thousands of pounds of NHS resources?

KILL THE FETUS: SAVE THE BABY

The Abortion Act 1967 (as amended by the Human Fertilization and Embryology Act 1990) in effect permits the destruction of embryos and fetuses up to 24 weeks' gestation at the doctors' discretion. The 1967 Act does not sanction abortion on request. Where the pregnancy is less than 24 weeks advanced, termination of the pregnancy is lawful if two medical practitioners are prepared to certify in good faith that the continuance of the pregnancy will involve either risk to the life of the pregnant woman, or risk of injury to her physical or mental health, or that of her existing children, greater than if the pregnancy were terminated. Many British gynaecologists are prepared to interpret those criteria in such a way that, at any rate in the first trimester of pregnancy, they will always declare that termination is the safer option. Even beyond 12 weeks of pregnancy little hard evidence of risk to the woman's health may be required. The distress of an unwanted pregnancy may suffice. There is only one fully reported judgment of a successful prosecution under the 1967 Act (*R.* v. *Smith (John) 1974*). A second prosecution succeeded in 1992. In both cases a single doctor engaged in a degree of fraud and obvious malpractice.

The Abortion Act 1967 set no time limit of its own on abortion in England. It left intact the provisions of the Infant Life (Preservation) Act 1929, prohibiting child destruction. That Act made it a criminal offence to destroy the life of any child 'capable of being born alive'. Section 37 of the Human Fertilization and Embryology Act 1990 amended the Abortion Act. Abortion beyond 24 weeks is lawful if either the termination of the pregnancy is necessary to prevent grave permanent injury to the physical or mental health of the mother, or its continuation threatens the life of the mother, or there is a substantial risk of serious fetal handicap. Only a risk to the life of the mother justified destroying the fetus 'capable of being born alive' under the 1929 Act. A doctor acting lawfully under the amended provisions of the Abortion Act is now immune from prosecution under the 1929 Act.

Professor Campbell welcomes the amendment of the Abortion Act. In so far as the statutory phrase 'capable of being born alive' had proved difficult to interpret he is right to do so (*C.* v. *S.* 1987; *Rance* v. *Mid-downs Health Authority* 1990). He notes the anomaly that a perfectly normal fetus who may be capable of surviving birth can now be destroyed up to 24 weeks of gestation. But he regards the removal of an upper time-limit for cases of severe fetal abnormality as sensible. In popular perception at the time of the debate on time-limits for abortion much was made of the cruelty of requiring a woman to continue a pregnancy where the fetus was grossly deformed or, as in the case of an anencephalic fetus, would at best survive no more than a few weeks after birth. The amended Abortion Act simply specifies that handicap must be severe. The wording of the Act is no different from the original provisions of that Act that since 1967 have always permitted abortion earlier in pregnancy on grounds of fetal handicap. Under those provisions fetuses diagnosed as likely to be suffering from spina bifida, hydrocephalus, or Down syndrome of whatever degree have been destroyed. No challenge has ever been made to the doctors' definition of what may constitute *severe* handicap.

The amended Abortion Act in England has this consequence. A potential Down syndrome child may lawfully be destroyed at any time up to birth. Yet a similar, perhaps more severely affected, child who escapes pre-birth termination may be made a ward of the court and operated on directly in opposition to both her parents' wishes (*Re B*. 1981) A gynaecologist who kills the fetus by whatever means acts lawfully. A pediatrician who does not actively treat the child may face trial for murder (*R* v. *Arthur* 1981; Gunn and Smith 1985). The paradoxical nature of the fetus–child distinction is further highlighted if we examine court-ordered interventions in pregnancy. In a number of jurisdictions in the USA women have been required to undergo surgery or other interventions to preserve the viable fetus (Gallagher 1989). In 1988 the English Court of Appeal refused to make a fetus a ward of court (*In re F. (in utero)* 1988). Yet in October 1992 the President of the Family Division issued a declaration authorizing a cesarean section against the mother's will (*In re S*. 1992)

Court-ordered interventions to protect the fetus are particularly anomalous in England, where in other circumstances abortion laws allow the deliberate destruction of the fetus. Perhaps it is foolish to seek for consistency in the law. Maybe in amending the Abortion Act 'pro-choice' campaigners 'won'? Whereas in the court cases on enforced cesarean surgery a 'pro-life' view prevailed? Such an explanation is over-facile. The paradoxes inherent in our differential treatment of the viable fetus and the born infant derive, I would suggest, from unwillingness to address directly the proper moral status of those entities. For those on the extremes of the debate life is much simpler: the fetus either has, and has had since fertilization, the same moral rights as you and I; or it is morally irrelevant. Consensus between these two standpoints is impossible. But I would suggest that until the 1990 amendment of the abortion legislation and the judgment in 1992 *in re S*, the common law in England at least operated a coherent compromise.

Before 1992 the English courts consistently held that the fetus had no independent legal personality (*Paton* v. *BPAS* 1978; *C* v. *S* 1987). The law conferred on the fetus no rights exercisable against the mother (*In re F (in utero) 1988*). The Congenital Disabilities (Civil Liability) Act 1976, granting rights to compensation for pre-natal injuries, specifically exempted mothers from general liability under that Act, and made any tort against the child derivative on a tort against the mother (Eekelaar and Dingwall 1984). The mother was restrained only from any direct attempt to destroy the fetus she carried. Even so, where the continued existence of the fetus threatened her life or health such a direct 'attack' on the fetus to preserve the mother was permitted both by the Infant Life (Preservation) Act and by the common law (*R. v. Bourne* 1938). With the exception of the novel provision allowing abortion on ground of fetal handicap the 1967 Act pursued the same policy. In cases of conflict between maternal rights and fetal interest, the maternal rights prevailed. Once the fetus was capable of an independent existence, though, that existence could be terminated only on evidence of an exceptionally serious threat to the mother's welfare.

The underlying policy of the pre-1990 law could be explained in the following manner. The nature of the developing fetus, its true moral status and significance, can never be resolved. The mother's moral status is beyond doubt (Brazier 1988). For so long as the fetus is inescapably dependent on the mother for survival, her welfare and rights must prevail over those of the fetus. As the fetus matures, so the balance begins to tip somewhat in its favour. Grounds justifying destruction of the fetus in the interests of the mother must be of much greater substance once the fetus could survive outside the womb, and once the burden we ask the mother to bear is lessened, at least in terms of the weeks of pregnancy still to be endured. But, right up to birth, in the rare situation where the choice is quite starkly mother or fetus, the mother's interests must still be preferred.

The law designated birth as the crucial watershed, not because the fetus lacked moral significance prior to birth, but simply because until birth the mother's interests in her own bodily welfare and autonomy prevailed in any case of conflict. Such a policy is not necessarily inconsistent with recognition in principle that the developing fetus shares the same moral status as his mother. Courts in the USA and now in England exercising a purported jurisdiction to compel the mother to undergo invasive procedures to benefit the fetus are exercising a power almost certainly not available for the benefit of a born child. Once delivered, the parental responsibilities devolving on both parents demand that those parents provide appropriate care for the infant. But under what power could either mother or father be ordered to undergo invasive medical treatment to save the child? Parents cannot be ordered to donate blood or bone marrow even if their child's life is forfeit. Special legislation has been required wherever we have sought to justify derogation from an adult's autonomy over her own body. The common law has never compelled its subjects to be Good Samaritans. We are enjoined from harming other persons. We are not compelled to help them. Before the 1990 amendment of the Abortion Act and the controversial judgment *In re S.* pregnant women were enjoined from harming the viable fetus, but could not be compelled to undergo procedures others judged to be in the interests of the fetus. Today a pregnant woman can arrange the destruction of a viable fetus deemed to be at risk of handicap, yet may be ordered to undergo surgery to preserve the life of its healthy brother. The law in England at least appears tacitly to have accepted that the handicapped fetus is of lesser moral value than its siblings.

PARENTAL RIGHTS AND THE NEWBORN INFANT

If a fetus survives the perils of gestation and birth itself, then from the moment he has an existence separate from the mother, the moment he has an independent circulatory system, he is in the eyes of English Law as much a person as you or I. Any act designed to hasten his death by however short a time constitutes murder, punishable by a mandatory term of life imprisonment. Moreover should any person subject to a duty to provide care for the child withhold appropriate care, be that food, warmth, or medical aid, intending that the child should die, that too constitutes murder (*R.* v. *Gibbins and Proctor 1918*). The newborn infant's parents and the team of health professionals caring for him are indubitably subject to such a duty of care to the child, however profound his handicap. The crucial question becomes, in the light of that handicap, what form of medical aid is called for to discharge that duty. Does it necessarily require that parents authorize and professionals carry out active treatments to prolong life? Does there come a point where even feeding is not mandatory? Professor Campbell has outlined the series of cases in which the English courts have tussled with these questions. Can any coherent conclusions be drawn from them in 1994?

In 1981, commenting on the trial of Dr Leonard Arthur, an editorial in the *British Medical Journal* forthrightly declared that parents should be the primary decision-makers. The parents should be seen as the instruments through which the baby accepts or rejects treatment (*British Medical Journal* 1981). Perhaps the only incontrovertible statement which can be made relating to the law and perinatology in the United Kingdom is that that view, of parents as *primary* decision-makers, does not represent current legal practice. Parents cannot require doctors to treat an infant where the latter deem such treatment futile (*Re J.* 1992). Nor do they have an absolute right of veto over treatment, as the Baby Alexandra judgment so amply demonstrates (*Re B.* 1981). The primary decision-makers are the professionals assessing and judging the infant's condition, prognosis, and needs. The parents' opinions and readiness to care for the child form a greater or lesser part of that judgment, depending on the circumstances of the child and the family, and the latter's relationship with the professionals. Parents dissatisfied with the professionals' judgment can resort to the courts to assert their 'right' to determine the child's fate. Both professionals and patients operate within constraints laid down by the courts, requiring them to accord the child respect as a fellow-person and to reach their respective collective or separate judgments in the 'best interests of the child'.

But should parents be afforded clearer and greater rights in relation to the infant? Is the current state of English Law too much an endorsement of medical paternalism? Have the courts any business compelling the parents of a Down syndrome infant to allow her to have surgery when a few days before, while she was still *in utero*, her mother could have had her killed? I remain uncertain about how far parents can in reality take on the primary role in decisions concerning their handicapped infants. But I am certain that the law is justified in imposing constraints on how such infants should be cared for, whether professionals or parents have made the initial decisions on treatment or non-treatment.

As I understand the position, in a significant number of cases, where a baby is born with potentially serious handicap, there is little if any time for reflection or consultation. A baby is delivered very prematurely and at a very low birthweight. An instant judgment must be made whether to resuscitate her and rush her to the special-care baby unit. A child is born with hydrocephalus. If he is to survive and to be spared agony, a shunt must be inserted more or less straight away. Can any parent make an informed judgment in these circumstances? (Morley 1991). The mother, if she has been delivered by cesarean under general anaesthetic, may still be unconscious. The father, if present, is asked to make a decision about a child who may be biologically his offspring but with whom he has as yet no substantive parental relationship. In another context the English Court of Appeal has declared that in any case of doubt as to whether or not to intervene to preserve a human life that doubt should be resolved in favour of preserving life (*Re T*. 1992). The infant should be given the benefit of the doubt. His parents' effective inability to play much of a role in the decision-making relating to those first moments of life should never prejudice his survival.

Of course, there is a major difficulty ensuing from the above argument. Once Baby X is in the Special Care Baby Unit attached to a ventilator, being fed by tube, and Baby Y's shunt has been inserted, the legal conundrum of what to do next is exacerbated. The initial decision to treat gains time— time to assess the baby's condition fully, to make a proper prognosis as to his future. The mother recovers from the birth, and both parents gain time to understand their, and their baby's, dilemma. But if the collective judgment of professionals and parents becomes that the child's profound handicap is such that he would be 'better off dead', then what may have to be contemplated is not simply withholding further treatment, but withdrawing existing treatment—turning off the ventilator; removing the naso-gastric tube. And then the question surfaces where such conduct amounts to an impermissible *act*, hastening death and so constituting murder.

Three judgments of the Court of Appeal chart a way through these troubled waters, *Re B*. (1981), *Re C*. (1989), and *Re J*. (1990). The acquittal of Dr Arthur after a bungled trial by a jury unwilling to equate a much-respected doctor with a vicious murderer tells us little if anything of substance about legal constraints on the treatment of the newborn. In *Re B*, the baby Alexandra case, the Court of Appeal made it clear beyond doubt that handicap of itself did not justify withholding the treatment to prolong an infant's life that would unhesitatingly have been given to a non-handicapped sister. Down syndrome *per se* is no reason to deny the infant any form of treatment or surgery necessary to preserve life or health. And I would argue that the same is true of any form of mental or physical handicap, however profound, and whatever the impact of that handicap on the child's family. Only if the child's life will be 'demonstrably awful' can she, in the words of Templeman, LJ, in effect be 'condemned to die'.

In *Re C.* in 1989 a baby girl had been made a ward of court at birth, and immediate authorization was given by the court to insert a shunt. She suffered from acute hydrocephalus, with only rudimentary brain formation. She appeared to be blind and virtually deaf. The expert evidence was that she could not survive for more than a few months whatever was done for her. At 16 weeks, when a further application was made to the court, she was the size of a 4-week infant, save for her enlarged head. Nurses were attempting to feed her painstakingly by spoon and syringe. She did not seem to be absorbing more than minimal nourishment. The questions for the court were whether the staff caring for C. were obliged to resort to naso-gastric feeding if other means failed; and, if C. developed an infection, must she be treated with antibiotics? The Court of Appeal confirmed the original judge's finding that no such obligation existed. C. was dying; her quality of life was 'demonstrably awful'. In addition to her multiple physical handicaps, she was incapable of even 'limited intellectual function'. The staff caring for C. owed her a duty to ensure she could die peacefully with ' . . .the greatest dignity and the least of pain, suffering and distress'.

What *Re C.* establishes is this. An infant born with multiple handicaps and at best a lifespan of some months need not be actively treated so as to extend that lifespan to its absolute maximum. Where ordinary feeding, as part of loving nursing care, is not possible, staff are not required to resort to artificial means of nutrition and hydration. The comfort of the child must be their primary consideration. *Re C.* invites one further question. C. was not in the care of her parents. What if a child in C.'s condition, with loving parents, were the subject of a dispute between the professionals and the parents, the latter wished their infant to receive all available means of prolonging her life. It is by no means certain in England that the parental wish would prevail. In *Re J.* (1992), remember, the Court of Appeal refused to order doctors to ventilate a child treatment of whose condition the doctors judged to be futile.

The criteria for withholding/withdrawing treatment from sick infants were taken a stage further on from *Re C.* in the other *Re J.* judgment, *Re J.* (1990). J. had been born 13 weeks premature, with a birthweight of 1.1 kg. He had nearly died several times, suffered from extensive brain damage, and was said to be likely to develop paralysis, blindness, and probable deafness. However, he was not imminently dying, and the medical evidence was that, given all available care when he developed, as he was likely to, intercurrent illnesses, he might well survive into his mid-teens. He had already suffered episodes of cyanosis and collapse. If such an episode recurred must J. be resuscitated? The Court of Appeal said no. Lord Donaldson, the President of the Court of Appeal, treated *Re B*. (1981) as requiring the court to conduct a 'balancing exercise' between the infant's interest in survival and the quality of his life. Was that life likely to be so 'demonstrably awful' as to outweigh the desire for life? And as Professor Campbell has noted, Lord Donaldson added a new twist to the tale. The decision must seek to act on the 'substituted judgment' of the child, to assess how he would, if he could, judge his fate. Once again the parents are not perceived as primary decision-makers, but together with health professionals and, in this case, the court, their role is to attempt to stand in the child's shoes and take for him a decision he cannot take for himself.

Re B., Re C., and *Re J.* pose three questions. (1) Just what role do parents play in the decisions to be made about their baby? (2) Have the courts paid due regard to parental rights? (3) Have the courts themselves got the 'balancing exercise' right? Answering the first question is not quite as straightforward as it might appear. It is clear the parents do not enjoy any sort of absolute right to determine the child's future. Withholding treatment is lawful only if on objective criteria the 'demonstrably awful' future of the child outweighs his interest in life. The child's perspective on that equation must be explored. Yet it is equally clear that it is not mandatory in every case to seek judicial sanction for withholding treatment. If doctors and parents agree on the equation there is no requirement that a court approve that joint decision. However, if parents want their mentally handicapped daughters sterilized, the approval of the court is mandatory, or doctors and parents may be liable for assault (*Re. B.* 1987). Parents of newborn infants, if in agreement with their professional advisers, and confident that the case of their child does fall within the broad parameters of permissible decisions as defined by the courts, do seem to have some greater power over their child than later in life.

Parents alone have limited power. They cannot in effect override the opinions of the professionals; only in certain limited circumstances may they endorse those opinions. The Children Act 1989 following on from the judgment of the House of Lords in *Gillick* v. *West Yorkshire and Wisbech A.H.A.* (1985) established that in England parents do not enjoy rights as such. They are subject to parental responsibilities, and parental rights exist to enable the parent to fulfil those responsibilities. Where a judgment has to be made relating to a child *prima facie* the parent may be considered best able to act for the child, to determine her 'best interests'. Should my teenage daughter be injured in an accident and I come to her finding her unconscious in the local hospital, the fourteen-year history of our relationship equips me to some extent to make decisions for her. I know her likes and dislikes, her fears, and her hopes for the future. Years of love and care, I trust, would enable me to put her first even if necessary at my and her father's expense. No such history underpins the relationship of parent and newborn infants. Parents have no equivalent knowledge of the child's character and desires. The interests of older siblings may quite naturally take priority in the parental mind. I would suggest that the younger the infant the less compelling is the parental claim to act for the child. Externally imposed constraints are right and proper.

Are those constraints rightly drawn in England? While I recognize that Lord Donaldson in *Re J.* directing that the 'substituted judgment' of the infant be considered was motivated by entirely proper concerns, I believe 'substituted judgment' in such cases is a fiction. Lord Donaldson was seeking to avoid the danger that in judging the interests of the child, healthy adults assess his quality of life from *their* perspective. What may seem intolerable to a person who has known no other life than one of good health and intellectual stimulation will be very differently perceived by another individual who has never himself enjoyed a life other than that constrained by his disability. In attempting the 'balancing exercise', that factor must always be borne in mind. None the less, the perspective of that particular child, of J., or B., or C., cannot in reality be determined. 'Substituted judgment' requires evidence of an individual's prior wishes and values. Handicapped newborn infants have never been able to articulate such wishes or values.

A much larger question arises, however, than any quibble over the nature of 'substituted judgment', should the treatment/non-treatment of newborn infants be subject to principles any different to those pertaining later in life? In the wake of the trial of Dr Arthur, proposals were advanced for legislation specifically directed at infants under 28 days (Brahams and Brahams 1981). Mason and McCall Smith in the first edition of *Law and medical ethics* advanced the case for legalizing active measures to terminate life of an infant less than 72 hours old where' . . .further life would be intolerable by virtue of pain and suffering or because of severe cerebral incompetence; and the underlying condition is not amenable to reasonable medical treatment' (Mason and McCall Smith 1983). They have since amended that proposal to delete both any provision for active 'euthanasia' and the 72-hour limit (Mason and McCall Smith 1991). The underlying issue remains: should we treat newborn infants differently from the rest of us? Is neonaticide distinguishable from homicide? Is the neonate less of a person than his six-year-old sister? It should be noted that, if the term neonate conventionally refers to an infant less than 28 days old, neither J., nor C., who were both about 16 weeks old, qualify as neonates.

ARE BABIES DIFFERENT?

In December 1992 the House of Lords was asked to rule on whether naso-gastric feeding could be withdrawn from Anthony Bland. Anthony Bland, by the time of the proceedings aged 21, had suffered devastating injuries in the disaster at the Hillsborough football ground in April 1989. Since that day he had lain in a hospital bed in a condition known as persistent vegetative state (PVS). He could breath unaided, and his brain stem remained alive. He was incapable of any voluntary movement; he could not swallow, nor could he see or hear. The cortex of the brain had lost its function. The courts were asked to decide whether naso-gastric feeding could be discontinued and whether, if Mr Bland developed an infection, he must be treated with antibiotics (*Airedale NHS Trust* v. *Anthony Bland* 1992).

I do not propose to analyse the Bland judgment in detail, but the case of Anthony Bland raises two important issues.

1. The media greeted the case as a British 'first'. The courts were to be asked for the first time to judge where doctors could lawfully decide to let a severely damaged patient, incapable of making any decision for himself, die. Yet on two previous occasions, *Re C.* and *Re J.*, the Court of Appeal had already addressed that question. The Court of Appeal in *Bland* recognized the importance of its earlier judgments. Sir Thomas Bingham MR (the new President at the Court of Appeal) applied much the same 'balancing exercise' to Anthony Bland's predicament as his predecessor had applied to C. and J. The judgment of the Court of Appeal was ultimately confirmed by the Law Lords, albeit on rather different reasoning.

    There seem to be two key differences in the manner in which the 'balancing exercise' was applied to Anthony Bland. First, the Court of Appeal and the Law Lords both ruled that feeding should not be withdrawn without the authorization of the court at least until such time that '. . .a body of experience and practice will build up which will obviate the need for application in every case'. Second, it is unclear whether an adult patient with multiple disabilities such as J., but not suffering from PVS, would be treated as J. was. In the case of Anthony Bland their Lordships stressed the total absence of any intellectual function in Mr Bland, the loss of all cortical activity. J. was, despite his profound handicap, in less desperate plight.

2. The ruling in the *Bland* judgment contains another issue of significance to the care of all severely handicapped patients. The Law Lords authorized the cessation of naso-gastric feeding, the removal of the naso-gastric tube. Their Lordships rejected submissions that such an act equated to administering a lethal dose of drugs to kill the patient. Discontinuing treatment, whether by deciding not to replace a defective naso-gastric tube or withdrawing a tube in place, did not attract criminal liability. Artificial means of nutrition and hydration constitute treatment just as much as the administration or drugs or any form of physical therapy. Artificial distinctions between acts and omissions, between 'initiating a new regime of artificial feeding and discontinuing an existing regime', should not be the basis for determining criminal liability.

Where does the *Bland* judgment leave the law relating to the care of handicapped infants? One matter is clarified. If criteria for not instituting artificial feeding, for not ventilating the child are met, existing regimes of treatment may also lawfully be withdrawn. How far identical criteria apply to devastatingly injured adults and severely damaged babies remains unclear. I would contend that the law and professional ethics should make no difference between the two. Once an infant is safely delivered the common law accords her full legal personality. Her status is the same as Anthony Bland's. Thus either society must accept that a degree of profound handicap short of the persistent vegetative state justifies cessation of treatment of *all* those injured by disease or trauma, be they child victims of meningitis, teenagers injured in road accidents, or elderly patients in the final stages of dementia; or infants such as J., handicapped but still with a functioning cortex, should be preserved. I suspect that the proposition that older children and adults who are neither terminally ill nor in PVS should have treatment discontinued would not meet with judicial or popular approval. Distinctions based on age are none the less illogical. They derive, I would suggest, from three sources. (1) Society's attitude to the newborn has been influenced by our attitude to the unborn. Proposals for legalized neonaticide are in effect an extension of abortion laws, granting parents a further period of 'grace' before they lose the ability to decide whether to accept or reject the infant. (2) The older the person, the greater we perceive his emotional claim on family and society. We assume that with an older child the harm to others occasioned by his death will be greater. Therefore greater reflection on the decision to escape treatment is called for. (3) Then there is the vexed question of resources. Hoffman, LJ in the *Bland* judgment commented 'one is bound to observe the cost of keeping a patient like Anthony Bland alive is very considerable and that in another case the health authority might conclude that its resources were better devoted to their patients'. The younger the patient the greater the potential drain on health-care resources. Are damaged babies too expensive to keep alive?

That crude, cruel question has received an affirmative answer from the British think-tank, the Office of Health Economics. A report published early in 1993 suggests that constraints on available resources should prompt a review of policy in relation to the resuscitation and care of premature low-birthweight infants. Can society bear the cost of first providing intensive care for these babies, and then in many cases shouldering the long-term burden of looking after those who survive but suffer from varying degrees of handicap? The logic of the report is this. Either society accepts that babies are different—to put it provocatively, the baby is not fully human, and lacks the same moral status as you and I—or a similar economic analysis is applied to all patients regardless of age. Can society properly bear the cost of caring for demented elderly patients, sometimes for decades?

CONCLUSIONS

No 'outsider' who, neither as a mother or a doctor, has had to take the painful decisions daily confronting those who work with sick newborn infants should lightly pronounce on the ethics of perinatology. I do not seek to do so. I do believe that at the heart of the debate on the management of severely handicapped infants one simple principle should be pre-eminent. If respect for human life is to retain any meaning, that respect must be accorded whatever the age of the human entity. Once safely delivered, the baby enjoys the same moral status and legal personality as any of us. Ethical and legal principles which in effect allow termination of an infant's existence where in similar circumstances treatment of an adult would continue seem to me to tread on dangerous ground.

REFERENCES

Airedale NHS Trust v. *Anthony Bland*. [1993] 2 Weekly Law Reports 316, C. A. and H. L.

Brahams, D. and Brahams, M. (1981). 'Limitation of Treatment Bill'. *Law Society Gazette*, **78**.

Brazier, M. (1988). 'Embryos' "rights". Abortion and research.' *Medicine, ethics and the law* (ed. M. D. A. Freeman). Stevens, London, 1988.

Brazier, M. (1992). *Medicine, patients and the law* (2nd edn). Penguin, London, 1992.

British Medical Journal (1981). 'Medical news'. **283** *British Medical Journal*, 567.

B. (a minor) (wardship: medical treatment) [1981] 2 Weekly Law Reports 1421 C. A.

B. (a minor) (wardship: sterilisation) [1989] 2 All England Reports 206 H. L.

C (a minor) (wardship: medical treatment) [1989] 2 All England Reports 782, C. A.

C V S [1987] 1 All England Reports 1:

Eekelaar, J. M. and Dingwall, R. W. J. (1984). Some legal issues of obstetric practice. *Journal of Social Welfare Law*, 258.

In re F. (in utero) [1988] 2 All England Reports 193 C. A.

Gallagher, J. (1989). Fetus as patient. *Reproductive laws for the 1990'* p.y 185 Humana Press, Totowa, New Jersey, 1989.

Gillick v. *West Norfolk and Wisbech A. H. A.* [1985] 3 All England Reports 402 H. L.

Glover, J. *Causing death and saving lives*. Penguin, Harmondsworth, 1977.

Gunn, M. and Smith, J. C. (1985). Arthur's case and the right to life of a down's syndrome child. *Criminal Law Review*, 705.

Harris, J. M. (1985). *The value of life*. Routledge, London, 1985.

J. (a minor) (wardship: medical treatment) [1990] 3 All England Reports 930 CA.

J. (a minor) (wardship: medical treatment) [1992] 4 All England Reports 614 CA.

Mason, J. K. (1988). *Human life and medical practice*. Edinburgh University Press.

Mason J. K. and McCall Smith, A. (1983). *Law and medical ethics* (ist ed). Butterworth, London.

Mason J. K. and McCall Smith, A. (1991). *Law and medical ethics (3rd edn)*. Butterworth, London.

Morley, C. (1991). Without their consent: working with very premature babies. In *Protecting the vulnerable: autonomy and consent in health care*. Routledge, London, 1991.

Paton v BPAS [1978] 2 All England Reports

R. v Arthur. The Times 6 November 1981.

R. v Bourne. [1938] 3 All England Reports 615.

R. v Gibbins and Proctor. (1918) 13 Criminal Appeal Reports 134.

R. v Hamilton. The Times 6 November 1983.

R. v Smith (John). [1974] 1 Weekly Law Reports 1510 C.A.

Rance v Mid-Downs Health Authority. [1990] 3 All England Reports 930 C. A.

S (adult: refusal of medical treatment). [1992] 4 All England Reports 671.

T (adult: refusal of medical treatment). [1992] 4 All England Reports 649 CA.

Towers, B. (1979). The trials of Dr Waddell. *Journal of Medical Ehics*, **5**, 205.

12

The economics of perinatal care in the United States

12A FINANCING HEALTH CARE FOR PREGNANT WOMEN AND NEWBORNS IN THE US

Birt Harvey

Appropriate prenatal and newborn care should minimize low birthweight, lower newborn mortality and morbidity, and—consequently—decrease subsequent chronic illness and handicapping conditions.

Barriers to appropriate prenatal and newborn care are not only financial; but lack of financial access is a major deterrent. Insurance coverage (status) influences both quality of care and outcome.

Prenatal care is cost-saving, and, for most sick or small newborns, neonatal care is cost-beneficial. Essentially all public-policy leaders profess to believe that governmental resources should be used to ensure that all children start life in the healthiest condition possible. In 1990 the Bush administration proposed and Congress accepted a plan to fund infant mortality-lowering projects in 10 cities. Yet many pregnant women and newborns still lack health insurance.

HEALTH CARE FUNDING AND EXPENDITURES

During the 1980s, national health expenditures increased dramatically, from $250 billion in 1980 to $666 billion in 1990. This increase caused the percentage of Gross National Product consumed by health care to rise from 9.2 per cent to 12.2 per cent. On an individual level, per caput expenditures rose from $1063 to $2566.[1]

Causes of this rapid rise are many. Even after adjusting for general inflation, which was responsible for almost half the rise, the average personal health-care expenditures still rose an average of 4.4 per cent during each year of the 1980s because of inflation in medical prices over and above general inflation. Thus, medical inflation accounted for 22 per cent of the total rise.[1] Other factors contributing to the rise in personal health-care costs included increased population, increased use of technology, population aging, and an increased number of services provided to each individual.

In 1990, 58 per cent of health-care funding came from private sources, including private insurance, and 42 per cent came from Government. Although this 42 per cent a dramatic change from the Government's 25 per cent share in 1960, the percentage that Government contributed to national health care has remained constant since 1980. From the Government's perspective, the picture is different. The percentage of total Government expenditures going into health care was not constant during the 1980s. The per centage of the Federal budget spent on health care increased from 11.7 per cent in 1980 to 15.3 per cent in 1990, and the share of health-care expenditures in State and local government budgets rose from 9.1 per cent to 11.4 per cent. Most of State health expenditures are consumed by Medicaid, the cost of which rose from 24.8 billion in 1980 to 71.3 billion in 1990.[1] Ohio provides an example of the continuing impact on States. In 1986, Medicaid accounted for 10.9 per cent of the State budget; by 1993, it was projected to account for 15.6 per cent.

In 1990, private health insurance funded 32.5 per cent of health care, an increase of 3.5 percentage points over 1980. Total premiums paid in 1980 were $73 billion. By 1990, total premiums amounted to $217 billion, with $186 billion paid out in benefits. The $31 billion difference remained with the insurers.[1] About 29 per cent of the population was covered in 1990 under employee benefit plans, and an additional 28 per cent as dependants of employees.

The rapid rise in the cost of care has been the primary reason, but not the only reason, for an explosion in the cost of private insurance.

GOVERNMENT AND EMPLOYER RESPONSES TO RISING COSTS

To limit expenditures, the Federal Government attempted to control Medicare costs by instituting in 1983 a Diagnostic-Related-Group (DRG) payment system for hospital care and by controlling payments to physicians for their services. Hospitals and physicians responded by shifting some costs to privately insured patients.

Federal and State governments controlled Medicaid expenditures by restricting eligibility, limiting benefits, and keeping reimbursement to providers at artificially low levels. Again, in response to low reimbursement, physicians and hospitals either discontinued providing care for Medicaid patients or attempted to shift the cost of doing so to privately paying patients and their insurance carriers.

Increasingly limited benefits for recipients of Medicaid, and the elimination of Medicaid insurance for many recipients in the early 1980s, resulted in an increase in uncompensated care and further added to the cost shift.

The resultant cost-shifting burden, added to increased cost of medical care, led to premium increases that became an intolerable burden for some employers. Employer responses included discontinuation of insurance; increased reliance on managed care and employer self-insurance plans; constriction of benefits; and increased deductibles, coinsurance, and premiums.[2] In 1990, only 33 per cent of employers paid the full cost of dependant insurance, whereas in 1980 40 per cent had done so.[3]

Increasing numbers of people without health insurance, either governmental or private, have increased the cost-shifting to private-sector purchasers of insurance. Thus the cycle of increasing costs and decreasing coverage and benefits goes on in an ever-expanding manner.

IMPACT ON WOMEN AND CHILDREN

During the past twenty years, employment has shifted from high-paying manufacturing firms with large numbers of employees to lower-paying service firms with fewer employees. The former are likely to offer health insurance; the latter are likely to offer no health insurance, or health insurance with premiums that their low-wage employees can ill afford.[4] Women are disproportionately likely to hold jobs that do not offer health insurance.[4] Consequently, by 1990 over 35 million US residents, including over 12 million children, were uninsured. Approximately 9 million women of childbearing age had no insurance to cover prenatal and delivery care.[5] Although Federal law requires that group health plans covering more than 15 employees provide maternity benefits, these services are often limited, or they have high coinsurance or deductible requirements.[6] Maternity care now accounts for almost 40 per cent of uncompensated inpatient care.[7]

Children in two-parent families with one employed parent suffered a decline in private health insurance coverage from 71 per cent in 1977 to 47 per cent in 1987.[8] Yet insurance problems for children living in two-parent families are fewer than for those living in single-parent households. Children who live in single-parent families increased from 17 per cent in 1977 to 26 per cent in 1987.[8] The percentage of these children who were uninsured rose from 14 per cent to 22 per cent during that decade. In spite of Medicaid expansion during the last half of the 1980s, 21 per cent of children in single-parent families remained uninsured in 1990.[4] Single mothers are more likely to be unemployed or to work part-time[8] and to work in lower-paying service industries. Two-thirds of children in single-parent families live in poor or low-income households.[8] Thus, changes in occupation, decreasing employer-based insurance, increasing premiums, and growth in single-parent families all contribute to an expanding problem: pregnant women and their newborn children who are uninsured or underinsured. Between 1982 and 1986, a study of uninsured and underinsured pregnant women in Northern

California showed a 45 per cent increase in the number of newborns without insurance.[9] In 1990, almost one-quarter of infants living in families just above the poverty level were without insurance, and over one of every six infants in the country had no health-care insurance.[4]

MEDICAID CHANGES

Lack of health insurance results in less preventive care (including prenatal care), delays in care for acute illness, and increased use of emergency departments for primary medical care.

In response to these and other problems associated with lack of insurance, Congress enacted a series of laws, starting in 1984, to expand Medicaid eligibility. One such law, OBRA 1986, gave States the option of expanding eligibility to pregnant women with family incomes below the US poverty level but above the State Aid to Families with Dependent Children income level. By 1988, 26 States had exercised that option.[6] As of April 1990, as a result of further Congressional action, States were required to cover pregnant women and children to the age of six with family incomes below 133 per cent of the Federal poverty level, and States had the option of covering these groups up to 185 per cent of poverty level. There is no evidence, however, that expanding Medicaid eligibility *per se* will improve birth outcomes and health status in young children.[10, 11]

As a result of Medicaid eligibility expansion, major groups without insurance for prenatal and newborn care are female employees or dependants of male workers who earn low salaries in service industries, but who earn more than 133 per cent of the poverty-level income.

RELATIONSHIP OF PRENATAL CARE TO LOW BIRTHWEIGHT AND INFANT MORTALITY

Although several investigators have concluded that an increase in the proportion of women offered insurance to cover care during the first trimester or actually receiving such care does not result in the expected decline in low-birthweight babies,[11, 12] many more studies summarized in a report from the Office of Technology Assessment (OTA) have shown that receipt of prenatal care is inversely related to low birthweight and neonatal mortality.[6] In 1988, 9 per cent of white women and 19 per cent of black women who had little or no prenatal care had low-birthweight babies, compared with 5 per cent and 12 per cent, respectively, of women who began prenatal care during the first trimester.[13]

To demonstrate conclusively that low birthweight and high infant mortality rate are caused by—rather than associated with—lack of prenatal care, a randomized, prospective, controlled study with defined frequency and content of care would be required. Because such a study is not feasible, the alternative is to utilize non-randomized observational studies and retrospectively collected data comparing women receiving or not receiving prenatal care. Such studies can be controlled for many demographic and medical risk factors; alternatively, the instrumental variable technique can be used to attempt to correct for selection bias.

Self-selection is a bias inherent in all studies—a bias that theoretically can cut both ways. Women who seek early prenatal care may have inherently different and lesser social and behavioural risks for adverse outcome than do those who seek late or no prenatal care. Conversely, women with greater medical, familial, or past pregnancy risks may seek care earlier than those without known medical risk.

Most studies based on birth and death records—with adjustments for confounding variables—show a positive and often strong association between prenatal care and birth outcomes. Eighteen of 21 multivariate studies demonstrated significantly improved outcomes in some groups of women receiving prenatal care, and 11 of 15 controlled studies found a significant relationship between neonatal survival and the receipt of prenatal care.[6] Similarly, five studies using the instrumental variable technique, which attempts to correct for biases unknown to persons conducting the study, all showed a significant relationship between lower neonatal mortality and receipt of prenatal care.[6] Further, the number of prenatal visits correlated positively with newborn health status.[14]

According to the OTA, receipt of prenatal care is associated with a 50 per cent reduction in low birthweight,[6] which appears to be a major factor in the positive relationship between prenatal care and pregnancy outcome. In another study, women who did not receive prenatal care were two-thirds as likely to deliver a normal-weight infant as those receiving prenatal care.[15]

Among 4653 infants delivered at Parkland Hospital in Dallas during a 6-month period, delivery of infants born with a weight less than 2250 grams occurred in 14 per cent of women without prenatal care, in contrast to 4 per cent of women receiving prenatal care.[16] Low-birthweight babies make a disproportionate contribution to neonatal mortality rates. Two-thirds of all neonatal deaths occur in infants with a birthweight less than 2500 grams.[17] Low-birthweight babies are almost 40 times more likely to suffer a neonatal death and two to three times more likely to have a lifelong disability than are normal-birthweight babies.[13] In the Parkland study, the perinatal mortality rate among women without prenatal care was over four times that of those women receiving prenatal care.[16]

RELATIONSHIP OF INSURANCE TO PRENATAL CARE AND MATERNAL HEALTH STATUS

Women without private health insurance are more likely to go without prenatal care or to seek it later in pregnancy and to have fewer prenatal visits than those with insurance.[18]

In our current health care-system, multiple factors influence access to prenatal care. They include the capacity and the organization of the system, as well as cultural and personal barriers. The various problems preventing access to care have been determined in a number of studies. A 1988 Institute of Medicine (IOM) report that evaluated 15 studies listed specific barriers.[19] Obstacles to receipt of prenatal care included a low value placed on prenatal care, transportation difficulties, inhospitable delivery of care, lack of provider availability, dislike or fear of prenatal services, and denial of pregnancy. The major obstacle, however, was financial; inadequate or no insurance. The report concluded that a fundamental restructuring of the nation's maternity-care system is needed. First on their list of recommended actions was removal of financial barriers to care.

Also in 1988, the American Academy of Obstetricians and Gynecologists (ACOG) issued a report citing essentially the same barriers to care as those described in the IOM report. They identified and analyzed five programs that might ameliorate the problem and that might impact positively on low birthweight and infant mortality rates. All five programs placed major emphasis on removing financial barriers to access.[20]

Subsequently, the Federal Government in a 1990 internal document that received wide circulation—even though it was never officially released— agreed that lack of insurance, whether private or public, is one of the most serious barriers to care.[5] This report implies Government acceptance of multiple studies demonstrating that financial barriers are the primary cause of failure to obtain or delay in obtaining prenatal care.[21-23]

Insuring more pregnant women by increasing eligibility to Medicaid has been the primary method of addressing financial barriers to care for families of the working poor or the unemployed. Unless such issues as appropriate provider reimbursement, increased availability of services, and successful encouragement of women to use services are addressed, insuring more women through Medicaid may not lead to increased appropriate use of prenatal services,[11] and may actually lead to a decrease in the adequacy and availability of care, with a resultant negative impact on birth outcomes. For example, State financing of increased numbers of eligible pregnant women, if it is financed by decreasing provider reimbursement by 10 per cent, is projected to result in the average birthweight of Medicaid babies decreasing by 165 grams.[10] This neonatal mortality loss would be four times greater than the predicted gain from the increase in the numbers of uninsured women eligible for Medicaid.[10]

A 1989 report by Hadley et al.[24] of over 200 000 hospital discharge records of pregnant women showed that the health status of these women and the hospital care they received were both positively related to having health insurance. Evidence suggesting that lack of maternity insurance results in poor health status in a pregnant women was reflected in an increased likelihood of pyelonephritis and diabetes and a decreased likelihood of toxemia among uninsured pregnant women compared with insured women. Toxemia may increase because of an association with larger babies and with full-term pregnancies, both of which are less common among uninsured women. Correcting for frequency of occurrence, insured women were still significantly more likely to be hospitalized with a secondary diagnosis of toxemia.

The Hadley study also noted that uninsured pregnant women had significantly shorter hospital stays for normal deliveries and lower rates of cesarean section. These findings—controlled for age, type of hospital, and secondary diagnoses—held true for both white and black women. These data do not address the questions of the appropriate length of stay or the appropriate rate of cesarean section, but they do provide evidence that insurance coverage influences the use of resources.

Although this study does not show that prenatal insurance would improve pregnancy outcomes for both mother and infant, it does demonstrate that a difference currently exists between those with and those without insurance, and that provision of insurance should be considered as one possible means of addressing the issue.

Availability of maternity insurance does not necessarily result in appropriate utilization of prenatal services.[11, 25] The removal of financial barriers to care in England failed to reduce the differential in infant mortality rates among different socioeconomic classes. The infant mortality rate of the lowest socioeconomic group was double that of the highest group before the introduction of national health insurance, and it remains so.[26] Thus, factors beyond maternal health insurance impact on the receipt of prenatal care and subsequent pregnancy outcome. Facilitating entry into the medical care system by removing financial barriers is but one step.

To address issues other than insurance, a number of programs have sought to augment utilization of prenatal care. These programs are designed to impact either on the delivery system by increasing its capacity or by making it more friendly or to impact on the individual by case-finding and social supports. The success of such programs is best measured by changes in low birthweight, infant mortality, and infant morbidity. Primarily because numbers of women are limited in most studies, data demonstrating the effectiveness of these programs are tenuous at best.[6, 10, 27, 28] In France, however, a large government-and industry-financed national program designed to prevent premature delivery by educating women about the advantages of prenatal care and appropriate lifestyle, by financing prenatal and delivery care, and by providing and financing necessary support services—including work leave with pay and home bed rest when indicated—appears to have decreased low-birthweight rates significantly.[29]

RELATIONSHIP OF INSURANCE TO NEWBORN HEALTH STATUS

Data on the relationship between hospital outcomes and insurance are minimal for both children and adults. Available evidence does show, however, an inverse relationship between health outcomes, including mortality, and private insurance status.[30]

A study of over 60 000 newborn hospital records[9] in eight Northern California counties in 1986 showed a significantly greater likelihood of an adverse outcome for uninsured compared with privately insured newborns. The risk of adverse outcome associated with a lack of newborn health insurance showed a significant increase between 1982 and 1986, and it was present in each of the 5 years. Factors other than lack of insurance may have contributed to the increased risk of adverse outcomes, but the increased risk remained significantly greater when controlled for low birthweight, fetal malnutrition, and ethnicity.

A 1987 study of over 150 000 newborn hospital discharge records showed that insured newborns had a significantly lower in-hospital mortality rate than did the uninsured. The data were corrected for condition at birth, sex, race, health status of the mother, birthweight, congenital anomalies and other clinical diagnoses, and type of hospital.[24]

RELATIONSHIP OF INSURANCE TO CONSUMPTION OF RESOURCES BY NEWBORNS

With evidence of a greater likelihood of adverse outcomes for uninsured newborns, the issue to be addressed is whether or not these infants are allocated resources equivalent to or greater than those supplied to insured newborns.

That sick people,[30, 31] including children,[32] who have no insurance receive fewer services when they are hospitalized is established. Most in the medical community, the public, and public policy leadership believe, however, that all newborns receive equal hospital care. The data refute this assumption.

Braveman and colleagues studied hospital records of 29 751 California newborns in 1987.[33] All of these infants had serious problems. Sick newborns without insurance, when compared with those with private insurance, had significantly shorter lengths of stay (16 per cent), total charges (28 per cent), and charges per day (10 per cent). The same data showed that the uninsured were at significantly higher medical risk, and therefore they would have been expected to consume more rather than fewer resources.

Privately insured sick newborns are unlikely to have received unnecessary and excessive care, because newborns with indemnity or prepaid insurance utilized equal resources. Physicians who cared for sick newborns whose care was capitated would have an incentive to avoid unnecessary services; but they utilized resources to the same extent as physicians caring for newborns with indemnification insurance, and utilized significantly more resources than physicians caring for uninsured newborns.

In other studies[14, 24] fewer hospital days, consultations, and procedures—in spite of health status worse than that of insured newborns—accounted for less use of hospital resources by uninsured infants.

COST-EFFECTIVENESS OF PRENATAL CARE

Applying more financial resources to prenatal care can be justified on humanitarian grounds if newborn morbidity or mortality rates are thereby reduced. The issue becomes one of deciding which among multiple prenatal care programs should be funded. To those allocating funds for various prenatal care programs, justifying health insurance for all pregnant women becomes more persuasive if the result is more cost-effective than allocation of resources to other programs that may affect newborn morbidity and mortality to a similar extent.

The cost-effectiveness ratio of a prenatal care program is expressed in terms of the additional costs of the program divided by the additional reduction of newborn mortality or morbidity. It is a ratio of cost per life saved or morbidity averted, and it is most meaningful when it is compared with how much alternative programs would cost to achieve the same decrease in morbidity or mortality. For example, one could also estimate the cost per additional life saved by the special supplemental food program for women, infants, and children (WIC). By this measure, among six programs evaluated, investing in prenatal care received during the first trimester is more cost-effective in reducing infant mortality rates than is teen family planning, WIC, abortion, neonatal intensive care, or community centers for maternal and infant care projects.[34] A similar pattern of cost-effectiveness holds true when the denominator is reduction in low birthweight rather than mortality or morbidity. Neonatal intensive care is the least cost-effective strategy among these six programs, but it is three times as effective in averting neonatal mortality.[34] Conclusions must be qualified: the projected improvement in outcomes is based on an outcome comparison with women who start care during the first trimester, and factors other than financial access to care are involved in the early initiation of prenatal care. Evidence suggests, in spite of selection bias inherent in practically all studies, that almost half of poor pregnant women without insurance who do not now initiate prenatal care during the first trimester would do so if financial barriers were removed.[6]

Other studies have looked at cost savings from removing financial barriers to prenatal care. The OTA evaluated the cost of expanding Medicaid to cover prenatal care for all pregnant women in poverty and the savings that would be expected from the resultant decrease in the number of low-birthweight infants. Although their study considered a limited number of factors, they concluded that such an expansion would result in net savings to the health care system.[6]

Another way to evaluate prenatal care is to compare dollars saved after delivery with dollars invested prenatally. Using this method, several studies have quantified the cost savings from receipt of prenatal care. Best known is the IOM study, which provided this oft-quoted figure: for every $1.00 spent on prenatal care for high-risk women, $3.34 could be saved through decreased neonatal intensive care.[35] A study in New Hampshire, using more conservative projections than the IOM analysis, calculated a $2.57 savings for each $1.00 spent on prenatal care.[36] An American Academy of Pediatrics report noted a savings of $2.00 to $10.00 in neonatal care for every $1.00 spent on prenatal care.[37] In Texas, lack of prenatal care was associated with a 50 per cent increase in newborn care costs.[16]

Schwartz[38] studied a stratified sample of neonatal intensive care units (NICUs) in urban hospitals. Slightly over half of all low-birthweight infants in the United States were cared for in these hospitals. Infants between 500 and 2500 grams consumed 57 per cent of NICU costs, whereas they constituted only 9 per cent of the infants. Schwartz estimated that providing prenatal care for all women delivering these babies would have increased the average birthweight enough to produce immediate savings of between $9 and $28 million.

COST-BENEFIT OF NEONATAL INTENSIVE CARE

In comparison with other means of producing healthy infants, neonatal intensive care is the least efficient use of resources; but it too can be evaluated from a cost-benefit perspective. Cost-benefit is (1) the monetary gain from children who survive and who are not chronically ill and who, therefore, consume fewer health resources, plus (2) their lifetime earnings during the years of productive life gained. This analysis, unlike cost-effectiveness analysis, can be viewed in absolute terms of net benefit of neonatal intensive care, without comparison with alternative resource expenditures.

In viewing cost-benefit, going one step further by looking at quality-adjusted years of life gained is particularly valuable. Compared with adults, when viewed in terms of productive years of life gained, the value of neonatal intensive care can be considerably more easily justified for those over 1000 g birthweight than for lower-birthweight infants.[39, 40] As data become available on more recent graduates of neonatal intensive care units, the birthweight at which intensive efforts become easier to justify may become lower.

Prediction of outcome based upon factors in addition to birthweight may be appropriate. Stevenson et al.[41] determined that birthweight was a poor predictor of care costs among infants who weighed between 500 and 1500 grams, and that birthweight as a single characteristic should not be used to determine allocation of resources. An evaluation of infants needing ventilatory assistance[42] demonstrated that expending resources on newborns of less than 28 weeks' gestation was extremely cost-ineffective in improving survival when compared with newborns of more than 28 weeks' gestation who required assisted ventilation, or when compared with infants of 24 to 28 weeks' gestation who did not require assisted ventilation.

Thus from a societal perspective we can decide in which programs we wish to invest. Prenatal care and care of newborns of some undetermined birthweight over 1000 grams can be justified on an economic basis. There is no rational economic reason for our government not to assure financial access to care for these infants and for all pregnant women.

For infants with certain complications or with a birthweight too low for a positive cost-benefit analysis, ethical issues become more important. How much is society willing to pay to decrease morbidity and mortality among the smallest and sickest premature infants? With limited resources, how should allocation be determined? Should we continue to ration resources on the basis of whether infants are fortunate enough to have insurance, or should rationing be implemented on another basis? The physcan responsible for providing care to sick very-low-birthweight infants, to children, or to young or elderly adults should not be required to decide which patients should be treated aggressively.

Our resources are not sufficient to meet all the health-care needs of everyone. In competing in a global economy, allocation of a considerably greater percentage of our gross domestic product to health care will result either in non-competitive prices for our products or in the need to forgo other amenities of life: high wages, leisure time, and generous benefits, including retirement benefits.

If our nation limits health expenditures as industry and public policy leaders and the people all seem to desire, then we must determine how best to allocate limited resources. Do we provide unlimited resources to achieve the lowest possible mortality and morbidity for the smallest of newborns? For whom do we offer organ transplants? How much do we expend on prolongation of life when death is at hand? These societal issues can be determined rationally by cost-effectiveness and cost-benefit analysis; but we have yet to address them.

Rationing decisions do not belong in the hands of the individual physician. Physicians should do all they can for the individual patient within the constraints imposed by society. It is the responsibility of society through elected policy-makers to make programmatic decisions that provide the boundaries within which the physician may provide diagnosis and treatment services, and which the patient must ultimately accept.

REFERENCES

1. Levit, K. R., Lazenby, H. C., Cowan, C. A., and Letsch, S. W. National health expenditures, 1990. *Health Care Financing Review.* 1991; **13**: 29–54.
2. Sullivan, C. B. and Rice, T. The health insurance picture in 1990. *Health Aff. (Millwood).* 1991; **10**: 106–15.
3. National Commission on Children. *Beyond A New American Agenda for Children and Families.* Washington, DC, 1991.
4. Employee Benefit Research Institute. *Sources of health insurance and characteristics of the uninsured, analysis of the March 1991 Current Population Survey,* Special Report and Issue Brief 123. EBRI, Washington, DC, February 1992.

5. Report of the White House Task Force. *Infant mortality in the United States.* Govt Printing Office, Washington, DC, 30 November 1989.
6. Minor, A. F. *The cost of maternity care and childbirth in the United States, 1989.* Health Insurance Association of America, Washington, DC, December 1989.
7. Sloan, F., Valvona, J., and Mullner, R. *Identifying the source of uncompensated care: a statistical profile.* Vanderbilt University, Nashville, 1983.
8. Cunningham, P. L. and Monheit, A. C. Insuring the children: a decade of change. *Health Aff. (Millwood).* 1990; **9**: 76–90.
9. Braveman, P., Oliva, G., Miller, M. G., Reiter, R., and Egerter, S. Adverse outcomes and lack of health insurance among newborns in an eight-county area of California, 1982–1986. *New Engl. J. Med.* 1989; **321**: 508–13.
10. Schlesinger, M. and Kronebusch, K. The failure of prenatal care policy for the poor. *Health Aff (Millwood).* 1990; 9: 91–111.
11. Piper, J. M., Ray, W. A., and Griffin, M. R. Effects of Medicaid eligibilty expansion on prenatal care and pregnancy outcome in Tennessee. *JAMA.* 1990; **264**: 2219–23.
12. Taffel, S. Prenatal care, United States, 1968–1975, DHEW publication no. (PHS) 78–1911. National Center for Health Statistics, Hyattsville, MD, 1978.
13. The Robert Wood Johnson Foundation. *Challenges in health care: a chartbook perspective, 1991.* The foundation, Princeton, NJ, 1991.
14. Hadley, J. *The effects of medical care on mortality and morbidity: selected analyses with secondary data.* Center for Health Policy Studies, Georgetown University, Washington, DC, March 1989.
15. Schwartz, R. and Poppen, P. *Measuring the impact of CHC's on pregnancy outcomes.* Abt Associates, Cambridge, MA, October 1982.
16. Leveno, K. J., Cunningham, F. G., Roark, M. L., Nelson, S. D., and Williams, M. L. Prenatal care and the low birth weight infant. *Obstet. Gynecol.* 1985; **66**: 599–605.
17. Shapiro, S., McCormick, M. C., Starfield, B. H., Krischer, J. P., and Bross, D. Relevance of correlates of infant deaths for significant morbidity at 1 year of age. *Am. J. Obstet. Gynecol.* 1980; **136**: 363–73.
18. Oberg, C. N., Lia-Hoagberg, B., Hodkinson, E., Skovholt, C., and Vanman, R. Prenatal care comparisons among privately insured, uninsured, and Medicaid-enrolled women. *Public Health Rep.* 1990; **105**: 533–5.
19. Brown, S. S. (ed.). *Prenatal care: reaching mothers, reaching infants.* National Academy Press, Washington, DC, 1988.
20. Committee on Health Care of Underserved Women. *Strategies and options for improving access to maternal health care: the obstetrician–gynecologist as advocate.* The American College of Obstetricians and Gynecologists, Washington, DC, September 1988.
21. Fingerhut, L. A., Makuc, D., and Kleinman, J. C. Delayed prenatal care and place of first visit: differences by health insurance and education. *Fam. Plann. Perspect.* 1987; **19**: 212–14.
22. Schwarz, R. H. Infant mortality and access to care. *Obstet. Gynecol.* 1989; **73**: 123–4.
23. Gold, L. B., Kenney, A. M., and Singh, S. *Blessed events and the bottom line:*

financing maternity care in the United States. Alan Guttmacher Institute, New York, 1988.

24. Hadley, J., Hoffman, J., and Feder, J. *Relationships between health insurance coverage and selected health and hospital use characteristics of newborns and pregnant women.* Center for Health Policy Studies, Georgetown University, Washington, DC, November 1989.

25. Murray, J. L., and Bernfield, M. The differential effects of prenatal care on the incidence of low birth weight among blacks and whites in a prepaid health care plan. *New Engl. J. Med.* 1988; **319**: 1385–91.

26. Fuchs, V. R. National health insurance revisited. *Health Aff. (Millwood).* 1991; **10**: 7–17.

27. McLaughlin, F. J., Altemeier, W. A., Christensen, M. J., Sherrod, K. B., Dietrich, M. S., and Stern, D. T. Randomized trial of comprehensive prenatal care for low-income women: effect on infant birth weight. *Pediatrics.* 1992; **89**: 128–32.

28. Korenbrot, C. C. Risk reduction in pregnancies of low-income women: comprehensive prenatal care through the OB access project. *Möbius.* 1984; **4**: 34–43.

29. Papiernik, E., Bouyer, J., Dreyfus, J., *et al.* Prevention of preterm births: a perinatal study in Haguenau, France. *Pediatrics.* 1985; **76**: 154–8.

30. Hadley, J., Steinberg, E. P., and Feder, J. Comparison of uninsured and privately insured hospital patients: condition on admission, resource use, and outcome. *JAMA.* 1991; **265**: 374–9.

31. Weissman, J. and Epstein, A. M. Case mix and resource utilization by uninsured hospital patients in the Boston metropolitian area. *JAMA.* 1989; **261**: 3572–6.

32. Gordon, T., DeAngelis, C., and Peterson, R. Capitation reimbursement for pediatric primary care. *Pediatrics.* 1986; **77**: 29–34.

33. Braveman, P. A., Egerter, S., Bennett, T., and Showstack, J. Differences in hospital resource allocation among sick newborns according to insurance coverage. *JAMA.* 1991; **266**: 3300–8.

34. Joyce, T., Corman, H., and Grossman, M. A cost-effective analysis of strategies to reduce infant mortality. *Med. Care.* 1988; **26**: 348–60.

35. Committee to Study the Prevention of Low Birth Weight, Institute of Medicine. *Preventing low birth weight.* National Academy Press, Washington, DC, 1985.

36. Gorsky, R. D. and Colby, J. P. The cost effectiveness of prenatal care in reducing low birth weight in New Hampshire. *Health Serv. Res.* 1989; **24**: 583–98.

37. American Academy of Pediatrics. *Child health financing report.* The Academy, Evanston, IL, Spring 1984.

38. Schwartz, R. M. What price prematurity? *Fam. Plann. Perspect.* 1989; **21**: 170–4.

39. Torrance, G. W. Measurement of health state utilities for economic appraisal: a review. *J. Health Econ.* 1986; **5**: 1–22.

40. Boyle, M. H., Torrance, G. W., Sinclair, J. C., and Horwood, S. P. Economic evaluation of neonatal intensive care of very-low-birth-weight infants. *New Engl. J. Med.* 1983; **308**: 1330–7.

41. Stevenson, R. C., Pharoah, P. O., Cooke, R. W., and Sandhu, B. Predicting costs and outcomes of neonatal intensive care for very low birthweight infants. *Public Health.* 1991; **105**: 121–6.
42. Doyle, L. W., Murton, L. J., and Kitchen, W. H. Increasing the survival of extremely immature (24- to 28-weeks' gestation) infants—at what cost? *Med. I. Aust.* 1989; **150**: 558–63.

12B   ECONOMICS AND ETHICS

Eugene Lewit

INTRODUCTION

In his companion piece in this volume, Birt Harvey has documented some important problems the US perinatal health-care system faces, including high costs and rates of infant mortality and low-birthweight births which appear high in international comparisons, particularly in comparison with the level of expenditures on perinatal care. In addition, a substantial proportion of pregnant women (433 000, or almost 9 per cent of all pregnant women) in the US do not have health insurance coverage to help defray the considerable costs of pregnancy, and thus face significant financial barriers to timely access to medical care.[1] The present state of perinatal care in the United States may not be supportable for too much longer, and may be viewed by many as being unfair and inconsistent with the often-stated national goal of equality of opportunity. Birt Harvey presents a number of arguments, economic and ethical, for removing financial barriers to prenatal care as a step towards resolving the dilemma.[1] Although this recommendation appears attractive, it may, for reasons discussed below, have only a limited impact on the problems the US faces in the delivery of perinatal care. Many of the current problems of high costs and poor outcomes are likely to persist, and will be debated as part of the process the US is likely to follow in attempting to make health care more affordable.

Because rising health-care costs are acknowledged to be at the heart of the chronic crisis of the US health-care system, economic considerations have taken center-stage in the current public debate over how to reform the health-care system. In this process of reform, economic considerations may lead to ethically difficult decisions. This paper attempts to inform the decision-making process by exploring how economic analysis interacting with ethical considerations may facilitate decision-making. We begin with a review of recent estimates of the costs of perinatal care, and then examine the economic point of view as it relates to health care and perinatology. Some arguments for expanding access to prenatal care are examined in the context of clarifying how cost–effectiveness and cost–benefit analysis may inform the debate. Then the critical decision-making role of physicians is explored from the perspective of the different incentives they face. Because physicians have repeatedly expressed discomfort or dismay with being asked to allocate health-care resources among patients explicitly, the Oregon proposal to ration health care via a prioritized list of conditions and treatments which would be eligible for reimbursement under Medicaid is briefly examined as an alternative resource-allocation device. Since this procedure appears to have several serious shortcomings, not the least of which is its inability to account for individual preferences in making treatment decisions, alternative procedures for making resource-allocation decisions, which would more directly involve the patient as well as the physician, are explored. Finally, some implications of the interaction of economics and ethics for national health-care reform are considered.

COST OF PERINATAL CARE

Although aggregate health-care cost data are not routinely reported for specific subcategories of care, such as perinatology, there is good reason to believe that this area of health care has been affected by exploding costs. Recently, Lewit and Monheit[2] estimated that health-care expenditures for children in their first year of life totaled $12.6 billion or $3271 per infant in 1987. Since only 10 per cent of total expenditures, or $312 per infant, were spent on health care not requiring hospitalization, it is likely that 85–90 per cent of expenditures, or approximately $11 billion 1987 dollars, were spent on the initial hospitalization and inpatient physician care of newborns. Such expenditures would have exceeded $15 billion in 1992 if per infant expenditures increased at the same rate as health-care expenditures generally between 1987 and 1992.

Lewit and Monheit[2] also estimate that expenditures on obstetrical care, excluding care for miscarriages and stillbirths, abortions, and family planning, totaled $14.7 billion, or $3872 per live birth in 1987. Hospital charges accounted for 54 per cent of these expenditures and professional fees for about 35 per cent of costs, and the balance represented separately billed tests and diagnostic services. Combining the estimates for expenditures on infants and obstetrical care suggests that total expenditures on perinatal care were approximately $26 billion, or $6826 per live birth in 1987. In that same year, the median income of married couple families was $34 879, and the poverty threshold for a three-person family was $8319.[3] Thus it appears that, on average, health-care expenditures on pregnancy childbirth, and infancy would loom large in the budget of even the average family, and would be virtually impossible to finance out-of-pocket for those families living in poverty.

Not only is perinatal care costly, but expenditures on pregnancy and infancy appear to have experienced the same kind of explosive growth as the rest of the US health-care system. For example, the estimate of expenditures on obstetrical care in 1987 prepared by Lewit and Monheit was almost 85 per cent higher than one reported by Fuchs and Perreault[4] for 1982. Although increases in the number of births, the frequency of cesarean deliveries, and a change in data reporting accounted for approximately 10 percentage points of this increase, most of the increase was the result of substantial increases in physican fees and hospital charges over the five-year period.

Lewit and Monheit also report that expenditures on health care for infants seem to be increasing even more rapidly than expenditures on obstetrical care or health-care expenditures generally.[2] A previously unpublished comparison of per caput health-care expenditures for those 0 to 2 years old suggests that expenditures on this age-group increased by 510 per cent between 1977 and 1987. This rate of increase substantially exceeded the growth in expenditures for children of other ages and for adults less than 65 years of age. It appears that most of this rapid growth (73 per cent) was due to changes in the intensity of service delivery to this age-group, and in particular to a very large increase in expenditures on inpatient hospital care. It is tempting to speculate that rapidly growing expenditures for the 0 to 2 age-group reflected the rapid rate of technological advance in the care of high-risk, very-low-birth weight babies in neonatal intensive care units (NICUs), and the proliferation of these units throughout the hospital system. The increase in the level of real medical care services received by these infants and young children may also reflect the increased health-care needs of high-risk infants who survive the neonatal period.[5] At this point in time, however, data at a level of detail which would allow full investigation of these hypotheses are not available. Regardless, however, of what further analyses may show, it is fairly clear that expenditures on perinatal health care have probably been growing more rapidly than expenditures on most other areas of health care. This observation combined with the fact that cost considerations have taken center-stage in the current debate over how to reform the US health-care system underscores the timeliness and importance of examining the relationships between economics and ethics in perinatology, and sets the stage for a brief consideration of how an economic perspective may facilitate decision-making in perinatology.

THE ECONOMIC PERSPECTIVE

Economics is the study of the allocation of scarce resources to satisfy competing wants. It assumes that resources are scarce relative to wants, that these scarce resources have alternative uses, and that people have diverse wants. The basic economic problem is then to allocate and combine resources so as to satisfy wants best. This problem is faced by individuals, families, communities, and Society.[6]

There are several economic maxims that follow from the scarcity assumption. First and foremost is the maxim that 'There is no free lunch.' This maxim does not deny that goods may be provided to individuals at no cost to them personally; rather, it emphasizes the importance of the alternative uses to which resources may be put. Resources engaged in one activity are forgone to another. A second maxim is that there are alternative ways to accomplish a given end. Each way may require different combinations of resources and have different consequences. How we feel about specific ends and the consequences of the alternative roads to those goals will influence our choices. Given the constraints and alternatives individuals face, economics relies on the concept of equality at the margin to describe how optimal decisions can be made. Following this rule, optimal states are achieved by trading off along a continuum of alternatives until the benefit of a small increment in one good is exactly equal to its opportunity cost—the small benefit of other goods forgone in the trade-off.

Economics, as it is being characterized in this discussion, is relatively value-free. This is not to say that economic analysis is amoral, but rather that economic analysis accepts the values, preferences, and physical and psychological needs of individuals as given in the decision-making process. Furthermore, while economists may posit that people try to do the best they can when faced with constraints of money, time, energy, and information, it does not follow that the result of each individual's attempt at optimization results in the best of all possible worlds—if this were true, economists would be out of work.[a]

Ethical considerations can enter into economic deliberations because the real cost of any particular activity is measurable in terms of other activities forgone. Thus, even though the sanctity of human life may be a key ethical value,[7] it should be recognized that to employ scarce resources to keep a particular person alive may have measurable costs in terms of other lives. In essence, as Marcia Kramer has observed, to treat without regard for cost is similar to treating without regard to side-effects-costs are one side-effect of expensive medical treatment.[8]

VALUES AND THE FINANCING OF PERINATAL HEALTH CARE

Some of the difficulties the US currently faces regarding reform of the health-care system generally and the provision of health care for newborns particularly stem from a tension between different ethical perspectives.[9] For example, it is possible to consider much health care as essentially similar to other important goods (like food and shelter). Accordingly, access to health care would be determined by individuals' income and wealth, their taste for health, the price of health care, and their state of health. Much research suggests that by and large this perspective explains individuals' demand for health care. For example, people buy more health care when its price is low than when its price is high, and, other things being equal, people with large incomes buy more health care than people with small incomes.[10] The

---

[a] Although economics is built on the paradigm of the rational individual who attempts to use his stock of resources to maximize his satisfaction, it is most concerned with behavior in the aggregate, and although economists do have things to say about how things should be, economics is more useful in describing how people make choices than in prescribing what choices are to be made.

three peculiar phenomena in the market for health care that distiguish it from other goods are that individuals rely heavily on agents—health-care professionals—to advise them on what they should buy; that health care is characterized by substantial uncertainty at all levels—ranging from the randomness of individual illness to the understanding of the outcomes of therapeutic interventions; and that as a consequence of the probabilistic nature of the demand for health care, much of health care is paid for through a complex third-party payment system which for most individuals reduces the cost of care to them at the time when they receive care.

The second perspective views health care as a right, which should not depend on individual income or wealth.[9] This perspective, which may justify government intervention to facilitate access to health care by those unable to pay for it, has strong appeal. Dougherty argues that it is based on the moral principle that each person has an inherent value beyond 'the contingencies of supply and demand'.[7] Cuyler, however, while adopting this perspective, points out that it need not create an open-ended claim on society's resources, since resources are limited and health is not the only 'good thing'.[9, b]

When it comes to health care for children, and particularly perinatal care, two other competing elements enter the social calculus. One is the notion that parents are responsible for the care and well-being of their children— including providing for their material, emotional, and health-care needs. The second is the notion that extremely vulnerable and innocent children require special consideration when parents do not or cannot provide for their needs.[6] The dependency of the fetus and newborn is complete—the newborn cannot survive long without external support, and the nature of the support it receives will have a significant impact on its overall development. For this reason, an agency relationship is said to exist between an infant and its mother. The well-being of the child depends critically on the choices made by its mother: how well she takes care of herself before, during, and after pregnancy; the care she provides for the infant; her genetic make-up; and even the degree to which she practices effective family planning.[6]

The symbiotic relationship between the mother and infant has several implications for the economics and ethics of perinatology. It suggests that, on average, expensive, heroic medical care may have little impact on population-based infant-health levels when compared with the effects of maternal behavior. Also it creates an ambivalence about the appropriate response of society to maternal behaviors which jeopardize infant health. Ambivalence about women's rights vs. fetal and infant rights is most obvious in the heated debate about abortion, but also enters into areas of perinatology. Consider, for example, the debate as to the appropriate response to drug-exposed

---

[b] An additional reason why society may have an interest in promoting health results from the possible externalities associated with contagious diseases. If individuals go untreated for certain contagious diseases, other people may become ill. The interdependency of individual health states in such situations has been used to justify public-health measures; but these considerations are less important in perinatology, except for the relation between the health of an infant and the health of its mother, which is explored at length below.

infants—a complex problem frequently characterized by images of severely
compromised newborns struggling for life in NICUs and caught indefinitely in
hospitals as boarder babies in the foster-care bureaucracy—their educational
and overall development jeopardized perhaps for years to come.[11] In these
circumstances, the human costs of maternal substance-abuse are high; but
so are the economic costs for intensive care, extended hospitalizations, and
special education. Society has responded to this problem through the legal
child-protective services and health-care systems; but the results have been
far from satisfactory, and very costly.[12]

Although the exposure of infants to controlled substances has been the
focus of much national attention recently, other maternal behaviors may take
a bigger toll on infant health and society's resources. Consider the impact of
maternal smoking on neonatal care. Women who smoke during pregnancy
are twice as likely as non-smokers to have low-birthweight babies, and low
birthweight is one of the strongest predictors of the use of neonatal intensive
care. Manning *et al.* estimate that if one-third of pregnant women smoked,
then smoking may have been responsible for as much as one-quarter of all
NICU costs for low-birthweight babies in 1986 ($652 million).[13] This estimate
excludes other likely additional health-care costs of low-birthweight babies
whose mothers smoked during pregnancy, as well as the costs of special
education and other services disproportionately consumed by low-birthweight
babies as they get older.[14]

Because of the dependency of the fetus and infant on the mother, many
activities may place maternal prerogatives in conflict with fetal and infant
well-being. This may give rise to complex ethical problems which are beyond
the scope of this paper. Here we only want to emphasize that these conflicts
frequently have economic consequences when resources are diverted from
other worthwhile endeavors to compensate infants for the deleterious results
of parental risk-taking during pregnancy.

The potential conflict between maternal prerogatives and infant health
also implies that improving infant health by providing limited inducements
to their mothers, such as free prenatal care, may not always be very effective.
Unless mothers act as perfect agents for their children, they may not seek
care, even if it is free. Given that some mothers knowingly engage in risky
behaviors, it is doubtful that they are acting as perfect agents for their
children.

PRENATAL CARE AND ECONOMIC ANALYSIS

The primary thrust of the analysis by Birt Harvey in this volume is that
government should act to remove all financial barriers to prenatal care in the
US. He also feels that 'care of newborns of some undetermined birthweight
over 1000 grams can [also] be justified on an economic basis'. Accordingly,
'there is no rational economic reason for our government not to assure
financial access to care for these infants and for all pregnant women'[1] Yet

a peek below the surface, reinforced by recent reports that expanding access to prenatal care may not improve pregnancy outcomes,[15] reveals that there are a number of important caveats attendant on the actual implementation of the policies implicit in these conclusions.

First, although questions of access, utilization, and efficacy of prenatal care have dominated the infant-health policy agenda, until recently little attention has focused on the actual content of prenatal care.[16] For example, standard guidelines for prenatal care as recommended by the American College of Obstetricians and Gynecologists call for care to begin early in the first trimester of pregnancy and then continue periodically for a total of 13 to 15 visits over a normal pregnancy.[17] In contrast, the Public Health Service Expert Panel on the Content of Prenatal Care recommends only 7 visits for healthy women who have previously had uncomplicated deliveries, and 9 visits for first-time mothers.[18] The Panel recommends that one of the 7 or 9 recommended visits should be a pre-conception visit, to identify problems before pregnancy. The Panel's report also focuses on the identification and management of high-risk pregnancies through such auxiliary services as home visits, case management, and treatment for substance-abuse. At this point in time, studies have not been performed to evaluate the costs and effectiveness of the alternative approaches to prenatal care; but to the extent to which costs and outcomes differ with the actual content of care delivered, discretion should be exercised in drawing sweeping conclusions about the 'rationality' of expanding access to care.

In a similar vein, some have argued that many of the components of prenatal care delivered to well-insured women in low-risk pregnancies are of little value.[19] Such services include routine ultrasound imaging and electronic fetal monitoring, which can add hundreds of dollars to the cost of a normal delivery. Recently, tocolytic therapy to avert premature labor also generated much controversy. This procedure, which combines ambulatory monitoring of pregnant women to detect the early onset of premature labor with aggressive drug therapy to postpone the onset of full labor and delivery, has not been demonstrated to be effective in several well-designed studies, but is being aggressively promoted by entrepreneurs seeking to develop a market for the components of the intervention.[20,21] On the other side of the coin, several studies have suggested that the less technologically intensive care provided to women of lower socioeconomic status in neighborhood health centers may be more effective for that population than care by private, fee-for-service obstetricians.[22] Many other examples of real uncertainty concerning how best to use limited resources to expand access to prenatal care could be cited. For example, should limited resources be spent increasing the proportion of women who get early care by encouraging women who start care during their second trimester to start earlier, or should women who would otherwise get late or no care be encouraged to start in their second trimester? Should expansion of public financing for prenatal care include funding for transportation, child care, and interpreters to help reduce what appear to be 'non-financial' barriers to care? Should publically financed care for low-income women include expensive services of little or no established value which are available to women with private health insurance? Since a blanket recommendation to expand access to prenatal care can have widely varying resource costs, and perhaps different effects on outcomes, addressing these issues should be an important part of any effort to expand access to care.

Just as there are many unresolved issues as to how best to expand access to prenatal care, there are also unresolved issues regarding the analytic concepts of cost-saving, cost-effectiveness, and cost-benefit which have been used to bolster the argument for expanding health-insurance coverage for pregnant women. First, strictly speaking, most economic analyses of medical interventions such as prenatal care focus on small changes around current circumstances. As one moves away from current levels of activity, another economic law, that of diminishing returns, suggests that eventually it will become increasingly expensive to achieve a particular increase in benefits. In the case of expanding the utilization of prenatal care, this may mean that it may become increasingly expensive to enroll additional women in prenatal care programs as non-financial barriers, such as lack of awareness, geographic remoteness, cultural isolation, ambivalent feelings about the pregnancy, and destructive behaviours, such as substance-abuse, are encountered. In addition, since the costs and benefits of treating many of the high-risk women who might be brought into an expanded prenatal care system have yet to be determined, it is hard to speculate about the possible net payoffs of increased access for this group of women.

Moreover, whether prenatal care is, in fact, cost-saving reflects, in addition to purely technical issues, the decisions made about treatment for low-birthweight infants. To a large extent, the cost savings attributed to early prenatal care reflect decisions that have been made regarding the intensive and expensive treatment of low-birthweight infants. Accordingly, for example, among populations in remote areas that have limited access to expensive neonatal care the cost savings that are attributable to reductions in the utilization of such care will not be realized. On the other hand, if decisions are made for economic or other reasons to restrict treatment for certain very sick infants, cost savings will be realized regardless of whether more prenatal care is in fact utilized.[c]

There are even several scenarios under which expanded access to prenatal care might not result in any significant cost savings. For example, if there is undercapacity in the provision of intensive care for sick infants, costs might not fall if infants who previously would not have been treated intensively receive treatment as aggregate demand for the service declines

[c] See Garber and Phelps (*Economic foundations of cost–effectiveness analysis*, NBER Working Paper series, No. **4164**, 1992) for a discussion of the effects of the interdependence of intertemporal care decisions on cost–effectiveness analyses. See also Braveman *et al.* (Differences in hospital resource allocation among sick newborns according to insurance coverage. *JAMA*, **266**(23), 3300–7, 1991) for evidence that health-insurance status affects the intensity and hence the cost of care for high-risk infants.

as a consequence of an effective prenatal care program. This might arise if heavier, lower-risk babies are admitted to NICU beds made available by the reduction in demand from smaller infants, or if released capacity were used to treat very small, higher-risk infants who might not have been previously considered viable. In fact, considering the entire distribution of birth outcomes to be a continuum, including fetal deaths and stillbirths, it is conceivable that more effective prenatal care could shift the entire distribution of pregnancies toward increased viability. As a result, some infants who would have previously been candidates for NICU care would no longer need it, but others who would have previously been considered too sick to benefit from NICU care may become candidates for care. The net effect on the demand for NICU care will depend on the relative shifts into the bottom end of the range and out the top end of the range. It is possible, however, that the number of infants who might benefit from expensive neonatal care may not change very much.

Most analysts would agree that, as is illustrated by the preceding discussion, the criterion that an intervention should be cost-saving may be both too restrictive and too loose to serve as the primary basis for decision-making.[23] The cost-saving criterion may be too restrictive because it ignores the fact that interventions may provide valuable benefits other than cost savings. More pertinent decision criteria have to do with recognizing these benefits and whether they are worth the cost and/or whether alternative, less costly strategies exist to achieve similar health outcomes. Cost-saving criteria may also be unsatisfactory because they are frequently technical criteria which ignore the way the health system functions. At present the US health-care system appears to respond to many technical attempts to reduce costs by uncovering new ways to soak up resources. Ambulatory care has been substituted for inpatient care and lengths of hospital stays have been shortened without substantial cost savings being realized on an aggregate level. Whether, therefore, we will be able to realize any significant cost savings by expanding access to prenatal care remains to be seen. That we may in this manner improve the overall health of infants and their mothers should also be an important consideration. If we can only accomplish one of these goals (cost savings with an equal health outcome or improved health at no additional cost) it seems compelling to move ahead. If, however, we can only achieve improved health status by spending more or realize cost savings by sacrificing a health benefit, then it will be appropriate to ask whether the additional expenditures are worthwhile, given the alternatives.

THE ROLE OF PHYSICIANS

Even if the US is successful in removing financial barriers to prenatal care, we will not eliminate the need to make difficult and critical choices involving lives and resources in perinatology. If no women faced financial barriers to access to prenatal care, other kinds of barriers would limit the effective utilization of prenatal care by some. Still other women would suffer bad pregnancy outcomes although they receive adequate or even extraordinary care, because prenatal care, and indeed all medical care, does not gurantee a healthy baby, but operates primarily to reduce the probability of an undesirable outcome. In these circumstances, physicians and other caregivers may be called upon to help make decisions which are difficult and which many would rather not contemplate. Birt Harvey echoes the feelings of many physicians and others when he writes 'The physician responsible for providing care to sick very-low-birthweight infants, to children, or to young or elderly adults should not be required to decide which patient should be treated aggressively.'[1]

Yet, many physicians make such resource-allocation decisions regularly. Consider, for example, the triage function in a busy emergency room or trauma facility. When, at times, many seriously injured patients present almost simultaneously, decisions must be made regarding which patient to treat first and who can wait. Effective decision-making in these difficult circumstances balances the benefits from immediate attention with the dangers of delay. Patients who have little or no chance of recovery despite heroic efforts may be shunted aside in favor of those for whom quick attention may make a difference between successful recovery and substantial morbidity or death. Uncertainty regarding the prognosis of each individual and the value of therapy may be high, but decisions are made which result in the allocation of scarce resources among competing wants.

Before rejecting this triage example as an invalid counterfactual to Harvey's position, consider that the absolute resource constraint physicians face in these situations arises because of prior decisions to limit the size and staff of trauma facilities. As an alternative to medical triage activities, trauma facilities could be expanded and more widely disseminated, creating sufficient slack in the system that difficult patient-care decisions do not have to be made.

Doctors make similar resource-allocation decisions in many less dramatic situations. Consider, for example, the obstetrician who leaves a room full of pregnant women waiting for routine prenatal care at his office while he attends the delivery of another patient. Earlier that day, that same physician may have decided to see his ambulatory patients for routine care, even after receiving a call that the woman he was to deliver later was in labor and on her way to the hospital. These and hundreds of other decisions physicians make routinely are resource-allocation decisions—time, attention, and energy are devoted to one patient at the expense of another. Similarly, physicians who decide not to treat Medicaid patients or not to practice in areas where need is great but where remuneration is likely to be low are making resource-allocation decisions which may seriously impact on the health and well-being of many, while perhaps adding little marginally to the health of those well-doctored, well-insured patients whom they choose to serve. Here economics, with its emphasis on rational responses to incentives, can guide us in predicting, if not evaluating, the resource-allocation decisions of physicians and other providers of medical care. Faced with strong incentives to deliver medical care to those who can pay, economists would argue that we should not expect physicians to do otherwise.[24] Birt Harvey implicitly acknowledges the ability of incentives to facilitate access to necessary medical care by emphasizing the importance of financial barriers to the receipt of effective and timely prenatal care.[1] Physicians may complain that the new cost-consciousness constrains their freedom to practice as they see fit; in many situations, however, the inability of patients to pay for care may prove an even greater constraint on medical decision-making.

In fact, a multiplicity of factors, including physicians' self-interest, their role as patients' advocates, and their concern for social good, influence medical decision-making.[25] Economists, in particular, have been interested in studying the problems that may arise when physicians' self-interested conflicts with their role as patient advocates. There has been much discussion of the extent to which physicians are able to induce demand for their services in order to enhance their incomes.[26] Such practices are regarded by the medical profession itself and by society at large as 'unethical'. The first code of ethics adopted by the AMA in the late 1840s affirmed that physicians should avoid unnecessary visits to patients in order that their motives might not be questioned.[27] Despite repeated official pronouncements over the years, the issue of professional financial conflict of interest resulting from physician referrals of Medicare patients to clinical laboratories in which they had a financial interest culminated in restrictive legislation in 1992.[27]

There is also evidence of conflicts of interest on the part of physicians in the perinatal arena. Many observers feel that the recent steady increase in the frequency of cesarean deliveries reflects, in part, concern about exposure to malpractice litigation, physician convenience, and the higher fees associated with the procedure.[28] Similar conclusions have been drawn with regard to the routine use during pregnancy of ultrasound and electronic fetal monitoring, costly procedures of dubious efficacy, but routinely ordered in most pregnancies.[19] Reports that physicians who self-refer for obstetrical ultrasonography were 4.5 times as likely to order the examination as physicians who referred patients to radiologists,[29] and that cesarean deliveries are more common among insured than uninsured patients, despite evidence that the uninsured are at higher risk,[30] suggest that financial incentives can have a strong impact on the practice of medicine in this area. In addition, to the extent that financial incentives encourage clinical practices which are not cost-effective, they make it more difficult for physicians to act as effective agents for their patients or for the social good.

Although physician behavior in the presence of different financial incentives may pose an ethical dilemma for the profession, physicians may rationalize their behavior with the thought that they are not violating their trust with patients because there is substantial uncertainty concerning the utility of various clinical activities in specific cases; most of the procedures may do no harm and may do some good; and some third party to the doctor–patient relationship is paying the bill.[25] However, the true costs of unproductive medical care are the beneficial purposes to which the resources used in that care might better be put. In this social context, the use of medical services of marginal value may precipitate an ethical dilemma, not only regarding physician responsibilities *vis-a-vis* current patients and third-party payers, but also with patients as yet unseen and those who may never be seen because resources available for medical care are wasted.[9] This consequence of wasted resources may be most visible in public programs which operate under tight budgetary constraints.

The principal–agent relationship which underlies the patient–doctor relationship requires that, in the best of all worlds, physicians should be indifferent to all interests other than those of patients, and particularly indifferent to the impact of the physician's practice style on the physician's income. The principal–agent relationship that exists between mother and fetus or infant may also pose difficult ethical problems for the physician and other health-care providers, who must decide who is the 'patient' when the interests of parents and child are in conflict. These difficult decisions may also have economic overtones. For example, questions of whether and how to intervene with, or report to law-enforcement authorities, mothers whose drug-taking during pregnancy puts their infants' health at risk also carry implications for the cost of perinatal care. Is the physician's responsibility to intervene greater because they are aware of the drain of high neonatal care costs on the health-care system? Does it make a difference if the mother is insured or uninsured, or whether mother and baby are enrolled in a capitated health plan in which the high costs of neonatal care may jeopardize the financial solvency of the plan?

What responsibility does the physician have after birth to resuscitate very-low-birthweight infants and others born with significant anomalies who will prove costly to care for during the neonatal period, who may die despite heroic medical efforts, and who may survive only with significant impairments? Does it matter if the infant is covered by health insurance or not? How do the wishes of parents and other family members fit into the decision-making calculus? Clearly the potential for conflict exists when the wishes of parents and medical staff are not in agreement. In cases where intervention is costly but the likelihood of survival and normal development low, the physician is faced with the dilemma that the cost of whatever is done with therapeutic resources is the best of all the other things that the resources could have been used for. Recognizing this fact, can or should the physician resist parents' desire for high-tech, high-cost rescue therapy? How should physicians respond if parents favor withholding intensive therapy because of their reluctance to be financially responsible for the cost of care in an NICU or for the cost of care for a child who survives with a high likelihood of a permanent disability? Do the hypothetical wishes of the child enter into the decision-making calculus? Should the willingness and ability of parents to care for seriously impaired infants be considered?[31]

The advance of neonatal technologies which have significantly lowered

Table 12.1. Handicap rates in very low birthweight infants, 1975–85

Birthweight group in grams	Survivors followed after hospital discharge		
	Total number per cent	Per cent with serious handicaps	Per cent with serious or moderate handicaps
Under 800	290	26	41
750–1000	434	17	31
1000–1500	1215	11	16

Source: Pooled as reported in OTA 1987, tables 10–12.[32]

the birthweight/gestation age-threshold of survivability has highlighted the dilemmas faced in perinatology. Between 1961–5 and 1981–5, neonatal mortality rates for infants 1001–1500 grams at birth declined from over 500 per 1000 births to just under 99 per 1000 births. Among infants under 1000 grams, the rates declined from 939 deaths per 1000 births to 520 deaths per 1000 births.[32] Yet, as the data in Table 12.1 demonstrate, surviving infants, particulary those at the lowest end of the birthweight continuum, experience a high frequency of mental retardation (IQ below 80), significant cerebral palsy, major seizure disorders, and blindness.

Clearly, the physician has an ethical responsibility to inform parents of the prognosis for each sick infant and to weigh parental input in making treatment decisions. In the light of anecdotal evidence of costly physician decisions to treat very immature infants aggressively that appear to conflict with parental wishes,[33] one may question the basis for some decision-making. Society also has asserted its prerogatives in this intimate decision-making process through the 'Baby Doe' decision and the abuse and neglect system.[34] Again, economic questions arise when decisions to sustain life in a seriously impaired infant may impose costs on the family, the community, and the health-care system.[31] These decisions may be further complicated by the recent enactment of the Americans with Disabilities Act, which restricts discrimination among patients on the basis of health status, and may mandate a minimum level of benefits for all, regardless of health status prior to or following therapy.[35]

THE TECHNOLOGIC IMPERATIVE

Studies of clinical decision-making within NICUs suggest that it is largely driven by the technologic imperative: 'delivering the best care that is technologically possible without regard to costs'. As Guillemin and Holmstrom point out in *Mixed blessings: intensive care for newborns*, virtually unlimited medical options combined with strong protective sentiments for newborns are two key components promoting aggressive intervention in the NICU.[34] They describe providers in the NICUs that they studied as being driven in part by a strong desire to succeed with each infant.[d] Decisions are frequently made incrementally, so that one intervention leads to another, and the staff develops a strong feeling of having invested in a particular infant. Decision-making in this highly technical environment has several consequences—Guillemin and Holmstrom express concern that it deflects attention from 'a broader calculation of the patients' chances for a meaningful life'. In addition, it can lead to a cascading effect, wherein efforts and costs escalate as an infant's condition deteriorates and the likehood of a good result rapidly declines.[34]

Ironically, lack of health insurance or ability to pay for medical care does not appear to be a substantial barrier to the extremely expensive care provided in the typical NICU. Although inability to pay for care may present an important barrier to obtaining adequate prenatal care for many pregnant women, once a low-birthweight infant is in a Level III facility access to aggressive neonatal intensive care is almost assured.[32] Like so many studies of the US health care system, the report by Braveman *et al.* on the differences in intensity of care experienced by sick neonates in California according to insurance status presents a picture of a cup which is half-full as well as half-empty.[36] For while many would be concerned to learn that the level of care received by uninsured infants was below that received by insured infants, others would be reassured by the very substantial level of expenditure on sick neonates for which no direct compensation was forthcoming. The patch work arrangement of the financing of health care for the indigent in the US may reflect ambivalence about whether health care is to be paid for by individuals, like other goods, or is a right to be guaranteed by society, and whether in the case of extremely vulnerable infants, only the latter consideration applies.[e] However, politically expendient reliance on extensive cross-subsidization of health care to create a safety-net for society's most vulnerable citizens may create its own set of inefficiencies, which need to be addressed if the delivery of health care is to be improved.[f] Such a patch work system may rely excessively on the 'Rule of Rescue'—people's perceived duty to save endangered life whenever possible—to legitimize interventions where the patient is unable to demand and pay for services in the traditional way.[37] Having invoked the rule of rescue as a justification to initiate an expensive course of therapy, it may be hard to draw the line as costs increase.

[d] Silverman reports similar experiences from the physician's perspective.[31]
[e] Concern for equality of opportunity may also be a strong factor motivating health care for uninsured infants.
[f] As a result of cost-shifting, private-paying patients are 'taxed' to pay for the indigent patients. If demand is at all elastic with respect to price this means that private patients will receive less treatment than they would had prices been set at the cost of their treatment. If cost-shifting occurs on to patients with all diagnoses then this has implications for the treatment received by all patients in the health system beyond the NICU population.

SOCIETAL GUIDELINES

Rapidly escalating health-care costs in the United States have focused attention on policies designed to control costs and make health care more accessible and affordable. In this cost-conscious environment, there has been interest in explicit rationing as a way of limiting health-care expenditures. Rationing is generally defined as deliberately withholding effective medical care in order to conserve scare resources for other purposes. Hence, public rationing explicitly recognizes that the total amount of resources devoted to health care needs to be limited. To the extent that the concept of rationing health care merely refers to a procedure for allocating scarce and/or limited resources, it is not new—the price system under which much of the economy functions is itself a rationing system which uses market prices to allocate scarce goods among individuals according to their ability to make purchases (their income and/or wealth) and their personal preferences. Attention has focused, however, on non-price rationing for health care, because of a reluctance to allow access to health care to be determined solely by an individual's ability to pay for it and because of concern that in the absence of the restraints traditionally imposed by individual's ability to pay for health care, controlling the rate of expansion in the health-care system will be very difficult.

In the US the idea of rationing health care has been most openly debated in regard to the proposal by the State of Oregon to cover all poor people on a limited budget under its Medicaid program by explicitly limiting their access to certain effective health-care services. Much has been written about the Oregon proposal, so it will only be briefly described here.[38-40] Essentially, Oregon attempted to establish coverage for payment, and hence spending priorities, by using a cost-effectiveness analysis to rank health-care services according to their costs and the benefits they provide. Using the prioritized list, the costs of providing each service to the eligible population were to be determined actuarially, and by matching the cost of coverage for each prioritized category of service with a fixed budget for the program, the extent of coverage determined. Thus, once the list of services is prioritized, the budget appropriations process would set the limits of coverage under the State's Medicaid program.

The original priority-setting procedure followed by the Oregon Health Services Commission was almost universally criticized as being too mechanical and as undervaluing high-cost, high-benefit procedures relative to low-cost, low-benefit procedures. In its second attempt at ranking health services, the Commission established 17 general categories of conditions and treatments, placed 709 condition and treatment pairs into one of the 17 categories, and then ranked each of the 709 within the category to which it was assigned. Finally, certain pairs were moved up and down the list individually when the Commissioners felt that they had been improperly ranked initially. From the perinatal perspective this procedure had the effect of ranking prenatal care high on the priority list, thus assuring its being covered under the Medicaid program, while ranking intensive care of some critically ill very-low-birthweight infants near the bottom of the list—thus effectively denying reimbursement for their care.

The Oregon proposal was hailed by many as a bold attempt to address the problems of escalating health-care costs and limited access by bringing the issue of the rationing of health care out of the closet and into the public-policy debate on the future of the health-care system. It was most vigorously critized by those who saw it as an attempt to introduce explicit rationing for the poor as a substitute for an expansion of resources to meet their needs.[41] Because features of the Oregon plan were inconsistent with provisions of Federal Medicaid legislation the State needed a waiver from the Federal government to implement the plan. This waiver was denied in August 1992, primarily on the grounds that the plan violated provisions of the Americans with Disabilities Act of 1990. The legal memorandum which supported this denial alleged that the quality-of-well-being measures used to prioritize condition–treatment pairs illegally discriminated against the disabled.[42] One of the two condition–treatment pairs specifically singled out in the memorandum was life-support for low-birthweight babies under 500 grams and under 23 weeks' gestation—the second lowest item (708) on the priority list.[g] In contrast, life-support for low-birth weight infants of at least 500 grams ranked high (22) on the priority list. While some may view this objection as a political maneuver in an election year, the debate over the attempt to measure quality of life and use it as a basis for the allocation of scarce health-care resources has been informative and has highlighted important conceptual and methodologic issues.

With a change in the administration in Washington DC, the continuing pressures of rising health-care costs, and a growing population of uninsured, Oregon may yet be able to obtain the federal wivers it needs to implement its Medicaid reforms. Whether the program goes forward or not, it can still be regarded as an interesting experiment in public policy-making. Without the opportunity to implement the demonstration, however, it is difficult to judge whether it would have been socially acceptable in actual practice and whether it is possible to build a consensus about an 'adequate level of care' and about trading off increased access for 'basic services' for controls on utilization.

Given the complexities of applying medicine to the variety of possible individual cases, many have questioned whether a single priority list, which reduced all possible clinical scenarios to 709 condition-treatment pairs, would in practice be an acceptable basis for clinical decision-making.[43] The greatest limitation of this process arises in its application to individual cases. From the clinical perspective, it is not uncommon for patients to present with a combination of conditions. Are these patients to be prioritized by the highest-ranking or lowest-ranking condition on the list? Should only conditions above

---

[g] For almost two decades, 500 grams and 23 weeks' gestation have been regarded as the boundary of viability among high-risk neonates. Anecdotal evidence suggests, however, that today neonates below these cut-points are being aggressively treated at some centers.

the cut-point be treated, even if failure to treat a lower-ranking condition increases the likelihood of a poor outcome? In many cases, the simultaneous presentation of several medical problems in a single patient may increase the cost of caring for that patient while decreasing the likelihood of a good outcome. If all these conditions rank 'high' on the priority list, such a patient may receive a costly mix of medical therapies before some other patient whose single condition placed him lower on the priority list.

In addition to clinical considerations, economists would emphasize the importance of individual preferences in making treatment decisions and the variety of therapeutic and palliative alternatives which might be involved in many situations.[39] A physician, John Wennberg, has observed 'Rational choices among treatments require that individual patients understand the predicaments they face ... there is seldom a single correct answer to a medical problem. Patients will be shown to differ in their degree of concern about their predicament and the outcomes they want will differ accordingly; they will also differ in the risks they are willing to take to get what they want'.[44] In reviewing the the Oregon proposal, Schwartz and Aaron, who were themselves responsible for encouraging discussion of the rationing of medical care with their 1984 book, *The painful prescription*,[45] agree that 'the meat-ax approach of denying payment for treatments of a given condition makes no sense.'[46]

Although the process of prioritizing medical interventions could be improved by assessing costs and benefits for more individuals and for a longer list of treatment–condition categories, by improving and expanding medical outcomes research, and by seeking input from individuals on their valuation of risks and benefits, it is unlikely that a priority list will be able to take account of the special preferences of individual patients. Accordingly, it may be necessary to recognize the pivotal role health-care providers, especially physicians, can play in the resource-allocation process, and to design programs which encourage their active participation as guardians of the public good and as advocates for their patients and for themselves.

There are several tested mechanisms that might be relied upon to achieve this end. One approach would be to reconstruct the immediacy of the resource constraints experienced in crowded trauma facilities by making the hard decisions 'upstream'. It may be easier to make trade-offs when decisions are being made about construction of facilities, development and diffusion of new technologies, and training and employment of personnel.[47] The actual experiences of patients and physicians should be important inputs into the upstream decision-making process. But when resource decisions have been made far in advance, it may make it easier to justify difficult allocation decisions when there are few alternatives. Patients' and physicians' acquiescence in the allocation of scarce resources when the alternatives are fairly apparent suggests that this process may be an acceptable way to approach the problem of scarcity. Advance planning may also increase the likelihood that appropriate decisions about the alternative uses of resources are incorporated into the decision-making process.

Alternative procedures which rely on capitation-based reimbursement and/or global budgeting to set resource limits may also be an effective way of limiting the cost of care while allowing for the flexibility in decision-making that can take into account unusual needs and individual preferences. Unlike a process which relied on priority lists or limitations on physical capacity to control costs, a capitated system which set boundaries on total resources available to treat a population of patients would create incentives for experimentation with alternative forms of care-delivery so as to minimize the costs of satisfying patients within the prescribed budgets. With regard to perinatal care, this would probably require that all aspects of care, from family planning through to prenatal care, delivery, and neonatal care, should be reimbursed at a preset comprehensive rate. Paying for all perinatal services by a prospectively determined fee should encourage providers to deliver services at low cost and to attempt to minimize the likelihood of poor and costly outcomes. There is increasing evidence that traditional private insurers and at-risk providers, such as HMOs and public programs, will attempt to deliver enriched prenatal care if they believe that it will reduce the costs of other care (especially NICU care for very-low-birthweight infants) for which they are responsible.[48]

To be sure, any system that relies on prospectively determined fixed budgets to control costs runs the risk of creating incentives to control costs in any way possible, so it will be necessary to monitor such systems to make sure that they are serving enrollees adequately. One alternative to formal monitoring is to encourage competition among providers so that patients may choose those providers who do a better job of satisfying their wants. Ultimately, however, because of the complexity of medical science and the health-care system, and of the fact that many patients do not pay directly for their care or even their health insurance, it may be appropriate to invoke a form of public decision-making and oversight to set prospective budgets and/or capitation rates and assure reasonable value for resources spent. Such public oversight may be particularly appropriate for perinatal care, where the preferences of the individual unborn and infant child are unknown and may conflict with the preferences of parents and providers.

CONCLUSION

There is a lot of work to be done if the United States is to reform its health-care system to be efficient, equitable, and ethically sound. Right now concerns about rapidly growing costs dominate the public debate. Attempts to control costs, however, may lead to difficult choices, because expansion in medical technology has failed to stem the escalation in costs even while it has pushed back the frontier of feasible interventions. No where is this dilemma more clearly evident than in the perinatal arena. Rapid technologic progress has increased survival rates among seriously compromised infants, but at substantial cost per survivor, not only during the immediate perinatal period but in many cases over a lifetime, as the number of survivors with moderate or severe handicaps has also increased.[5]

The explosions in medical technology and medical costs have, in some sense, left traditional social institutions in their wake. It will probably take time for these institutions to evolve and to develop new norms and procedures for dealing with the problems created by expanding horizons and limited resources. Physician training will probably need to be modified to incorporate better resource-management skills, with reduced reliance on the technologic imperative. Patients' expectations may also need to be modified, and reimbursement schemes which encourage resource-conservation and discourage waste may need to be implemented.

The need for reform is not limited to perinatology. Consider this quotation from a man asked to evaluate the cost of saving the life of a severely premature infant—'You are asking to save money by watching some premature infant die when he has a chance of being saved, while you are still wasting the kind of money we are throwing away. No way.'[49] It would appear that public perception of the efficiency and equity of the entire US health-care system will need to be improved before participants can feel more comfortable with the difficult allocation decisions that may be made.

Comfort with the decision-making process will depend, in part, on the value system underlying that process. Despite the current focus on the costs of health care, economic analysis by itself may be inadequate for successful decision-making. Economics, with its emphasis on making choices based on a full accounting of the consequences of the choices made and those forgone, can, however, facilitate decision-making. What choices should be made or policies should be followed is a matter of the values which we hold as a society and as individuals. These values implicitly underline all decision-making. Perhaps, if we make them more explicit, we will be able to improve the policy process.

Acknowledgements

This paper has benefited from thoughtful insights and helpful comments provided by Richard Behrman, Don Hoban, Jeffery Horbar, Theodore Joyce, Nancy Kerrebrock, Linda Quinn, and Jeannette Rigowski. Cheri Gaither prepared the manuscript and helped with the references. The usual caveats apply.

REFERENCES

1. Harvey, B. Financing health care for pregnant women and newborns. (This volume,) Chapter 12 A.
2. Lewit, E. M. and Monheit, A. C. Expenditures on health care for children and pregnant women. *The future of children.* 2(2), 95–114 (1992).
3. US Bureau of the Census. *Statistical abstract of the United States: 1992.* (112th edn). Govt. printing office, Washington, DC (1992).

4. Fuchs, V. R. and Perreault, L. Expenditures for reproduction-related health care. *JAMA* **255**(1), 76–81, (1986).
5. McCormick, M. C., Brooks-Gunn, J., Workman-Daniels, K., Turner, J., and Peckham, G. J. The health and development status of very low-birth-weight children at school age. *JAMA* **267** (16), 2204–8 (1992).
6. Fuchs, V. R. *Who shall live? Health economics and social choice.* Basic Books, New York (1974).
7. Dougherty, C. J. Ethical values at stake in health care reform. *JAMA*. **268**(17), 2409–12 (1992).
8. Kramer, M. J. Ethical issues in neonatal intensive care: an economic perspective. In *Ethics of newborn intensive care* (ed. A. R. Jonson and M. J. Garland) Health Policy Program, School of Medicine, San Francisco CA. (1976).
9. Culyer, A. J. The morality of efficiency in health care—some uncomfortable implications. *Health Economics.* **1** (1), 7–18 (1992).
10. Pauly, M. V. Fairness and feasibility in national health care systems. *Health Economics.* **1**(2), 93–104 (1992).
11. *Drug-exposed infants*, Larson, C. S. and Behrman, R. E. (eds) *The Future of Children.* **1**(1), 1–120 (1991).
12. Larson, C. L. Presentation at Pediatric Grand Rounds, University of California at San Francisco, 15 October 1992.
13. Manning, W. G., Keeler, E. B., Newhouse, J. P., Sloss, E. M., and Wasserman, J. (1991). *The costs of poor health habits.* Harvard University Press, Cambridge, Massachusetts.
14. Chaikind, S. and Corman, H. The impact of low birthweight on special education costs. *Journal of Health Economics.* **10**, 291–311.
15. Haas, J. S., Udvarhelyi, S., Morris, C. M., and Epstein, M. The effect of providing health coverage to poor uninsured pregnant women in Massachusetts. *JAMA* **269** (1), 87–91 (1993).
16. Racine, A. D., Joyce, T. J., and Grossman, M. Effectiveness of health care services for pregnant women and infants. *The Future of Children.* **2** (2), 40–57 (1992).
17. Freeman, R. K., and Poland, R. L. (1992) *Guidelines for perinatal care* (3rd edn). American Academy of Pediatrics, Washington DC.
18. Public Health Service, US Department of Health and Human Services (1989). *Caring for our future: the content of prenatal care.* Washington, DC.
19. Rosenblatt, R. A. The perinatal paradox: doing more and accomplishing less. *Health Affairs.* Fall, 158–68 (1989).
20. Chalmers, I., Enkin, M., and Keirse, M. J. N. C. (1989) *Effective care in pregnancy and childbirth.* Oxford University Press.
21. Eichenwald, K. Market place: new troubles for tokos. *The New York Times*, 2 December 1992.
22. Institute of Medicine (1985). *Personnel needs and training for biomedical and behavioral research.* National Academy Press, Washington, DC.
23. Doubilet, P., Weinstein, M. C., and McNeil, B. J. Occasional notes: use and misuse of the term "cost effective" in medicine. *New Engl. J. Med.* **314** (4), 253–6 (1986).
24. Relman, A. S. and Rheinhardt, U. E. Debating for- profit health care and the ethics of physicians. *Health Affairs* pp. 5–31, (Summer 1986).

25. Eisenberg, J. M. (1986) *Doctors' decisions and the cost of medical care.* Health Administration Press, Ann Arbor Michigan.
26. Phelps, C. E. (1992). *Health economics.* Harper Collins Publishers, New York.
27. Rodwin, M. A. The organized American medical profession's response to financial conflicts of interest: 1890–1992. *The Milbank Quarterly.* **70** (4), 703–41 (1992).
28. Sachs, B. P. (1989). Is the rising rate of cesarean sections a result of more defensive medicine? In *Medical professional liability and the delivery of obstetrical care.* (eds V. P. Rostow and R. J. Bulger) Vol II, pp. 27–40. National Academy Press. Washington, DC.
29. Hillman, B. J., Joseph, C. A., Mabry, M. R., Sunshine, J. H., Kennedy, S. D., and Noether, M. Frequency and costs of diagnostic imaging in office practice—a comparison of self-referring and radiologist-referring physicians. *New. Engl. J. Med.* **323** (23), 1604–8 (1990).
30. Hadley, J., Hoffman, J., and Feder, J. *Relationships between health insurance coverage and selected health and hospital use characteristics of newborns and pregnant women.* Center of Health Policy Studies, Georgetown University, Washington DC, 1989.
31. Silverman, W. A. Overtreatment of neonates? A personal retrospective. *Pediatrics.* **90** (6), 971–6, (1992).
32. Office of Technology Assessment. *Neonatal intensive care for low birthweight infants: costs and effectiveness, Health technology case study 38.* Congress of the United States, Washington DC, 1987.
33. Harrison, H. (1983). *The premature baby book.* St. Martin's Press, New York.
34. Guillemin, J. H. and Holmstrom, L. L. *Mixed blessings; intensive care for newborns.* Oxford University Press, New York (1986).
35. Gostin, L. O., and Roper, W. L. Update: The American with Disabilities Act. *Health Affairs* **11** (3), 248–63 (1992).
36. Braveman, P., Egerter, S., Bennett, R., and Showstack, J. Differences in hospital resource allocation among sick newborns according to insurance coverage. *JAMA.* **266** (23), 3300–7 (1991).
37. Handom, D. C. Setting health care priorities in Oregon: cost effectiveness meets the rule of rescue. *JAMA.* **265** (17), 2218–25 (1991).
38. Wiener, J. M. and Hanley, R. J. Winners and losers: primary and high-tech care under health care rationing. *The Brookings Review.* 46–9 (1992).
39. Grannemann, T. W. Priority setting: a sensible approach to Medicaid policy? *Inquiry* **28**, 300–5 (1991).
40. Eddy, D. M. Oregon's methods: did cost-effectiveness analysis fail? *JAMA.* **266** (15), 2135–41 (1991).
41. Rosenbaum, S. Poor women, poor children, poor policy: the Oregon Medicaid experiment. In *Rationing America's medical care: the Oregon plan and beyond* (eds. M. A. Strosberg, J. M. Wiener, R. Baker, and I. A, Fein) pp. 91–106. The Brookings Institution, Washington, DC (1992).
42. Capron, A. M. At law—Oregon's disability: principles or politics? *Hastings Center Report* **22** (6) 18–25 (1992)
43. Aaron, H. J. The Oregon experiment. In *Rationing America's medical care:*

the Oregon plan and beyond (eds. M. A. Strosberg, J. M. Wiener R. Baker, and I. A. Fein) pp. 107–11. The Brookings Institution, Washington, DC, (1992).

44. Wennberg, J. E. Outcomes research, cost containment, and the fear of health care rationing. *New Engl. J. Med.* **323** (17), 1202–4 (1990).
45. Aaron, H. J. and Schwartz, W. B. *The painful prescription: rational hospital care.* The Brookings Institution, Washington, DC. (1984).
46. Schwartz, W. B., and Aaron, H. J. The Achilles heel of health care rationing. *New York Times* 7 July 1990.
47. Fuchs, V. R. *How We live.* (1983). Harvard University Press, Cambridge, MA.
48. Sheils, J. F. and Wolfe, P. R. The role of private health insurance in children's health care. *The Future of Children.* **2** (2), 115–33 (1992).
49. Bales, S. N. Public opinion and health care reform for children. *The Future of Children* **3** (2), 184–97, 1993.

13

The economics of perinatal care in the United Kingdom

13A   THE ECONOMICS OF PERINATAL CARE IN THE UNITED KINGDOM

Richard C. Stevenson

Only a few years ago some clinicians were willing to question the whole morality of economic intrusions into medical matters. Is it right, they would ask, to place a value on the life of a baby? Is it proper, or even conceivable, that an infant might not be treated for want of funds? These questions, understandable in a National Health Service (NHS) when clinicians were not expected to count costs, now seem almost antediluvian. Resources were always limited, and difficult choices had to be made between and within specialties; but these choices were made implicitly. For better or worse, the application of economics to health-care issues has tended to make costs and choices explicit. It can also be argued that health economics has added a dimension to medical ethics.

This part of the economic contribution discusses the economic appraisal of perinatal care in the UK, and comments on moral and ethical issues which have arisen. Reference is made to several areas of perinatal medicine; but the emphasis is on the evaluation of neonatal intensive care (NIC) for low-birthweight (LBW) infants. This narrow focus is justified partly because LBW infants, being a small proportion of all births, are thought to provide an efficient means of monitoring changes in neonatal and perinatal care. The emphasis on NIC is also a fair reflection of the literature. Moreover, problems which arise in the evaluation of NIC encapsulate many issues which are of general concern in perinatal care, and indeed throughout medicine.

ISSUES

From the economic point of view, NIC is not very different from other medical specialties; but it is politically sensitive, and has attracted more than its share of attention from health economists. In part this is because new technologies, perceived to be expensive, are much more likely to be evaluated than older technologies, which are perceived to be cheap. It is also the case that neonatology is a relatively new specialty, which has been forced to fight for budgets, and neonatal clinicians therefore welcomed both clinical and economic appraisal some years before this became standard procedure.

The issues most at stake have been, and are, as follows:

1. Do the benefits of NIC exceed its cost when account is taken of the increased prevalence of impaired children?
2. How much NIC should be made available in a NHS which has to choose between many competing claims on its budget?
3. If it is not possible to provide NIC for all infants who could conceivably benefit, is it possible and legitimate to identify and treat those who would benefit most? In particular, is birthweight a good predictor of medical outcomes and costs?
4. Planning issues, which include the optimum size and geographical distribution of specialist units and making provision for the education, training, and long-term care of impaired survivors.
5. Under the new arrangements for the NHS, local health authorities enter into contracts with hospitals for the provision of care. In an attempt to mimic market processes, the system aims to curb rising costs by encouraging competition between providers. At present there are too few providers to create a proper market environment; but hospitals need to predict the costs of NIC for the purpose of making contracts. This problem is akin to those encountered in operating the Federal neonatal diagnosis-related group-pricing system in the United States.

THE PURSUIT OF EFFICIENCY AND ITS IMPLICATIONS

In the most recent of a long line of reports on the organization and scale of perinatal services in the UK, the Royal College of Physicians drew attention to what it regarded as a serious under-provision of resources for the care of the newborn.[2] In part, the report explained deficiencies in neonatal services by a failure of capacity to grow in line with the demand for specialist care. For more than a decade there has been an increase in the number of liveborn LBW infants and in the prevalence of multiple births. Both of these categories of infants place disproportionately high demands on neonatal services.

Technological development has also been influential in creating demand for extra resources. Improvements in NIC have made it possible to treat infants who in earlier times might have been classed as stillbirths or abortions. Better nutritional support, drug therapies, and diagnostic and surgical techniques have increased survival rates, but neonatal care has become more complicated and costly. Most recently, the use of surfactants to improve respiratory function has further lowered the threshold for admission to NIC, so that smaller babies are being treated for longer periods.

All these developments have occurred during a period when the whole of the NHS has been subject to financial strain. Budgetary stringency is, however, fundamental to the NHS rather than peculiar to the 1980s, or to the policies of a particular government. Lives could be saved, improved, and extended in many ways. The problem is to assess conflicting claims within a given budget. In adjudicating between alternative uses of resources, equity competes with efficiency as the guiding principle. Equity was uppermost in 1947, when the NHS was founded; but definitions of equity are numerous and difficult to apply in practice.[3] Everyone agrees that fairness in the distribution of health care is important; but it is important in different degrees to different people. For these reasons, economists are inclined (perhaps too readily) to try to separate issues of efficiency and equity. Very frequently, equity objectives tend to be regarded as (ill-defined) politically determined constraints on the main business of health economists, which is the pursuit of efficiency.

For health services to be efficient, each therapy or procedure should meet three basic criteria:

(1) it should be demonstrably effective in improving patients' health;
(2) it should be performed at the least possible cost i.e. cost-effectively; and
(3) the size of the program ought to be determined by a comparison between marginal (extra) cost and marginal benefits. (The logic is that if the expenditure of an extra £1 on care creates benefits which society values at more than £1, the expenditure is justified. If it results in benefits worth less than £1, the expenditure is not justified. At the margin, a programme will be efficient if marginal benefits equal marginal cost.

These three propositions are necessary but not sufficient for efficiency in the whole system. All procedures may be effective, and cost-effective and of the optimum scale, but it may still not be possible to accommodate all the desirable programmes within a global budget. In choosing between technically efficient programmes an additional criterion is needed. One such criterion which commands fairly wide approval is that an NHS should manage resources so as to achieve the maximum possible improvement in the health of the nation.

If the impact of a given budget on health is to be maximized, resources need to be concentrated on those therapies which produce the most benefits. It follows that some treatments which could benefit some patients may not be offered, and some treatments which are available will not be offered to all patients. The Oregon experiment to set priorities for its Medicaid programme was based on this principle.[4]

The acceptance of efficiency criteria for health systems is bound to offend against some people's notions of fairness. It also has implications for clinical practice, and for this reason it was suggested earlier that economics has

added a dimension to medical ethics.[5] The strong implication is that depar-
ture from efficiency is unethical. If medical practices are not cost-effective, a
procedure could be performed equally well by other means at lower cost, and
more resources would be available for other patients. Similarly if the costs of
a programme exceed the value of its benefits, some of those resources would
be better employed in other activities.

The issue at stake is 'who is the patient?'. This question is discussed
further in a later section, but the suggestion here is that clinical responsibility
is not limited to the patient being treated, but extends to other patients who
might be on waiting-lists, or whose illness has still to be diagnosed.

EVALUATION TECHNIQUES

Methods of economic evaluation are designed to make efficiency criteria
operational, and in their various forms involve weighing costs against
benefits. The ideal method is cost–benefit analysis, which takes a society-
wide view of welfare, and attempts to quantify all costs and benefits
to all parties, including those persons who might have been treated if
health-care resources had been differently distributed. This is a tall order,
and few, if any studies can claim to have come close to a full evaluation of
this sort.

The hardest problem in health-care appraisal is to put a value on the
benefits. Many studies try to avoid the difficulty by using cost–effectiveness
analysis (CEA), which seeks the least-cost method of achieving a well-defined
objective. CEA has been used in the evaluation of pre-natal screening for
Down syndrome and neural tube defects—but the method is best-suited to
relatively simple procedures, for which it can be shown that an alternative
therapy reduces costs without effecting outcome.[6] It is not readily applicable
to the comprehensive appraisal of complex therapies, such as NIC, which
have a wide range of possible outcomes.

Cost–utility analysis (CUA) is perhaps the most powerful and flexible evaluation technique. It was developed in Canada, and has become familiar to clinicians in the UK through the work of Alan Williams and his colleagues at York
University.[7,8] CUA is similar to CEA, but focuses directly on the welfare of the
patient by measuring the cost of producing a quality-adjusted life-year (QALY)
where the quality of life is measured on a 0–1 scale on which 0.00 is dead,
and 1.00 is well. An early application of CUA, influential in UK research,
was a Canadian study of NIC for very low birthweight (VLBW) infants.[9]

The remainder of this paper reviews some UK economics literature and
takes the ingredients of an economic evaluation as an organizing principle.
The main elements are: (1) identifying some meaningful alternative to a
particular therapy against which costs and benefits can be measured; (2)
discounting; (3) measuring costs; and (4) measuring benefits. A final section
comments on ethical and moral issues.

SELECTION BIAS, CONTROL GROUPS, AND EFFECTIVENESS

Selection bias and the choice of a control group are problems common to all evaluation. Selection bias can be avoided in geographically defined populations, such as the studies of LBW children in Aberdeen and neonates on Merseyside; but it remains a problem in evaluations conducted at regional NIC Units which receive referrals from local hospitals.[10,11] It is thought that, in the early days, local hospitals were disposed to refer only those infants with relatively good prognoses. Even so, in children transferred to the Liverpool NIC Unit in 1979-81 by special ambulance or *in utero*, outcomes were worse and costs were 25 per cent greater than for children born in the unit.[12] Most local hospitals now have intensive-care cots, and are more likely to refer only the sickest infants to specialist centres.

The costs and benefits of a particular medical intervention can best be compared in randomized controlled trials (RCTs). Many have been carried out in perinatalogy, and a few have some economic content; but a survey of economic aspects of the care of neonates found only one such trial of NIC, and that was conducted in Australia between 1966 and 1970.[13,14] In more recent times, clinical trials of the major components of NIC have not been a realistic option—probably they would not be approved by the ethical committees which supervise medical research in the UK.

An alternative approach is to make use of historical control groups. In the Canadian study, Boyle and his colleagues were able to estimate the impact of NIC by comparing geographically defined samples of LBW infants born before and after the introduction of modern techniques.[9] This method requires retrospective costing, a hazardous process seldom attempted in the UK because historical records are insufficiently detailed. Economists have therefore been forced to make assumptions about the likely consequences of not treating LBW infants in specialist units. One study assumed that if infants born in 1979–81 had not received respiratory support, they would most probably have died, so all of the QALYs gained could be attributable to NIC.[12] At the time this was considered to be a good working assumption, since all the infants in the study were very sick; but now it would no longer be defensible. The expansion of NIC facilities has allowed more infants to be treated, and some babies would undoubtedly survive without intensive care.

The problem of defining a control group has not been satisfactorily solved, but it is perhaps not as critical as it once was. Early studies needed the 'before and after' method to establish the effectiveness of NIC. The effectiveness of NIC in reducing infant mortality now seems well established.[15] Most of the remaining issues concern the epidemiology of morbidity and impairment and their long-term costs.

DISCOUNTING

Most medical interventions give rise to a stream of costs and benefits over long time-periods. Medicine is not peculiar in this respect. The same problem arises in all sorts of investment appraisal which require comparisons to be made between alternative projects which differ in the timing of their costs and benefits. The way in which costs and benefits are aggregated is a technical issue of particular importance in the evaluation of perinatal medicine.

Most treatments involve initial costs, and sometimes, as in the case of an impaired child, a stream of expenditure which may extend over many years. It is likely that costs will rise over time owing to inflation; but this is taken into account by expressing future cost estimates in constant prices. It is still, however, not legitimate to add up costs incurred at different points in time. A pound today is not the same as a pound tomorrow or forty years hence; and for this reason the technique of discounting is widely used as a means of reducing flows of expenditure to a common base.

The technique of discounting applies compound interest in reverse to calculate the present discounted value (PDV) of a stream of costs or benefits. If the discount rate is 6 per cent the PDV of £100 to be received in 1 year's time is the amount which, invested at 6 per cent, will yield £100 at the end of the year. It is £94.30. Discounting a stream of costs reduces a whole treatment to its PDV, which can be thought of as the amount of money which the NHS would need to set aside to cover the lifetime costs of, for instance, caring for a disabled child.

Where time-horizons are short, as in the valuation of care for the elderly mentally ill, the choice of a discount rate may not be critical to the outcome of an economic appraisal; but PDVs are highly sensitive to discount rates over long periods, such as those contemplated in perinatal medicine. The longer the time-horizon and the higher the discount rate applied, the less is the value attached to future costs and benefits.

For the purpose of health-service appraisals, the UK government recommends a standard discount rate, which since 1989 has been 6 per cent in real terms. There is, however, no correct rate, and the best studies apply sensitivity analysis to show how findings would differ if alternative discount rates were applied. In the Canadian study, it was shown that NIC for infants in the 1000–1499 g birthweight range resulted in an economic gain if costs and benefits were discounted at rates up to 5 per cent. Economic losses resulted if rates higher than 5 per cent were applied.[9]

Discounting costs is fairly uncontroversial; but economists are by no means agreed on the desirability of discounting benefits when these are expressed in terms of life-years or QALYs. In favour of discounting life it can be said that benefits are put on an equal footing with costs. It is also argued that faculties diminish with age, and one year's life is less productive of both income and enjoyment in forty years' time than at the present. However, powerful arguments have been raised in opposition which suggest that there is no reason to think that the value of life declines with age.[16] The promise of an extra year of life in forty years' time ensures that parents will see how their children turn out and get to know their grandchildren (which might be a mixed blessing). Furthermore, if the wealth of nations grows over time, the opportunities to enjoy old age may expand, and technical advance in medicine may ease the problems of ill health in old age.

These arguments are receiving serious consideration in UK government departments. A decision to discount the non-monetary benefits of health care at a zero rate would have powerful implications for the productiveness of perinatal medicine relative to treatments for adults. The present practice of discounting QALYs can be said to discriminate against perinatal care because it attaches only negligible value to life produced in the distant future. Discounted at 6 per cent, 1 year of full-quality life in 40 years' time has a PDV of only 0.097. If life-years and QALYs were discounted at a zero rate, the benefits of all medical interventions would increase, but the impact would be greatest on those therapies which produce the most life. The effect would be to alter the ranking of treatments on an 'Oregon-style' list which orders therapies according to the cost of producing a QALY.[16] The principal beneficiaries would be perinatal and paediatric specialties, and might include NIC for even the smallest infants.

COSTS

Costs should be as comprehensive and as specific as possible to the therapy being appraised, and are defined with reference to a budget centre. The measurement of costs is therefore by no means an entirely objective exercise. Costs will differ according to whether they are viewed from the NIC Unit, the hospital in which it is contained, the health authority, central government, or the family of the patient. Changes in medical policy frequently alter the distribution of these costs. The most obvious example is a reduction in the length of hospital stays, which reduces hospital costs, but causes patients to recuperate for longer at home, and imposes extra costs on families and community medical services.

Some economic studies are designed to provide quite specific information on costs from the viewpoint of a single centre, usually a hospital; but comprehensive evaluations try to give a rounded view by measuring all possible costs, and leaving decision-makers to place appropriate weights on the different categories. This comprehensive approach is particularly necessary in perinatal medicine, because interventions made in early life have cost (and benefit) implications for families and for health, education, and social services over many years. Economic evaluation therefore needs to take a long-term view of costs, and must be subject to considerable uncertainty. Crude outcomes of care can be measured at discharge from hospital; but late-infant mortality and long-term morbidity will only be revealed over time. It follows that full evaluation is a long-term process, made all the harder by the rapid change in medical technology. A picture of the medium-term consequences of LBW has only recently begun to emerge for infants born in 1980; but the techniques by which these children were treated have long since been overtaken.

NEONATAL COSTS

Careful costings of NIC units start with the so-called 'top down' method, which allocates the whole budget among all the activities of the unit, which include teaching and postnatal clinics as well as the care of infants and the counselling of parents. Most published work is concerned specifically with the evaluation of intensive care for very-low-birthweight (VLBW) infants (≤1500 grams); but NIC units treat a heterogeneous patient group, most of whom are not of VLBW, and some of whom are not ventilated. An important preliminary, therefore, is to define intensive care and to apportion the total costs of care between infants to be studied and others.

NIC units usually share premises with maternity hospitals, and receive services from a wide range of pathology and other departments. Hospital overheads have to be apportioned (heating, lighting, and portering and catering for staff rather than infants); and special care is needed in the costing of diagnostic tests, which can differ according to the laboratory in which they are performed and the time of day. The methods of costing are not controversial, but findings differ according to the comprehensiveness of individual studies. Nevertheless all studies show that medical and nursing costs are the largest cost category, amounting to between 45 per cent and 70 per cent of total costs.

Having established the total cost of the care for VLBW infants receiving intensive care, further distinctions are necessary, because, in so complicated a process, inpatient days are not an adequate measure of the treatment received. Following more or less closely the guidelines of the British Paediatric Association,[17] UK studies in Liverpool and Birmingham have defined three levels of care and calculated a cost per day at each level.[18,19] A Leeds study used two levels.[20] On average, the most intensive level of care costs 2–3 times more than the intermediate level, which is about 3 times the cost of the lowest level.

Using medical records to find the number of days which each infant spent at each of the levels and multiplying by the unit costs gives a total cost for each child. The Liverpool costing was made more baby-specific by costing tests individually for each infant.[18] Account also has to be taken of the cost of care for non-survivors. This is usually incorporated into results by presenting the average cost of producing a survivor, which is the total cost of care for survivors and non-survivors divided by the number of survivors.

Most data sets show at least a superficial negative correlation between BW and cost; but this finding needs cautious interpretation. Data are usually presented grouped into BW ranges—often above and below 1000 g. Costs within BW broad ranges have a very high variance, and this is greatest in the lowest ranges. Extremely LBW infants who survive for a short period cost very little, but all of the 6 cohorts examined at Liverpool contained at least one infant who survived at great expense for a matter of months. There is a temptation to exclude these cases as 'statistical outliers', but to do so would be to misrepresent the nature of intensive care, which is inherently uncertain in its outcomes.

It has been suggested that the association between cost and BW is in part a statistical artefact dependent on the grouping of data.[18] The relation between BW and cost has been shown to vary with the BW groups selected. Using ungrouped BW data, the influence of BW on costs was shown to be statistically significant ($P<0.05$), but its predictive power was very low ($R=0.04$). Furthermore, no structural break could be detected in the data at 1000 g, or any other conveniently round number.

In an attempt to improve predictions of cost, the number of weeks' gestation and dummy variables for survivors/non-survivors, inborn/outborn infants, and in utero transfers were added to regression equations; but these added virtually nothing to the explanatory power of the equations. In another paper, the inclusion of four clinical conditions predicted 60 per cent of the variance in neonatal costs ($P<0.05$), and it was concluded that the medical condition of the infant was far more important than BW.[21]

From an ethical and NHS management point of view, the most interesting finding from the UK data comes from a comparison between units of the cost of care shown in Table 13.1. Wide variations in costs, not explained by differences in admission criteria or regional epidemiology, are commonplace in the NHS; but the striking feature of Table 13.1 is the difference between costs for survivors and non-survivors. The approximate ratios are 6:1 (Birmingham); 2:1 (Leeds); and 4:3 (Liverpool). Conclusions must be tentative, since the studies differ somewhat in their methods; but the strong implication is that hospitals differ in their management of very sick infants with poor prognoses.

Detailed data on outcomes for two of the three centres have not been published, so a proper evaluation of management policies is not possible. However, the cost data alone lead one to wonder whether a policy which allows very sick infants to die relatively cheaply represents an efficient use of resources, or whether the extra cost of more enthusiastic treatment is justified in terms of better outcomes, or the satisfaction which parents derive from knowing that all possible measures have been taken. From an ethical point of view, it might also be asked whether parents have a right to know that professional opinion and management policy differ on matters which have an important bearing on their welfare.

As always in perinatal care, the clinician treats not only the infant but also the family, which bears substantial psychological costs. NHS care for infants is free of charge, so, compared with the situation in the United States, economic costs to UK parents at the neonatal stage are fairly marginal. They are not, however, insignificant, in view of the high proportion of parents from lower socioeconomic groups with no earned income. The only UK study to investigate costs to parents of visiting NIC units found that travel costs were a significant expense, and 24 per cent of families were experiencing financial difficulties.[22]

The issue of whether specialist facilities should be large and regionalized, or smaller and more widely dispersed, is mainly an efficiency concern; but it also has access-cost implications for families. A recent study of 17 hospitals in a single region found clear evidence of the existence of economies of scale in the provision of intensive care; but these diminished at around the 13–14 cot level.[23] The authors concluded that concentration of facilities beyond this level might not be adequate to offset the extra costs of travel, especially in sparsely populated areas.

LONG-TERM COSTS

Most longitudinal studies of LBW infants do not deal in detail with economic issues, so much of the following is based on published and unpublished data from the Merseyside studies. A geographically defined sample consisted of all children born in 1980–1 of BW≤1500 g together with a 10 per cent sample of children in the BW range 1501–2000 g. All unimpaired children were followed up at age 8–9, and matched with a control child attending the same school. Impaired children were assessed individually.

The objective of the study was to investigate physical and educational development in unimpaired LBW children, and to estimate the extra cost of educating and caring for an LBW child as compared with a normal child. In tests of motor impairment, IQ and reading ability, the LBW infants performed significantly worse than the control children, and there was a much higher prevalence of behavioural disorders as perceived by both teachers and parents. Striking differences were also found in health-service usage. Unimpaired LBW children consulted family practitioners far more frequently than the control children, and the cost of hospitalization was approximately 10 times greater, as a consequence of more frequent admissions and longer stays.

An earlier study conducted at age 4 predicted that, as the children aged, the long-term costs of LBW would become dominated by the cost of caring for those who were impaired. Even if still more recent developments in NIC are not associated with an increase in impairment, larger numbers of survivors will impose an increasing cost on families and the Exchequer.[12] In a study of 52 impaired survivors, it was found that the cost of hospital care up to age 8–9 years was approximately 3 times greater than for an unimpaired LBW child, and 30 times greater than for the control children. Recent work in the United States has estimated the extra cost of special education for LBW survivors at £370.8 million (1989–90).[24] No similar figure has been calculated for the UK; but of the 52 impaired survivors in the Merseyside study, 45 attended a variety of special schools which, at a conservative estimate, cost 4 times more

Table 13.1 Comparison of costs (£) for care of VLBW infants at 3 UK centres

	Birmingham*	Leeds**	Liverpool*
Cost per patient	4850	6979	4159
Cost per survivor	6220	8192	4490
Cost per non-survivor	1081	4169	3446

* 1984 pay and prices
** 1985 pay and prices

than normal schools, making the incremental annual cost about £3000 a year for each pupil (1991).

Translating these findings into lifetime costs for LBW survivors is fraught with uncertainty. Morbidity is found to decline towards normal levels as LBW children reach the age of nine; but slow educational development and physical clumsiness could have implications for social integration and future employment. More seriously, mildly and moderately impaired children impose large costs on families, and in the worst cases life-long institutional care may be needed. Costs to families can be estimated by pricing the services provided in the home at market rates. An alternative is to suppose that although most severely impaired LBW survivors will receive some care at home, the cost imposed on families will be of a similar magnitude to the cost of institutional care, which in a Merseyside institution amounts to £24 000 per year in 1991 prices.

BENEFITS

Some medical interventions can be justified in pure economic terms. Improved therapies for low back pain could 'pay for themselves' in terms of a reduction in working days lost, and the same might be claimed for a malaria eradication programme which increased agricultural productivity. Similarly, the expected future earnings of LBW infants have been used in two North American studies as one measure of the benefits of NIC.[9, 25] Although earning potential remains a useful part of some studies, economists have never been happy with a measure of benefits which seems to suggest that man is made mainly to earn and consume. Furthermore, this method is difficult to apply in the presence of widespread unemployment, and cannot be used to justify treatment of the elderly or the disabled.

Also less than fully satisfactory is the method used in some studies of prenatal screening which measure the benefits in terms of the costs averted by terminating a pregnancy which might have resulted in an impaired child. This may be legitimate where the evaluation is concerned only with

RICHARD C. STEVENSON

Exchequer costs; but the real benefit of screening is to be found in the value of reassurance and reduction in anxiety to mothers. More recent work is attempting to reveal the preferences of women, and to take account of what has been called 'deprivation disutility', which arises from the knowledge that tests exist which are not offered to all women.[26]

It seems most natural to express benefits of perinatal care in terms of lives, or life-years, gained; and these then may, or may not, be adjusted for perceived differences in quality. NIC compares well with most adult therapies because it generates a large quantity of life. It is also possible that in some areas perinatal care is more productive than adult care, because some children respond better than do some adults. To take one example, drug-addicted infants are weaned from heroin addiction in a matter of days, presumably because there is no psychological dimension to their addiction.[27] By contrast, the dropout rate from adult drug therapy programmes is about 75 per cent.

If lives or life-years gained are taken as a yardstick, the largest gains will be found in the lowest-birthweight groups, where mortality has decreased most in recent years. There is, however, a complication. Provided that parents are capable of having other children, a perinatal intervention which saves the life of an infant might displace another child. The replacement demand for children has not been discussed in the context of NIC, but it has been considered in the economics of prenatal screening.

Alternatively, outputs may be measured in quality-adjusted life-years. This will reduce the value of NIC according to the prevalence of impairment and the disutility which is attached to it. The estimation of QALYs is still in its infancy, and many conceptual and practical problems remain unsolved.[28] Perhaps the central issue is whose opinion should count in the valuation of alternative states of health. Some studies take the opinion of clinicians and other health professionals; the Oregon experiment consulted public opinion; and in the evaluation of NIC, Boyle and his colleagues interviewed a panel of Canadian parents.[9] In the Canadian study, utility values, conventionally scaled from 1.00 (normal health) to 0.00 (dead), were extended from 1.00 to − 0.39 because parents rated some chronic dysfunctional states as worse than death.

The only published UK study which takes account of long-term costs and estimates outcomes in lives, life-years, and QALYs gained, reports on VLBW infants born in Liverpool between 1979 and 1981.[12] It was estimated that the average lifetime cost for 40 survivors in 1981 was £20 574. Quality-adjustment for the impaired survivors reduced the lives gained to 37.0 and raised the average cost to £22 242 per quality-adjusted life. Life expectancy was assumed to be normal for the unimpaired and mildly impaired survivors, but only 45 years for those infants who were severely impaired. Adjustment for quality and life-expectancy gave the number of QALYs gained as 2572, at an average cost of £1152. All costs were given in terms of 1984 pay and prices. This finding supported the view of the report of the Royal College of Physicians, which concluded that the outcomes of NIC, expressed in terms of the cost of gaining a QALY, 'appear to compare very favourably with other forms of treatment available to adult patients, and with certain screening programmes'.[2]

ETHICS, HEALTH ECONOMICS, AND PERINATALOGY

It remains to draw together the ethical issues to discuss their implications; but first, a brief account of the way in which economists view the professions.

Medicine is one of the licensed professions which has privileges in law. Membership of the profession is restricted to the holders of certain qualifications, which are in the gift of the profession and are expensive to acquire in terms of money and time. Admission to medical schools and fellowships of the Royal Colleges are examples. In addition, licensed professions are to a large extent self-regulated by written, or unwritten, codes of professional ethics. However, professional ethics are expensive to enforce, and some sorts of 'cheating' are difficult to detect. Therefore acceptable professional conduct depends not only on the ethical code, but also on morality derived from individual consciences. By way of an example, probably rather few perinatalogists would detect that some of the points contained in this section are derived from R. C. O. Matthews's 1989 Presidential Address to the Royal Economic Society, but it would be immoral and unethical not to mention it.[29]

The feature which unites professions of different sorts, and is of special interest to economists, is the agency relationship, which exists between doctors and patients, teachers and pupils, and stockbrokers and their clients. In professional transactions, information is said to be asymmetrically distributed between the parties. Patients know less about medicine than doctors, and are ill equipped to judge the quality of the service received. They depend, therefore, on a relationship in which professional ethics require the doctor to consult the best interests of the patient. If an agency relationship were perfect, the doctor would select for the patient the type and quantity of treatment which an equally well-informed patient would select for him- or herself.

In this way professional ethics may be seen as a *quid pro quo*, by which a profession offers assurances of high standards in return for privileges which it receives from the State. However, in transactions of this kind many opportunities exist for the professional to pursue self-serving objectives. This has caused economists to view the professions with deep misgiving. Special rights in law, barriers to entry, and self-regulation can all be used to restrict competition to the disadvantage of the consumer. This view has come to prominence in the UK during the past decade, and has resulted in wide-reaching legal changes, or proposals for change, which would alter the status of professions in the law, stockbroking, education, medicine, and even the Church. The aim is to increase efficiency and standards of service to the consumer by promoting competition. Or, as Matthews puts it, 'to try to make the professions more like business'.

This policy has already made a distinct impact on the medical profession in the UK. Clinicians are being obliged to manage in a more 'businesslike' manner, which involves closer attention to financial budgeting and to clinical audit. These concepts come together in the economic evaluation of health care.

It has been suggested at various points that health-care evaluation is by no means a mechanical and value-free procedure. In the selection of techniques, and at every stage in the process, judgements have to be made which influence outcomes and may have bearing on professional conduct. Perhaps the central issue is the extent to which economics should be allowed to intrude on the doctor–patient relationship.

In perinatology the agency relationship is peculiarly complicated, because the preferences of the patient cannot be consulted. Clinicians treat infants; but they have to deal with parents. In many circumstances, parents can be regarded as perfect agents for the infant, or the fetus; but this is not always the case. If the life of a mother is at stake, or if the effect of the birth of an impaired child could have an unfavourable effect on siblings, the interests of the family could conflict with those of an unborn, or newly born, child. In this context, it will be remembered that, in Canada, some parents regarded some impaired states as worse than death.

The situation is further complicated because neonatal medicine is inextricably linked to the 'right to life'. In the UK there is nothing equivalent to the 'Baby Doe' rule, which impinges on clinical freedom in the United States.[30] Nevertheless, this is a area in which Society may wish to express a view and, in some circumstances, overrule the opinions of both doctors and parents.

The weights which are attached to the views of parents, doctors and Society at large will affect resource allocations. A significant amount of clinical time is spent in counselling parents, and it was suggested that increased concentration of NIC facilities might not be justified if the cost of access is taken into account. In a world of scarce resources, trade-offs exist, and better services for parents may be bought at a cost to infants.

Attention has also been drawn to UK cost data, which show significant differences in the cost of NIC between hospitals. Medical outsiders are frequently puzzled by the persistence of wide cost variations, which, to an economist, seem most 'unbusinesslike'. In a competitive environment businesses seek the most cost-efficient technology. Those firms which get it right get rich, or, at least, they stay in business. Firms which get it wrong go broke. This mechanism does not operate in publicly financed industries such as the NHS. Nevertheless clinicians are gregarious, and information-flows in medicine are good. Is it not therefore surprising that best-practice medicine is not more readily identified and applied more widely?

The cost data also revealed what seem to be differences in policy in the management of LBW infants with poor prognoses. In a health service which claims to be national, it might be expected that policy should be fairly uniform throughout the country. If policy variations exist, it might be asked whether they can be justified on ethical, moral, or resource-management grounds. It has also been suggested that professional ethics might require parents to be better informed about management policy.

In private health-care systems, where the family pays the bill, financial considerations enter automatically into the agency relationship, since it would be futile to recommend a course of action beyond the means of the family. Insurance systems and national health services allow the clinician to select on behalf of the family the best treatment, rather than the best which can be afforded. It might therefore be argued that from a purely medical point of view, an insurance scheme or an NHS allows a more perfect agency relationship than does a private system.

This proposition depends on how widely the clinician is prepared to extend his or her responsibilities. In the presence of scarcity, the failure of the clinician to take economic considerations into account will increase premiums for other policy holders or, in an NHS, leave fewer resources for other patients. For these reasons it has been suggested that departures from efficiency are unethical. In other words, a wide view of professional ethics, which takes account of economic issues, requires the clinician to act as an agent not only for the patient and the family, but also for the NHS and ultimately the taxpayer.

Health-care evaluation is intended to provide guidance on making decisions of this sort; and, disagreeable though it may be, health-care evaluation does place a value, at least implicitly, on the life of a child. This is not specially shocking: the international community declines to 'purchase' a large number of very cheap lives in Africa. Nevertheless, if choices are to be made on the basis of what economists call efficiency, it is as well to know that apparently technical matters, like discounting or the choice of a control group, can affect outcomes.

Economists in the UK are not so naïve as to suppose that the results of the sort of evaluations which have been described above will be translated immediately into policy. In fact, medical decisions at the margin seem to be based on the principle that, if a procedure is possible, it should be performed, and no quantity of journal articles will (or necessarily should) prevent neonatalogists from honing their skills and extending the realms of the possible. However, over time the absolutely unavoidable need to limit the liability of the NHS will cause economists and managers to seek rules by which to ration scarce resources, and these will limit clinical discretion.

It might therefore be concluded that clinicians ought to know at least enough economics to protect themselves from economists. Without that knowledge doctors are at a disadvantage in representing the interests of patients. If clinicians try to stand aside from the economic implications of their work, decisions affecting clinical practice will be made by managers, economists, and accountants—a prospect which not every potential patient will relish.

Nevertheless, one sympathizes with the view that in a complex world, it is unreasonable, and perhaps impossible, for the clinician to act as an agent for the whole of Society in the management of scarce resources. We should also think carefully before doctors are asked to behave like businessmen. It might be unsafe to conclude that Hippocrates was an economic illiterate. It could be that his failure to mention cost-effectiveness specifically reflected the view that, by and large, good medicine is cost-effective, bad medicine seldom is, and that the best that can be expected is that a doctor will 'first, do no harm', and second, consult the best interests of patients and their families.

REFERENCES

1. Resnick, M. B., Ariet, M., Carter, R. L., Fletcher, J. W., Evans, J. H., Furlough, R. R., Ausbon, W. W., and Curran, J. S. Prospective pricing for tertiary neonatal intensive care. *Pediatrics* 1986; **78** (5): 820–36.
2. Royal College of Physicians of London. *Medical care of the newborn in England and Wales*. Royal College of Physicians, London, 1988.
3. Culyer, A. J and Wagstaff, A. *Need, equality and social justice*, Discussion paper 90. Centre for Health Economics, York, 1992.
4. Hadorn, D. C. Setting health care priorities in Oregon: cost-effectiveness meets the Rule of Rescue. *JAMA* 1991; **265**: 2218–25.
5. Culyer, A. J. Morality of Efficiency in health care: some uncomfortable implications. *Health Economics* 1992; **1**: 5–18.
6. Henderson, J. B. The economic efficiency of prenatal screening. In *Chorion villus sampling* (ed. D. Liu, E. Symonds, and M. S. Gollus), pp. 245–53. Chapman and Hall, London, 1987.
7. Torrance, G. W. Measurement of health state utilities for economic appraisal. *Journal of Health Economics* 1986; **5**: 1–30.
8. Williams, A. Economics of coronary artery bypass grafting. *British Medical Journal* 1985; **291**: 326–9.
9. Boyle, M. H., Torrance, G. W., Sinclair, J. C., and Horwood, S. P. Economic evaluation of neonatal intensive care for very-low-birthweight infants. *New Engl. J. Med.*, 1983; **308**: 1330–7.
10. Powell, T. G., Pharoah, P. O. D., and Cooke, R. W. I. Survival and morbidity in a geographically defined population of low birthweight infants. *Lancet* 1986, March 8: 539–43.
11. Illsley, R. and Mitchell, G. R. (eds). *Low birth weight: a medical, psychological and social study*. Wiley, Chichester, 1984.
12. Pharoah, P. O. D., Stevenson, R. C., Cooke, R. W. I., and Sandhu, B. Costs and benefits of neonatal intensive care. *Arch. Dis. Childh.* 1988; **63**; 715–18.
13. National Perinatal Epidemiology Unit, World Health Organization. *A classified bibliography of controlled trials in perinatal medicine 1940–1984.* Oxford University Press, 1985.
14. Mugford, M. A review of the economics of care for sick newborn infants. *Community Medicine* 1988; **10**; 99–111.
15. Stewart, A. L., Reynolds, E. O. R., and Lipscomb, A. P. Outcome for infants of very low birthweight: survey of the world literature. *Lancet* 1981; **1**: 1038–41.

16. Parsonage, M. and Neuberger, H. Discounting and health benefits. *Health Economics* 1992, 1; 71–9.
17. British Paediatric Association and British Association for Perinatal Paediatrics. *Categories of babies requiring neonatal care.* BPA/BAPP, London, 1984.
18. Sandhu, B., Stevenson, R. C., Cooke, R. W. I., and Pharoah, P. O. D., Cost of neonatal intensive care for very low birthweight infants. *Lancet*, 1986; 1, 600–3.
19. Newns, B., Drummond, M. F., Durbin, G. M., and Culley, P. Costs and outcomes in a regional neonatal intensive care unit. *Arch. Dis. Childh.* 1984; 59: 1064–7.
20. Ryan, S., Sics, A., and Congdon, P. Costs of Neonatal care. *Arch. Dis. Childh.* 1988; 63: 303–6.
21. Stevenson, R. C., Pharoah, P. O. D., Cooke, R. W. I., and Sandhu, B. Predicting costs and outcomes of neonatal care for very low birthweight infants. *Public Health*, 1991; 105: 121–6.
22. Smith, M. A. and Baum, D. Cost of visiting babies in special care baby units. *Arch. Dis. Childh.* 1983; 58: 56–9.
23. Fordham, R., Field, D. J., Hodges, S., Normand, C., Mason E., Burton, P., Yates, J., and Male, S. Cost of neonatal care across a regional health authority. *Journal of Public Health Medicine* 1992; 14: 127–30.
24. Chaikind, S. and Corman, H. The impact of low birthweight on education costs. *Journal of Health Economics* 1991; 10: 291–311.
25. Walker, D. B., Feldman, A., Vohr, B. R., and Oh, W. Cost–benefit analysis of neonatal intensive care for infants weighing less than 1000 grams at birth. *Pediatrics*, 1984; 74: 20–5.
26. Mooney, G. and Lange, M. *Economic appraisal in pre-natal screening: reassessing the benefits, 1991*, Discussion Paper 08/91. Health Economics Research Unit, University of Aberdeen.
27. Shapiro, H. *Drugs, pregnancy and child care.* Institute for the study of Drug Dependency, London, 1990.
28. Loomes, G. and McKenzie, L. The scope and limitations of QALY measures. In *Quality of life: perspectives and policies*, (ed. S. Baldwin, C. Godfrey and C. Propper). Routledge, London, 1990.
29. Matthews, R. C. O. The economics of professional ethics: should the professions be more like business? *Economic Journal*, 1991; 101: 737–50.
30. Stevenson, D. K., Ariagno, R. L., Kutner, J. S., Raffin, T. A., and Young, E. W. D. The 'Baby Doe' rule. *JAMA*, 1986, 255: 1909–12.

13B ECONOMIC ISSUES IN THE UNITED KINGDOM: COMMENTARY ON THE ECONOMICS OF PERINATAL CARE IN THE UNITED KINGDOM

Miranda Mugford

INTRODUCTION

In this discussion I shall try, with reference to the issues raised by Richard Stevenson, to throw further light on the problems of arriving at the best use of resources for perinatal health care in the UK. I shall also make reference to some international comparisons. First, I shall consider what evidence there is about available resources and benefits in maternity and neonatal care, what evidence there is for the relationship between resources and outcomes of care, and what evidence there is in particular about practice which is demonstrably relatively inefficient. Then I shall discuss the obstacles to moving towards a more efficient and equitable use of resources.

VARIATIONS IN PROVISION OF CARE

There are wide geographical variations in the provision of care in maternity and neonatal health services that cannot be explained by indicators of need for such interventions. For example, in many countries nearly all deliveries take place in hospital, but in some there is a high rate of home delivery which is not associated with elevated perinatal mortality rates.[1] Caesarean section rates vary more than twofold between industrial countries, but again there is no apparent correlation with crude infant mortality rates.[2] In English health districts there is a persistent variation in the per cent age of liveborn babies who are admitted to neonatal paediatric care in different maternity units. In 1978 the admission rate varied from 9.1 per cent to 21 per cent in various English Health Regions.[3] More recent data for 1986 show a difference in admissions to neonatal units between 11 per cent in England and Wales and 22 per cent in Scotland.[4] This difference does not reflect indicators of need such as the number of low-weight births, and may only partly be accounted for by differences in the amount of care given to smaller or sick babies in postnatal maternity wards. There are clear cost implications of all of these variations: care during delivery for women at low risk of problems can be less costly in settings other than specialist obstetric units [5, 6], Caesarean delivery doubles the cost of the hospital delivery episode[7], and admission to neonatal special care could add considerably to the cost of caring for a newborn baby with minor health problems. Whatever the cost differences, the cost-effectiveness, and ultimately the efficiency, or otherwise, of such variations would need to take account of the contributions of the different policies to the mothers' and babies' health.

THE RELATIONSHIP BETWEEN PROVISION OF CARE AND OUTCOMES

Observational studies of outcomes of health interventions are always subject to the difficulty of making causal inferences relating observed events. Differences in outcome can result either from treatment and/or from prior health status. No amount of multivariate analysis will be able to disentangle completely the relative contributions of these explanations, although it can help to explore relationships between variables. A series of studies of the relationship between access to health-care facilities at the time of birth and neonatal mortality have been published which use this approach. Such studies lead to conflicting views. Two studies[8, 9] done in Norway and the United States respectively, find that, for the lower-birthweight babies, lower mortality was associated with birth in more highly equipped centres. Stilwell and his colleagues[10, 11] observed that babies of low birthweight had higher mortality in units with fewer paediatricians; but a study in Sweden found that babies born in hospitals with no paediatric department were less likely to die.[12] As mortality rates have fallen, any relationship becomes harder to separate from chance variation due to the small number of deaths, and this is one possible explanation of the results from two studies in England and Norway, which showed that in more recent years there was no significant association between outcome and resources for care.[10, 11, 13] There has also been an increase in resources for neonatal care in many countries, and this may have resulted in a smaller variability between units in the amount of resources. Once again, this would make it more difficult to identify any relationship if it did exist. Whatever relationships are found in observational data, we cannot conclude that there is a direct cause and effect. By that token it would be possible to 'prove' that storks bring babies in Sweden.[14] Therefore, such studies do not allow conclusive statements about the relative efficiency of maternity and neonatal services. But practical decisions have to be taken in spite of the difficulties of interpreting the research evidence; judgements about quality of care have to be made, and there is therefore continuing debate in the UK about the relative efficiency of different patterns of neonatal intensive care provision,[15, 16] and about the appropriate setting for low-risk birth.[1, 6]

Randomized controlled trials give the least biased estimate for the additional effect on health outcomes conferred by a particular intervention. As has been pointed out, the time has passed where the whole package of neonatal intensive care could be regarded as experimental for most pre-term babies, and it is difficult to imagine circumstances in which randomized allocation of a sick baby to care that did not include the life-support technology of neonatal intensive care would now be considered ethical or practicable. However, there is a large and growing body of data from randomized controlled trials of particular forms of care during pregnancy and childbirth. These data have recently been synthesized and critically reviewed as a result of work originated in the National Perinatal Epidemiology Unit in Oxford, UK, by Iain Chalmers, in collaboration with many others. A series of these systematic reviews of different aspects of maternity and neonatal care based on meta-analysis of randomized trials have now been published in two books.[17, 18] The reviews are regularly updated in electronic form as the Pregnancy and Childbirth Module and the Neonatal Care Module of the recently established Cochrane Collaboration, set up to foster the systematic review of existing research on the effectiveness of health care.[19]

With knowledge from overviews of randomized trials about the effects of interventions on pregnancy outcomes, and with information about the inputs required by different care policies, it is easier to draw conclusions about the importance of variations in care for health outcomes, and for the efficiency of health services.

For example, lung immaturity in pre-term babies is one of the major causes of neonatal death. Because these babies need ventilatory support, mechanical ventilation, and supplemental oxygen, they are among the most costly to care for in neonatal units.[20, 21] Interventions that could reduce mortality, morbidity, and the costs of care would be important for those concerned with increasing the efficiency of the health services. Two treatments which clearly reduce both mortality and respiratory problems in pre-term babies are giving women corticosteroids where pre-term delivery is anticipated, [22] and surfactant given to the baby at birth or soon afterwards. [23] The effects of the different interventions are striking and are of similar magnitude. But surfactant costs about £1000 per baby at 1992 prices, whereas it only costs between £10 and £15 per woman to give steroids before pre-term delivery. As a result, improved outcomes for pre-term babies could be achieved at relatively low cost by giving steroids antenatally, and may even be accompanied by resource savings in neonatal care. However, in practice, surfactant use is now widely disseminated, whereas only a minority of mothers of preterm babies in the UK have been given corticosteroids.[24, 25] Knowing about the relative costs and outcomes from the research that has been done, it seems reasonable to conclude that, in the UK, provision of care for women who give birth before term and for their babies is not as cost-effective as it could be.

OUTCOME MEASUREMENT FOR COMPARISONS BETWEEN HEALTH PROGRAMMES

The example of antenatal corticosteroid use in the UK lends support to those who point to variations in health practice as evidence of possible inefficiency: this can sometimes be the case. The issue still remains that the effects of interventions in health care in general, and in perinatal care in particular, are very difficult to measure. In the example of prevention of respiratory distress in pre-term babies, the measure of health improvement was the number of babies discharged alive from hospital. As Stevenson has pointed out, the need for a generic measure of health gain that can be used to compare health programmes has generated the concept of quality-adjusted life-years (QALYs). Care in the perinatal period has a very wide range of outcomes. While preventing the deaths of the mother and baby is certainly the underlying aim of care, there is a very low risk of such an outcome in most births. Prevention of morbidity in both mother and baby is also an important aim of care, and many would also aim to allow women to have as good an experience of birth as is possible. The possible longer-term psychological effects of birth on mothers and their family relationships add to the complexity of finding a simple measure of outcome for comparing perinatal interventions. Several approaches to health-status measurement and relative valuation have been put forward, but have not been widely applied in the perinatal field.

The QALY has been used in economic studies of neonatal care, [26] but it does have shortcomings. Firstly, it is not clear whose values should be reflected in the weights used to assess the value of different health outcomes. Secondly, the measure does not include outcomes for more than one individual. Although the mother is often still a recipient of health care when a newborn baby is treated, the interaction between her health and that of the baby is not measured in neonatal quality-of-life measures. It is possible that separation of a sick newborn from a mother who has had a difficult delivery might have long-term repercussions.[27] Even a relatively well mother's ability to breast-feed and her confidence in caring for her child can be influenced by the type of care she receives during pregnancy and labour.[28–30] So far, it does not seem possible to simplify these factors into a single measure of health gain. Therefore the decisions that are made about the appropriate division of resources between low and high-risk perinatal care, for example, or between maternity and other forms of health care, are made intuitively, and are based on partial information, and on different values.

The differences in the values applied to neonatal outcomes become clear when comparisons are made between economic studies of antenatal screening for congenital anomalies and of neonatal intensive care. Studies of antenatal screening often start with the assumption that women would choose to end a pregnancy if the fetus were to be diagnosed to have Down syndrome or a neural tube defect.[31-33] These studies have not been based, as some neonatal studies have been, on actual measurements of parents' or other peoples' valuations of the relative quality of life for them and the baby, of any disabling condition. The different approach taken by economists to the evaluation of prenatal screening and neonatal care reflects two things. First, the economic evaluations of antenatal screening were early examples of health-economic evaluations, done before the concepts of quality-adjusted life-years and cost–utility analysis had filtered into health-economics research. Second, economic evaluations reflect the values local to the context of the study: therapeutic termination of pregnancy is a legal and, for many, an ethical option in England, Wales, and Scotland. In other countries the situation is very different. A recent European workshop on the role of economic evaluation in the diffusion of technologies for antenatal screening considered these issues, and recognized that there needs to be an advance in the measurement of the benefits of screening.[34] The ethics of life-and-death decisions after live birth are far less clear, and therefore most economic studies of neonatal care, with one exception, [26] have not addressed the possibility that in some cases the severe disability of a surviving baby is valued as worse than death by parents.

MEASURING THE COSTS OF PERINATAL CARE

Measurements of outcomes in perinatal care give an incomplete picture, and are some way from providing the simple overall measure of utility or social welfare gain that economists envisage for comparison with other uses of society's resources. The same is true of costs, not least because in economics a cost is a benefit forgone, with all the attendant problems of measurement of benefits.

The principles and methods for cost measurement used in health-economics studies have already been outlined by Stevenson. As he points out, the financial valuation of the resources required varies over time and between countries. In addition, market prices or charges for health care or diagnostic tests are the result of a compromise between supplier and purchaser, and take account of many factors beyond the value of the resource inputs required. Some inputs are not even valued at market prices, and are frequently left out of health-cost studies. For example, in neonatal units, most babies receive a certain amount of care from their parents, and women giving birth in the UK are usually accompanied by a relative or partner. In both cases, this can release staff, even if briefly, from the obligation for one-to-one nursing care. In hospital costing studies of neonatal care, the 'informal' care input is not usually measured, even though, it may add to the resources of the ward and result in loss of earnings. Where such inputs are measured, as is increasingly done in studies of community care, the valuation of the time given voluntarily is debatable. On one hand, the value could be estimated as the cost of buying in the skills provided free. Another approach is to use current average wage levels to estimate the earnings forgone by the informal carer; but because women earn less than men, informal care from women would be given a lower value than that given by men. A further difficulty for economic studies is how to include the value of medical equipment and other items donated by charitable organizations or for promotional purposes by commercial companies, which do not appear in the hospital accounts but which provide service and may require maintenance or monitoring.

In any detailed study of resource inputs, there is a problem of ascribing resource inputs to particular recipients of care. A nurse may give attention to more than one patient at a time or in a short period, and this fact could only be detected in very detailed observation. Patient-care also requires staff to spend time away from the patient, and this cannot easily be observed and ascribed to particular cases. Different approaches to measurement of ward costs can require very different levels of research input, and may also have quite different implications for the cost estimates that result for particular cases.[35, 36] It is perhaps surprising in the light of these issues that there is so much consistency between the estimates that have been made of the relative costs of neonatal care for babies at different birthweights reported in studies from around the world.[37]

Even though there are variations in the methods used for measurement, hospital costs have been the basis for most cost-effectiveness work. Health-care costs outside hospital, and non-health-sector costs are much less frequently measured. This approach parallels the perspective of clinical evaluations of effectiveness, which have tended to be short-term studies of hospital interventions. There is no doubt that such studies are necessary; but they are not sufficient to answer the question about the costs and benefits of the interventions that policy-makers need to ask. There is a problem in adding together estimates for hospital and non-health-sector costs in studies using widely differing methodologies, however. This would for example be the case in studies using a ward-costing approach to hospital inpatient costs, and survey methods to gather data about patients' costs.

It is the basis of neoclassical economic theory that optimal benefits are obtained for society when an additional unit of input to production would provide the same amount of benefit wherever it was applied. This 'marginal' approach puts a different perspective on the relative importance of particular policies for care, and helps to make decisions about the right amount of care to provide. If, for example, it were known that a certain level of funding for a neonatal intensive-care service is currently preventing 100 neonatal deaths annually, the important question for economists is whether the cost of preventing an additional death (or gaining an additional quality-adjusted life-year) is greater or less than would be the case for other health programmes. The calculation is not to find out the average cost per desirable outcome, but the additional cost of increasing the desirable outcome. In the case of screening programmes, the incremental or marginal approach has a striking impact, as was shown in an analysis of costs and benefits of screening for colorectal cancer.[38] Apart from the Canadian neonatal care study, [26] very few perinatal studies have adopted this approach.

DECISIONS ABOUT THE ALLOCATION OF RESOURCES

However much information is available about the costs and effectiveness of different aspects of care, and however completely social and long-term costs and benefits are measured, cost–effectiveness analysis does not make decisions about the best use of resources. That is done by decision-makers with or without access to evidence about costs and effectiveness. Somewhere in the process of decision-making choices are made about what forms of care to provide, how much to provide, and to whom the care will be given.

Stevenson has given reasons why neonatal care has been under the microscope of health economics for longer than most aspects of health care. This is less true of maternity care, and reflects the interests of funding agencies in expensive technologies with dramatic effects. Most maternity care is given to women in good health, and the different effects of alternative types of care on mortality or serious morbidity are difficult to detect unless extremely large trials are set up. Because birth is a frequent event, however, large amounts of health-care resources are used in maternity care. As a result there is the potential for ineffective routine procedures to absorb significant amounts of resources. As much of neonatal care is funded from the same budgets as maternity care in the NHS, the expansion of resources for neonatal care has to some extent been taken from other aspects of maternity care. For example, in the late 1980s the numbers of midwives employed in English neonatal units have increased, but the overall number of midwives has remained more or less constant, while the number of births has increased.[4] Wherever choices have to be made in health care, they are usually presented in terms of the costs and outcomes that have been measured. The dominance of what is known over the unknown could lead to distorted priorities in the provision and use of health resources. The aim of perfect information is obviously impossible, and would probably be more costly than beneficial for health care; but a very low priority is given to the critical use of existing and available data to assess the probable costs and benefits of different policies.

Much of the debate on the ethics of health decision-making centres on the individual doctor–patient relationship. Although individual clinical decisions inevitably affect how resources are used at health-provider level, decisions affecting the amount of resources available for perinatal care are also made at national, regional, and local health-service levels, by managers, public health departments, and lay representatives, few of whom are elected. The responsibility for particular budgets, and division of responsibilities within health care, may influence decisions, as may many apparently extraneous factors.

There has been heated debate about the relative efficiency of different ways of financing health care.[39] Adam Smith spoke of the 'hidden hand' that guided a market towards a solution to competing uses for society's resources.[40] He did not, as is commonly thought, suggest that this process would be ideal, depending as it does on the imperfections of the combined moralities of the traders in the market. The latest reorganization of the National Health Service[41] has introduced explicit elements of market trading, by requiring District Health Authorities and some general practitioners to contract with health providers for their services. Previously, District and Regional Health Authorities were responsible for the whole process of assessing health-care needs and providing services. The change has created concern that the regional organization of services such as neonatal and high-risk obstetric care will not survive, and that competition between providers of care will not lead to a more efficient service. In attempt to answer this criticism, the UK Health Departments have set up a committee on clinical standards to assess the impact of the NHS reorganization on health care for rare conditions, including care of pre-term newborn babies.[42]

The process of health-resource allocation plainly does not follow a model of rational, once-and-for-all decision-making. Knowledge of who is responsible for which resources can help us to understand why apparently irrational and inefficient care persists. For example, although it is clear that giving women prophylactic antibiotics at the time of Caesarean section would be cost-effective, [43] the policy has been slow to catch on in the UK. Many reasons for resistance to change have been put forward, but one may be that although specialists in obstetrics may be seen as the target for this policy, hospital pharmacists and microbiologists must also be part of the decision to change hospital policy about antibiotic use. In the case of giving corticosteroids where pre-term birth is anticipated, the potential resources affected are those under control of paediatricians; however, it is not they, but obstetricians, who are responsible for the intervention.

A well-recognized source of conflict in decision-making is the difference between individual and group interests. Even at the individual level it has been demonstrated that different clinical decisions for the same health problem are taken depending on whether the clinician is given a name for the patient, or merely a scenario with an unnamed patient.[44]

Given the agency relationship between doctor and patient, it would also seem that clinicians act as advocates for the whole group of their patients in competition with other specialties or group practices. Health funders do not see named patients, but must consider overall needs in the population and provide services accordingly. They have to make choices between providing funds for different areas of health care. In setting policies for health spending, there is increasing interest in seeking lay opinion about the priorities for health spending, and the Oregon exercise is given as an example. There are many models of lay involvement in health decision-making, from full democratic representation on health management bodies, to customer-satisfaction surveys, to empowerment and advocacy for patients in contacts with the health services. All of these have been advocated at different times and places as solutions to the failure of the perfect agent-relationship.

CONCLUSIONS

Although, as Stevenson points out, Hippocrates was not a health economist, he did give some advice on financial aspects of a doctor's work:

There should be no discussion of fees during the illness, for that will suggest you will leave the patient if no agreement is reached, or at least neglect to propose immediate treatment. Such a worry will be harmful to the patient, particularly if the disease is acute. It is better to reproach a man whom you have cured than to extort money from a man mortally sick.[45]

Papers on the economics of neonatal care have generated an indignant response from those who feel economists threaten medical freedom. It is not economists who impose this limit, but the nature of the world. Decisions have to be made between alternative treatments for particular patients, about the priority to give to different patients, and about the level of different health services to provide. Economists are the unpopular messengers who point out that the way these decisions are made could affect the overall benefits that could be gained from health care. The problems arise in defining and measuring these benefits, and the resources that produce them. The application of existing definitions and data to health decision-making has fuelled the worry about the ethics of using economic evaluation in priority-setting. It does not seem to me to be impossible that, even when following Hippocrates' advice, an individual clinician who knows what overall resources are available to her, and who knows what is the most effective form of care, will use her skill to greater benefit than one who takes no interest in costs.

REFERENCES

1. Campbell, R. and Macfarlane, A. J. Place of delivery: a review. *British Journal of Obstetrics and Gynaecology*, 1986; 93: 675–83.
2. Macfarlane, A. J. and Mugford, M. An epidemic of caesarean sections? *Journal of Maternal and Child Health*, 1986; 11: 38-42.
3. Macfarlane, A. J. and Mugford, M. *Birth counts: statistics of pregnancy and childbirth.* Vol. II, p. 252. HMSO, London, 1984.
4. Macfarlane, A. J., Johnson, A., and Mugford, M. Epidemiology. In Roberton, N. R. C. (ed.). *Textbook of neonatology*, 2nd edn, pp. 3–27. Churchill Livingstone, Edinburgh 1992:
5. Stilwell, J. A. Relative costs of home and hospital confinement. *British Medical Journal*, 1979; **2**: 257–9.
6. Mugford, M. Economies of scale and low risk maternity care: what is the evidence? *Maternity Action* 1990; **46**: 6–8.
7. Clark, L., Mugford, M., and Paterson, C. How does the mode of delivery affect the cost of maternity care? *British Journal of Obstetrics and Gynaecology*, 1991; **98**: 519–23.
8. Paneth, N., Kiely, J. L., Wallenstein, S., Marcus, M., Pakter, J., and Susser, M. Newborn intensive care and neonatal mortality in low birthweight infants. *New England Journal of Medicine, 1982;* **307**: 149–55.
9. Bakketeig, L. S., Hoffman, H. J., and Sternthal, P. M. Obstetric service and perinatal mortality in Norway. *Acta Obstetrica Gynecologica Scandinavica*, Supplement 77, 1978.
10. Stilwell, J., Szczepura, A., and Mugford, M. Factors affecting the outcome of maternity care. I. Relationship between staffing and perinatal deaths at

the hospital of birth. *Journal of Epidemiology and Community Health*, 1988; **42**: 157–69.

11. Mugford, M., Szczepura, A., Lodwick, A., and Stilwell, J. Factors affecting the outcome of maternity care. II. Neonatal outcomes and resources beyond the hospital of birth. *Journal of Epidemiology and Community Health*, 1988; **42**: 170–6.

12. Eksmyr, R. Early neonatal deaths in geographically defined populations with different operation of medical care. *Acta Paediatrica Scandinavica*, 1985; **74**: 848–54.

13. Forbes, J. F., Larssen, K., and Bakketeig, L. S. Access to intensive neonatal care for low birthweight infants: a population study in Norway. *Paediatric and Perinatal Epidemiology*, 1987; **1**: 33-42.

14. Lane, P., Galway, N., and Alvey, N. *Genstat 5: an introduction. Clarendon Press, Oxford, 1987.*

15. Roper, H., Chiswick, M., and Sims, D. Referrals to a regional neonatal intensive care unit. *Archives of Disease in Childhood*, 1988; **63**: 403–7.

16. Field, D. Survival and place of treatment after premature delivery. *Archives of Disease in Childhood*, 1991; **66**: 410–11.

17. Chalmers, I., Enkin, M., and Keirse, M. J. N. C. (eds). *Effective care in pregnancy and childbirth.* Oxford University Press, 1989.

18. Sinclair, J. C. and Bracken, M. B. *Effective care of the newborn infant.* Oxford University Press, 1992.

19. The Cochrane Centre. NHS Research and Development Programme. The Cochrane Centre, Oxford, 1992.

20. Phibbs, C. S., Williams, R. L., and Phibbs, R. H. Newborn risk factors and costs of neonatal intensive care. *Pediatrics* 1981; **68**: 313–21.

21. Mugford, M., Piercy, J., and Chalmers, I. Cost implications of different approaches to the prevention of respiratory distress syndrome. *Archives of Disease in Childhood*, 1991; **66**: 757–64.

22. Crowley, P., Chalmers, I., and Keirse, M. J. N. C. The effects of cortico-steroid administration before preterm delivery: an overview of the evidence from controlled trials. *British Journal of Obstetrics and Gynaecology*, 1990; **97**: 11–25.

23. Soll, R. F., and McQueen, M. C. Respiratory distress syndrome In Sinclair, J. C. and Bracken, M. B. (eds). *Effective care of the newborn infant,* pp. y 325–58. Oxford University Press, 1992.

24. Donaldson, L. J. Maintaining excellence: the preservation and development of specialised services. *British Medical Journal, 1992;* **305**: 1280–3.

25. OSIRIS Collaborative Group. Early versus delayed neonatal administration of a synthetic surfactant—the judgment of OSIRIS. *Lancet* 1992; **340**: 1363–9.

26. Boyle, M. H., Torrance, G. W., Sinclair, J. C. and Horwood, S. P. Economic evaluation of neonatal intensive care for very low birthweight infants *New England Journal of Medicine*, 1983; **308**: 1330–7.

27. Richards, M. Possible effects of early separation on later development of children—a review. In Brimblecombe, F. S. W., Richards, M. P. M. and (Roberton, N. R. C. *Separation and special Care Baby Units*, Clinics in Developmental Medicine No 68. SIMP, London, 1978.

28. Hodnett, E. D. General social support from carers during pregnancy. In Chalmers, I. (ed.) *Oxford database of perinatal trials*, Version 1. 3, Disk issue 8, November 1992. Record number 4169.

29. Hodnett, E. D. Social support during labour. In Chalmers, I. (ed.) *Oxford database of perinatal trials*, Version 1.3, Disk issue 8, November 1992. Record number 3871.

30. Martin, J. and Monk, J. *Infant feeding 1980, OPCS Social Survey Division Report SS 1144. OPCS, London, 1980.*

31. Hagard, S. and Carter, F. A. Preventing the birth of infants with Down's syndrome: a cost benefit analysis. *British Medical Journal* 1976; **1**: 753–6.

32. Henderson, J. B. An economic appraisal of the benefits of screening for open spina bifida. *Social Science and Medicine* 1982; **16**: 545–60.

33. Hibberd, B. M., Roberts, C. J., Elder, G. H. Evans, K. T., and Laurence, K. M. Can we afford screening for neural tube defects? The South Wales experience. *British Medical Journal* 1985; **290**: 293–5.

34. Mooney, G. *Report of the working group on the review of established technology: prenatal screening.* Health Economics Research Unit, University of Aberdeen, 1992.

35. Walker, A. R. and Whynes, D. K. The costing of nursing care: a study of 65 colorectal cancer patients. *Journal of Advanced Nursing, 1990;* **15**: 1305–9.

36. Jenkins-Clarke, S. *Measuring nursing workload; a cautionary tale.* Centre for Health Economics, University of York, 1992.

37. Mugford, M. A review of the economics of care for sick newborn infants. *Community Med.* 1988; **10**: 99–111.

38. Neuhauser, D. and Lewicki, A. M. What do we gain from the sixth stool guaiac? *New England Journal of Medicine*, 1975; **293**: 226–8.

39. Culyer, A. J. Maynard, A. K., and Posnett, J. W. *Competition in health care. Reforming the NHS.* Macmillan, London, 1990.

40. Smith, A. *An enquiry into the nature and causes of the wealth of nations*, Ed. R. H. Campbell, Skinner, and W. B. Todd. Clarendon Press, New York, 1976.

41. *Parliamentary Acts. National Health Service and Community Care Act 1990.* HMSO, London, 1990.

42. Department of Health. Clinical Standards Advisory Group. *DH Press Release 26 Mar 1991 H91/136.* Department of Health, London, 1991.

43. Mugford, M., Kingston, J., and Chalmers, I. Reducing the incidence of infection after caesarean section: implications of prophylaxis with antibiotics for hospital resources. *Br. Med. J.* 1989; **299**; 1003–6.

44. Redelheimer, D. A. and Tversky, A. Discrepancy between medical decisions for individual patients and for groups. *New England Journal of Medicine* 1990; **322**: 1162–4.

45. Phillips, E. D. *Greek medicine.* Thames and Hudson, 1973.

14

Pediatric nursing ethics

14A NURSING ETHICS IN PERINATAL CARE

Joy Hinson Penticuff

INTRODUCTION

In approaching nursing ethics in perinatal care, it is useful to take a broad view, because many of the factors that bear on nurses' ethical reasoning and actions are influenced by the context of the hospital environments in which they practice and nurses' close interactions with patients. Nursing ethics is an ethics of obligations within practice environments—environments that impose some degree of constraint on nurse autonomy. Within this milieu, nurses, expectant families, pregnant women, infant patients and their parents, the medical team, and administrative personnel are in dynamic interaction.

Nurses' ethical reasoning and action take into account obligations not only to the patient—the pregnant woman or infant—but also obligations to patients' families and obligations as hospital employees and interdependent members of the health-care team. Essentially though, nurses' ethical reasoning and actions are influenced by the degree to which each nurse defines her/himself as someone who is morally accountable for the effect of personal actions and (less directly) team or institutional actions on patients' well-being, regardless of the characteristics of the practice environment. For the nurse who by self-definition is morally accountable, the ethical push and pull of multiple loyalties and institutional constraints sometimes make ethical action seem tantamount to crossing a minefield. But the effects on conscience of not acting can be as devastating as tripping the mine itself.

A number of factors affect the extent to which nurses perceive themselves as moral agents in health care. Individual nurse characteristics—amount of education, number of years in practice, courses in ethics, level of clinical competence, and perceived influence in nurse–physician and nurse–administration interactions—have been found to affect nurses' ethical decision-making. The contribution of moral development to moral action, although extensively researched, remains unclear.[1-3]

It is likely that moral sensitivity and commitment go into moral self-definition, and that these are derived from what one is taught in the way of beliefs and values, and from role models and life experiences. The individual brings to any professional ethical code his or her own view of what we owe others.

Characteristics of the practice environment also play a large role in nurses' ethical reasoning and action. The NICU practice environment will be described in some detail later; but, in both neonatal intensive care and obstetrics, nurses are much more likely to participate actively in preventing or resolving ethical dilemmas when they perceive themselves as having both autonomy and influence within the practice setting. Perceived autonomy and influence are enhanced when nurses' contributions to patient well-being are recognized and valued by physicians and administrators. This is especially true if recognition and valuing translate into nurse–physician collaborative practice and administrative policies that facilitate shared governance.[4, 5]

It may not at first be clear why collaborative practice is relevant to nursing ethics. The reason is that within hospitals nurses occupy two different roles *vis-à-vis* physicians and administrators. They are *independent clinicians* because some patient care is uniquely within the purview of nursing— assessing skin condition or anxiety level, for example. And nurses are *subordinate* to hospital rules that hold them responsible for carrying out the tasks ordered by the patient's physician. Thus nurses who disagree on ethical grounds with medical treatment plans will have difficulty fulfilling what they see as their ethical obligations to patients unless their concerns are taken seriously.

There are many barriers to appropriate nurse–physician collaborative practice. Probably the most important one is the physician's evaluation of the nurse's clinical competence. Part of the confusion about nurse competence is the fact that when you meet a nurse in a hospital hallway, little in the way of labels gives you clues as to this nurse's training or level of experience, and there are widely varying programs of preparation for registered nurses. The nurse you meet may have graduated from a two-year community college with an associate degree, a three-year hospital training program, or a four-year university with a baccalaureate degree. In addition to these basic preparations, the nurse may also have had in-hospital clinician training for expanded practice, or university graduate preparation for advanced practice at the master's or doctoral level. It is no wonder that physicians and families must interact over a period of time with each nurse before trusting the nurse's expertise.

Physicians (and families) are understandably reluctant to accept input if they think nurses' judgments are not relevant to patient benefit. Most nurses are highly competent; but if there is frequent turnover of nurses in a unit, then nurses with less experience in specialized OB or NICU practice will make up an increasing proportion of the total nursing staff, and, with inexperience, mistakes occur. If nursing staff do not demonstrate mastery of the nursing and technical aspects of patient care, it is unlikely that physicians will view them as moral agents, since preventing patient harm is a foundational principle of health-care ethics.

On the other hand, where nurses are not only competent but also are expert, physicians are often pleased to embark on collaborative practice, because they see clearly the benefit to patients that excellent nursing care can produce. Such nurses are respected by physicians because they have demonstrated their ethical commitment to the welfare of patients through diligent efforts, and because their observations and interventions can markedly influence the patient's outcome. These nurses are usually eager to work closely with physicians, and they can have significant positive influence in hospitals that value nursing excellence. It must be noted, though, that nurses who strive for excellence and hold themselves morally accountable for patient benefit are very unlikely to remain in hospitals where their contributions are not recognized or where they are unable to influence what happens to patients.

This discussion of nursing ethics will attempt to provide an account of background as well as situational elements that nurses see as relevant to the ethics of providing nursing care for pregnant women, imperiled newborns, and their families. While nursing ethics and medical ethics are seen as having substantial overlap, nursing ethics is taken as having also areas of unique obligation and values that arise from the distinctive nature of nurse–patient interactions and nursing's institutional roles. Some of the more important elements that I take to be morally relevant in perinatal nurses's ethical decision-making are discussed below.

NURSING PERSPECTIVES ON OBSTETRICAL DILEMMAS

Today the traditional American family—mother, father, and children—might be considered an endangered species. At least two-thirds of families in the United States are either headed by a single adult or are childless. Many expectant families are blended—having children from previous marriages, or the pregnancy is to a woman out of wedlock, or the marriage is a common-law arrangement. Our prevailing stereotype of *the family* is often inaccurate, and may result in flawed assumptions about what families ought to do and what values they ought to have in the face of perinatal crisis. The structure, functioning, and values of patients' families may be different from that of middle-class, work-focused health-care professionals' families. Yet there are universal human experiences—hopes for the unborn infant, anxiety about labor, and fears if the newborn infant is imperiled—that we often can comprehend from the family's perspective if we take the time to ask and to listen to them as they describe their circumstances, values, and purposes.

Characteristics of pregnant women

> ... Some things ... arrive on their own mysterious hour,
> on their own terms and not yours,
> to be seized or relinquished forever
> —Gail Godwin, American writer.

Each woman has become pregnant for reasons that are unique to her own life. She may be joyously pregnant, regrettably pregnant, resentfully pregnant, fearfully pregnant, or some combination of these. Upon first meeting her, nurses do not know whether her pregnancy is intended, supported by mate or family, or—depending on time since conception—whether she plans to abort or carry the fetus to term.

Prevailing societal attitudes about pregnant women are complicated, reflecting our country's division over abortion. Attitudes toward pregnant women are derived from our pluralistic beliefs about the moral status of the fetus, moral obligations of the pregnant woman to the fetus, and the lay public's idealized expectations surrounding pregnancy. The 'hopes and fears of all the years' converge, symbolically, within the womb of each pregnant woman.

When possible, obstetrical nurses seeking employment select hospitals in which the institutional philosophies regarding pregnancy termination and about the extent to which it is taken to be morally justifiable to benefit the fetus through forced treatment are congruent with the nurse's personal values. Many hospitals make their policies explicit in pre-employment interviews so that nurses will not be confronted with the ethical problem of a duty to participate in care that goes strongly counter to the nurse's personal moral views. Thus nurses with strong views against abortion will seek hospitals that do not perform abortions. Sometimes, however, employment choices are limited.

We now turn to discussion of factors that influence nurses' ethical reasoning about the pregnant woman's obligations to the fetus. The general societal view—shared by most perinatal nurses—is that if a woman does not terminate a pregnancy within the first trimester, she has a moral obligation not to endanger the fetus by her actions. Of course, the flaw in this reasoning is that not all women who want to terminate their pregnancies are able to obtain first-trimester abortions, and other women do not view abortion as an option because of their moral values or the moral views or interests of others with whom they have significant relationships.

Attitudes of obstetrical nurses toward a woman who experiences complications of pregnancy—gestational diabetes, for example—are generally that she ought to minimize risk to the fetus by complying with the medical treatment plan, especially if compliance is not unduly burdensome to her and does not threaten her own health. Most nurses believe that a women who is pregnant should refrain from behaviors, such as drug use, promiscuous sexual activity, drinking or smoking, workaholism, or strenuous sports, that might jeopardize fetal well-being.

I think it is accurate to say that the general public and many health-care professionals—perinatal nurses included—have strongly condemning views of the woman whose behaviour endangers the fetus. She is seen as selfish, callous, irresponsible, even slatternly. But this punitive view denies a number of harsh realities about the lives of many women in today's society. What is omitted from the equation is consideration of the adequacy of the woman's sources of emotional and material support and the fact that the male sex partner (not the sperm donor) has moral obligations to the fetus that, one might conclude, are just as binding as those of the pregnant woman. Each has engaged in the same sexual activity; but it is the woman who, literally, bears the consequences.

When obstetrical nurses are confronted with ethical dilemmas, they bring their holistic understanding of pregnant women into their deliberations. They may not articulate their reasoning in the same manner that bioethicists would, but usually they do consider significant general issues: the moral status of the fetus, obligations of the pregnant woman to the fetus, and professional obligations to the pregnant woman, the fetus, and the family. In addition to these somewhat abstract philosophical considerations, obstetrical nurses bring their understanding of the physical, psychological, and sociological aspects of pregnancy. Further, since most obstetrical nurses are women, they have often had personal experiences that may influence their moral reasoning.

Nursing curricula emphasize the comprehensive view of the patient noted above. Nurses assume her to be a member of a family and community, an individual with values and purposes that we are morally obliged to respect, and a person attempting to make the best choices she can. Nursing curricula also typically include study of family dynamics and family pathology, with attention to such topics as family violence, addictions, teen pregnancy, and incest. Thus obstetrical nurses assess not only the blood-sugar levels of the pregnant woman; they are also concerned with her expectations, her level of stress, her understanding of what she faces, her sources of support, and other factors that influence her overall well-being and the well-being of the fetus she carries.

Nurses in obstetrics usually have been exposed to theories of women's psychological adaptation in pregnancy, and will consider as morally relevant factors that can impair the woman's psychological commitment to a pregnancy. In weighing these factors, nurses may reason that some women's moral culpability for fetal endangerment is mitigated because they are not free to choose a different life course.

Ambivalence about being pregnant is normal for women in the first trimester, even if the pregnancy is intended. The patient is concerned about being pregnant, about how her life will change. Bechtel's[6] qualitative study of pregnancy experiences provides the following quotation from a 19-year-old married woman who was pregnant with her second child.

When I first found out I was pregnant I was shocked. It was upsetting in the beginning because I have one at home and we had planned on not having any more children. And when I found out, it was like my heart was taken out. It was real depressing.

In the second trimester, most women feel fetal movement, and the pregnancy by then is usually seen as a reality, for better or worse. The woman begins to ponder what the unborn child will be like. However, if her own well-being is endangered by the pregnancy, or complications threaten the healthy development of the fetus, pregnancy adaptation may be disrupted. Bechtel notes that pregnancy may trigger feelings in some women that their lives are out of control, and that they must somehow take back their lives. One of Bechtel's study participants, a 23-year-old unmarried woman pregnant for the fourth time, said

You know, people around me, my kids ... a lot of things have happened, so it's kind of hard to concentrate on being pregnant when your mind is on other things. I was going through so much that I was doing things, drug wise, that I wasn't supposed to be doing. So I had to get out of that before I couldn't get out anymore. So I decided, well I'm pregnant and I have got to get away from the people I was with and get my life back. Just start trying to do everything right.[7]

When there are pregnancy complications, the woman may continue to be ambivalent because she fears that the hoped-for child will never come to be, or she superstitiously dreads that her wish not to be pregnant has resulted in fetal threat. When the woman endeavors to work for the best pregnancy outcome she can achieve, she becomes occupied with making preparations and a physical space for the child who will soon be born. Women with continuing ambivalence or little material support may not prepare for the infant's birth until very late. In medically normal pregnancies and with a basic level of emotional and material support, most women plan for delivery and make a place for the infant during the third trimester. Premature labor or any other complication of pregnancy disrupts the anticipated trajectory of childbearing, producing revived ambivalence, anxiety, and a sense of vulnerability.

I think that public attitudes and social policy are based on erroneous assumptions about pregnant women. These assumptions are that women are pregnant by choice, and that if they did not wish to become pregnant, they should have forgone sexual activity. Such a view denies the fact that sexual activity may not always be voluntary. Condemnation of women who engage in behaviors that risk fetal well-being is based on the myth that, once pregnant, 'maternal instinct' prompts the woman to adhere to a straight and narrow path, as though pregnancy is discontinuous with the rest of her life. We need to have the insight that pregnancy does not turn the woman into the virtuous—if not virginal—Madonna, mother of a savior. We see the pregnant woman in two polarized ways: virtuous Madonna or slut Madonna. It is intriguing that the popular rock star Madonna, in her artistic presentation of herself, repudiates society's deeply held views of the Madonna as Mother of Christ. She is symbolically the slut Madonna, the antithesis of sacred maternity. What is needed is an understanding of the circumstances of each pregnant woman who comes to us for care. Our moral obligation is to set aside our assumptions and views, to accept her as she is and to attempt to weave together a plan of care that assists her voluntarily to forgo those things that put the fetus at risk.

Even though nurses may believe that, given her life circumstances, the pregnant woman's culpability for fetal harm is limited, this does not mean that interventions that limit her liberty are necessarily thought to be ethically reprehensible. If the pregnant woman is impaired in her pregnancy adaptation by forces beyond her control (for example, incest or addiction), nurses may view paternalistic interventions as morally justifiable. The moral issue often turns on whether the intervention is effective in persuading the patient that limitation of her liberty is ultimately a good *for her* as well as for the fetus. Such interventions affirm our intent to do good for her as an individual deserving of benefit. In weighing how far to go if a pregnant woman refuses to forgo risk behaviours or refuses treatment necessary for fetal health, Obade's[8] summary of morally relevant factors is helpful and seems congruent with the views of many obstetrical nurses: 'Providers should analyze each case in light of fetal age, maternal risk, fetal risk, and the degree of proposed bodily invasion'.

Paternalistic interventions that involve coercion or force are not likely to be considered ethically justifiable by obstetrical nurses. If we forcibly do good for the fetus in spite of the mother's non-consent, we treat the pregnant woman as a means, an instrument that makes babies and has no other important purposes. Nurses may be morally outraged at the harm done to the fetus of a cocaine-addicted woman; but often at some level, being women, they recognize, 'There, but for the grace of God, go I.' Obstetrical nurses want to intervene in ways that prevent fetal harm by addressing factors that disrupt normal psychological adaptation in pregnancy: lack of pregnancy prevention programs, lack of culturally sensitive prenatal care, lack of emotional and material support, lack of access to drug treatment programs, and lack of shared responsibility for the pregnancy.

We turn now to the other side of perinatal nursing, care of the newborn. The moral dilemmas there usually occur when infants are born at the edge of viability or with profound impairments. The ethical question is, to what extent are we justified in applying a life-sustaining technology that is burdensome to the infant and can be ultimately futile in preventing death, or can maintain a life of suffering or one devoid of even the most basic human communication?

Characteristics of infant patients

Moral worthiness of infants

Neonatal nurses typically do not question whether they have moral obligations to prevent harm and to do good for the infant patients in their care. They usually do not debate the philosophical question of whether the newborn infant is a person in the philosophical sense, with rights or claims. They see the infant admitted to neonatal intensive care as worthy of attempts at a chance for a life. The infant is a baby, a member of the human community, a newborn son or daughter within a specific family. On the whole, nurses' views are similar to those expressed by Jecker[9] that the moral status of the infant is not based on intrinsic qualities such as self-consciousness and rationality, but that extrinsic qualities—'standing in an intimate interpersonal relationship, . . . belonging to a family, being a patient, or filling a particular role in a social group suffices to establish personhood'.

Neonatal nurses initially assume that application of life-sustaining technology will sustain a life that the infant will experience as a good. Even though therapies may be invasive and cause pain and disruption of normal comforting interaction, if the ultimate outcome is relatively intact survival, NICU nurses see therapy as morally justifiable. When burdensome therapies seem either futile or likely to sustain lives of profound impairment, nurses begin to question the morality of aggressive treatment. For neonatal nurses, withholding life-prolonging therapies is morally correct if continued life is perceived by nurses and families as not a benefit for the infant. We do not make quality-of-life judgments on the basis of whether the infant has the potential to make societal contributions. Rather, we view the infant as a valued member of the human society whose moral demand on us is that we use medical technology to do good, rather than harm.

Jennings[10] deals with the question of our ethical orientation toward prolonged, aggressive treatment for infants who fall within an ethical 'gray zone' of neonatology—for example, infants of less than 27 weeks' gestation and birthweights less than 750 grams. He states 'most available outcome statistics suggest that aggressive treatment of infants below about 750 grams should receive very strict ethical scrutiny' because of the significant iatrogenic consequences and disabilities that accompany survival following aggressive therapy in this group.

The NICU's mandate to provide emergency life-saving treatment combines with the field of neonatology's research mission to initiate treatment in cases once considered hopeless. With no external limit on referrals or admissions, each unit has the flexibility to experiment without a scientific protocol and without rigorous inquiry into the long-term outcomes of drastic intervention. In those NICUs associated with research-oriented medical centers, drawing the distinction between routine and experimental cases is often difficult. This line can never be rigidly fixed as long as we value advances in neonatal medicine. As Guillemin and Holmstrom[11] note

The storming of the 500 gram barrier to neonatal survival may be an agenda that society and parents accept. However, the option for parents and the public to choose is present only when the experimental nature of the quest is openly communicated. The same is true for the treatment of infants with serious anomalies.

Some infants need to be protected from unduly burdensome, extraordinary medical interventions. Jennings[13] states:

They need to be rescued from the cascade effect that so often marks neonatal intensive care when incremental interventions, each justified if looked at in isolation, pile one upon the other to create a totality that is brutal and grotesque. They need to be rescued from a futile course of repeated painful and debilitating surgeries; rescued from a life prospect of perpetual, interminable patienthood in the NICU, forever dependent on a ventilator or some other life-sustaining apparatus, never to learn, never to speak, never to develop psychologically or socially much beyond the point at which they were when they were first saved.

Jennings also notes the difficulty physicians, nurses, and families have in deciding to withhold or withdraw life-sustaining therapy and allow an infant to die. 'Surrendering goes against the impulse of most parents and against the grain of neonatologists who for years have been trained to *do*, not to stand aside'.

Burden of NICU treatment

Infants in intensive care are subjected to multiple daily invasive procedures. Before the mid-1980s little attention was given to the burden of neonatal therapies. It is now evident that premature infants respond to painful stimuli, and may in fact be more sensitive to painful stimuli than adults.[14]

Butler[15] has argued that the driving concepts of neonatology—the mandate to save infants' lives, the view of the infant as 'an extremely complicated set of mechanical systems that can be affected positively with a combination of drug, surgical, and technological interventions', and the focus on the underdevelopment of the patient—tend to exclude infant pain as a priority (p. 184). She develops this argument by noting that most physicians are so focused on preventing death that pain-control is not a significant concern. She quotes one physician as saying, 'Of all the issues I deal with, whether or not I'm hurting a child is probably the least worry because I don't do anything I don't think is necessary for their survival' (Butler,[16] quoting from Gustaitis and Young 1986, p. 65).

Frank[17], in a national survey of neonatal intensive-care units, found that staff did not adequately assess or manage pain in critically ill infants, particularly those who were intubated and paralyzed. Premedication of the infant for procedures such as arterial puncture, line-placement, and chest-tube insertion was not common practice in the majority of the 76 NICUs surveyed. Agitation was identified as a problem in almost every NICU surveyed, occurring with diverse medical conditions, but most frequent in infants with chronic bronchopulmonary dysplasia. Agitation usually is produced by some combination of air-hunger, pain, discomfort, and overstimulation. Franck also found that of the 21 medications administered to relieve infant pain in the survey, only 11 have true analgesic properties.

The widespread use of muscle paralytics often masks signals the infant may give to indicate pain and discomfort. Medication for pain or sedation is not routinely administered to infants who are paralyzed—often the most critically ill and the most subjected to invasive procedures. Franck[18] notes 'Nurses should be concerned about the lack of analgesia provided to paralyzed infants since sensation remains intact in neonates receiving neuromuscular blocking agents'.

Owens[19] offers an interesting explanation for care-providers' lack of attention to patients' pain. He cites Hoffman's review of studies which indicated that one who witnesses another person in distress experiences an affective response accompanied by physiological changes, and findings that observers who are prevented from going to the aid of a victim often engage in cognitive restructing of the situation to justify inaction. Owens notes that Hoffman's theory of altruism

has two implications for the researcher interested in neonatal pain. First, it suggests the relevance of the adult observer's emotional response to an infant experiencing noxious stimulation ... Second, it suggests an explanation for adults who assume that neonates do not experience pain. Physicians who routinely perform noxious procedures may reduce their own sympathetic distress by a cognitive restructuring expressed as a disbelief in the subjective distress of the infant. Unfortunately, this cognitive restructuring may subsequently result in a disinterest in distress-reducing procedures.

The infant as end or as means

A subtle aspect of the NICU context has to do with valuing the advancement of technology in relation to valuing avoiding infant harm in the NICU, and the seeming inability to further one goal without impeding the other. Breshnahan[20] describes this as valuing of the instrumentalist versus the personalist perspective:

The instrumentalist perspective focuses on the instrument and its development and on the experimental method that has produced it and will make it possible to perfect it further. The patient is certainly not forgotten, but is viewed first in relation to the intensive care instrumentality and to the experimental task. The personalist outlook focuses on the patient's suffering not only due to disease and injury but also due to the medical power focused on this patient. The real possibility of iatrogenic sickness or injury is vividly imagined. The predicament of the patient cannot be slighted from this perspective.

A disturbing account of the potential iatrogenic effects of life-sustaining NICU technology is Perlman and Volpe's[21] description of a previously unrecognized extrapyramidal movement disorder characterized by rapid, random, jerky movements (similar to chorea) and 'restless' movements (similar to akathisia) of the extremities, neck and face, and 'darting' tongue movements in ten infants with severe bronchopulmonary dysplasia. These infants were chronically air-hungry, with recurrent episodes of bronchospasm and marked oxygen desaturation. The investigators suggest that pathogenesis was due to chronic hypoxemia, hyperbilirubinemia, hypercarbia, acidosis, and/or treatment with medications such as theophylline. Three infants died; of the remaining seven, three have no symptoms of the disorder at 15, 18, and 30 months of age, and four infants continue to have the disorder at 21 months of age. These cases demonstrate that for the smallest and sickest patients in the NICU, aggressive therapies are not only highly iatrogenic, they also involve prolonged suffering.

Characteristics of families

Vulnerability and crisis

Parents have intense feelings when birth is a crisis event. Most parents experience a profound sense of loss—the loss of the fantasied perfect infant—and intense anxiety, anger, denial, and depression. Parents face a number of challenges: to understand their infants' condition and prognosis realistically, to plan and carry out appropriate action on the infant's behalf, to handle feelings in an emotionally healthy manner, and to seek and accept offered help[22]. The uncertainty of outcome is one of the most anxiety-producing aspects facing parents. Fleischman[23] notes

The question all parents of low birthweight infants ask is:[1] Will he live or will he die; and which is the better alternative?' Understandable thoughts that the child might be better off dead are frequently felt to be unacceptable. Parents try to push them out of their minds but they continue to intrude ... The ambiguity of outcome, the fear of what the baby's living will mean and the equal fear of the baby's death frequently result in terrible feelings of helplessness and loss of control. In addition, parents have little sense that this baby is really theirs, so completely has its care been handed over to physicians, nurses, technicians and machines.

Deference in decision-making

The initial posture of most parents in the NICU is one of handing over their infant to the care of experts. They rely on the knowledge of physicians and nurses and assume that what is done is best for their infant. Pinch's research found that parents assume a passive role; they are overwhelmed by the technology, the apparent unapproachability of busy professionals, the critical illness of the infant, and their own emotional upheaval. The initial passivity, however, takes a toll, and is often later regretted.[24, 25]

Foreclosure of decision-making prerogative

Robert and Peggy Stinson[26] published a book about the prolonged suffering of their extremely premature infant son, and their own frustration and helplessness as parents who opposed life-prolonging therapy, but were unable to influence treatment decisions.

The sad list of Andrew's afflictions, almost all of which were iatrogenic, reveals how disastrous this hospitalization was ... He was 'saved' by the respirator to endure countless episodes of bradycardia and cyanosis, countless suctioning and tube insertions and blood samplings and blood transfusions; 'saved' to develop retrolental fibroplasia, numerous infections, demineralized and fractured bones, an iatrogenic cleft palate and finally, as his lungs became irreparably diseased, pulmonary artery hypertension and seizures ... We think the question must be raised as to whose interests were really served by this six months of imposed hospitalization. Certainly not Andrew's. He had the misfortune of being declared 'salvageable' (the NICU's word) by people who knew neither how to salvage him nor when or how to stop. Certainly not ours. Those six months were for us a nightmare of anguish, frustration and despair. It seems clear to us that all the benefits in this case went to Pediatric Hospital and its staff. The medical residents got a chance to broaden their education by working with a baby with malfunctions of virtually every system of his body, the specialists took part in some 'interesting consults' and gathered some data and the hospital collected the mind boggling sum of $102 303.20 from the insurance company.[26] [That sum would probably exceed $250 000 today.]

DYNAMICS WITHIN NICU PRACTICE ENVIRONMENTS

Each nurse has ethical obligations that are met or failed within a context of organizational realities. The extent to which a professional role for nurses is valued within the NICU, the influence of nurses in the design of patient-care, representation of a nursing perspective in policy-making and patient-care decisions, all affect nurses' abilities to meet their ethical obligations to infant patients.

The amount and quality of communication between nursing and medical staff in the NICU is significant to nurses' involvement in resolving ethical dilemmas. In fact, where there is a sense of mutual respect, collegiality, and ample discussion of clinical problems on a day-to-day basis, many ethical dilemmas can be prevented. It can, therefore, be problematic when physicians and nurses do not have adequate time to talk about individual patient problems or ongoing concerns.

Nursing influence

Where nursing occupies an influential position within the hospital, and within the NICU, neonatal nurses are more likely to request medication to alleviate infant pain and air-hunger, and changes in the routine of the unit to allow for periods of undisturbed infant rest. Additionally, they frequently request team conferences which include the attending neonatologist for the purpose of reviewing an infant's responses to therapy and questioning whether additional aggressive therapies will be a good for the infant[27, 28].

Staffing patterns, rotations, resources

When nurses from outside agencies supplement the specially trained nurses in neonatal intensive care to provide adequate staffing, or when many of the staff are part-time, consistent communication and cohesive action on behalf of infants and families may be impaired. If residents, medical students, and attending pediatricians rotate frequently, this may disrupt the process by which nursing input can influence medical planning. When staffing is inadequate, nurses must focus on completion of essential safety measures and may be unable to attend to the more emotional/psychological aspects of the infant's response to illness and therapy.[29] Each of these structural aspects of the practice environment can have an important influence on the extent to which nurses are involved in prevention or resolution of ethical dilemmas.

The experience of giving hands-on care

Because of their close, prolonged work with infants, NICU nurses are vulnerable to emotional attachment and feelings of anxiety and loss as they deal with the uncertainty and possible death or profound disability of infants in their care[30]. This attachment may enhance realistic appraisal of the infant's response to therapy, or it may distort appraisal, because the nurse may be unwilling to support a decision to withhold or withdraw aggressive therapies. Parents may feel displaced by their infant's nurses, especially if the parents are inexperienced and the nurses do not encourage their involvement in care and decision-making.

NEONATAL DILEMMAS

Ethical dilemmas in neonatal intensive care often arise because of the power of medical technology to produce double effect: intended good and unintended harm. As Bush[31] notes, 'Technology always raises issues of values, equity, and power and involves historically and culturally situated human beings who decide whether, how, and to what ends they will invent, disseminate, and apply devices and techniques'.

Infants born at 24–30 weeks' gestational age and those with serious anomalies present perinatal caregivers with troubling questions about the ethical use of life-saving technologies. Families and clinicians must decide whether to initiate and how long to continue treatment that can save some lives, and also can inflict harm and suffering on others. A major factor in these dilemmas is the uncertainty of prognosis in life-threatening illness of the newborn, as discussed elsewhere in this text. Some infants will not survive the first year of life, some will experience relatively intact survival, and some will endure agonizing treatment only to survive with profound impairment.

In ambiguous cases, where treatment is burdensome and outcomes are unclear, nurses' conflict over inflicting pain and the inability to provide comfort result in a sense of guilt and frustration. Most nurses acknowledge a duty to alleviate infant suffering, but typically only more experienced nurses are likely to question attending physicians about whether continued life-prolonging treatment is a good for specific infants in their care. Less experienced nurses are likely to talk with other staff nurses or the head nurse. At each level, nurses' ethical practice is facilitated when their concerns are appreciated.

The fact that neonatal intensive care may prolong dying or produce survivors whose lives are filled with suffering has forced parents and care-providers to recognize that the continuation of futile therapy—treatment that prolongs the process of dying but offers no realistic chance of improvement—is not appropriate. Young and Stevenson[32] ask 'Is it possible to develop a more rational view of stopping aggressive therapy once having started?' There is some consensus among bioethicists that, at birth, there is a moral obligation to attempt to save the life of each infant born with a heartbeat. This approach gives the infant a chance to survive. The difficulty with it, however, is that there are no criteria or standards by which to determine when life-prolonging intervention has become death-prolonging intervention.

Ethical dilemmas require us to analyze the morally relevant elements of the situation, and then to weigh the principles, values, rights, and obligations involved. But we weigh them within moral frameworks that lack directions as to hierarchical order[33]. Nurses weigh moral imperatives as carefully and comprehensively as they are able, but seldom are they certain that they have made the morally right decision, and usually they feel lingering doubts. The less certain nurses feel, the more likely they are to experience a sense of ethical anguish[34, 35, 36]. If nurses are faced with multiple cases in which they experience intense uncertainty about what is morally right, or think that they are inflicting harm, their ethical anguish may become so great that they leave nursing practice or abandon their personal sense of ethical integrity[37].

GOOD, HARM, AND QUALITY OF LIFE

Good and harm are defined by most neonatal nurses in terms of the infant's present and future experiences, within the context of the values and prerogatives of the infant's caring family. Nurses recognize that each infant's future flourishing is dependent upon a present that nurtures and protects intact his or her potential for future growth and development. With this general framework in mind, good for infants encompasses: (1) comfort; (2) opportunities for parental affectionate interaction that promotes infant–parent emotional bonding; and (3) protection and nurturance of the infant's future emotional, cognitive, and physical development. Harms, then, are: (1) unpleasant or painful sensory experiences (for example, air-hunger, painful procedures, muscle spasms); (2) deprivation of affectionate interaction and bonding (for example, restriction of parents' access to the infant or constraints to parental holding, soothing, or feeding behaviours; and (3) treatments that iatrogenically damage neurological, motor, or organ systems, and thereby limit the infant's inherent development potential. Most neonatal nurses believe that parents should have considerable discretion in judging whether treatment for their infant constitutes good or harm within this general framework of an infant-centered perspective.

Nursing values

One of the most important reflections of neonatal nurses' values is their acknowledgement of parental prerogatives in NICU ethical decision-making.

Unless parents are unable to comprehend the infant's condition and prognosis, or unable to put the best interest of the infant above competing interests,
or unable to agree on a course of action, most nurses feel that parents should
have substantial input in decisions about infant treatment. There are certain
cases— specifically, when life-prolonging aggressive therapies are judged by
experts as likely to produce questionable ultimate benefit, as is typically the
situation for infants with birthweights of less than 1000 grams or those with
severe anomalies—in which families' values should be the most important
factor in decisions about life-sustaining treatment.

On the other hand, if therapies do not subject the infant to suffering over
a prolonged time-period, and treatment is very likely to result in intact or
nearly intact survival (for example, a 72-hour course of ventilation for a
34-weeks' gestation infant with respiratory distress syndrome), decisions to
apply aggressive therapies are usually morally justifiable, even over parental
objections. In such cases, nurses and physicians are seen as morally obliged to
do all that they can to persuade the parents that treatment is clearly in their
infant's best interest, and to avoid coercive actions that have the potential of
creating an enduring resentment of health-care authorities and a barrier to
development of parent–infant attachment.

Related to the value of parental prerogative is the consideration given to
quality-of-life judgments in ethical decisions. The infant's present and future
quality of life are usually important to nurses, and they are often sympathetic
to the idea that caring families are rightfully the infant's surrogate in making
these judgments. Benner[38] suggested, 'Quality of life can be approached from
the perspective of quality of being, and does not need to be approached merely
from the perspective of doing and achieving'. The notion of quality of life
incorporated in the best-interest standard does not mean social worth, but
only the value that the life has for the infant.

The work of Oleson[39] is relevant to nurses' understanding of their own
and parents' judgments about infants' quality of life. To understand parents'
definitions of their infant's present and future quality of life, we must identify
the attributes that parents perceive as being critical to their judgment.
Parents' subjective quality-of-life judgment is determined primarily by their
perception of the infant's level of satisfaction and/or happiness relative to the
various life domains of importance to infants and children. Level of happiness
reflects the extent to which positive feelings outweigh negative feelings. Thus,
when therapies in the NICU are perceived by nurses or parents as being
burdensome to the infant, this factor is weighed in relation to possible
ultimate benefit. When infants are thought to be suffering, the potential
benefit of therapy should be of large magnitude to justify the continuation
of burdensome therapy.

Ferrans and Powers[40] categorized the major quality-of-life domains identified in an extensive literature review as follows: health and functioning,
socioeconomic factors, psychological/spiritual factors, and family. Families
and nurses evaluate the infant's current level of comfort or distress and
the infant's potentialities in each of the areas identified above. Ultimately,

quality-of-life judgments reflect parents' and nurses' values, and quality-of-life considerations then weakly or potentialy influence decisions to withhold or withdraw aggressive therapy in the NICU.

As presented in Oleson's model, a positively perceived quality of life is necessary to free the individual (in this case, the infant) to expand available resources for personal growth. Gillingham[41] referred to the consequence of a positively perceived quality of life as the opportunity for creative fulfillment by choosing one's own path through life and developing it fully. We in health care may find that understanding the values on which parents make quality-of-life judgments about their infants and our scrutiny of the bases for our own judgments may be important if we are to work in concert with parents in decisions about aggressive treatment.

NURSING AND INSTITUTIONAL CONSEQUENCES OF IGNORING ETHICAL DILEMMAS

When the actions of health-care personnel result in consequences for patients that nurses view as harmful, and nurses are unable to influence resolutions for these problems, they are at risk of becoming overwhelmed with frustration and ethical anguish. Prolonged frustration and ethical anguish are significantly related to burnout—physical, emotional, and attitudinal exhaustion associated with workers' loss of concern and emotional feelings for the people they are helping. Burnout occurs when the nurse's best efforts are ineffective in achieving valued goals. One nurse put it this way

We're not getting anything we value accomplished; we're just spinning our wheels. We become more and more frustrated, then we do become burned out. And it's really a shame if you become burned out and yet you can't leave that situation. You can actually turn into something like a zombie.

Some of the institutional consequences of ignoring nurses' ethical dilemmas are erosion of staff performance, burnout, and high staff turnover[43]. Each of these consequences is expensive for institutions in terms of legal risk, training costs, and patient jeopardy. If nurses' perspectives in ethical dilemmas are not heard, their loyalty to the institution erodes and they begin to wonder whether their effort is justifiable. Another consequence can be distorted communication, because when nurses consistently have frustrating or confrontational interactions with physicians or administrators they may lose their motivation to voice ethical concerns.

NURSING PERSPECTIVES ON NEONATAL DILEMMAS

Philosophy of care

A shared philosophy of care that articulates the purposes of nursing specific to each NICU is an important foundation for nurses' ethical decision-making.

Within the culture of each unit, such a philosophy often evolves when nursing staff do not experience high rates of turnover or part-time personnel, and nurses, families, and physicians work collaboratively to agree on what is good for infants. The extent of pain-relief; evaluation of the burdens and benefits of therapies; the influence of quality-of-life judgments as well medical indicators; the amount of uncertainty that is allowed in treatment decisions; and the degree of acceptance of parental prerogative in NICU decision-making are all derived from the unique philosophy of care of each NICU.

An ethic of the good

Jennings[44] proposes an ethic of the good for neonatal dilemmas that seems congruent with the perspective of many neonatal nurses. Such an ethic promotes the infant's human flourishing, and takes into account

... such factors as the relief of suffering, the preservation or restoration of functioning, and the quality as well as the extent of life sustained. An accurate assessment will encompass consideration of the satisfaction of present desires, the opportunities for future satisfactions, and the possibility of developing or regaining the capacity for self-determination. We need a more nuanced and flexible understanding of what it means to promote the infant's good in the context of its future family life and in terms of its potential for development and self-realization. We have to think in terms of what the good life for this particular baby might be ... recognizing that in some cases the infant's good is best served not through aggressive rescue ... even if that means a foreshortened life.

Family histories and values

Most nurses concur with Duff's[45] view that the infant's caring family provides the most practical religious, humanitarian, and philosophical values needed to deal with the complex decisions that are necessary in the NICU, and that only if the family goes too far towards sacrificing their infant's interests and seeking their own should their decision-making prerogative be overridden. In acknowledging the complexity of these decisions, he notes 'Of course, what is "too far" is a very difficult assessment to make'. Stinson and Stinson also state, 'We believe there is a moral and ethical problem of the most fundamental sort involved in a system which allows complicated decisions of this nature [whether or not to resuscitate the Stinsons' infant son] to be made unilaterally by people who do not have to live with the consequences of their decisions'.[46]

Moral prerogative of parental decision-makers

The family is the source of the basic sustenance and nurturance of its children, and it is through the intimate interactions within the family that

422   JOY HINSON PENTICUFF

society's most deeply held beliefs and values are transmitted. Legal tradition recognizes the rights and obligations of parents to control their children's health and medical care.

Limits to parental prerogative

When therapies are not clearly beneficial, parental decisions should be followed unless it can be convincingly shown that parents do not meet the three criteria below. Parents must be able (a) to put the welfare of the child ahead of their own and others' welfare; (b) to comprehend the essential facts of their child's condition and prognosis; and (c) to make rational decisions about how burdensome and how useful medical treatments will be for their child.[47, 48]

ORGANIZATIONAL ETHICS RESOURCES

Nursing representation on hospital ethics committees

In the United States, large hospitals have ethics committees, and usually there is nurse representation. The nurse representatives are in an important position to articulate a nursing perspective on ethical dilemmas, and should be influential, well respected, and willing to assert a nursing viewpoint. They should go into the clinical areas and talk with the nurses involved in problem cases, find out what the nursing perspective is, and represent it at the meetings of the ethics committee. It is often appropriate for two or three of the key nurses involved in the infant's care also to come to the ethics committee meeting, to talk about their specific nursing perspectives on the case. Nursing representation on the Hospital Ethics Committee is an important organizational factor in whether resolution processes include rather than exclude nursing.

Nursing ethics council

Some hospitals have instituted a Nursing Ethics Council to develop ethics expertise among nursing staff. It is usually open to any nurse interested in ethical issues, is chaired by a nurse, and meets regularly to discuss cases and elements of ethical reasoning and action. Speakers with bioethics expertise are often invited to present ethics theory and analyze cases. Through the Council, as issues arise, they can be dealt with, and nurses can continually improve their understanding of how to recognize and be involved in resolving dilemmas.

Nurses who attend the Council meetings usually become known as in-unit resource persons to whom other staff can go for informal consultation about dilemmas. In this way, the Council provides staff nurses with peers in their units who can help them in their decision-making about ethics concerns. An essential part of the success of the Council is the relationship between the chairperson of the Nursing Ethics Council and the chairperson of the Hospital Infant Ethics Committee. These two people need to have an excellent collegial relationship. Their cooperative work can mean that when team members have a concern involving a patient's medical treatment plan, the two chairpersons can discuss the case and decide on the strategy most likely to resolve the problem in a way that enhances rather than disrupts team relationships. Very often unit dilemmas can be resolved without resorting to outside intervention when nurses and physicians each respect the other discipline's perspectives and have the goal of joint responsibility for decisions.

Finally, if a dilemma cannot be resolved within the unit, then, with the consultation and support of the Nursing Ethics Council, the nurses involved can feel more comfortable in going to the Hospital Infant Ethics Committee to request formal consultation for the case.

Ethics rounds

In hospitals that hold ethics rounds, it is important that nursing staff should be included in case discussions so that bioethical deliberations can take into consideration the data that nurses may have regarding the patient's response to therapy, family concerns that may not have been communicated to physicians, and nursing values and perspectives. Typically, nurses are not invited to attend ethics rounds, and they often mistakenly conclude that they have no role in ethical discussions and actions.

CONCLUSIONS

Perinatal nursing ethics focus on the good or harm done in health care to the pregnant woman, the fetus, the newborn, and the family. Ethical obligations in perinatal care are among the most complex of all health-care dilemmas. The explosion of reproductive technologies; the fact that fetal therapies necessarily affect the pregnant woman; the philosophical uncertainty of the moral status of the fetus and thus our obligations to it; the sometimes brutally traumatic iatrogenic consequences of neonatal intensive care and its frequent double effect; and issues of when the pregnant woman's autonomy or parents' autonomy should be respected in fetal or neonatal treatment decisions—all contribute to ethical quandaries in perinatal nursing.

I propose that nursing ethics in perinatal care should emphasize two heuristics for reasoning and action in ethical dilemmas. The first is our recognition that persons are whole beings, not merely organ systems whose physiological functioning we seek to alter. The second is acknowledgement of our moral obligation to attempt to understand the values, circumstances, and life goals of the pregnant women and families who come to us for care,

424   JOY HINSON PENTICUFF

and to use that understanding to provide care that is truly a benefit and not a harm.

REFERENCES

1. Crisham, P. Measuring moral judgment in nursing dilemmas. *Nursing Research* **30**, No. 2, (1981), p. 104–10.
2. Ketefian, S. *Moral reasoning and ethical practice in nursing: an integrative review.* New York: National League for Nursing Publication #15-2250, (1988).
3. Ketefian S. Critical thinking, educational preparation, and development of moral judgement among selected groups of practicing nurses. *Nursing Research,* **30**, No.2 (1981), p 99–103.
4. Penticuff, J. H. Principal Investigator. Nurses' ethical decisionmaking in perinatal settings. Research funded by the National Center for Nursing Research, NIH (1990).
5. Kramer, M. The Magnet Hospitals: excellence revisited. *Journal of Nursing Administration,* **20**, No. 9 (1990), p 35–44.
6. Bechtel, D. A. *The experience of prenatal care in women of childbearing age: an interpretive interactionist approach.* Unpublished dissertation, The University of Texas at Austin School of Nursing, (1993), p 48.
7. Bechtel, D. A. *The experience of prenatal care in women of childbearing age: an interpretive interactionist approach.* Unpublished dissertation, The University of Texas at Austin School of Nursing, (1993), p 65–6.
8. Obade, C. C. Compelling treatment of the mother to protect the fetus: the limits of personal privacy and paternalism. *The Journal of Clinical Ethics.* **1**, No. 1, (1990), p 87.
9. Jecker, N. S. Commentary: the moral status of patients who are not strict persons. *The Journal of Clinical Ethics.* **1**, No. 1, (1990), p 35.
10. Jennings, B. Beyond the rights of the newborn. *Raritan* **7**, No. 3, (1988), p 84.
11. Guillemin, J. H. and Holmstrom, L. L. *Mixed blessings: intensive care for newborns.* Oxford University Press,: New York (1986).
12. Jennings, B. Beyond the rights of the newborn, *Raritan* **7**, No. 3, (1988), p 85.
13. Jennings, B. Beyond the rights of the newborn. *Raritan,* **7**, No. 3, (1988), p 86.
14. Fitzgerald, M. The developmental neurobiology of pain. In Bond, M. R., Charlton, J. E., and C. J. Woolf (eds.) *Proceedings of the Sixth World Congress on Pain.* Elsevier, New York, NY (1991).
15. Butler, N. C. Infants, pain and what health care professionals should want to know now—an issue of epistemology and ethics'.' *Bioethics* **3**, No. 3, (1989), p 184.
16. Butler, N. C. Infants, pain and what health care professionals should want to know now—an issue of epistemology and ethics. *Bioethics* **3**, No. 3, (1989), p 181–99.

17. Franck, L. S. A national survey of the assessment and treatment of pain and agitation in the neonatal intensive care unit. *JOGN Nursing*, **16**, No. 6, (1987), p. 387–93.

18. Franck, L. S. The influence of sociopolitical, scientific, and technologic forces on the study and treatment of neonatal pain. *Advances in Nursing Science* **15**, No. 1, (1992), p. 11–20.

19. Owens, M. E. Pain in infancy: conceptual and methodological issues. *Pain*, **20**, (1984), p. 222.

20. Breshnahan J. F. Suffering and dying under intensive care: ethical disputes before the courts. *Critical Care Nursing Quarterly* **10**, (1987), p. 13F.

21. Perlman, J. M. and Volpe, J. J. Movement disorder of premature infants with severe bronchopulmonary dysplasia: a new syndrome. *Pediatrics* **84**, No. 2, (1989), p. 215–18.

22. Caplan, G. Patterns of parental response to the crisis of premature birth. *Psychiatry*, **23**, (1960), p. 365–74.

23. Fleischman, A. R. The immediate impact of the birth of a low birth weight infant on the family. *Zero to Three: Bulletin of the National Center for Clinical Infant Studies.* **6**, No. 4, April, (1986), p. 1–5.

24. Pinch, W. J. Ethical decision making for high-risk infants: the parents' perspective. *Nursing Clinics of North America* **24**, No. 4, (1989), pp. 1017–23.

25. Pinch, W. J. and Spielman, M. L. The parents' perspective: ethical decision making in neonatal intensive care. *Journal of Advanced Nursing* **15**, (1990), p. 712–19.

26. Stinson R. and Stinson P. On the death of a baby. *Journal of Medical Ethics*, **7**, (1981), p. 5–6.

27. Penticuff, J. H. Principal Investigator. Reactions of care providers to federal guidelines on care of handicapped newborn infants after the case of Baby Doe. Research conducted as Visiting Scholar, The Hastings Center: Institute for Ethics, Society and the Life Sciences, Hastings-on-Hudson, New York, (1983).

28. Penticuff, J. H. Principal Investigator. Nurses' ethical decisionmaking in perinatal settings. Research funded by the National Center for Nursing Research, NIH, (1990).

29. Hinshaw, A. S. and Atwood, J. R. Nursing staff turnover, stress, and satisfaction: models, measures, and management. In Werley, H. H. and Fitzpatrick, J. J. (eds.) *Annual Review of Nursing Research Vol. 1*, Springer Publishing Co., New York, (1983).

30. Savage, T. and Conrad, B. Vulnerability as a consequence of the neonatal nurse–infant relationship. *Journal of Perinatal Neonatal Nursing*, **6**, No. 3, (1992), pp. 64–75.

31. Bush, C. G. Women and the assessment of technology: to think, to be; to unthink, to free. In Rothschild, J. (ed.) *Machina ex dea: feminist perspectives on technology.* Pergamon Press, New York (1983), pp. 151–70.

32. Young, E. W. D. and Stevenson, D. K. Limiting treatment for extremely premature, low-birth-weight infants (500 to 750 g). *American Journal of Diseases of Children*, **144**, (1990), pp. 549–52.

33. Clouser, K. D. and Gert, B. A critique of principlism. *The Journal of Medicine and Philosophy.* **15**, No. 2, (1990), p. 219–36.

426   JOY HINSON PENTICUFF

34. American Hospital Association. Moral distress in nursing, *Hospital Ethics* **3(4)**, (1987), pp. 1–4.
35. Cameron, M. The moral and ethical component of nurse burn-out, *Critical Care Management Edition* **17(4)**, (1986), pp. 42B–E.
36. Wilkinson, J. M. Moral distress in nursing practice: experience and effect, *Nursing Forum* **23(1)**, (1986), pp. 16–29.
37. Mitchell, C. New directions in nursing ethics. *Massachusetts Nurse* **50**, No. 7, (1981), pp. 7–10.
38. Benner, P. Quality of life: a phenomenological perspective on explanation, prediction, and understanding in nursing science. *Advances in Nursing Science.* **8**, No. 1, (1985), p. 5.
39. Oleson, M. Subjectively perceived quality of life. *Image: Journal of Nursing Scholarship*, **22**, No. 3, (1990), pp. 187–90.
40. Ferrans, C. E. and Powers, M. J. Quality of life index: developmental and psychometric properties. *Advances in Nursing Science*, **8**, (1985), pp. 15–24.
41. Gillingham, F. J. The quality of life. *Australian and New Zealand Journal of Surgery*, **52**, (1982, October), pp. 453–60.
42. Wilkinson, J. M. Moral distress in nursing practice: experience and effect, *Nursing Forum* **23(1)**, (1986), pp. 16–29.
43. Hinshaw, A. S. and Atwood, J. R. Nursing staff turnover, stress, and satisfaction: models, measures, and management. In Werley, H. H. and Fitzpatrick, J. J. (eds.) *Annual Review of Nursing Research Vol. 1*, Springer Publishing Co., New York (1983).
44. Jennings, B. Beyond the rights of the newborn. *Raritan*, **7**, No. 3, (1988), pp. 91–2.
45. Duff, R. S. Counseling families and deciding care of severely defective children: a way of coping with medical Vietnam. *Pediatrics*, **67**, No. 3, (1981), pp. 318.
46. Stinson, R. and Stinson, P. On the death of a baby. *Journal of Medical Ethics* **7**, (1981), p. 8.
47. Veatch, R. M. Limits of guardian treatment refusal: a reasonableness standard. *American Journal of Law and Medicine* **9**, No. 4, (1984), pp. 427–68.
48. Penticuff, J. H. Neonatal intensive care: parental prerogatives. *Journal of Perinatal and Neonatal Nursing*, **1**, No. 3, (1988), pp. 77–86.

14B PAEDIATRIC NURSING ETHICS

Andrew L. Jameton

Not for the good that it will do
But that nothing may be left undone
On the margin of the impossible.
—Agatha, in *The Family Reunion*, by T. S. Eliot

INTRODUCTION

Penticuff outlines very well some of the main perinatal ethical concerns to which nurses attend. In so doing, she has made important observations about nurses' roles and their perceptions of perinatal issues. She makes it clear that nurses tend to be intensely involved in the ethical issues of pregnancy, birth, and neonatal care. She observes that nurses normally accept all infants as persons and do not distinguish, as some philosophers have, between infants who are persons and infants who are not. Nurses tend to make moral judgments about parents, especially mothers; to emphasize communication with parents; and to involve them in conversation and decisions about infant care. In the NICU, nurses tend to be strongly aware of the suffering of and burdens on infants; they are intensely involved in providing infant care and responsible for it.

I am going to focus my comments on issues that arise for nurses in NICUs, and set aside issues surrounding pregnancy and birth. I will comment occasionally on Penticuff's discussion, but this will not be my main purpose. Nor will I attempt to represent a nursing perspective, partly because I am not a nurse, and partly because I believe that many nurses would disagree with what I have to say in this essay. Nevertheless, much of my discussion arises from talking with nurses and attending to their concerns in NICUs. Also, I will be discussing the roles of nurses in NICUs as one major theme.

Penticuff's discussion focuses largely on what nurses see as being needed in ethical perinatal care. Her discussion thus has a normative tone in contrast to a descriptive one. My belief is that if one were to attempt a description of NICUs in relationship to the ethical concerns of nurses that Penticuff discusses and which I outline briefly above, one would find that NICUs tend to engage in practices far from satisfying to a nursing ethical perspective. This is at least my impression from my limited work observing in NICUs and consulting on ethical issues in these units; this is also my impression derived from reading a variety of studies of NICU life and decision-making.[1–4]

In my commentary below, I outline a perspective on NICUs as a way of using social resources to save lives; I then discuss nursing roles in NICUs in a little more detail; and in so doing, I draw a few connections between the perspective and the nursing roles.

MYTHICAL ELEMENTS IN NICU ETHICAL DECISION-MAKING

I think that one of the most interesting areas of ethical questioning arises from tensions between overall judgments concerning large enterprises and day-to-day judgments regarding work on smaller tasks within large enterprises. These sorts of tensions arise when a worker is daily doing good and dedicated service, but the overall meaning and value of the larger enterprise can be questioned. Such tensions might arise for a soldier fighting in a dubious battle, a waitress working in a restaurant that serves unhealthy food, or a citizen paying taxes for unjust government activities. Moral questions about our responsibility for participation in such larger enterprises arise endemically for people of good will. When professionals encounter elements of these larger questions in their daily work, these elements may pose questions about specific acts, but may also pose larger questions about an enterprise as a whole.

In order to discuss ethical aspects of NICU nursing work, it is thus important to set it in the larger context of moral questions about the nature of the NICU as an enterprise as a whole. This will help us better to appreciate the nature of ethical questions that nurses and others face, and to make explicit the conflict of respecting the moral genuineness of the work of individuals working in NICUs while at the same time experiencing a sense of strangeness, irrationality, and illusoriness about the NICU as a social enterprise and a commitment of resources.

To set the context, I want to make compelling for the reader the feeling I have that the NICU is something of an illusion—a ritual hallucination of the most respectable sort, but nevertheless surely a brief historical aberration and surely not an institution that will endure the ages, much less the next half-century. I will not attempt to argue the position thoroughly, largely because I am not myself convinced that the perspective is a valid one; but since it has some power for me and others, I will at least strive to make it vivid.

Questioning the rationality of NICUs

The NICU is usually presented as a rational enterprise: it saves lives; it prevents long-term handicaps; it serves the needs of parents and children; it reduces infant mortality rates; and it applies amply the techniques and equipment of the most advanced medical sciences. Through objective observation and experiments it also continues to improve its work, to increase the range of infants it can help, to stabilize the process of care, and gradually to improve outcomes.

But this is not the only way to see it; there are elements of illusion that halo these truths. We need to look beyond the concrete day-to-day services of the NICU to the symbolic meanings of its activities, meanings which foster our extensive cultural investment in it.

As an institution, as an image, the NICU seems to say to us: 'Every baby will live; everyone will live because science will learn to save all babies, and science is the key to the survival of all of us.' But, the truth is that many babies die around the world—indeed, more babies die around the world than ever before, and many more will die. Even though babies die, people and families survive and continue to have babies—indeed, people survive and increase their population without much help from medicine and science.

Moreover, health care makes only a minor contribution to public health. Despite maintaining the most expensive medical care system the US, for instance, has high infant mortality rates and other poor public-health statistics as compared to other first-world nations.[5] NICUs do little to improve the basic health of mothers and their infants. NICUs thus save a few lives with extravagant use of resources and attention while, as a culture, we do not show much respect for life in other major respects, not in our own nation, and certainly not in the world at large.

This is of course not the direct fault of NICUs or the people who work in them. People who work in NICUs generally would like to see public health improved; if nothing else, sound public-health policies would create less egregious work for them. But NICUs are part of a larger public economic and health strategy that uses its resources for the extravagant benefit of a few without much attention to the many in the background. And, in so doing, NICUs symbolize and make concrete national cultural values concerning life and infancy. NICUs seem to say that what counts is saving *this* baby. What matters is whether *this* baby lives. But, the truth is that it does not matter that much that this baby lives. Statistical survival is the key to survival; not individual survival. In fact, everyone dies, but humanity continues to survive. Indeed, statistical survival is key to our investment in the NICU. NICUs survive as enterprises despite the deaths of many individual infants in them, in part, because they so fully express the fundamental commitment of our culture to the individual.

In struggling so hard to save individual babies, we invest heavily in a philosophy of individualism that emphasizes individual birth and death, not the survival of the community or society. But new babies are, of all age-groups, the least individualized, the least invested with personality, individuality, and interests.

To express our striving for individual survival, we invest extravagant resources in NICU rescue work. These resources involve more than money; they include skilled labor and education, time, transportation, disposables, paper, electricity, metal, plastic, intricate equipment, complex chemicals, and so on. In so doing, the NICU fosters an illusion that resources are not scarce; the NICU lives as if there were no budget, no global population and resource conflict, and no end of our ability to extend the use of these means to save all infants victimized by poor public health, unfortunate genetics, and the accidents of fate. The truth is that there must increasingly be a sense of concrete resource limitations—not just fiscal limitations—in using resources to save individual lives. Indeed, while we use science to build a consumer-based society that destroys natural resources on a global scale, the NICU seems to say that, in the future, we will have more resources to spend on more units to save more babies; when in fact, humanity faces an urgent need to use science to reduce resource-use and to improve public health during another doubling of the human population expected in the next fifty years.[6-8] In short, the irony is that, while the products of science are being used to destroy humanity and the natural world, the NICU says that science will save us if we simply focus it on a few individuals.

Indeed, by saving so few babies at such great expense while so many babies die, the NICU represents an 'island' mentality, suggesting that economic development improving the lives of a few people while neglecting a vast peripheral population is a sound strategy of coping with the global crisis of resources and population. But no enterprise can be long isolated from the natural processes of the earth as a whole: a nurse who checks a baby's oximeter has driven to work in a car that releases carbon dioxide to the detriment of future generations of babies. The fracture of attention between babies in the unit and discharged babies that go to homes with inadequate resources for their care also illustrates an island mentality. The NICU clinician consistently shuts out consideration of the parent's perspective and problems of long-term outcome for patients (Guillemin and Holmstrom 1986, p. 43).[1]

The NICU must be a temporary historical phenomenon. Looking ahead fifty years to a world of a doubled population and even more greatly stressed world resources, it is incredible to think that we will continue to invest social resources in such an extravagant and unbalanced way; and, if we do, we may well be charged by the next generations with inhumanity for our devotion.

The clinician of today may take comfort in what is before him or her: 'There are infants who wouldn't be alive now if we hadn't started this unit' (Guillemin and Holmstrom 1986, p. 25).[1] But future generations may instead count the lives that were not saved because our culture neglected the larger picture of life and death, and count those good-hearted souls who have worked so hard to build the NICU enterprise as complicit in this shocking failure. Moreover, those saving lives in NICUs believe that their life-saving work is independent of the larger loss of life in the background. They thus feel that their life-saving at least rescues a few infants from death without harm to other infants. But wealth and extravagant resource use do not exist independent of poverty; they cause poverty by appropriating concrete resources that could be used elsewhere.[9] The hands of those saving lives are thus not quite clean; they work as part of a pattern of wealth that deprives people around the world of life and health.

NICUs are also places of unique values and ethical perspectives. In few other places do we strive so hard to save lives; we see no similar focused and extravagant social investment to reducing the homicide rate among children, to cleaning up neighborhoods, to seeing that families have educations, housing, jobs, and healthy diets. Indeed, the dedication to life-saving in such units is so strong that parents joke of trying to have their infants in the wilds of Canada, so that, if there were a problem, there would be no danger of being forced by law and seduced by medicine or driven by parental passion into sending one's baby to such a unit for rescue.

Penticuff rightly notes that nurses in NICUs are concerned for the pain and discomfort of infants, while many physicians deny that these infants feel pain and fail to use anesthetics. NICUs thus deny that there is pain and suffering, when in fact there is (see, for example, Perri Klass's vivid description of causing pain in 'Hurting babies'[10]). Nor do NICUs prevent the long-term pain and suffering of the infants who otherwise would have died, that are saved, with a heavy burden of chronic health problems. And the concerns of parents for their own welfare, the welfare of their other children, and the welfare of others' children are often dismissed under cloak of an ethos of exclusive devotion to the interests of the infant patient. Such negative consequences are often not looked at closely, and so long-term pain and suffering are denied by NICUs. Thus, even with all the cost expended, less is gained than is often believed.

The mythical foundations of NICUs

If the NICU is not a rational enterprise, but only seems to be, and we invest so much in it, why then does it have such a strong appearance of rationality? I want to suggest that it acts out deep and ancient mythical motifs about birth and life. When consulting in the NICU, I happened to read part of Sir James George Frazer's classic and questionable history of ideas, The golden bough.[11] Something in Frazer's account of the myth of the unsleeping priest and murderer who guards the sacred grove of Diana at Nemi seemed compellingly to suggest the atmosphere of the work of the NICU physician. Like the priest, eternal wakefulness is the fate of the NICU physician. Like other physicians, neonatologists regard the sixty-hour week as a normal minimum, are constantly on call, and follow their patients closely. The residents have 'no break in their work schedules to allow formal reflection on either their feelings or ethics' (Guillemin and Holmstrom 1986, p. 42).[1] The Frazer myth that the priest must ward off being murdered by his would-be successor conjures up the physician as fighting against death in the NICU and the commonly conflictual nature of relations among physicians. And, by ritualizing the caring role of the mother and protecting the lives of infants in the unit, the nurses seem to suggest the myth of Egeria, the goddess of easy birth related to the goddess Diana (Guillemin and Holmstrom 1986, p. 135).[1] The Golden Bough itself, which the challenger must seize, represents the next scientific discovery to be wielded magically in the name of life.

Parents, in this mythological picture, become the hesitant human visitors to fairyland. They venture in to the unit to bring back their baby, stolen by the fairies. They must tread carefully and follow strange rules only vaguely grasped by them. They feel as though, should they step off the path, they may be punished, or may never get their baby back. Alluding to the Christian images, they often speak of their infant as 'our miracle baby'.

When we perceive the NICU as expressing mythical themes to which we respond deeply, we recognize that we do not save these lives for the sake of the babies. The babies are more like fetishes or amulets. Like holding an amulet in one's hand to keep one safe from dangers and the unknown, we hold babies in the hands of science in the belief that these rituals will keep our culture safe from starvation, poverty, and misery. The baby is thus an amulet of life and wealth in the face of vast changes on a global scale that may well overwhelm our culture; the NICU is like the Indian Ghost Dance—a ritual of obeisance to the old gods on the threshold of a future that is dangerous, frightening, and inevitable. Babies, by symbolizing illusory hopes for life and the future, thus become the objects of extreme devotion in a vast, magical process of social homeopathy.

THE NURSES' SITUATION

I doubt that more than a few nurses (maybe, two) see the NICU as pictured above. My impression is that nurses regard NICUs highly as a place to work. NICUs allow nurses to 'blend technology with personal knowledge'. They enjoy the involvement with the infant; they enjoy providing ritual and routine to help the infant to adjust to the alien environment. They like the sense of empathy for the needs of infants, who 'cannot ring a bell for the nurse'.[12] Whether the nurses are men or women, they have ample opportunity to express the maternal values of protecting life and fostering growth.[13] And, the architecture of the units—the grouping of many small beds into one room—allows an easy flow of community and shared information among nurses, and among nurses and patients.

But, when nurses are challenged and morally distressed by what they witness or participate in, they are often troubled because they see past the illusions mentioned above. Miya supplies quotations from nurses that resonate with what I have heard from informants, for instance: 'I find it difficult to understand why so much time and effort is spent on babies that cannot possibly live. It is painful to watch and must be painful for the babies.'[3]

In nursing school, students are usually taught to be concerned for public health and prevention and to look closely at the social aspects of patients and their families. This holism fosters an ability to set saving lives in a broader context and to focus less on the individual.[14] So, when things turn bad on the unit, nurses tend to question the meaningfulness of the enterprise as a whole rather than look for solutions by defining specific principles for distinguishing one case from another.

Nurses also perceive and connect with infants and their parents in ways very different from physicians, so that their experience of caregiving is different. Nurses touch infants; physicians are rarely seen holding babies (Guillemin and Holmstrom 1986, p. 59)[1]; physicians look at the charts; nurses look at the babies. Nurses touch and comfort patients; they sit with them; they attend the funerals more than busy physicians do; sometimes, they visit the babies after they go home. Nurses touch and feel suffering that is not measured in the numbers, and that suffering counts in the larger balance against NICUs; this also challenges the loyalty of nurses to the enterprise as a whole.

PUZZLES ABOUT PROFESSIONALISM

The roles and concerns of neonatal intensive-care nurses also provide a context for raising some interesting and complex issues surrounding the concept of professionalism, especially as it applies to nurses. I will discuss four areas of tension here: emotionality in competition with technology, the person in conflict with the professional role, process and participation, and the decisional authority of the nurse.

Emotions and technology

A nurse recently told a story of her unsuccessful attempts to have her hospital include a measure of time spent with patients in needed teaching and interviewing as one of the indicators of the intensivity of nursing labor. She was told by her CEO to do her talking while doing procedures; a practice she felt was not always possible, since both talk and procedures each often required full attention. This rejection of talk as a separate and important service marks an important focus of tension about the role of the nurse. Increasingly, nurses must play 'beat the clock' in accomplishing a list of procedures for patient care (Reverby 1987, p. 204).[15]

Nurses strongly value their relationships with patients; patients are also supported, strengthened, and educated by their relationships with nurses. As a hospital poster for the annual nursing week said, 'Nurses are the heart of health care.' Although traditional medical roles have emphasized detached concern and equanimity as emotional models,[16–17] the education of nurses tends to foster more attention to empathy, care, and touch.[18–19] Many nurses seem to regard emotional labor—the management of their feelings and those of patients to produce a supportive atmosphere[20–21]— as an essential part of nursing practice. If I am right in my discussion of the mythological foundations of NICUs, the emotional drama of the unit is much more important than is usually supposed in philosophical discussions. Although feelings are less visible and less studied, they provide the narrative and satisfactions that make NICU practices feel justified. As Callahan notes, emotions as well as reason are 'tutors' of ethics.[22]

Yet not everyone supports an emphasis on the emotive aspects of nursing care. A recent survey by Zussman suggests that patient stays are now normally so short that the relational aspects of care are much diminished.[23] Hospitals are reluctant to treat emotion work as explicit labor because it is so hard to measure, although they often emphasize a positive emotional atmosphere and the supportiveness of nurses in their advertising. Women rightly view emotional work with caution, since it represents traditionally exploitative aspects of women's work.[20]

In the NICU, it is perhaps somewhat easier than on other units to talk to the infant while doing procedures (since conversations with infants tend not to be very demanding), and the long stays of some infants and their developmental level tend to keep emotional labor central. The great stress of the unit on parents also requires extensive emotional support and communication from nurses. However, the intensity of the technology in the NICU creates tensions between conceptions of the nurse as skilled technician and the nurse as a builder of relationships. Some NICU technology directly conflicts with caring attention, as do painful procedures. Other NICU technology nurses feel they can master and combine with a sense of caring: 'machines used routinely can become an extension of the nurse and can result in a type of symbiotic relationship (between nurse and machine)'.[12]

Some new technology fosters connections with patients; other technology, by replacing touch, vision, and contact, separates practitioners from patients. Certainly the barriers of the isolettes and the delicacy of the tubing and instruments, not to speak of the delicacy of the infant, make the handling of infants a challenging matter. But being handled gently and comforted is one of the essential caring processes for infants, and when it cannot be done effectively, nurses become justifiably distressed.[24] As a heuristic, I sometimes imagine what it would be like if nurses or physicians were replaced by gentle, sophisticated robots (consider also the potential replacement of parenthood by technology[25])—one or two steps beyond the Cyborg vision of Bosque above. Would something essential to health care be lost? I think so; thus, only if nurses have substantial input into new infant-care technology and if the emotional and touch aspects of basic care are recognized and acted upon by developers of new technology can nurses feel that the progress of technology will be to improve their ability to feel and provide care rather than create barriers to it.

The person and the professional role

Doing emotional work does not make the person playing the professional role identical to that professional. Even though I may use my emotions in my work to support others, I may hold substantial feelings in reserve that reflect my real feelings as a person. In so far as emotionality is part of a professional's work, the professional must cope both with maintaining a professional demeanor and with handling his or her own feelings. Emotion work, especially on matters of such importance as saving the lives of infants, brings the two close together. Doing work that is very like mothering in such close intimacy with the infant, and holding views about parents, nurses are tempted to step beyond the role, to become the mother, and even to adopt infants. Doing the deep acting that is required to present consistently in a personal manner,[21] one will inevitably call upon a broad range of one's personality, including one's values and one's opinions of others.

As Penticuff notes, nurses make judgments about mothers. As one physician invidiously put it 'Nurses talk about "liking". They like a patient or a patient. Or they don't like them. That's not what physicians do. We stick to the facts.'[1] Nurses will become very concerned about the backgrounds of patients, and wonder about their moral responsibility for harm done to their infants, and about the personalities and abilities of parents to provide care for their infants after leaving the unit. Parents are also often judged strongly on how often they visit and how they handle the infant and talk to staff; a parent wise about impression-management in the hospital will be careful neither to visit too little nor too much.

The physician speaking in the paragraph above has encapsulated in a few words a long epistemological tradition of resolving value questions in medicine, as far as possible, by adhering as closely as possible to putatively morally neutral categories such as diagnoses and prognoses. This tradition has difficulty handling questions which involve predictions of patient compliance or where the health problems of patients are linked closely to patients' lifestyles,[26] and another approach may be useful here. Harding argues that 'standpoint logic' is an epistemologically more sound approach than 'objectivity' for understanding issues where social and cultural factors are involved.[27] Belenkey et al. also discuss 'connected knowing' as a mode of learning for women that proceeds carefully by building from particular and contextual features to conclusions, rather than moving quickly to broad principles.[28] While objectivity involves a rapid retreat from evaluative elements, situated knowing requires a careful dialogue among one's own views, others involved in culturally differing situations, and scientific explanations.[27]

To express more of a situated-knowing approach to issues in the NICU, the ways nurses look at patients and their families need to be more fully represented in NICU decision-making. Units would need greatly to improve nursing and parental participation in decision-making and to expand dialogue and process.

Process and participation

What is 'process'? Process requires all who are closely involved in a situation to discuss, and to listen respectfully and interestedly to, each other's openly expressed views, feelings, and reflections on the situation. This sort of process includes strong humanistic elements, requires sharing psychologically significant concerns, and distinguishes itself from legal conceptions of process requiring formal elements and order. Ordinarily, process leads to a consensual decision; and, if not, those involved who do not make the decisions feel that they participated in the decision.

Nurses tend to lack a sense of participation in the decisions in NICUs, as do parents. Martin describes nurses as feeling 'seldom involved' in treatment decisions, in contrast to their 'intensive and enduring contact with the infant'; nurses also felt that their opinions were generally 'not usually respected' or 'only minimally respected'.[4] Pinch describes parents as taking a 'passive role', as 'not involved' in decision-making, and feeling 'disconnected from the child'. She describes a 'chasm' between parental and professional perceptions of decision processes in NICUs.[2]

One source of these feelings is that some units do not allow enough time for engaging in process around decisions. Indeed, it is my impression that NICUs vary quite a bit in the degree to which they set aside time regularly to involve nurses and parents in decisions. In units where more commitment is made to process, nurses and parents feel more involved in decisions, even though their formal control over decisions is not much different. Indeed, although I sometimes argue that nurses should have a leadership role in making decisions in the NICU, most nurses I have talked with have a strong interest in participation and less interest in being the ones to make decisions.

In Gilligan's acute critique of Kohlberg's theory of moral development, she observed that young women tended to pay more attention to the relational qualities of discourse than to the principled qualities; in treating the Heinz case of the impoverished husband considering stealing cancer medications for his wife, Gilligan's respondents were more likely to puzzle over the relationship of the couple to the pharmacist and the community than to state the tension between respect for life and respect for property.[29] What Gilligan seems to suggest is that the process by which a decision is made is as important, and perhaps even more important, than the principles according to which it is made.

This may be a useful approach to debates about decision-making in NICUs. It may be more important to establish sound decisional processes in units than to state clear principles concerning the value of life, the rights of parents, and the role of developmental deficits in evaluating medical conditions. The 'principled' approach to evaluating life-saving decisions in the NICU has the problem that since the 'respect for life' principle is so strong, ethicists have tended to require that 'not human' conditions need to apply in order to discontinue therapy.[30] However, there have proved to be two major drawbacks to this approach. First, premature babies, who constitute the bulk of NICU clients, are not unhuman; they are merely 'unfinished' or 'incompletely integrated.'[31] Second, nurses and others very strongly perceive virtually all infants as persons. Nurses frequently discern the personalities of babies. Penticuff observes that nurses see infants as communicating preferences, trying to assert control, preferring one caregiver over another, and protecting themselves (p. 000).[32] When a baby lives or dies, it is common for staff to speak of the infant's 'deciding' whether to live or die—a phrase expressing the individualist mythology behind NICUs.

The 'principled' approach also requires that we make statements that apply very generally or universally. But politically we cannot expect to get universal agreement on any statement of principle concerning life, and disagreements are likely to be strong. But, if we emphasize process over principle, then we will be more concerned that we achieve local agreement— that is, agreement among those closely involved with the infant. It is possible to get local agreement when national agreement is impossible. Moreover, good process, by involving nurses, rests on the opinions of a wider range of individuals, and thus has potentially broader moral authority than a decision by a narrower range of professionals. This emphasis on process also respects, what Jonsen and Toulmin have observed, that moral consensus in particular cases tends to be achieved with a large degree of independence from stated disagreements on principles.[33]

When nurses feel moral conflicts about their work, they are challenged to find a resolution. They may turn to ethics as guidance, and, in such cases, may well regard their ethical concerns as merely personal ones, and may choose not to bring them into discussion on the unit. Regrettably, the 'principled' approach to ethics has tended to support, rather than to critique, the tendency of nurses to be excluded from ethical decision-making. Nurses concerned with moral questions continue to receive lectures on beneficence, autonomy, and justice when they raise ethical issues, when this vocabulary and the process of presenting it tend to alienate nurses from the learning process.[28] A process orientation ('Let's talk and see what we come up with'), besides being more inclusive and respectful, is also more likely to generate pertinent vocabulary and observations in particular cases.[34]

Indeed, stronger involvement of nurses in NICU decisions has the potential for making NICUs more humane. It is striking how nurses, who humanize infants so strongly, are also able to speak strongly for allowing infants to die. The personal willingness of nurses to see infants fully as persons and yet appreciate the limitations of life-saving convinces me that one can allow persons to die with integrity and respect, if one maintains a close and personal connection with the decision. Nurses who make such judgments thus exemplify the importance of connectedness and process that is being sought when ethicists criticize euthanasia decisions like those of Jack Kevorkian's work or the 'It's over, Debbie' case, where the physicians involved lacked adequate involvement with the patients.[35]

The 'process' approach may also permit parents a larger role in making decisions in units. A stronger sense that meetings and discussion are impor- tant may invite stronger participation by parents. Moreover, an atmosphere of permission to discuss feelings and doubts may allow parents to express their own concerns more actively, rather than being excluded by a 'right principles' approach ('If you don't agree with the right principles, you should not say anything'). Although Penticuff strongly supports greater parent participation, she sets up conditions of participation that require much more than parents can realistically or justifiably be expected to maintain (p. 000).[32] First, she requires that they put the child's interests before those of others, when they must also think of the interests of themselves and their other children. Second, she holds that parents must comprehend the essential facts, when in fact the full implications of these facts must stay well beyond them. For instance, Pinch notes that the 'full realization of the depth and breadth of child care' does not come upon parents until later (Pinch and Spielman 1990, p. 717).[2] And third, she holds that parents must make 'rational decisions' in a setting in which, as I have argued above, the real foundations are ritual and myth, not rationality. If 'rational' also means 'objective', this condition also disqualifies parents, since they are almost always deeply emotionally involved parties. Moreover, the principle of putting the child first pursues impossible ideals of parenthood characteristic of stereotypic traditions of parenthood.[36]

Let us consider process considerations in application to one of the most difficult cases for units to handle from the point of view of both process and principle. The child is premature and having serious difficulty. If he survives the unit, he will need close attention at home. The child's family is poor; the mother is fifteen years old, and not easy for staff to talk with. She lives with her parents, who are also very involved. The father, also fifteen, lives elsewhere, and seldom comes in. In the typical case I see in the unit, the nursing and medical staff tend to be very angry with the mother. They have trouble talking with her, and get poor information on what they need to know when they have to make decisions. They may treat the mother as a child ('These are children having babies,' is a common staff observation) and work with the grandparents, despite the legal concern that the grandparents lack standing. Staff are uncomfortable with the father. Staff also feel that intense care might be futile, as they lack confidence in the mother's ability to provide adequate support after the child leaves the unit.

I don't think process will resolve every problem in this type of case—the public-health reproach to the NICU; but it can do a lot more than principle has.[37] Rather than setting conditions on the mother's participation, the staff should openly and respectfully involve the mother, the father, and the grandparents. They may have to visit them at home. Staff should not expect a lot of rationality; everyone is in the same boat on this one. Indeed, they would learn, if they listened, that most fifteen-year-old mothers take their role as mothers very seriously, and dedicate themselves to giving excellent care to their babies.[38] In the long run, teen mothers and their children often fare better than staff imagine.[38-39] Also, staff would visit the home in a friendly, not inquisitorial way, and think with the family about what is and is not possible. Maybe, they would decide together that in this situation it would be best to stop care, because the situation at home really makes the future unsustainable. Or maybe they would decide to continue support because of the strong and involved commitment of the mother and grandparents. Thus, judgments about social conditions might be involved; but not in an angry, distant, way, without participation. Instead, social judgments by both parents and staff would be integrated into the conversation.

Such a process would take a lot of time; but infants often spend weeks or months on a unit—occasionally more time than they spent in the womb—and thus there is often ample time available for such decisions in typical cases of prematurity. The sense that time is lacking arises from our social investment in technology in relationship to social processes,[40] which arises from the mythology that life-saving is a matter of technological skill, not social relations.

The decisional authority of the nurse

In this paper, I have challenged the pose of rationality involved so much in the legal and ethical discussion of neonatal care. In so doing, I have been claiming that the actual political impact of this pose has been to exclude nurses and parents from the process of decision-making in NICUs. I think that Penticuff in general also calls attention to the importance of greater nursing and parental involvement, but she has not emphasized, as I have tried to do emphatically, how sorely the needed processes for involvement are lacking. I have also wanted to suggest that this lack tends to be supported by styles of philosophical thinking that use a vocabulary and argumentation style that tends to exclude nurses.

In my view, Penticuff is wrong in her paper at only two points. We have already discussed my view that her conditions on parental participation are too strong. The other point is her early contention that nursing involvement in decisions depends on their engaging in independent nursing practices in NICUs (p. 000).[32] However, the right to be involved in decisions does not depend on independence; instead, it rests on involvement with others. Because nurses are involved in medical care plans and in care consequential for parents, and because they have views on medical diagnoses and therapies, infants, and parents, they should be involved in making decisions.

Continuing practices that exclude nurses indicate continuing social practices that fail to show equity to both genders. It is true that more men are entering nursing and more women are entering medicine. But, the nurse–physician job-role division is an invention of Victorian times. Although both jobs have been greatly redefined, the Victorian gender-based assumption that the physician retains all the professional decisional power still stands. The bioethics revolution has tended to return decisional power to patients somewhat, but it has not at all addressed power inequities between nurses and physicians, who share different parts of one job of service to patients based on stale icons of gender. Consider an analogy of master to slave before the American Civil War. If equality were regarded simply as a question of equal opportunity among races, the solution to slavery would have been to ensure that blacks and whites had equal opportunity to get jobs either as master or slave. Similarly, equal opportunity of men and women to become nurses or physicians does not address the basic power inequalities between the two professions.

I recommend that nurses should have at least an equal role with physicians in making decisions in the NICU. Since three major parties would be involved in making decisions—physicians, nurses, and parents—good decisional processes would also be necessary to maintain conversation to reach consensus.

This would also certainly require that staff ratios and schedules should be shifted to allow more decisional process time; such a policy would therefore have economic consequences.

If there must be a dominant health professional, then I suggest that it should be the primary nurse, not the physician. The nurse has the right kind of involvement with the infant and parents to take the lead in setting objectives for care. Physicians, who are already used to consulting roles in relationship to each other, would act as consultants to define the medical care plan appropriately, subordinate to the overall life, social, and parental objectives. This would not restore maternal power to units. Ruddick rightly observes that it is disrespectful not to distinguish nursing from mothering (1989, p. 47).[13] But such a move would tend to reestablish the symbols of maternal power in medical child-care—power that was first taken from midwives by gynecologists, and is now being stolen from nurses in NICUs. (Remember that the priest at Lake Nemi was guarding a grove belonging to a goddess of birth.)

However, I prefer the suggestion that nurses and physicians take an equal standing in NICU decisions. Besides supporting the principles of gender equity, this would, by requiring strong decisional processes, tend to give principles their proper place in the midst of discourse, and not above it, as gods of the modern mythology of rationality.

CONCLUSION

In discussing the roles in the NICU of process and emotion, narrative and mythology, I don't wish to set up an incompatibility between reason and these other considerations. Like Callahan, I believe that emotion and reason work hand-in-hand. I trust that those engaged in process will address issues reasonably, and I think that reason is empty unless it is spliced to culture and a sense of larger meaning by which the elements of a reasonable position can be evaluated. The flavor of reasonableness depends on its cultural context; but the culture of nursing is not well enough represented in NICUs. If nurses were more in control, the economics, the pace, and the emphasis of NICU work would be different; certainly, there would be more communication among the parties involved.

I don't know what impact such changes would have on the future of NICUs or their role in society. Although I have tried to state a strong case against NICUs as a social policy for saving infant lives, I believe they may well have their place in policies respectful of life on a more global scale. I think that it would probably be a much more limited place, and I think that more conscious adoption of nursing-based values by such units would tend to reshape units toward a better fit in a global picture. Even if this does not occur, I believe that nurses are wronged when unit schedules, procedures, and systems of authority overly restrict the decision-making participation of nurses, who, as Penticuff has shown, maintain deep concern for the ethical issues of infant care. I think more nursing involvement in NICU treatment-planning decisions would also facilitate more active participation by parents in such decisions—a value on which there is much agreement, but which is in fact practiced very conditionally.

REFERENCES

1. Guillemin, Jeanne Harley and Holmstrom, Lynda Lytle (1986). *Mixed blessings: intensive care for newborns*. Oxford University Press, New York.
2. Pinch, Winifred J. and Spielman, Margaret L. (1990). The parents' perspective: ethical decision-making in neonatal intensive care. *Journal of Advanced Nursing* 15: 712–19.
3. Miya, Pamela A., Boardman, Karen K., Harr, Kathleen L. and Keen, Annabelle (1991). Ethical issues described by NICU nurses. *The Journal of Clinical Ethics* 2: 253–7.
4. Martin, Darlene Aulds (1989). Nurses' involvement in ethical decision-making with severely ill newborns. *Issues in Comprehensive Pediatric Nursing* 12: 463–73.
5. Shapiro, Andrew L. (1992). *We're number one: where America stands—and falls—in the New World Order*. Random House, New York.
6. Meadows, Donella H. (1991). *The global citizen*, pp. 37–8. Island Press, Washington, DC.
7. Meadows, Donella H. Meadows, Dennis L. and Randers, Jørgen (1992). *Beyond the limits*: confronting global collapse; envisioning a sustainable future. Chelsea Green Publishing Company, Post Mills, Vt.
8. Union of Concerned Scientists (1992). *World scientists' warning to humanity*. Union of Concerned Scientists, Washington, DC.
9. Gorz, André (1980). *Ecology as politics*, trans. Patsy Vigderman and Jonathan Cloud. South End Press, Boston.
10. Klass, Perri (1992). 'Hurting babies'. In *Baby doctor*, pp. 74–80. Random House, New York.
11. Frazer, Sir James George (1890, 1959). *The New Golden Bough*, ed. Theodor H. Gaster. New American Library, New York.
12. Bosque, Elena Marie (1993). Symbiosis of nurse and machine through fuzzy logic: improved specificity of a new neonatal pulse oximeter alarm. University of California, San Francisco, School of Nursing, Ph. D. dissertation.
13. Ruddick, Sara (1989). *Maternal thinking: toward a politics of peace*. Beacon Press, Boston.
14. Smith, Martha N. and Whitney, Gail M. (1991). Caring for the environment: the ecology of health. In Chinn, Peggy L. (ed.), *Anthology on caring*, pp. 59–69. National League for Nursing Press, New York.
15. Reverby, Susan M. (1987). *Ordered to care: the dilemma of American nursing, 1850–1945*. Cambridge University Press.
16. Osler, William (1991). Aequanimitas. In Reynolds, Richard and Stone, John (eds), *On doctoring*. Simon and Schuster, New York.
17. Hilfiker, David (1987). *Healing the wounds*. Penguin Books, New York.
18. Fry, Sara T. (1992). 'The role of caring in nursing ethics'. In Holmes, Helen

Bequaert and Purdy, Laura M. (eds), *Feminist perspectives in medical ethics.* pp. 93–106. Indiana University Press, Bloomington.

19. Gadow, Sally A. (1985). Nurse and patient. In Bishop, Anne H. and Scudder, John R., Jr. (eds), *Caring, curing, coping: nurse, physician, patient Relationships.* The University of Alabama Press.

20. Calhoun, Cheshire (1992). Emotional work. In Cole, Eve Browning and Coultrap-McQuin, Susan (eds), *Explorations in feminist ethics. Indiana University Press.*

21. Hochschild, Arlie (1983). *The managed heart: commercialization of human feeling.* University of California Press, Berkeley.

22. Callahan, Sidney (1988). The role of emotion in ethical decisionmaking. *Hastings Center Report* **18** (3): 9–15.

23. Zussman, Robert (1993). Life in the hospital: a review. *The Milbank Quarterly* **71**: 167–85.

24. Mitchell, Christine (1986). Caring for T. J.: a profoundly retarded infant. *Nursing Life* **6** (1): 20–3.

25. Ramsey, Paul (1970). *Fabricated man: the ethics of genetic control.* Yale University Press, New Haven.

26. Greiner, Carl (1991). Compliance: a new version of merit (abstract). Nebraska–Dartmouth 'Dilemmas in Organ Transplantation' conference, Omaha, Ne., October 25.

27. Harding, Sandra (1991). *Whose science? whose knowledge? Thinking from women's lives.* Cornell University Press, Ithaca.

28. Belenky, Mary Field, Clinchy, Blythe McVicker, Goldberger, Nancy Rule, and Tarule, Jill Mattuck (1986). *Women's ways of knowing: the development of self, voice, and mind.* Basic Books, New York.

29. Gilligan, Carol (1982). *In a different voice: psychological theory and women's development.* Harvard University Press, Cambridge, Mass.

30. Tooley, Michael (1974). Abortion and infanticide. In Finnis, John, Thomson, Judith Jarvis, Tooley, Michael, and Wertheimer, Roger (eds), *The rights and wrongs of abortion,* pp. 52–84. Princeton University Press.

31. Jonsen, Albert R. (1982). Ethics, the law, and the treatment of seriously ill newborns. In Doudera, A. E., and Peters, J. D. (eds), *Legal and ethical aspects of treating critically and terminally ill patients,* pp. 236–41. AUPHA Press, Ann Arbor.

32. Penticuff, Joy Hinson, this volume, Chapter 14-A.

33. Jonsen, Albert R. and Toulmin, Stephen (1988). *The abuse of casuistry: a history of moral reasoning,* pp. 18–19. University of California Press, Berkeley.

34. Friedman, Marilyn (1987). Care and context in moral reasoning. In Kittay, Eva Feder, and Meyers, Diana T. (eds), *Women and moral theory,* pp. 190–204. Rowman & Littlefield, Savage, Md..

35. Anonymous (1989). 'It's over, Debbie.' *JAMA* **259**: 272.

36. Firestone, Shulamith (1970). Down with childhood. In *eadem,* The *dialectic of sex: the case for feminist revolution,* pp. 72–104. Bantam Books, New York.

37. Miles, Steven H. (1992). What are we teaching about indigent patients? *JAMA* **268**: 2561–2.

38. Lamanna, Mary Ann and Langworthy, Nancy. *Talking to teens: a new*

understanding of young women's decision-making about sexuality and reproduction. National Council on Family Relations annual meeting. New Orleans, La., November 7, 1989.

39. Pope, Sandra K., Whiteside, Leanne, Brooks-Gunn, Jeanne, Kelleher, Kelly J., Rickert, Vaughn I., *et al.* (1993). Low-birth-weight infants born to adolescent mothers: effects of coresidency with grandmother on child development. *JAMA* **269**: 1396–1400.
40. Furstenberg, Frank F., Brooks-Gunn, Jeanne, and Morgan, S. Philip (1987). Adolescent mothers and their children in later life. *Family Planning Perspectives* **19** (4): 142–51.
41. Rifkin, Jeremy (1987). *Time wars: the primary conflict in human history.* Simon & Schuster, New York.

15
Religious influences on decision-making

15A RELIGIOUS INFLUENCES ON DECISION-MAKING I

David Harvey

The newborn baby presents a challenge to anyone concerned with the ethics of medical care. Whereas an adult can usually be asked to make rational decisions about her or his care, an infant is clearly unable to express views on such a decision.[1] This has been recognized for a long time; but modern advances in neonatal care now result in our having to make difficult decisions on an infant's behalf more frequently than in the past. This is because of the use of life-saving treatment such as ventilation and intravenous feeding. The use of such techniques has to be balanced against the suffering which can be produced by very prolonged intensive care when the prospects of survival are very slim or when the baby's brain has been damaged by a congenital malformation or a severe disorder arising after birth, such as periventricular leukomalacia. Therefore discussions about ethical conduct of neonatal care, particularly intensive care, are a daily activity in maternity and children's hospitals. The cultural and religious aspects of care are clearly very important in reaching a consensus decision by the parents, guardians, professional staff, and those, such as priests, who represent the religion to which the family belongs. These decisions are a source of potential conflict, particularly when the parents themselves have different religions and where these differ from the religions common in the country where they live or the religious persuasions of the professional staff.

All doctors and nurses need to be sensitive to the different views expressed by different religions and to take them into account when looking after a baby. The issues are further complicated by the fact that strong religious views are often written into the laws of nations, and they differ considerably from one part of the world to another.

I am writing this section of the chapter from the perspective of a paediatrician who has been involved in neonatal care for thirty years. I have seen the exciting advances that have allowed us to save many pre-term babies' lives, so they can grow up to be normal children. I have also observed the tragedy and distress caused by the birth of severely abnormal babies, and that prolonged neonatal care has sometimes caused extreme physical distress to babies and emotional distress to families and professional attendants. Christianity is the established religion of England, where I was born; here, the principles of the Protestant Reformation have often been regarded as fundamentally important. I was brought up in the Anglican tradition, and in my adult life have changed my religion from Christianity to Buddhism, which allows me to observe the problems from a different perspective.

Concern about the ethical limits of neonatal care is world-wide. This is shown by a literature search I performed on ethical problems in the newborn; it produced references for many articles in different continents.[2-4]

RELIGIOUS ADHERENCE IN BRITAIN

The pattern of religion throughout the world is well known, but there are constant changes. Christianity dominates in Western Europe and the Americas. There are major differences in religious traditions within the Christian family; this causes amazement to many observers outside Christianity, who sometimes believe that these traditions are almost different religions, because of the strongly held different views and the religious wars of the past. Islam dominates in the Middle East and North Africa. The rest of Africa and Asia is a patchwork of religions, including Islam, Buddhism, and Hinduism. In many countries there are important and vocal religious minorities, particularly Christians and Muslims. This pattern of religion is changing rapidly in many countries, as a result of various influences, including migration, a disaffection with religion in some populations, and conversion to old or new religions. One only has to note the advance in Islam in large parts of Africa to see how important these changes are. This means that the practising doctor is likely to be faced with families who have very different religious beliefs to those dominant in a given society in the past. It is critically important that we should understand the religious beliefs of the families whose babies need neonatal care and achieve a consensus about care which respects those beliefs as far as possible.

Britain represents a country where religious adherence has changed rapidly and dramatically. Anglicanism (the Church of England) has been the established and dominant religion in England since the Reformation. At one time, Roman Catholics and Jews were banned from worship or participation in public life. Anglicanism is still the official established (State) religion in England, although it has been disestablished in Wales. The Church of Scotland is Presbyterian. The tragic history of battles between Roman Catholicism and Protestantism in Ireland is well known, and unfortunately still persists in the north of the divided island.

A recent survey reported in *The Economist* demonstrates the religious changes in the United Kingdom.[5] It confirms what is common knowledge in

Britain; there has been a major reduction in attendances at religious services for many of the long-established religions, and an increase in attendances for others. Interestingly, many in Britain still believe in God—71 per cent of them said they did in 1990, which is only a small change from surveys a quarter of a century ago. However, the Church of England now contains only a fifth of all religiously active British citizens; that Church together with the Roman Catholic Church has only 41 per cent of regular worshippers among their adherents. Figure 15.1 shows on the left that the Christian churches still make up an important number of people, but only 1–2 million take part in religious activities out of a total population around 55 millions. There is an important change in other religions; there are now a million Muslims in the British population; many more than there are Jews, who number under half a million, but have contributed much to British social and cultural life. The right side of the figure shows the changes which have occurred in the latter half of the 1980s during the decline in attendances in the mainstream Christian churches. There has been very little change in Jewish religious observance, but a major increase in other religions. The increasing religions in Britain are in several categories: there has been a considerable increase in those religions observed by immigrants, partly because of high birth-rates. As can be seen from Fig. 15.1, there have been increases in Sikhism, Islam, and Hinduism.

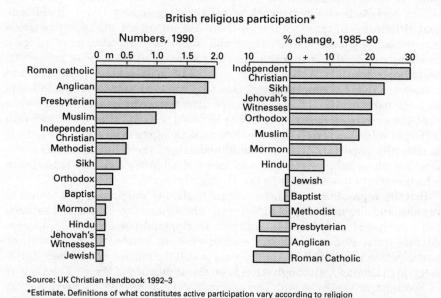

Source: UK Christian Handbook 1992–3

*Estimate. Definitions of what constitutes active participation vary according to religion

Fig. 15.1 Changes in religious participation in Britain, showing the numbers participating in religions and the per centage changes in the last half-decade (source: *The Economist*, 13 March 1993, p. 35). Reproduced with permission.

The Christians have also shown changes; although relatively small, Orthodox Christianity is growing; and there has been a big increase among the independent Christian churches. Some of these are within the historically familiar Christian sects and some are outside, among them the pentecostalists and charismatic Christians. Evangelical groups are playing a larger part in the Christian communities; many of their adherents have very strongly held views about the importance of strict adherence to the written word of the Bible, which may lead to equally strongly held moral views derived from the Bible's interpretation.

The figure shows clearly the increase in the numbers of Jehovah's Witnesses in Britain. Their views about the use of blood products are well known, and have caused difficulties in the medical care of young infants. Hidden amongst the changes is also an increase in small groups led by charismatic leaders that are loosely and inappropriately referred to as *cults*. Quite a lot is written about them in the newspapers, but one meets them in clinical practice relatively infrequently. 'New-age' religions are also becoming more important, and derive their beliefs from many sources.

What importance do these changes have for the practice of paediatrics in Britain? Religion is clearly still an important factor for many people in Britain. In any neonatal unit one can see religious objects placed by parents next to the babies in their cots or incubators. A simple tour around our unit would regularly show copies of the Bible, rosaries, portraits of Sikh holy men, and Muslim medals. It is, therefore, important that nurses and doctors working in neonatal units should understand as much as possible about the people from other cultures whose babies will be admitted. A number of useful articles have been written about such matters as naming systems, cultural behaviour, and religious practices.[6-9]

Seminars and teaching sessions should be instituted so that the staff not only have material to read but are also able to discuss problems and ask questions in an informative educational format. This can be particularly important where culture and food habits may appear strange to members of the professional staff.[10] Such seminars must be conducted very carefully. I had the experience of setting up a seminar to explain and explore Rastafarianism and its culture to the staff of a hospital in which I worked. This was somewhat misunderstood by local Rastafarians, who asked, at the seminar, why we were picking them out particularly; our attempts to inform ourselves of their beliefs and therefore improve the medical care of their children were seen as a threat to them. Discussions with local communities can get over these problems; and such initiatives need to be recommended and increased.

There are of course many texts available to explain the ethical basis of many religions in books on medicine[11] or specific religions.[12] It is important that the neonatal unit should not be seen as supporting one particular religion or tradition, but is open to care for people from every cultural background.

CONFLICT BETWEEN MEDICAL CARE AND THE BELIEFS OF CERTAIN RELIGIOUS GROUPS

Discussions of the ethics of neonatal care often stress major problems of conflict where a parent refuses treatment or insists upon treatment against the advice of the medical and nursing staff. Such areas of extreme conflict are in fact uncommon, but are remembered by the members of the staff because of the emotional pain caused by the turmoil. There are particular issues at stake in one or two religious positions. The most famous concerns Jehovah's Witnesses and their objection to the use of blood or blood products in medical treatment. This conflict is stressed in many texts, and may become a more common problem because of the increase in Jehovah's Witnesses in many countries around the world. In Britain, the legal position of a doctor is clear when treating a baby; the doctor must provide what is regarded as the best medical treatment in an emergency for a baby despite the parents' objections but it is always wise to obtain a second opinion from a senior colleague.[13] There is a legal procedure (the situation is probably similar in other countries) in less urgent situations which allows a doctor to make an application to a judge for treatment, including blood, to be given. This is regarded as permissible because the baby is unable to give an opinion, and may later have different religious persuasions from the parents. The baby can therefore be made a ward of court, so that the legal authorities are the guardian of the child instead of the parents. The need to use such a procedure is rare, and its use should be avoided wherever possible. Conflict between the professionals caring for a baby and the members of its family does not lead to good medicine in most cases, and a search should be made for a way round it. In the United Kingdom, there is a special committee of Jehovah's Witnesses concerned with hospital treatment; they have proved extremely helpful in the medical care of babies. Blood transfusions are a very common procedure in neonatal units; a newborn baby receiving intensive care is more likely to be transfused than any other person of any other age admitted to hospital. This is because samples of blood are taken frequently to monitor biochemical changes in a sick baby, and the baby may easily become anaemic in these circumstances. Small blood transfusions are used to keep the oxygen-carrying capacity of the blood at a reasonable level during respiratory illness, which often leads to low blood oxygen-saturation. Careful explanation of the problems, with the help of another Jehovah's Witness experienced in visiting hospitals, can avoid conflict. The parents may allow procedures to be performed when necessary without an outright ban which could result in the doctor's turning to the law; and the parents can recognize that the baby is not able to speak for himself or herself.

An insistence on obtaining permission for blood transfusion during an operation is often unnecessary. I can remember one case in which a baby with a very poor outlook for life required an operation, largely for cosmetic reasons, for hydrocephalus. The purpose of the shunt operation was to ensure that the head did not get very large and ugly; it would make nursing easier and relieve the child's distress. One consultant neurosurgeon refused to operate because the parents were Jehovah's Witnesses, and would not sign permission for blood transfusion to be used during the operation. Another consultant surgeon was found in another city; he was happy to do the operation without a blood transfusion, recognizing that, if there was a slightly increased chance of death, the operation was not to save life but to make the child's life more comfortable. On balance, the operation probably prolonged the baby's life, and the lack of a blood transfusion was not important.

There have been reports of ways of avoiding blood transfusions in babies of Jehovah's Witnesses. Cardiovascular operations have been performed safely without blood transfusions.[14] New medical treatment may allow blood transfusions to be avoided; a case has been reported in whom erythropoietin was used for anaemia.[15] A baby, born at 24 weeks gestation to parents who were Jehovah's Witnesses, was made a ward of court and treated against their wishes with blood products. However, erythropoietin, which promotes red-cell production in the marrow, was successfully used to treat the anaemia.

Sometimes parents may have such extreme views about the care of their children that this almost amounts to child abuse. An example is the use of extremely unusual diets, which can be insufficient to allow the baby to grow. Severe nutritional disorders, including kwashiorkor, marasmus, and rickets, as a result of parental food faddism were reported in four children seen in Britain[16]; this was regarded as a form of child abuse. Legal measures are needed for such problems if the parents cannot be persuaded to put their children on a normal diet. A Rastafarian couple who had refused, on religious grounds, to allow their diabetic daughter to have insulin were convicted of manslaughter in 1993.[17]

NEONATAL INTENSIVE CARE

There are considerable problems with some religious views when considering if intensive care should be instituted and when it should be stopped. Many of these problems surround the baby who is born extremely prematurely at 23–25 weeks' gestation.[18] Such children never survived two to three decades ago; they are very small, have limited chance of survival, and require many weeks of intensive care. On the other hand they do not appear to have a greater risk of handicap than children born at 26–28 weeks' gestation when the rate of disability is taken as a percentage of all live births at a particular gestational age or birthweight. Much more follow-up will be required to be certain that such babies are not severely damaged. It is now becoming clear that many of the survivors do have minor motor, behavioural, and learning difficulties when they are of school age.[19] However, many families do not regard such problems as major disabilities, and it seems clear that

most people—professionals and parents alike—regard the four main severe
disabilities (blindness, deafness, severe mental handicap, and cerebral palsy)
as the problems they would want to avoid. The decisions surrounding the
introduction of intensive care vary considerably from country to country and
culture to culture. In many parts of the world, such as much of Africa, where
children only have less than a dollar a year for the whole of their health
care, it would be inconceivable to consider intensive care for a baby under
1000 grams at birth. What is also true is that the cost of caring for very
pre-term babies in developed countries is also very high when they are
born very prematurely.[20] There is still very little prospect of preventing
pre-term birth; in some respects the problem is getting worse because of
the increased number of multiple pregnancies which have resulted from
treatment for infertility.[21]

The care of newborn infants has to be seen against the background of what
used to happen to miscarriages around 23 weeks' gestation—they almost all
died—and the present frequent practice of terminating pregnancy for social
reasons before 24 weeks' gestation. Different religious have strongly differing
views about whether abortions are justified or not, and this will be reflected
in their attitudes to the care of very pre-term babies. Families also have
very different views about whether intensive care is justified for babies who
are born very early, although most families are very keen that everything
possible should be done as far their baby is concerned. I have simultaneously
looked after two very pre-term babies of the same gestation, one of whom
had parents who were only 19 years old and were unmarried and said that
the baby had not been planned, whereas the other was the result of a tenth
pregnancy in a women in her early forties who had no living children. It is
understandable that people from many religions say that every baby's life
is equally valuable; but one can also understand those who feel that these
two situations are very different. One family might expect the baby to die as
a result of the miscarriage they thought was happening; whereas the other
family would want all possible medical care for their baby. It is difficult to
make a decision in this situation; but with the modern results of intensive
care it is our practice to resuscitate every baby born after 26 weeks' gestation.
At 22 weeks or less the outlook is still hopeless, and the baby is not usually
resuscitated; whereas resuscitation is performed for babies between 23 and
25 weeks' gestation only after discussion with the obstetricians and parents.
What is very unsatisfactory is to have reached a decision that resuscitation
should not be performed, but then to have this done 20 minutes or more after
birth when the baby is still breathing. This is likely to give the baby a very
bad start in life, since the period of asphyxia shortly after birth may well have
led to a greater risk of brain damage; it is a good example of the importance
of planning as far as possible before birth and making a decision about
whether intensive care is to be started or not. These are difficult decisions
for junior members of staff, and their best course, at an unexpected birth,
is to resuscitate the baby and then call a more senior member of staff who
will discuss whether resuscitation by ventilation should be continued or not.

It is common practice for these problems to be discussed at seminars and discussions within a neonatal unit and to involve representatives of certain religions. It is not usually possible to get the opinion of a religious leader at the time of crisis; but clearly the parents' religion will influence their views on whether life-saving resuscitation should be attempted or not.

WITHDRAWAL OF LIFE-SUPPORT

There are occasions where the continuation of intensive care appears to be inappropriate because the prognosis for the survival of an infant is very poor indeed or even hopeless. This can be a source of great anxiety and controversy for the neonatal staff and the family of the child. Brain-death criteria do not apply to the newborn at present, so withdrawal is usually done on the basis that medical treatment is no longer indicated. Some religions and cultures hold the view that life-support should be continued without regard to the prognosis of the infant. Personal reports from colleagues in countries as wide apart as Saudi Arabia and Japan indicate that it is their practice to continue life-support until death occurs; this is on religious grounds, often reflected in law.

It is of critical importance to take into account strong religious views held by parents or members of staff. In order to do this several consensus meetings need to be held to discuss the outlook for the baby, the views of the unit staff, and the views of the parents, and to bring all these discussions together. It is necessary to give an opinion on how effective the treatment is. As far as possible, standard treatment should today be based on studies from large numbers of infants and subjected to controlled trials and appropriate statistical analyses. These are now being brought together in such publications as the Cochrane Collaboration Database of Pregnancy and Childbirth and a book which has summarized in print the overviews from those trials.[22] Within the resources that are available, all pregnant women and newborn infants should be given the benefit of treatment which has been shown by analyses of data to be effective, and the corollary is that treatment should be avoided where there is no good reason for its use. There are wide areas of newborn medicine which have not been subjected to sufficient investigation, and it is vital that research should be pursued in those areas, so that resources are not wasted by using treatment which is not properly evaluated and may preclude the introduction of treatment which has been evaluated and is effective.

The statistical basis of the analyses which were done on trials relates the probability or chance with which a particular observation could have occurred. This implies that one is never certain of a particular outcome or result of treatment, but only of the probability of its occurring. This sometimes startles lay persons who attend ward rounds or seminars on

the ethics of the treatment or the withdrawal of treatment for a particular
infant or group of infants. They sometimes ask, 'When can you be absolutely
certain that the prognosis is hopeless?', and are surprised when the answer
is 'Never.' There is a saying, which is said to be Buddhist—it is also common
in other religions—'The only certainty is uncertainty'; unfortunately, I have
not been able to find the reference for it. It is the working basis for much of
neonatal medicine.

The practice on our unit when there is doubt about whether treatment
should be continued is to have a case discussion around the baby involving
all members of the neonatal professional staff. All are asked for their views,
even if they are very junior members of staff. It is important to have this
discussion before making a proposal to the parents that the treatment
might be discontinued. Members of staff often say that they want to hear
the parents' views. That is, of course, important; but the purpose of the
discussion is to find out whether any staff would object to a particular
action's being undertaken if the parents consented to it. It would be a
source of great confusion if a senior member of staff, after discussions
with the parents, agreed to the withdrawal of life-support only to find
that some members of staff were adamant that this was not justifiable.[23]
Some reports in this field have suggested that withdrawal of support should
only go ahead if all members of staff were united as to the justification for
the withdrawal. We have never felt constrained by this rule, as it would seem
unreasonable that a very junior and inexperienced professional might object
to withdrawal without understanding the problems of the future, which only
more professional experience would provide. However, this has never been a
problem in the cases that I have had to deal with. After having discussed
the case professionally and come to a view or a number of views about
possible action for the future, it is important to have a discussion, or a
number of discussions, with the parents to describe the options for the
future. Sadness that a hoped-for miracle is unlikely to occur means that it
will take many families some time to come to a decision about treatment; it
is critical that this whole procedure should not be rushed. It is at this point
that a priest, or other religious adviser, may be able to give very helpful
support; but parents request their presence less often than one might expect.
Sometimes, their role is to provide emotional support for the family without
being particularly involved in the difficult ethical decisions concerning the
use of treatment or not. It is our practice for a relatively senior person to be
involved in the withdrawal of treatment; it is only delegated when that more
junior professional feels happy about being involved in such difficult ethical
actions.

Great sympathy and kindness is needed in supporting the family while
the baby is dying. It is important to remember that the baby may not
die immediately, and could even live for a long period. Some parents
put the withdrawal in such terms as seeing whether nature, the baby,
or God will decide whether the baby lives or dies after ventilation is
stopped.

DECISIONS ABOUT WHETHER TREATMENT IS INDICATED OR NOT

Often, there is genuine doubt about whether treatment is indicated at all; this happens in extreme prematurity, but also in those babies who have severe congenital malformations. These are increasingly diagnosed before birth, so that there is time for discussion about what is to happen at the time of birth. The issues fall into two major categories: whether resuscitation, involving endotracheal intubation, is to be started at birth; and whether surgical procedures are indicated for the correction of a particular abnormality. Where parents, for particular religious reasons, wish treatment to be carried out there is usually no conflict between them, the staff, and the law; treatment will be pursued. One can put forward hypothetical occasions when treatment would be unethical. I have always regarded intubation of an anencephalic to be inappropriate treatment in the past; but this is of course not the case where the baby may have to be kept on a ventilator for the purpose of heart trasplant. It would be possible, although I have never met this in any professional life, to say to a parent that I think that such a course of treatment is quite unethical, and that they would have to choose another doctor to carry it out. This could put an intolerable burden on the parents, who would be left with the task of finding another physician or surgeon. There are a number of occasions where parents want to persist in treatment when the outlook seems hopeless. They may be influenced by those who feel that treatment should always be continued when there is any hope at all of a satisfactory outcome.

The conflict about whether to start treatment has often been presented in terms of the baby with a serious chromosome abnormality and a potentially curable congenital obstruction of the gut. I was involved in such a case about a decade ago; it is usually known in British law as *in re B*.[24,25] The facts of this case are well known. A baby was recognized as having duodenal atresia by antenatal ultrasound and, when the baby was born, there were signs of Down syndrome—a common association of duodenal atresia. The case occurred at a time when a well-known British paediatrician had been accused of murder of a child with Down syndrome—he was later acquitted. This increased the anxiety amongst the neonatal staff, and it was felt that a life-saving operation should be performed. The parents refused the operation, stating that they loved their child very much but believed that one did not have to interfere with nature by correcting a fatal abnormality in a child who had other serious problems. The local authority made an application for the child to be made a ward of court, and the judge agreed to an operation. All this was done in chambers, and there was therefore no publicity. The child was referred to a children's hospital for operation; but several consultant surgeons refused to operate, on the grounds that it was not common practice to do such an operation in a case of Down syndrome. The case went back to the judge, who felt he had not been completely informed of the facts of the case, and therefore the consent for operation was withdrawn. An appeal was made by the local authority, and the judges again gave permission for the operation, which was done. Because the appeal was public the newspapers took up the case world-wide, to the great distress of the parents and the neonatal staff. It has now been decided in Britain that such appeals need no longer be held in public.

It is interesting that a popular medical newspaper had several letters on the subject of the case. The religious polarization involved was shown by two letters in the same issue: one said 'What were the doctors doing, playing God by not performing a life-saving operation immediately?' and the other said, 'What were the doctors doing, playing God by not allowing a natural death to occur?'

The case changed medical opinion in Britain, and a baby with Down syndrome would now routinely have an operation for duodenal atresia. An interesting postscript is that I was asked to explain the facts of the case at a national committee concerned with medical ethics. Someone at the committee said that the problem arose because of advances in medical technology which had allowed us to keep babies alive. I pointed out that the operation for duodenal atresia was described at the beginning of the century; what had changed was not our ability to cure the condition, but our attitude to Down syndrome. We now expect children with the syndrome to have the same rights as other children.

RELIGIOUS CEREMONIES

Special religious ceremonies may be requested by parents; they should be allowed in hospital whenever possible. They often celebrate the birth and naming of the baby; others are concerned with death and bereavement. Staff should ask whether any special ceremony is needed. This should be done with sensitivity; at one time, I always asked Christian parents whether they wanted their seriously ill baby to be baptized. About a decade ago, I stopped asking this after several parents answered uncomfortably, 'No'. They had put Church of England as their religion on the hospital notes; but my question forced them to state publicly that they had no religion. This merely turned the knife in the wound at a time when they were trying to cope with the possible death of their baby. After that, I expected parents to tell us when they wanted a baptism. We are now returning to the question, since agnosticism and atheism are now so much more common and respected in our society.

A literature search using newborn infant and religion as keywords produced around 200 references; of these there were 21 on male circumcision alone. This procedure is performed in the neonatal period in a number of societies, including those of Jews, West Africans, and Muslims. It has produced a problem of discrimination against Muslim babies in Britain. There are many arguments against routine neonatal circumcision where it is not required by religious conviction,[26] with the result that it is not provided free in the health service in Britain. This is generally no problem, since Jews have a system of recognized *mohelim* who will perform the operation, usually at home. The rapid increase in Muslims in the UK has not been accompanied by a similar increase in the availability of local practitioners for the operation. This causes a problem for poor families who cannot pay for the operation[27]— another example of the importance of accommodating changing religious practices. Female circumcision is, of course, illegal in Britain, even though it is requested occasionally for strong cultural and quasi-religious reasons. It is interesting that there has not been a movement to oppose male circumcision on the grounds that it is also mutilating, although less so.

DEATH AND BEREAVEMENT

The death of a baby is a tragedy for the parents and a source of great emotional pain for the professional staff, who may feel that they have failed. It is sad that doctors and nurses sometimes feel that they must pursue intensive care at all costs, and forget their important role in allowing death to occur and to be dignified and peaceful. The principles of caring for families have been published;[28] a randomized trial made it clear that special help for parents who have lost a baby will ease their mental distress.[29,30] Giving the parents the time to hold the dead baby and start the grieving process is now widely recognized as essential.

This is a critical time to involve a priest or other religious leader. Every hospital should have a list of persons who can be contacted in an emergency. The priest will be able to comfort the family, perform important ceremonies, and advise the staff on what needs to be done about laying out the baby's body. There are often other important issues to be discussed, such as whether a post-mortem examination will be allowed, and whether the funeral must take place immediately.

All hospitals must have a place where the baby can be kept after death, before being sent to the mortuary. It should be nicely decorated, as a place where the parents can go to see and hold the baby; they may request to do this several times, and this wish should be respected. This place is often called 'the chapel'; but it is obvious that it should not be seen only as a Christian place. All staff should be reminded to remove Christian symbols from the chapel when the family who are about to use it have a different religion.

CONCLUSION

The different religions of the world influence the values and decisions of families who have sick babies in hospital. Their views should be respected, and every effort should be made to avoid conflict in making decisions about

care. All of us need to learn more about other religions and to realize that
the pattern of beliefs in the world is becoming more complex.

REFERENCES

1. Campbell, A. G. M. (1992). Ethical problems in neonatal care. In *Textbook of neonatology*, 2nd edn (ed. N. C. R. Roberton), pp. 43–8. Churchill Livingstone, Edinburgh.
2. Ho, N. K. (1992). Resuscitation of the small baby. *Singapore Medical Journal*, **33**, 595–6.
3. Sauer, T. J. (1992). Ethics decisions in neonatal intensive care units: the Dutch experience *Pediatrics*, **90**, 729–32.
4. Nishida, H., and Sakamoto, F. (1992). Ethical problems in neonatal intensive care units: medical decision making on the neonate with poor prognosis. *Early Human Development*, **29**, 403–6.
5. Anonymous. (1993). Religion: worship moves in mysterious ways. *The Economist*, **326**, 13th March, pp. 35–6.
6. Black, J. (1985). Paediatrics among ethnic minorities: contact with the health services. *British Medical Journal*, **290**, 689–90.
7. Black, J. (1985). Paediatrics among ethnic minorities. Asian families I: cultures. *British Medical Journal*, **290**, 762–4.
8. Black J. (1985). Paediatrics among ethnic minorities: families from the Mediterranean and Aegean. *British Medical Journal*, **290**, 923–5.
9. Black, J. (1985). Paediatrics among ethnic minorities: Afro-Caribbean and African families. *British Medical Journal*, **290**, 984–8.
10. Springer, L, and Thomas, J. (1983). Rastafarians in Britain: a preliminary study of their food habits and beliefs. *Human Nutrition and Applied Nutrition*, **37**, 120–7.
11. Campbell, A. G. M. (1988). Ethical issues in child health and disease. *In Child health in a changing society* (ed. J. O. Forfar), pp. 215–53. Oxford University Press.
12. de Silva, M. W. P. (1991). Buddhist ethics. In *A companion to ethics*, (ed. P. Singer), pp. 58–68. Blackwell, Oxford.
13. British Medical Association (1988). *Philosophy and practice of medical ethics*. BMA, London.
14. Ott, D. A. and Cooley, D. A. (1977). Cardiovascular surgery in Jehovah's Witnesses: report of 542 operations without blood transfusion. *Journal of the American Medical Association*, **238**, 1256–8.
15. Davies, P., Herbert, M., and Verrier Jones, E. R. (1992). Case study: erythropoietin for anaemia in a preterm Jehovah's Witness baby. *Early Human Development*, **28**, 279–83.
16. Roberts, I. F., West, R. J., Ogilvy, D., and Dillon, M. J. (1979). Malnutrition in infants receiving cult diets: a form of child abuse. *British Medical Journal*, **1**, 296–8.
17. Brahams, D. Religious objection versus parental duty. *Lancet*, **342**, 1189–90.
18. Stewart, A. L., Costello, A. M. de L., Hamilton, P. A., Baudin, J., Townsend, J., Bradford, B. C., and Reynolds, E. O. R. (1989). Relationship between

neurodevelopmental status of very preterm infants at 1 and 4 years. *Developmental Medicine and Child Neurology*, **31**, 756–65.

19. Marlow, N., Roberts, B. L., and Cooke, R. W. (1989). Motor skills in extremely low birthweight children at the age of 6 years. *Archives of Disease in Childhood*, **64**, 839–47.
20. Sandhu, B., Stevenson, R. C., Cooke, R. W. I., and Pharoah, P. O. D. (1986). Cost of neonatal intensive care for very low birth weight infants. *Lancet*, **1**, 600–3.
21. Griffin, J. (1993). *Born too soon*. Office of Health Economics, London.
22. Sinclair, J. C. and Bracken, M. (1992). *Effective care of the newborn infant*. Oxford University Press.
23. Whitelaw, A. (1986). Death as an option in neonatal intensive care. *Lancet*, **2**, 328–31.
24. Mason, J. K., and Meyers, D. W. (1986). Parental choice and selective non-treatment of deformed newborns: a view from mid-Atlantic. *Journal of Medical Ethics*, **12**, 67–71.
25. Anonymous. (1988). *In re B (a minor)*. *Medicine and Law*, **7**, 95–101.
26. Milos, M. F., and Macris, D. (1992). Circumcision: a medical or human rights issue? *Journal of Nurse-Midwifery*, **37** (2 Suppl), 87S–96S.
27. Madden, P. and Boddy, S. A. (1991). Should religious circumcisions be performed on the NHS [letter]? *British Medical Journal*, **302**, 292.
28. Forrest, G. C. (1992). Perinatal death. In *Textbook of neonatology*, (ed. N. R. C. Roberton), pp. 75–80. Churchill Livingstone, Edinburgh.
29. Forrest, G. C., Claridge, R., and Baum, J. D. (1981) The practical management of perinatal death. *British Medical Journal*, **282**, 31–2.
30. Forrest, G. C., Standish, E., and Baum, J. D. (1982). Support after perinatal death. *British Medical Journal*, **285**, 1475–9.

15B RELIGIOUS INFLUENCES ON DECISION-MAKING II

Ernlé W. D. Young

In his contribution to the subject 'religious influences on decision-making' Dr David Harvey has emphasized the importance of the cultural and religious aspects of care 'in reaching a consensus decision by the parents, guardians, professional staff, and those, such as priests, who represent the religion to which the family belongs'. He rightly reminds us that cultural values and religious beliefs 'are a source of potential conflict, particularly when the parents themselves have different religions and where these differ from the religions common in the country where they live or the religious persuasions of the professional staff'. He discusses various clinical ethical issues—such as blood transfusion, whether or not to initiate aggressive treatment, the withdrawal of life-sustaining treatments, and circumcision—in which the religious views of the family will affect the decision-making process, one way or another. He points out the danger of assuming that because a family professes to belong to a certain denomination, they will automatically want certain rituals, such as baptism. And he underlines the central role religion can play in times of death and bereavement.

In my own contribution to this subject, I intend to broaden the discussion, looking at beliefs and values more generally than in specifically religious terms.

Clinical ethical decision-making inevitably takes place within a fourfold grid or matrix. This includes the facts pertinent to the situation; rational biomedical ethical principles and duties; values (or beliefs); and extrinsic constraints or controls. The matrix may be illustrated as follows (Fig. 15.2):

This chapter will focus on the role values and beliefs play in the clinical ethical decision-making process. However, in order to set the stage for that discussion, a brief exposition of each of the other three quadrants in the grid may be helpful.

Database of factual information	Rational biomedical ethical principles and duties
Operative values or beliefs (essentially non-rational)	Extrinsic constraints or controls

Fig. 15.2 A clinical ethical decision-making matrix.

FACTUAL INFORMATION

Responsible decision-making requires a substantial basis in factual information. Although, in practice, it is not possible neatly to separate facts
from their interpretation (or from the values that inform our judgments
about which facts to include in our database), facts and values will be
treated separately for methodological purposes. Facts are elusive, and are
seldom incontrovertible. Nevertheless, sound decision-making begins with
the patient and often laborious task of accumulating such data as may be
available to shed light on the clinical situation. Obviously, medical facts will
be paramount, and will be elicited from the patient's history as well as from
different clinical and laboratory tests and studies. However, if the patient
is to be viewed holistically, various socio-economic, psychological, religious,
and familial data will also need to be sought. Beyond the facts pertaining
to the particular individual who is the focus of clinical attention, general
demographic, epidemiological, and genetic information may also be useful,
as will relevant facts about technology and outcome assessment. Until all
the pertinent data have been brought to light, no ethical problem can be
adequately or responsibly addressed. In arriving at a diagnosis, there will
be less reliance on beliefs (or intuition) than when offering a prognosis;
prognoses depend more on judgment, and are likely to be informed as much
by the clinician's beliefs as by solid empirical data.

PRINCIPLES AND DUTIES

The rational guiding biomedical ethical principles and duties have been
well delineated and discussed, for example, by Beauchamp and Childress.[1]
Their collaboration illustrates that these principles may be derived either
deontologically (Childress) or from a utilitarian approach (Beauchamp).
The principle of non-maleficence, probably the original biomedical ethical
guideline, requires the avoidance of harm (*primum non nocere*) and the
alleviation of suffering. The principle of beneficence, which came to predominate over non-maleficence once medicine entered the scientific era
and it became possible to benefit patients more predictably, requires the
attempt to preserve life using whatever technological means are at hand.
The principle of respect for autonomy emerged after the Second World War in
both the research and the therapeutic settings,[2] and, in the United States at
least, has brought the patient or the patient's surrogate as a full participant
into the decision-making process along with the physician. And the principle
of justice, distributively understood, has assumed increasing importance as
medicine has been compelled to come to terms with the finitude, and even
the shrinking nature, of societal resources.

    These four principles are ever in tension, and often in conflict, with one
another.[3] The tension between non-maleficence and beneficence gives rise

to the need to assess harms (or risks) versus benefits. Every medical intervention inflicts *some* harm, however minimal. Usually, this is offset by the hoped-for compensatory benefits. From an ethical standpoint, the harms of medical or surgical interventions ought never to be disproportional to the benefits they produce; once it becomes evident that this is happening, then the principle of non-maleficence trumps that of beneficence. The tension between beneficence and (distributive) justice provides the impetus for cost–benefit (or cost–effectiveness) calculations. Economic realities are pushing us in the direction of practicing cost-effective medicine; at the same time, at least in the United States, the threat of litigation nudges medicine in the opposite direction, that of practicing cost-ineffectively. And what patients (or their surrogates) autonomously demand may at times be in conflict with all three of the other principles: with beneficence (when what is wanted is not necessarily beneficial for the patient); with non-maleficence (when what is wanted may even be harmful to the patient); and with distributive justice (when what is wanted by or for a single individual may be detrimental to the common good). Part of the art of ethical decision-making consists of making the determination, in a given clinical situation, which of these four principles ought to take precedence over the others, and why.

The traditional duties devolving on physicians are veracity (truthfulness), privacy (defined by Beauchamp and Childress, quoting Ferdinand D. Schoeman, as 'a state or condition of limited access to a person'[4], confidentiality, and fidelity (the faithfulness of the physician to the patient). These duties are increasingly assailed by some of the realities of contemporary medicine.

There are cultural groups (Chinese, Japanese, and Vietnamese, for example) within which respect for the patient, especially the patient who is an elder, requires that the truth of a diagnosis or prognosis (and even about the potential harms of a proposed treatment) should be veiled; this presents the physician committed to veracity with an unavoidable and often uncomfortable conflict. Privacy and confidentiality are threatened, not only by computerized information banks, but by the rights others may have to privileged information—as was established in the Tarasoff case in psychiatry; with respect to the HIV epidemic, an urgent question is 'How far do the principles laid down in *Tarasoff* extend?' And the faithfulness of physicians to individual patients is being tested in managed care settings by the requirement that they should simultaneously be faithful to their group or institution, displaying as much solicitude for its financial health as for the medical health of individual patients. The physician as 'double agent'—committed both to the patient and to the solvency of the group or institution—is a relatively new phenomenon, one for which medical students are still largely unprepared.

The main point of this short discourse is that these principles and duties are ontologically rational. That is to say, not only their derivation but also their ranking in a given situation is essentially reasonable. As such, they contrast markedly with the values and beliefs (to be discussed below) that enter, as decisively yet more subtly, into the decision-making process.

EXTRINSIC CONTROLS AND CONSTRAINTS

A third element in the matrix is that of extrinsic controls and constraints. These have been described as 'contextual features'.[5] Either term signifies such things as regulatory stipulations, economic pressures, reimbursement mechanisms, legislative requirements, the threat of litigation, and political ideologies (as in the Bush–Reagan administration's ban on the use of fetal tissue in research or the introduction into the United States of RU 486). The clinician taking care of a patient may have little, or no, ability directly to change or modify these external variables, yet they impinge inevitably on the decision-makers, often and abruptly bringing the parties involved up against limits. Not to take account of them in clinical ethical decision-making may be not only idealistic but also foolhardy. Many of the chapters in this present volume address external constraints or controls impinging, one way or the other, on the decision-making process.

VALUES AND THE BELIEFS UNDERGIRDING THEM

This brings us to the fourth element in the grid, the one with which we will be primarily concerned in this chapter. In speaking of values, one has also to include, as correlates, such things as beliefs, biases, and even prejudices. These are essentially non-rational, which is not to say that they are irrational (they may seem perfectly rational to those holding similar beliefs, espousing like values, or compelled by the same biases or prejudices). It is to say that they may neither seem reasonable to those outside the group professing them (that is, be publicly defensible), nor be readily amenable to rational persuasion. Beliefs (and the values that stem from them) are held with deep feeling, even passion. People not only attempt to live by their beliefs, but, on occasion, are willing to die for them—Jehovah's Witnesses are a case in point. Expecting to change these beliefs by means of reasoned arguments may be an exercise in futility—as anyone knows who has attempted to obtain parental consent for blood transfusions for infants from staunch Jehovah's Witnesses.

Values and their correlate beliefs are held not only by individuals, but also by professions, institutions, and whole societies. Lynn Payer[6] illumines the way in which variations in preferred treatments between the United States, England, West Germany, and France are determined more by national cultural values than by any scientific rationale. In terms of institutions, those affiliated to the Roman Catholic Church, for example, may be expected to adopt different policies with respect to abortion and certain non-treatment decisions than, say, Protestant or secular hospitals;[7] major medical centers, equally, will be driven by different value systems (predominantly focused on research and teaching) than community hospitals (principally concerned with good clinical practice). As professionals, nurses and physicians are often described in the literature, albeit somewhat stereotypically, as being committed, respectively, to caring and curing.[8] And individuals' values and beliefs vary and differ, even within the same family or treatment team.

Values and their correlate beliefs are both universal and particular phenomena. They are universal, inasmuch as all human beings necessarily live with and by beliefs and the values to which they give rise. The basic scientist proceeds as much with certain fundamental beliefs as does the religious fundamentalist; the only difference between them is what they believe in *qua* basic scientist (about the essential orderliness of the observed world) or *qua* religious fundamentalist (about the derived nature of the observed world). This is where the particularity of beliefs must be taken into account. Values are particular (to individuals, institutions, or whole societies) in the sense that in each category belief has a different locus, and gives rise (often unconsciously) to different biases or prejudices.

There is a distinction to be drawn between professed values and operative values. The values individuals, institutions, or even societies profess are not necessarily those with which they actually function. 'Give us your tired, your poor, your hungry' is proclaimed at the base of the Statue of Liberty as the dominant value system of the great American nation; the fact that so many of our tired, poor, and hungry are homeless and sleeping in the streets suggests that another value system is actually operative in our common life. Neither institutions nor individuals always practice what they profess. In ethics, one is less interested in the values that are professed than in those that actually shape attitudes, actions, and the arguments employed in justification of these. Since individuals, institutions, and societies are both rational and non-rational, exercising both faith (beliefs) and reason, morality can never be confined to 'the limits of reason';[9] ethics, at times, must plunge into the murky waters beyond that boundary.

These waters can be murky indeed. Value conflicts frequently present an almost insurmountable barrier to decision-making by consensus in the perinatal setting. The phrase 'decision-making by consensus' requires some elaboration. Because of the importance the principle of respect for autonomy has come to assume in the contemporary practice of medicine, because 'managed care' is causing administrators to be involved more prominently in the clinical setting, and because of the way in which neonatal intensive-care nurses have claimed and are asserting their own professional identity, physicians can no longer engage in unilateral decision-making. Family members, nurses, institutional representatives (managers and legal counsel, for example), and even third-party payers, may also have a role in decisions either to continue to treat aggressively or to forego such treatment. This means that the goal of ethical decision-making is not necessarily to reach for absolutely right solutions to complex moral problems; more modestly, it may be simply that of building such a consensus as will represent the best possible solution at the time, in the discrete circumstances, and among the various individuals involved. Value conflicts can make arriving at this consensus difficult in the extreme. On occasion, it may be possible only to agree to disagree. When the inability to reach a consensus has negative implications for the care of the neonate, it may be necessary to have recourse to the courts as a means of furthering the infant's best interests.

The remainder of this chapter will be devoted specifically to religious influences on decision-making in perinatology. However, before turning to that task, let it again be noted that it is not always religious beliefs (and the values which are expressive of them) that give rise to value conflicts. Secular beliefs may be powerfully operative as well. The pediatric surgeon who advocates an aggressive series of surgical procedures for an infant born with hypoplastic left-heart syndrome may be operating (or wanting to operate!) on the basis of beliefs as powerful (and as impermeable to reason) as those of any religious believer. The nurse who resists attempts on the part of her fellow team-members to limit further aggressive therapy because she perceives the infant she is taking care of to be clearly 'a fighter' (who, by implication, will thus win his fight), is equally driven by powerful (though hidden) beliefs. Because of the universality of beliefs, as well as their particularity, one can never be certain that the decision-making process will proceed reasonably.

RELIGIOUS BELIEFS

Turning now to religious beliefs, one basic problem that will recur in our discussion of selected themes is that religious beliefs are not always expressed in a common language. That is to say, the vocabulary used to describe and express dogmas and doctrines may be perfectly understandable within the community holding them, yet entirely incomprehensible to those who stand outside that community. Even, say, within 'Christianity' the language of one group (based on a belief in the literal, verbal inspiration of the Bible) may be incomprehensible to others (whose approach to the Bible is historical and critical), and vice versa. As we shall see in our discussion of 'miracles', this can create difficulties, not only for those involved in the decision-making process who are atheists, agnostics, or secularists, but also for those who claim to be Christians as well yet employ different religious language and metaphors. The responsibility of believers is to make their beliefs comprehensible in a realm of public discourse, not merely within the community where these beliefs are nurtured and are thus well understood. Unfortunately, frequently this responsibility is neither recognized nor assumed. This can lead to alienation and polarization, rather than any meeting of minds.

This problem is pervasive, and will haunt us, if not in our discussion of several important themes, then certainly as we grapple with these in the clinical setting: 'quality of life' versus 'sanctity of life'; 'revealed' truth versus empirical evidence; realism versus hope; and the ability or inability to confront the reality of death.

'QUALITY OF LIFE' VERSUS SANCTITY OF LIFE

Those who readily allow quality-of-life considerations a place in the medical and ethical decision-making process and others who repudiate such criteria on sanctity-of-life grounds commonly find themselves in bitter and unresolvable opposition. The polarity of these two points of view can be particularly acute in the neonatal setting. Recently, I was involved as the ethics consultant in a case of an infant diagnosed with trisomy 13. The child had a cleft, not only of the palate, but of the entire face, and was in other ways severely deformed. The attending neonatologist, the residents working with him, the nurses, and the parents of the infant were unanimous in agreeing that aggressive interventions (nasogastric tube-feeding followed by a series of surgical procedures to attempt to remedy the cleft so as to enable the child eventually to swallow) were inappropriate, not only because of the low likelihood of long-term survival, but also because the quality of the infant's brief life was likely to be abysmally poor. The one dissenting view (which prevented us from arriving at a consensus) was that of the consulting geneticist, who opposed any consideration of the child's quality of life (and, at the same time, presented unusually optimistic morbidity and mortality data), for sanctity-of-life reasons. Because of her vigorous objections, a nasogastric feeding tube was inserted, to the dismay of the parents. Before the first scheduled surgical procedure, the child died, at two-and-a-half months of age.

I have no way of knowing whether the sanctity-of-life point of view of the geneticist in this case was religiously inspired. However, such views often are, and the weight of theological opinion, at least in the conservative Jewish, Roman Catholic, and Protestant communities favors a sanctity-of-life posture.

Howard Brody quotes this uncompromising statement by Moshe Tendler, an orthodox Jew and Professor of Talmudic Law at Yeshiva University:

... the ethical foundation of our society of Western civilization is a biblical one. ... There are certain indispensable foundations for an ethical system and one of them is the sanctity of human life. This concept has a corollary; that is that human life is of infinite value. This in turn means that *a piece* of infinity is also infinity and a person who has but a few moments to live is no less of value than a person who has 70 years to live.

And likewise a person who is handicapped and cannot serve the needs of society is no less a man and no less entitled to the same price tag—a price tag inscribed with an infinite price. A handicapped individual is a perfect specimen when viewed in an ethical context. *This value is an absolute value.* It is not relative to life expectancy, to state of health, or to usefulness to society.[10]

Ashley and O'Rourke elaborate a no less tenaciously held Roman Catholic point of view:

Physicians, nurses, and health care workers should give public witness to their belief in the sanctity of life, the integrity of every person, and the value of human life at every stage of its existence by their compassion and care for their patients.[11]

And the late Paul Ramsey, a conservative though by no means a fundamentalist, was nevertheless perhaps the most widely read recent Protestant advocate of the sanctity-of-life point of view. A somewhat defiant (1978) statement is typical of his stance:

I'd rather be charged with morally justifying first-degree murder ... than add a feather's weight on the balance in favor of quality-of-life judgements—unless these are part of a competent patient's balancing determination of goods and harms in his own case.[12]

Obviously, this excludes the newborn.

Against this inter-faith consensus in favor of the sanctity-of-life position, there are some few Reformed Jewish theologians who, in private conversation if not in their published writings, allow that quality-of-life considerations have a place in the decision-making process. A larger number of Roman Catholic theologians are prepared to do the same, both verbally and in writing.[13] And many liberal Protestant theologians are in their writings as outspokenly in favor of quality-of-life criteria having a legitimate role in decision-making as their more conservative colleagues are opposed to this. Joseph Fletcher may be allowed to speak for many:

The traditional ethics based on the sanctity of life—which was the classical doctrine of medical idealism in its pre-scientific phases—must give way to a code of ethics of the *quality* of life. This comes about for humane reasons. It is a result of modern medicine's successes, not failures. New occasions teach new duties, time makes ancient good uncouth, as Whittier said.

There are many pre-ethical or 'metaethical' issues that are often overlooked in ethical discussions. People of equally good reasoning powers and a high respect for the rules of inference still puzzle and even infuriate each other. This is because they fail to see that their moral judgments proceed from significantly different values, ideals, and starting points. If God's will (perhaps 'specially revealed' in the Bible or 'generally revealed' in Creation) is against any responsible human initiative in the dying process, or if sheer life is believed to be, as such, more desirable than anything else, then those who hold these axioms will not find much merit in any case we might make for ... [withholding or withdrawing treatments]. If, on the other hand, the highest good is personal integrity and human well-being, then [withholding or withdrawing treatments] could or might be the right thing to do, depending on the situation.[14]

The prevailing climate of opinion, at least in the United States, is against including the infant's quality of life as a licit criterion in decision-making. The so-called 'Baby Doe Regulations'[15] illustrate the widespread dominance (at least in the political arena during the Reagan–Bush years) of the sanctity-of-life point of view. A number of brief excerpts from the Regulations should make this evident:

Considerations such as anticipated or actual limited potential of an individual and present or future lack of available community resources are irrelevant and must not determine the decisions concerning medical care.

In cases where it is uncertain whether medical treatment will be beneficial, a person's disability must not be the basis for a decision to withhold treatment.

The physician's 'reasonable medical judgment' concerning the medically indicated treatment ... is not to be based on subjective 'quality of life' or other abstract concepts.

It is beyond the scope of this chapter to offer a theological, philosophical, and ethical critique of the absolutist sanctity-of-life position, although I have done this elsewhere.[16] For our present purposes it is sufficient to note that there are these two diametrically opposed points of view. Both represent divergent value systems, and both are founded in differing beliefs—held with equal tenacity despite all reasoned argument to the contrary. As in the case of the infant born with trisomy 13 mentioned above, these divergent values frequently make it impossible for the members of the treatment team and the family to arrive at a consensus about treatment and non-treatment decisions. In the United States, at least, to proceed to limit therapy in the absence of unanimity among the caregivers, within the family, and between caregivers and family members, can be hazardous in the extreme. The Barber case[17] is a stark reminder of this. In situations where vigorous objections are registered against quality-of-life considerations, it may be more prudent to found non-treatment decisions either on the best-interest standard or on a perceived disproportionality between the harms of continued aggressive interventions and the hoped-for benefits.

'REVEALED' TRUTH VERSUS EMPIRICAL EVIDENCE

Some years ago, in the Stanford University Hospital Intensive Care Nursery, an extremely premature (25 weeks' gestational age), small for gestational age (475 gram) infant developed hyaline membrane disease[18] and became chronically ventilator-dependent. For five months, before he died, this infant continued to receive aggressive neonatal intensive care (at a cost to the State of California of more than $560 000)—only because the parents claimed to have received a divine 'revelation' in which they were promised that their child would be fully healed, provided he stayed in the hospital and continued to receive maximal ventilatory support. After the infant had been in the nursery for two or three months, the staff were unanimous in the opinion that he had no hope of any meaningful recovery, that he was not benefiting from ventilatory therapy, and that he was even being harmed by the continued aggressive regimen (the nurses involved were more explicit; it was their conviction that we were 'torturing' this child).

Although it is impossible for clinicians to offer parents a prognosis that is absolutely sure, there are times when the empirical evidence points so clearly in a definite direction that the probability of a particular outcome approaches certainty. This was one such case. (At other times, where the empirical evidence is more ambiguous, the intuitions of parents or, indeed, of nurses and other caregivers, may turn out to be correct.)

The parents of this particular infant, as is often the case when children are in a regional neonatal center, lived 150 miles away and came to visit their baby only infrequently. Whenever they did so, they would exclaim over the marked 'improvement' they were able to discern in his condition—notwithstanding the nurses' protests that the child was not merely no better but was clearly much worse. Whenever the subject of discontinuing aggressive therapy was broached, the parents' response was to insist on staying with the present course, appealing to the 'vision' in which they had been promised healing. So far as could be determined, they belonged to no organized church or sect. Their beliefs were entirely idiosyncratic.

Here we have an extreme example of how 'revealed' truth can sometimes fly in the face of empirical evidence. Had these parents belonged to an identifiable religious group, one strategy for attempting to resolve the impasse would have been to appeal to their minister or pastor—as one who both shared their belief system and was more likely to be receptive to recommendations based on objective empirical data—eliciting his or her support in the attempt to make the parents more cognisant of the clinical facts staring them in the face. In this case, that option was not available. Nor was it possible, after five months, to demand either that the parents transfer their child to another facility or that they begin to assume a fraction of the cost of their child's care, on the assumption that footing even a small percentage of the bill might inject a note of realism into their thinking.

What finally broke the deadlock was the team's insistence that the parents spend one week in the nursery, participating fully in the care of their child. Reluctantly, they agreed to do this. After three days, they came round to the view that their infant was indeed being tortured, and that the time had therefore come to allow him a natural and peaceful death. He was extubated, and died minutes later in his mother's arms.

In cases that are not as clear-cut as this, where the empirical evidence favoring a prognosis is less unambiguous, different belief systems may end up being opposed to one another. The parents' belief that their infant will recover (which can be reinforced by what is sometimes referred to as 'denial', but may, in fact, be nothing other than their stubborn refusal to give up the fight for their child's life) may be in conflict with the belief of the team (based, perhaps, on insubstantial empirical or historical evidence) that she will not. Just as parents' positive beliefs may have to be challenged on the basis of convincing empirical evidence, so, too, may the clinicians' negative beliefs at times have to be called into question by the lack of hard data. It is easier to dismiss parents' confidence in a certain outcome as non-rational than it is to recognize the same reliance on belief in ourselves.

REALISM VERSUS HOPE

A similar issue is the sometimes wide discrepancy between a realistic medical prognosis, on the one hand, and, on the other, the parents' religiously grounded hope for a miracle. No prognosis can be completely certain. At most, it offers a prediction of the infant's probable future course, as informed by the weight of empirical data and historical and statistical evidence. There are always individual variables (such as the quality of the relationship between the parents and their infant) that can affect the probable outcome—one way or the other. This is why hope assumes such importance in most cases in keeping up the parents' spirits and in motivating them to continue surrounding their child with love and affection. Unfortunately, however, hope often takes the quite specific form of expecting a miraculous physical restoration, rather than that of looking for healing in more general terms—and serves to reinforce the parents' denial of facts that seem self-evident to all others involved in the case.

The distinction between hope for healing in general terms and longing for a specific outcome requires some explanation. With respect to Christianity (about which I am better qualified to speak than about other religions) the four Gospels report numerous healings by Jesus of sicknesses of every kind,[19] three raisings of the dead,[20] and seven nature miracles.[21] When subjected to a critical literary and linguistic analysis, the content of the miracle stories diminishes considerably; the material is reduced yet further if these stories are compared with Rabbinic and Hellenistic sources; and a form-critical analysis of the miracle stories of the Gospels helps to distinguish a later Hellenistic stratum of tradition from an earlier Palestinian one.[22] Nevertheless, as Jeremias puts it,

even when strict critical standards have been applied to the miracle stories, a demonstrably historical nucleus remains. Jesus performed healings which astonished his contemporaries. *These were primarily healings of psychogenous suffering*, especially what the texts described as the driving out of demons, which Jesus performed with a brief word of command.[23]

Clearly, there are no stories at all of amputees miraculously being given new limbs: psychogenous, or as we might put it, psychosomatic, healings predominate.

In general terms, healing is hoped for holistically in the major religious traditions. That is to say, what is encouraged is the hope that the entire person will move towards wellness and fullness of being, not merely that some (more limited) physical restoration or regeneration will occur. There is also the hope that this process of journeying towards wellness and fullness of being will be completed, if not in time, then in what is referred to symbolically as 'eternity'; it is something for which we are invited to hope, not necessarily in this life, but in a life beyond death. Hoping for miracles in this dual sense—holistically and within the larger context of eternity— allows for the possibility that people may not recover from their illnesses and may actually die, without hope necessarily being destroyed. Hoping for miracles in the more limited and specific sense of physical restoration or regeneration can lead, ultimately, to disappointment, and, in the meantime, to a conflict between the realism of the treatment team, committed to its empirically-founded prognosis, and the confidence of the parents that there will be a certain desired outcome.

How is the clinician to proceed in the face of such an impasse? Three suggestions may be apposite. The first is to enlist the help of a chaplain, priest, minister, or rabbi, preferably one sharing the same religious beliefs as the family, in all discussions with them. Such a religious representative is likely to be perceived by the family as their ally, rather than as being opposed to them; at the same time, it is possible that such a person will be able to bring more balance, objectivity, and theological sophistication to the situation than the family members themselves. Second, it is essential that different members of the treatment team repeatedly reinforce the same message to the parents from their respective disciplinary vantage points. However differently they may express it, each member of the team should consciously strive to deliver the same information. Unless, in matters of diagnosis and prognosis, the team members speak with a common voice, family members are likely to seize upon and exploit (for the purpose of sustaining their own denial and hope) any discrepancies they may be hearing in the pronouncements of various team members. And third, without discounting the possibility that miraculous events do sometimes happen, and even (if this is consistent with the clinician's own religious beliefs) while affirming one's own personal faith in 'miracles', it is at the same time important to disclaim any knowledge of how to produce this kind of longed-for result. Ultimately, miracles are a gift from God—not the result of human manipulation, either by means of faith or prayer. Therefore, faith as trust or as entrusting is called for, rather than faith construed as belief in a desired outcome. This type of faith can be encouraged by all members of the treatment team, whatever their own beliefs (or lack of them).

THE ABILITY OR INABILITY OF THE FAMILY TO CONFRONT THE REALITY OF DEATH

Our American culture is characterized by a pervasive denial of death.[24] In part, this is a result of increasing urbanization in the post-industrial era. In rural communities, death is experienced by children growing up as an inherent part of life—as are birth, sickness, and aging. Urban children are unlikely to know where milk comes from, let alone to witness the death (and birth) of animals and of humans. Television trivializes death; people die so frequently on the screen that the enormity and horror of what is depicted as happening fade. The denial of death is also a reflection of our American preoccupation with youth and vitality. And, additionally, the denial of mortality is fostered by the advertising industry: health and beauty sell products on television and in glossy magazines; the depiction, for advertising purposes, of disease, disability, and death is likely to have little or no commercial value. Hence there is a tendency to ignore the reality of these darker and less optimistic aspects of the human condition.

The denial of death (or the stubborn refusal to give up the fight for a child's life), as we have seen, can lead parents with infants in the intensive-care nursery to cling to unrealistic hopes—the empirical evidence underlying dire prognoses notwithstanding. Those who have come to terms more fully with death as a fact of life—for themselves as well as for their children—will be better able to let go of unrealistic expectations than those who have not yet confronted existentially their own mortality. Furthermore, those who have religiously grounded beliefs in life beyond death may be more prone to accept reality than those who are agnostic or frankly disbelieving on this score. Incidentally, there is a difference between extrinsic and intrinsic religious beliefs that is pertinent to this point; it is similar to the difference between professed and operative values. Intrinsically religious people, who not only profess but actually operate on the basis of deeply held beliefs, are likely to be better able to accept reality and look beyond death to a larger, hoped-for life, than those whose religion is merely extrinsic.

Christianity from its beginnings has fostered at least five fundamental categories of hope in life beyond death. These have been lucidly delineated by Jaroslav Pelikan.[25]

Justin Martyr and his pupil, Tatian (second century C. E.), set forth what is essentially a Jewish view of death. This life is all we can be sure of; anything beyond death is speculative; therefore the emphasis needs to be on living in the present moment rather than on hoping for future immortality.

Clement of Alexandria (second century C. E.) inherited a doctrine of pre-existence as part of his Platonic tradition. He posited an immortal soul, united with the body at birth and then separated from it at death, which then continues to exist in a realm beyond death. This view lends itself readily to belief in reincarnation; the soul, being immortal, can be 'recycled' over and over again in different physical bodies.

Cyprian (third-century Bishop of Carthage) developed a view that reso- nates well with those of modern fundamentalists. The soul is not naturally immortal; immortality is a gift of God conferred on the faithful. Resurrection to the life of eternity is the reward of those who, in time, faithfully follow and serve Jesus Christ. This view tends to be judgmental and exclusive: only 'true believers' (as defined by the 'in' group), will inherit God's promises. Others can be sure only of life in this world.

Origen (third century, C. E.), like Clement, subscribed to an essentially Hellenistic belief in the pre-existence of the soul. Between birth and death the soul is joined to the body and leads an individual, historical existence. As the soul takes its origin from God, so Origen also envisions its destiny beyond death as being in God and with God. Death is inevitable, but it is but a doorway to the fuller life of eternity. This is a view warmly embraced by liberal Protestant Christians in the twentieth century.

Irenaeus (second-century Bishop of Lyons) is responsible for the view that 'in the midst of life we are in death, for death is the end of life. Yet in the midst of death we are in life, for life is the end of death.'[26] Irenaeus encourages us to experience dying (with a lower-case 'd') in little ways throughout life and, at the same time, to discover the new beginnings (resurrections, with a lower case 'r') that are possible as we confront loss creatively and with courage. This prepares us for Dying (with a capital 'D') and for the Resurrection life of eternity (with a capital 'R'). Death interrupts, but does not end, a process of transformation that begins in time and will continue throughout eternity. In Irenaeus' view, death and resurrection (in time as in eternity) make possible a process of divinization. This process is dynamic, not static. It accords well with modern developmental theories of human nature.

These types of hope in a life beyond death are by no means exhaustive. They illustrate the wide variety of eschatological points of view, even within a single religious tradition. Those who hold strong beliefs (of whatever type), and who hold these intrinsically, not merely extrinsically, are likely to be able better to overcome the tendency to deny the reality of death that is endemic in our culture and to let go of their child, entrusting him or her to the love of God and to a larger (and eternal) destiny. Again, enlisting the support of religious leaders who can reinforce such beliefs can facilitate (even expedite) decisions to forgo life-sustaining treatments.

This completes our summary review of four important themes that illustrate the force of beliefs (and the values to which they give rise) in clinical ethical decision-making: belief in the sanctity, as opposed to the quality, of life; 'revealed' truth versus empirical evidence; realism versus hope; and the parents' ability or inability to confront the reality of death.

Enough has been said to illustrate how powerfully the rational decision-making process can be complicated, if not subverted, by non-rational factors. In clinical ethical decision-making, no less than in medicine itself, much art is required in addition to all that science can offer. This art will be challenged (and possibly improved!) by the religious influences on decision-making that have been examined, as well as by beliefs (and the values deriving from them) that are more secular in nature.

NOTES AND REFERENCES

1. Beauchamp, T. L. and Childress, J. F. *Principles of biomedical ethics* (3rd edn). Oxford University Press, New York and Oxford, (1989).

2. See Rothman, D. J. *Strangers at the bedside: a history of how law and bioethics transformed medicine*. Basic Books, New York, (1991).

3. Young, E. W. D. *Alpha and omega: ethics at the frontiers of life and death*, pp. 27–40. Addison-Wesley, Reading, Mass. (1989).

4. Beauchamp and Childress, *op. cit.*, p. 319.

5. Jonsen, A. R., Siegler, M., and Winslade, W. J. *Clinical ethics* (3rd edn), pp. 121–59. McGraw-Hill, New York. (1992).

6. Payer, L. *Medicine and culture*. Penguin Books, London, (1989).

7. Marty, M. E. and Vaux, K. L. *Health/medicine and the faith traditions: an inquiry into religion and medicine.* Fortress Press, Philadelphia (1982).
8. Benjamin, M. and Curtis, J. *Ethics in nursing* (2nd edn). Oxford University Press, New York. (1986).
9. Hardin, R. *Morality within the limits of reason.* The University of Chicago Press, Chicago and London (1988).
10. Brody, H., *Ethical decisions in medicine* (2nd edn), p. 75. Little, Brown and Company, Boston (1981). Italics added.
11. Ashley, M. A. and O'Rourke, K. D. *Health care ethics: a theological analysis,* pp. 242f. The Catholic Hospital Association, St. Louis, Missouri (1978).
12. Ramsey, P. *Ethics at the edges of life: medical and legal intersections,* p. 225. Yale University Press, New Haven and London (1978).
13. McCormick, R. A. The quality of life, the sanctity of life. *Hastings Center Report,* Vol. **8**, No. 1. February, 1978. pp. 34 ff
14. Fletcher, J. Ethics and euthanasia. In Williams, R. H. (ed.) *To live and to die: when, why, and how,* p. 114. Springer-Verlag, New York, 1973.
15. *The Federal Register,* Vol. **49**, No. 238, Monday, December 10, 1984. Proposed rules, p. 48160.
16. Young, E. W. D. *Faith reason, and biomedical ethics.* Concordia Publishing House Saint Louis, Missouri (in process of publication).
17. *Barber* v. *Superior Court,* 147 Cal. App. 3d 1006, 195 Cal. Rptr. 484 (1983), aff' g *People* v. *Barber,* No. A025586 (Los Angeles Mun. Ct. Mar. 9, 1983).
18. Hyaline membrane disease is also known as respiratory distress syndrome. It is a developmental disorder causing the premature lungs to have difficulty coping with a gaseous environment; in attempting to do so, the lungs undergo severe stress.
19. Possession (Mark 1: 21–8 and parallels; 5:1–20 and par.; 7: 24–30 and par.); fever (Mark 1:12–19 and par.); leprosy (Mark 1:40–5 and par.; Luke 17: 12–19); lameness (Mark 2: 1–12 and par.; Matt. 8: 5–13 and par.; John 5: 1–18); consumption (Mark 3: 1–6 and par.); haemorrhage (Mark 5: 25–34 and par.); deafness and muteness (Matt. 9: 32–4; Luke 11: 14 and par., Matt. 12: 22, where he is blind in addition); blindness (Mark 8: 22–6; 10: 46–52 and par.; Matt. 9: 27–31; 12: 22; John 9: 1–34); epilepsy (Mark 9: 14–29 and par.); deformation (Luke 13: 10–17); dropsy (Mark 14: 1–6); sword wound (Luke 22: 51).
20. Mark 5: 35; Luke 7: 12 f.; John 11: 39.
21. Walking on the water (Mark 6: 45–52); cursing the fig-tree (Mark 11: 12–14, 20 and par.); the coin in the fish's mouth (Matt. 17: 24–27); Peter's catch (Luke 5: 1–11); the stilling of the strom (Mark 4: 35–41 and par.); the feeding in the wilderness (Mark 6: 34–44 and par.; 8: 1–9 and par.); and the water into wine (John 2: 1–11).
22. Jeremias, J. *New Testament theology: the proclamation of Jesus,* pp. 86–91. Scribner, New York, 1971.
23. Jeremias, *ibid.,* p. 92, italics added.
24. Becker, E. *The denial of death.* Macmillan, New York, 1973.
25. Pelikan, J. *The shape of death: life, death, and immortality in the early Fathers.* Macmillan, London, 1962.
26. Quoted by Pelikan, op. cit., p. 101.

Glossary*

Alpha-fetal protein. First of a group of substances constituting the greater part of the nitrogen-containing components of animal and vegetable tissues in the fetus, increased in women carrying fetuses with abnormal openings in their central nervous systems.

Amicus curiae. An impartial expert adviser called in to assist a court of law (fr. Lat., literally 'friend of the court').

Amniocentesis. Procedure in which aminotic fluid is removed by inserting a needle through the pregnant mother's abdominal wall and into the uterus. The fluid is often used to determine whether fetal chromosomes are normal.

Anencephaly (adj., anencephalic). Congenital absence of the vault of the skull, with the higher centres of the brain (Cerebral hemispheres) altogether missing or only present as small masses.

Aortography. Photographic examination of the aorta.

Ascites. Accumulation of clear fluid in the abdominal cavity.

Asystole [Gk. *a* priv. + *systole*, a contracting.]. Absence of contractions of the heart; cardiac standstill.

Cardiopulmonary bypass [Gk. *Kardiē*, heart, + L. *pulmo*, lung]. Exclusion of heart and lungs from the circulation by means of pump-oxygenator, employed during open heart surgery.

Cyclosporin. A potent immunosuppressive agent which prolongs survival of allogeneic transplants involving skin, heart, kidney, pancreas, bone marrow, small intestine, and lung.

Cystostomy. Creation of an artificial channel to the bladder by surgery.

'Double-blind' trials. Trials of treatments in which neither the treating physicians nor their patients know which of two or more treatments is being supplied to any particular patient.

Down (also Down's) syndrome. A congenital condition usually caused by an extra chromosome number 21. Associated with a characteristic facial appearance, and with usually severe mental deficiency.

Ductus arteriosus (ductus Botalli, Botallo's duct). A fetal vessel connecting the left pulmonary artery with the descending aorta. During the first two months after birth, it normally becomes changed into a fibrous cord, the ligamentum arteriosum.

Encephalopathy [Gk. *enkephalos*, brain, + *pathos*, suffering]. Any disease of the brain. (Hypoxic encephalopathy—brain injury secondary to inadequate oxygenation.)

Epidemiology. The study of the relationships of factors determining the incidence and distribution of disease in a population.

Gastrostomy. The surgical creation of an artificial passage into the stomach.

Gynecology. The branch of medicine dealing with diseases of the genital tract in women.

Hyaline membrane disease. Also known as respiratory distress syndrome. A developmental disorder causing the premature lungs to have difficulty coping with a gaseous environment; in attempting to do so, the lungs undergo severe stress.

Hydrocephalus. Accumulation of cerebrospinal fluid within the skull, usually with enlargement of the head, a prominent forehead, brain atrophy, mental deterioration, and convulsions.

Hypoplastic left-heart syndrome. Defective formation of left side of heart; incomplete development of the left side of the heart, in which the left ventricle is so small that it is unable to support the systemic circulation of the blood; a life-threatening congenital anomaly found in infants.

Hypoxic Ischemic insult. An injury or trauma resulting in a decreased amount of oxygen delivery to organs and tissues and a reduced amount of alkali reserve (bicarbonate) of the blood and other body fluids, with or without an actual decrease in pH.

Iatrogenic. Resulting from the activities of doctors. Used if any worsening of a patient's condition is brought about as a result of medical treatment prescribed by a doctor.

Inotropic [Gk. *is* (*in-*), fiber, + *tropos*, a turning, influencing]. Influencing the contractility of muscular tissue, including the heart.

Intraventricular hemorrhage [Gk. *haimorrhagia*, fr. *haima*, blood, + *rrhagia*, n. fr. *rhgnūmi*, breakout, break loose]. Bleeding, a flow of blood, especially profuse within a ventricle of the brain.

In utero (Lat). [Still] in the womb.

Ischemia (adj., ischemic). Lack of blood in part of the body because of constriction or obstruction of blood vessels

Kernicterus. Degenerated yellow pigmentation of nerve cells in the spinal cord and brain, manifesting itself about the second or third day of life by convulsions, drowsiness, and anorexia. Death may occur around the end of the first week, or in less severe cases cerebral palsy, spasticity, and mental defects may appear at a later date.

Laminectomy. The surgical removal of the posterior arch of a vertebra.

Myelomeningocele. A hernial protrusion of the spinal cord and its membranes (meninges) through a defect in the vertebral column.

Myocardial infarction. A condition in which a portion of the heart muscle dies as a result of blockage of the blood vessel supplying it. Commonly called a 'heart attack'.

Necrotizing enterocolitis [Gk. *nekroō*, to make dead, mortify]. The pathologic death to a greater or lesser extent of both small and large intestines.

Neonate. A newborn infant.

Neutropenia. A diminished number of neutrophils (cells for fighting infection) in the blood.

Norwood Procedures. Surgical procedures which are intended to provide an infant suffering from a hypoplastic left-heart syndrome with an adequate system for the circulation of blood.

Obstetrics. The branch of medicine dealing with pregnancy, labor, and childbirth.

Orthotopic organ [Gk. *orthos*, straight, correct, + *topos*, place]. An organ in the normal or usual position.

Pediatrics. The branch of medicine dealing with the child and its development and care, and with diseases of childhood.

Perinatology. The branch of medicine dealing with the fetus and infant immediately before and after birth; obstetrics and gynecology.

Phenytoin. A drug commonly used to treat epilepsy. It can cause birth defects if taken by the mother in early pregnancy.

Polyhydramnios. Excess of amniotic fluid.

Primum non nocere (Lat.). 'First of all, do no harm'. Part of the Hippocratic Oath.

Pulmonary Hypertension. High blood pressure in the circulatory system of the lungs. Women with this disorder tolerate the cardiovascular demands of pregnancy poorly.

Retrolental fibro-plasia. A condition in which blood vessels and fibrous tissue accumulate behind the lens of the eye, leading to detachment of the retina and arrest of the growth of the eye. It can be caused by the use of over-high concentrations of oxygen in the care of premature babies.

Reye's syndrome. A rare, acute, and often lethal brain disease of childhood, with acute brain swelling and liver disturbance, often leading to seizures. It often follows influenza or other viral respiratory infections.

Scleroderma nephropathy. A form of chronic kidney failure associated with scleroderma, a progressive disease of connective tissue that can affect many organs. The kidney involvement often progresses during pregnancy.

Spina bifida (Lat., literally 'split spine'). A congenital anomaly of development where the spinal cord is not fully enclosed in the bones of the spinal column.

Septicemia. A morbid condition produced by disease-causing bacteria and associated poisons in the blood.

Surfactant. A lipoprotein substance that normally coats the lining of the air sacs of the lungs and prevents lung collapse during expiration. The absence of surfactant in lungs of premature babies often leads to serious and sometimes fatal breathing difficulties.

Teratogen [Gk. *teras*, monster]. Something that causes physical defects in the developing embryo (teratogenic, adj.).

Thrombosis [Gk. *thrombosis*, a curdling]. The formation of a thrombus; the presence of a thrombus.

Thrombus [Gk. *thrombos*, a clot of blood or curdled milk]. A clot more or less completely occluding a blood vessel (here, the aorta) produced *in situ* by coagulation of the blood.

Tracheostomy. Creation of an artificial opening into the windpipe (trachea) through the neck by surgery.

Trisomy [Gk. *treis*, three; sōma, body]. Presence of an additional third chromosome alongside the usual pair, usually leading to some degree of congenital abnormality. There are various trisomies with different effects depending on which chromosome is triplicated, each known by the number of the chromosome involved—for example trisomy 21 (Down's syndrome).

*Sources consulted in compiling the Glossary: *Stedman's medical dictionary*, 21st edn, 1966, repr. August 1967; *PDR*, 46th edn, 1992; *Dorland's medical dictionaryt*, 23rd edn, 1982.

Index

DATE DUE